The Radiology of Emergency Medicine

Second Edition

The Radiology of Emergency Medicine

Second Edition

JOHN H. HARRIS, JR., M.D., D.Sc.

Professor and Chairman
University of Texas Medical School
Chief Emergency Radiology
Hermann Hospital
Houston, Texas

WILLIAM H. HARRIS, M.D.

Clinical Professor of Orthopaedic Surgery
Harvard University School of Medicine

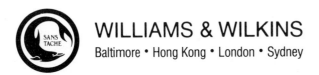

WILLIAMS & WILKINS
Baltimore • Hong Kong • London • Sydney

Copyright ©, 1981
Williams & Wilkins
428 E. Preston Street
Baltimore, Md. 21202, U.S.A.

Accurate indications, adverse reactions, and dosage schedules for drugs are provided
in this book, but it is possible that they may change. The reader is urged to review
the package information data of the manufacturers of the medications mentioned.

Made in the United States of America

First Edition, 1975
Reprinted, 1976
Second Edition, 1981

Library of Congress Cataloging in Publication Data

Harris, John Harold, Jr. 1925-
  The radiology of emergency medicine.

  Includes bibliographical references and index.
  1. Diagnosis, Radioscopic. 2. Medical emergencies. I. Harris, William Hamilton,
joint author. II. Title [DNLM: 1. Emergencies. 2. Radiography. WB105.H314r]
RC78.H33   1981   616.07'572   80-18944
ISBN 0-683-03883-4

Composed and printed at the   89   90   91
Waverly Press, Inc.   10

Dedicated to

JOHN H. HARRIS, Sr., M.D., M.Sc. (Rad)
father, friend and first teacher
and to
CATHERINE CONNELL HARRIS
without whose understanding, encouragement
and love this work would not exist.

Foreword
To the Second Edition

Seven years ago I was given the honor of introducing this book to the medical world. It was a personal pleasure for me, and it is doubly pleasurable now to introduce the second edition. This textbook has been so highly successful that most Emergency Departments throughout the English- and Spanish-speaking worlds contain a copy. Since the first edition, newer techniques such as ultrasound and CT have made giant strides, and examples of their application to Emergency Radiology are included in this edition. Many more excellent illustrations have been added, along with different concepts involving cervical spine fractures, pulmonary contusion and infarction, soft tissue signs of pelvic effusion, and a consideration of the soft tissue injury associated with ankle trauma.

I have been a very close friend of the authors and of their father, John Harris, Sr., a dedicated radiologist and community leader deeply concerned with people. This unusual family has contributed richly to medicine, the example of the father inspiring his sons, one now a "gowner" in orthopaedic surgery, and one, until recently, a "towner" in radiology.

The ties of this close family have held over the years and now the two brothers, working together, are able to offer this lucid and sophisticated revision of their contribution to Emergency Medicine. It pools their expertise in two disciplines.

My friendship with both authors and their father has been a privilege and a pleasure for me for many years. I encouraged the beginnings of this book; saw its original progress; and hope that my encouragement and support have contributed to its existence, its enthusiastic reception, and its revision.

It is a much needed work. Its revision keeps pace with new developments, capabilities, and insights. Completely practical, it avoids the distraction of esoteric disgressions to attack the immediate problem. As I originally expected, it has become indispensible in Emergency Departments and offices throughout the world.

You have in your hands a classic in the field of Emergency Medicine; now, in its revised form, it will enjoy many more years as a trusted handbook filling a constant need.

Jack Edeiken, M.D.

Preface
To the Second Edition

The decision to revise a textbook is usually motivated by a favorable reception afforded the original volume, new technical and scientific advances which have occurred since preparation of the original manuscript, and a desire on the part of the authors to improve the original version. All these factors played an important role in arriving at the decision to make revisions in the initial manuscript. The revisions have been so extensive as to warrant a new edition rather than simply another printing.

We are deeply appreciative of the reception that has been afforded the initial publication of *The Radiology of Emergency Medicine*. We are particularly indebted to the reviewers for their observations and constructive criticisms and to those of our readers who have taken the time to point out errors or to offer suggestions for improving the content and format of the original volume. Wherever possible, these suggestions have been incorporated into the second edition.

Radiology is, without doubt, the most rapidly advancing specialty in all of medicine. The most exciting advances in radiographic capability, such as computed tomography, interventive angiography, ultrasound, and nuclear medicine, as well as the recognition of Emergency Medicine as a distinct area of specialization, have all either emerged or undergone spectacular growth since 1974 when the manuscript for the first edition was submitted for publication. All of the developments just cited have resulted in dramatic changes in the field of Emergency Radiology. We have made a diligent effort to incorporate the indications for, and examples of, the applications of these new techniques, procedures, and diagnostic concepts into this second edition.

Even though this revision is as reflective of the contemporary practice of emergency radiology as possible, we recognize that currently emerging new imaging modalities, such as digital fluoroscopy, positron emission tomography, nuclear magnetic resonance, and newer techniques in interventive angiography are developing so rapidly that this edition may be out of date within two or three years of its publication. In spite of these dramatic and exciting technical advances, it is important to remember that the roentgen evaluation of the majority of acutely ill or injured patients still begins with the plain film examination. We predict that basic tenet will be true for the foreseeable future. Therefore, the major emphasis of this text remains with plain film radiography.

Since preparation of the original manuscript of *The Radiology of Emergency Medicine*, the authors have expanded their knowledge, have acquired greater understanding and clearer insight regarding the radiologic aspects of emergency medicine, and have accumulated a considerably greater caseload of material. All of these have resulted in significant revisions of all chapters and major revisions of the chapters dealing with the skull, spine, chest, abdomen, kidneys, pelvis, and the ankle.

It is our sincere hope that these substantial modifications will be of proportional value to those physicians involved in Emergency Medicine and that the second edition of *The Radiology of Emergency Medicine* will have, therefore, a direct and positive influence upon the management of the acutely ill or injured patient.

Preface
To the First Edition

Radiology, and the radiologist, can be of invaluable assistance in the assessment and management of the acutely ill or injured patient. The radiology of emergency medicine occupies a minor position in the curriculum of most medical schools and radiology training programs. Consequently, physicians involved in the care of emergency patients have varied experience and training in the radiology related to this aspect of medicine.

The purpose of this work is to describe the role of radiology in the appraisal of the acutely ill or injured patient, to emphasize and illustrate its value as well as its limitations, and to guide the physician in the roentgen diagnosis of the emergency patient. It is hoped that this will provide a better understanding of the appropriate roentgen examination to be requested and the information that the study can be reasonably expected to provide.

It is not our intent to present radiographic examples of every disease entity that might prompt an Emergency Department patient visit, nor is it our intent to present any entity described herein exhaustively. Many textbooks and articles exist which do provide such comprehensive roentgen descriptions.

Rather, it is our purpose to focus upon those radiologic aspects of emergency medical care which, in our experience, have acted as "pitfalls" to the examination, diagnosis, and understanding of emergency medical problems. Every illustration has been chosen from our personal practices to illustrate a point which, at some time or other, has presented some degree of difficulty. Emphasis has always been placed upon objective, although frequently subtle, changes which should lead to the correct radiographic diagnosis.

While the prime motivation for this effort has been a desire to be of assistance to Emergency Department physicians, it is hoped that the book will be of value to physicians of all disciplines involved in the diagnosis and management of the acutely ill or injured patient.

John H. Harris, Jr. M.D., D.Sc.
William H. Harris, M.D.

Acknowledgments

I acknowledge with deep appreciation that neither the first edition of *The Radiology of Emergency Medicine* nor this revision could have been completed without the unstinting support and assistance of many friends and associates. Through this mechanism, I am pleased to specifically thank those individuals who have contributed in a major and clearly identifiable fashion to this work.

Joan Frey Boytim, undaunted by the inconveniences inherent in my peripatetic meanderings of the past 18 months, has continued to provide concise, accurate, and illuminating drawings that contribute greatly to the understanding of several sections of this revision.

Jack Edeiken, M.D., Professor and Chairman of the Department of Radiology at Thomas Jefferson University in Philadelphia, has continued to provide stimulating new challenges and opportunities for me to learn and grow, while simultaneously, by his example, affording the encouragement and support so necessary to the completion of this work.

Many of the new prints contained within this edition, as well as many of those substituted for prints appearing in the first edition, are the work of James Steinmetz of Carlisle, Pennsylvania. Mr. Bert Pickens, of Aviso, Inc., Lansing, Michigan, worked with pleasantness and diligence in an area in which he had little previous experience, to provide other new prints that appear in this edition. Since the quality of the illustrations is a direct reflection of the quality of the prints produced by the photographer and supplied to the photoengraver, it is entirely appropriate to applaud the efforts of these gentlemen.

Noreen Roeske, of East Lansing, Michigan, provided badly needed and valuable assistance in collating and integrating the revised portions into the original manuscript.

Susan Westmoreland, my secretary and alter ego, has been of invaluable assistance in cheerfully tolerating the tedium required of careful and critical proofreading and index preparation while, at the same time, efficiently conducting the myriad activities of a very busy office.

The fact that *The Radiology of Emergency Medicine* came to fruition and that there is now a second edition is a tribute to Ruby Richardson's interest and support.

Alice Reid, editor, Carol Eckhart, production coordinator, and Sara Finnegan, editor-in-chief of Williams & Wilkins, have all provided professional assistance in the manner which is characteristic of, and which one expects from, this distinguished and prestigious publishing house.

A special expression of abiding gratitude is due Jane Lendvey Conley, my secretary of eight years, who was as essential to completion of this revision as she was to the preparation of the original manuscript. Mrs. Conley, working nights and weekends, typed and retyped manuscript revisions supplied to her by mail. She graciously provided of her own time, energy, and talent to the final preparation of the revised manuscript for submission to the publisher. This revision, like the original text, could not have been undertaken, let alone completed, without the promise of her interest, enthusiasm, support, and dedication.

John H. Harris, Jr., M.D., D.Sc.

Contents

chapter one

Skull

General Considerations

Injury to the skull, including the intracranial contents, may occur as an isolated event or in association with injuries of other body parts. The more numerous and severe the multiple injuries, the greater the probability of head injury. In an analysis of 146 fatal traffic accidents, 42% of the victims were found to have radiographically demonstrable head injuries ranging from simple linear fractures to massive skull damage (1).

The primary consideration in the management of the severely injured or unconscious patient must be directed toward hemostasis, the maintenance of an adequate airway, and prevention of cardiovascular collapse. When vital functions are stable, it is appropriate to consider the roentgen evaluation of the head and neck. In the severely injured patient, these anatomic regions should be considered as one, since Davis et al. (2), in a review of 50 patients who died of craniospinal injuries, noted that 61% of those with brain damage also had cervical cord injury and 25% of the victims had concomitant head and cervical spine injuries. Therefore, prior to performing radiographic examination of the head, a horizontal beam lateral radiograph of the cervical spine should be obtained to exclude an unstable lesion of the cervical spine. Unless there is a compelling clinical indication to do otherwise, the horizontal beam radiograph of the cervical spine should be obtained prior to endotracheal or nasogastric intubation (Fig. 1.1).

The philosophy and rationale regarding the radiographic examination of the skull for trauma has changed during the past 5 years largely as the result of the efficacy studies of Bell and Loop (3) and the work of Phillips (4) at the University Hospital and the Harborview Hospital in Seattle, Washington, and because of the increased availability of computed tomography. Bell and Loop, in a prospective study of 1500 patients who had skull radiographic examinations for trauma, identified 21 "high yield" criteria (Table 1.1) which resulted in the detection of 92 skull fractures in 1065 patients as compared to one fracture in 435 patients in the "low yield" group.

A modification of Bell and Loop's high yield criteria for the selection of patients to have skull radiographic examination following trauma (Table 1.2) led to an approximate 40% reduction in skull radiography and a significant improvement in the yield of positive findings.

It is important in the utilization of such stringent criteria for the selection of patients for post-trauma radiographic examinations of the skull to realize that linear or nondepressed fractures will be unrecognized in some patients. The adoption of the "high yield" criteria, therefore, requires good rapport between the attending physician and the patient, the realization (by the patient) that linear, nondepressed fractures do not, per se, alter medical management, and close supervision, or monitoring, of the patient by a responsible person.

In fact, the appropriatenesss of the high yield criteria in the roentgen evaluation of children with head trauma has been challenged by DeSmet et al. (5), who report that all the skull fractures which occurred in children in their series would have been undetected since none of the children met the high yield criteria. Regarding nondepressed, linear skull fractures, Pendergrass et al. (6) state that "a fracture of the cranium which does not involve a sinus and is not otherwise compound or depressed is, in itself, of no great importance. Harwood-Nash (7), in discussing skull fractures in children, states that "a simple fracture in an otherwise well child has as likely a chance of serious intracranial sequelae as a child without a fracture, and they should be treated in the same manner."

Computed tomography is recognized by many as the radiographic diagnostic procedure of choice in the evaluation of a patient with head trauma (8–11).

Many influences affect the attending physician's decision regarding the roentgen evaluation of the patient with head trauma. These include the condition of the patient, the physician's previous experiences, the demands of the patient or family, and, probably

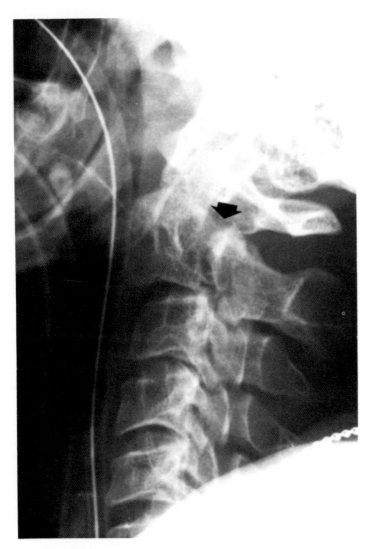

Fig. 1.1 This patient was unconscious upon admission to the emergency department and had multiple organ system injuries. He had not vomited and had a patent airway. A cervical spine injury was not considered and, consequently, the hangman's fracture of C_2 (*arrow*) was not recognized until the horizontal beam lateral radiograph of the cervical spine was obtained *following* the passage of the nasogastric and endotracheal tubes. Only the favorable spinal canal/cord ratio at the C_2 level and the decompression of the canal resulting from the bilateral pedicle fractures prevented cord damage during the manipulation of the cervical spine required during intubation.

Table 1.1
High-Yield Findings (3)

History	Physical Examination
>5 min of unconsciousness	Palpable bony malignment
>5 min of retrograde amnesia	Discharge from ear
Vomiting	Discharge from nose
Nonvisual focal symptoms	Eardrum discoloration
Accident at work or gunshot wound	Bilateral black eyes

Neurologic Examination	Physical Evaluation
Stupor, semiconsciousness or coma	Injury considered "severe"
Breathing irregular or apneic	Odds for fracture "50:50" or "9:1 certain"
Babinski reflex present	Examination because "fracture seriously suspected"
Other reflex abnormality	
Focal weakness	
Sensory abnormality	
Anisocoria	
Other cranial nerve abnormality	

Table 1.2
High-Yield Criteria

Historical Criteria
1. An established history of unconsciousness
2. Gunshot wound or skull penetration
3. Previous craniotomy with shunting tube in place

Physical Examination Criteria
1. Skull depression palpable or identified by probe in scalp laceration
2. Discharge from ear
3. CSF discharge from nose
4. Blood in middle ear cavity
5. Battle's sign
6. Racoon's eyes
7. Presence of coma or stupor (not related to alcoholic ingestion)
8. Focal neurologic signs

least significant, medicolegal implications. For these reasons, we do not believe it appropriate to set forth specific indications for the roentgen examination of the skull in instances of head trauma beyond those which are considered to be absolute, i.e., 1) localization of foreign bodies, 2) the detection of compound or depressed fractures, or 3) the localization of fractures. Efficacy studies are useful and, in the instance of head trauma, have provided valuable guidelines for the effective utilization of radiographic skull examinations. However, efficacy studies are not a substitute for value judgments. The latter are the result of individual patient-physician interaction, and it is at this level that the responsibility, and the decision, for the diagnostic evaluation of patients with head trauma rests.

Radiographic Examination

The routine, or basic, roentgen examination of the skull should include anteroposterior, posteroanterior, each lateral, and occipital projections. Stereoscopic examinations may be useful but are not essential.

The standard views may be obtained with the patient either erect or recumbent. When necessary, an adequate, diagnostic radiographic study of the skull may be obtained with the patient entirely in the supine position.

The base view of the skull (Hirtz) has little application in the evaluation of the patient with acute symptoms referable to the skull or its contents. This projection, which requires forced hyperextension of the cervical spine, is contraindicated in patients suspected of cervical spine or skull injuries because of the possibility of producing or exaggerating spinal cord or brain stem damage.

When the radiographic examination of the skull is made with the patient supine, a horizontal beam lateral projection must be included in order to record the presence of an air fluid interface.

The presence of an air fluid level in the sphenoid or maxillary sinuses, demonstrable only in this position, may be the most striking roentgen sign of fracture of the sphenoidal or maxillary bones.

Special projections may be suggested by clinical or routine radiographic findings. For example, in the presence of bleeding from the external ear or bluish discoloration behind the tympanic membrane, laminograms of the petrous pyramids or routine mastoid views may be indicated. The amount of depression of fracture fragments can frequently only be properly assessed by radiographs made with the skull rotated into an appropriate oblique position and with the central ray passing tangential to the involved arc of the skull.

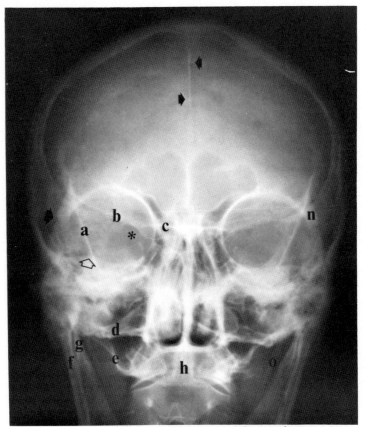

Fig. 1.2 Posteroanterior roentgenogram of the cranium. The vertically situated linear density in the midline of the skull indicated by the *two small solid arrows* is physiologic calcification of the cerebral falx. *a* is the greater sphenoidal wing; *b*, the lesser sphenoidal wing; *c*, the cribriform plate of the frontal bone; *d*, the occipital bone projecting through the maxillary sinus; *e*, anterolateral wall of the maxillary sinus; *f*, neck of the mandible; *g*, coronoid process of the mandible; *h*, odontoid process of C₂; *o*, styloid process. The *solid arrow* lateral to the lateral wall of the right orbit indicates the zygomaticofrontal suture and the *open arrow* the arcuate eminence.

Radiographic Anatomy

The posteroanterior roentgenogram of the cranium (Fig. 1.2) is, as its name states, made with the patient supine, the zygomatic arch perpendicular to the table top, and the central ray parallel to the arch. This projection, a variant of the posteroanterior study, has sufficient advantages to justify the time and radiographic exposure necessary to produce it. The skeletal anatomy of the skull and face are demonstrated in a slightly different, but significant, perspective. In Figure 1.2, *a* is the greater sphenoidal wing; *b*, the lesser sphenoidal wing; *c*, the cribriform plate of the frontal bone; *d*, the occipital bone; *e*, the anterolateral wall of the maxillary sinus; *f*, the neck of the mandible; *g*, the

coronoid process of the mandible; and *h*, the odontoid process of C₂. *o* is the styloid process. The *open arrow* indicates the arcuate eminence; the *solid arrow* at the lateral wall of the orbit, the zygomaticofrontal suture; and the *small solid arrows* in the midline of the calvarium, the calcified cerebral falx.

The posteroanterior projection of the skull (Fig. 1.3) is designed to demonstrate both the cranium (that portion of the head above the orbits) and the face. When properly positioned, with the patient prone, the forehead and nose resting upon the table, and the central beam directed slightly above the occipital protuberance, the petrous pyramids should be projected through the orbits sufficiently well to visualize the apices of the pyramids, the internal auditory mea-

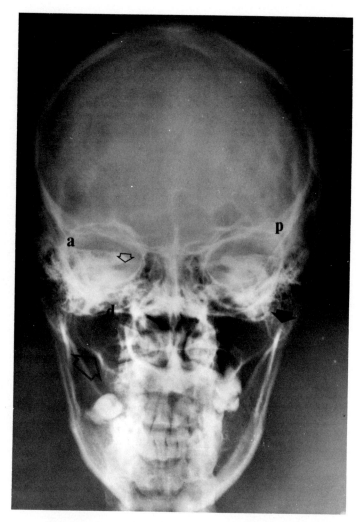

Fig. 1.3 Posteroanterior projection of the skull. The petrous pyramids are projected through the orbits. The *small open arrow* indicates the internal auditory canal; the *small solid arrow* indicates the coronoid process of the mandible; and the *large open arrow* the anterolateral wall of the maxillary sinus. *a* is the greater wing of the sphenoid which comprises the floor of the temporal fossa. *d* is the occipital bone projected through the maxillary sinus and *p* is the confluence of the lesser wing of the sphenoid with the orbital process of the frontal bone.

tus, and the internal auditory canal (*small open arrow*). This projection also provides clear visualization of the lateral margin of the greater wing of the sphenoid (*a*) which comprises the floor of the temporal fossa, the lesser wing of the sphenoid and its confluence with the orbital process of the frontal bone (*p*), and the anterolateral margin of the maxillary sinus (*large open arrow*). The occipital bone (*d*) is projected through the maxillary sinus. The *solid arrow* indicates the

coronoid process of the mandible. When calcified, the pineal gland or the cerebral falx identifies the position of the intracranial midline structures.

The lateral roentgenogram of the normal adult skull is seen in Figure 1.4. The purpose of examining the skull in each lateral position is to help locate intracranial calcifications or lateral cranial wall fractures that cannot be identified on sagittal projections. Radiographic images are smaller and more sharply defined on that lateral roentgenogram in which they are closest to the film. This difference in radiographic characteristics is real and recognizable, and, on the basis of the relative size of the image and sharpness of its margins, it is possible to "lateralize" the structure in question. Radiographic densities located in, or near, the midline have an identical appearance on each lateral roentgenogram.

The general appearance of the lateral radiograph of the skull is that of a midsagittal cross-section of the cranium. The anterior cranial fossa lies anterior to the anterior clinoids and the free margin of the lesser sphenoidal wings, the posterior fossa between the petrous pyramids and the occipital bone, and the middle cranial fossa between the two. The coronal (Fig. 1.4*a*) and lambdoidal (*b*) sutures are normally well seen in the lateral examination. The squamosal suture is commonly not visible on the lateral roentgenogram of the skull. The hypophyseal fossa (*) is bounded by the anterior (*small solid arrow*) and posterior (*large solid arrow*) clinoid processes. The floor of the hypophyseal fossa forms a portion of the roof of the sphenoidal sinuses (*d*). When sufficiently calcified, the pineal gland or the habenula (Fig. 1.5) is recognizable. The relationship of the groove for the anterior division of the middle meningeal artery (Fig. 1.6) as it parallels the coronal suture is of particular importance. The posterior branch of the middle meningeal artery (Fig. 1.7) crosses the squamosal portion of the temporal bone.

Several venous sinuses can be identified on the lateral radiograph. One of the largest and most constant of these is the transverse sinus (Fig. 1.8), which appears as a broad, smoothly margined band of decreased density extending from the region of the internal occipital protuberance in an obliquely downward course to the apex of the petrous pyramid. At this point, the sinus bends and parallels the posterior surface of the petrous pyramid (lateral sinus plate) as the sigmoid sinus.

The sphenoparietal sinus groove (Fig. 1.9, *solid arrow*) is frequently identifiable extending from above downward just posterior to the coronal suture.

Convolutional markings (Fig. 1.10) are focal areas of decreased density caused by thinning of the bones of the calvarium due to pressure of the cerebral gyri. The markings, which are variable in their incidence

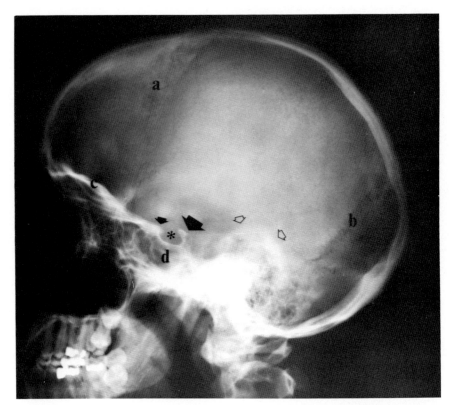

Fig. 1.4 Lateral projection of the adult skull. The *small solid arrow* indicates the anterior clinoid processes and the *large solid arrow* indicates the posterior clinoid processes. The hypophyseal fossa is indicated by the asterisk (*). The *open arrows* indicate the soft tissue density of the pinna of the ears. *a* is the coronal suture; *b*, the lambdoidal. *c* indicates the floor of the anterior cranial fossa (roof of the orbits). The sphenoidal sinus is indicated by *d*.

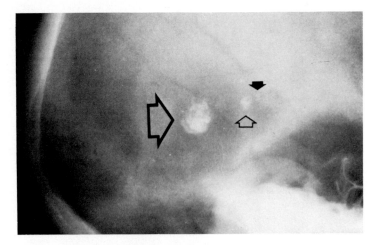

Fig. 1.5 Lateral radiograph of the posterior half of the skull. The faint crescentric density indicated by the *solid arrow* represents the habenular commissure; the *open arrow* designates calcification in the pineal gland. The *large open arrow* indicates superimposed calcifications of the choroid plexuses of the lateral ventricles.

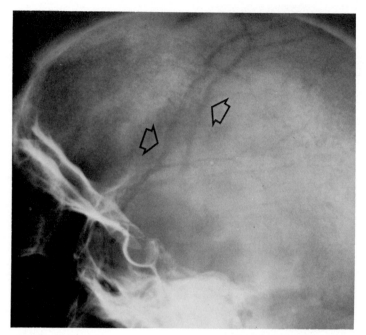

Fig. 1.6 The *arrows* indicate the groove for the anterior division of the middle meningeal artery. This artery is a bilateral structure and its course extends upward in the anterior portion of the parietal bone just posterior to the coronal suture. This vessel is frequently torn by a fracture involving this portion of the skull, resulting in an epidural hemorrhage or hematoma.

Fig. 1.7 The *arrows* indicate the groove for the posterior branch of the middle meningeal artery.

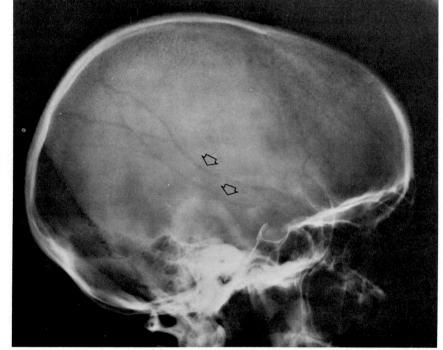

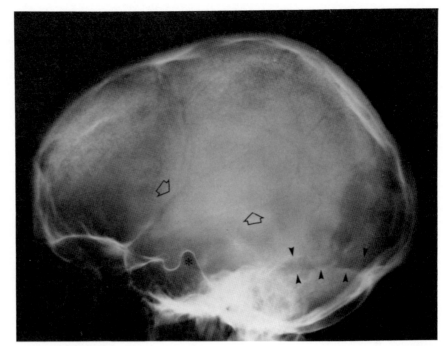

Fig. 1.8 The margins of the transverse sinus groove are indicated by the *arrowheads*. Grooves for the anterior and posterior divisions of the middle meningeal arteries are identified by the *open arrows*. Pneumatization of the sphenoidal sinus extends into the dorsum sellae (*).

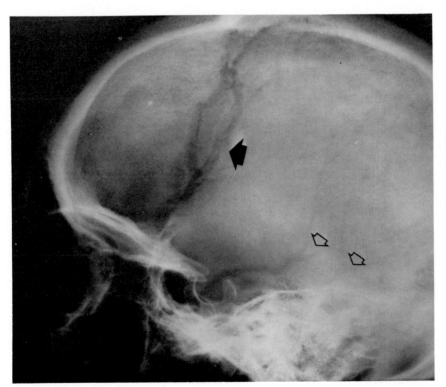

Fig. 1.9 The *open arrows* indicate the posterior branch of the middle meningeal arteries. The *solid arrow* designates the groove for the sphenoparietal sinus (middle meningeal vein).

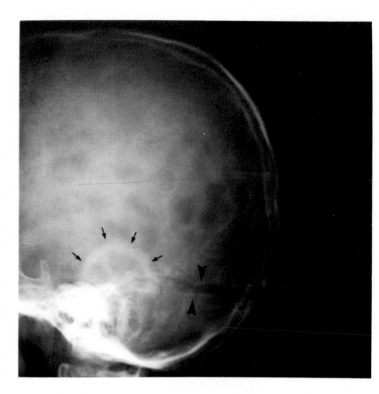

Fig. 1.10 The ill defined lucencies in the parietal bone represent areas of focal thinning of the calvarium which coincide with the convolutions of the cerebral cortex. The *arrowheads* indicate the groove of the transverse sinus. The pinna of the ear produces the broad curved density (*stemmed arrows*) above the density of the petrous pyramid.

and appearance and more common in infants and young children, are of no clinical significance.

Intradiploic venous lakes are small, irregularly outlined areas of decreased density situated in the diploe (Fig. 1.11, *solid arrow*). Characteristically, an intradiploid venous channel can be found leading into the venous lake. Vascular marks, which may be grooves either on the inner table of the skull or in the diploic channels, have characteristics that permit their distinction from suture or fracture lines. Vascular marks have faintly sclerotic, slightly irregular ("beaded"), parallel margins, are usually paired structures, and branch. Reflecting this normal arborization, the caliber of the arterial grooves on the inner table diminishes peripherally (Figs. 1.6, 1.7 and 1.9), while the caliber of the intradiploic venous channels increase as

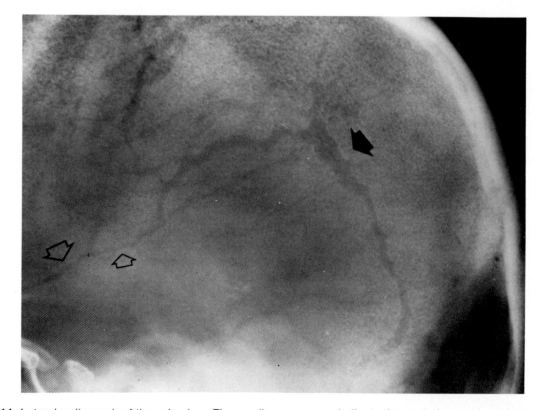

Fig. 1.11 Lateral radiograph of the calvarium. The *small open arrows* indicate the posterior meningeal artery and its branches. The *solid arrow* indicates an intradiploic venous channel.

these structures coalesce to form the vascular lakes (Figs. 1.11, 1.12). These features aid in the distinction between a vascular mark and a fracture line.

The occipital view (Fig. 1.13) is designed to portray the bony structures of the posterior cranial fossa. The posterior margin of the foramen magnum (*solid arrow*) is the most striking structure in the occipital projection. Depending upon the anatomy of the occipital bone and the angulation of the x-ray tube, the dorsum sellae (*a*) or the posterior arch of C_1 (Fig. 1.14) may be seen through the foramen magnum. The anterior rim of the foramen is obscured by the superimposed bony structures of the middle cranial fossa.

The petrous pyramids (Fig. 1.13*b*) are superim-

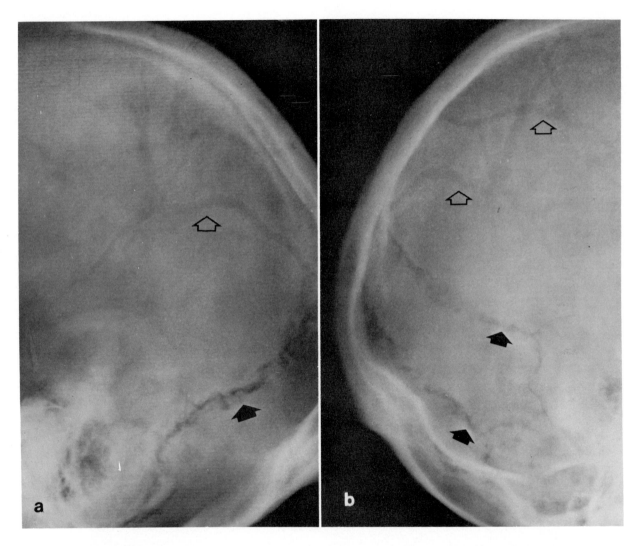

Fig. 1.12 (a) The *open arrow* indicates an intradiploic venous channel. These normal vascular structures are most frequently found in the frontal or parietal areas, and particularly in the region of the parietal eminence. Their number and extent is variable. They produce broad bands of decreased density with faintly sclerotic, somewhat indistinct, irregular margins. Irregular small areas of decreased density along the course of these channels or adjacent to them represent intradiploic venous lakes. The *solid arrow* indicates the lambdoidal suture. Notice that the suture line is serrated, its margins more sharply defined, and the suture line itself more radiolucent than the diploic vein. **(b)** A slightly obliqued lateral projection of the occipitoparietal portion of a normal adult skull. This technique was used to demonstrate that the diploic veins and the arms of the lambdoidal suture are paired structures and to facilitate recognition of the radiographic characteristics of a diploic vein (*open arrows*) and a cranial suture (*solid arrows*).

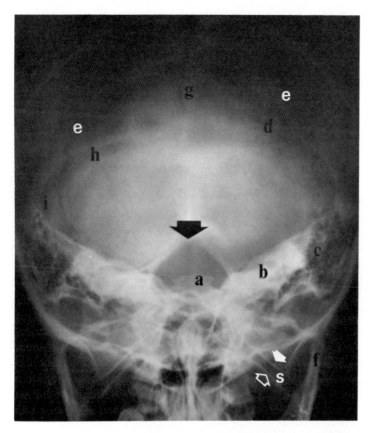

Fig. 1.13 Occipital view of the skull. The *large solid arrow* indicates the posterior margin of the foramen magnum through which is projected the dorsum sellae (*a*). *b* represents the petrous pyramid; *c*, air cells of the petrous pyramid and the mastoid process; *d*, the coronal suture; *e*, the lambdoidal suture; *g*, the sagittal suture; *h*, the groove for the transverse sinus; *i*, the groove for the sigmoid sinus. *f* represents the neck of the ascending ramus of the mandible. The sphenomaxillary fissure (*s*) is formed by the sphenomaxillary surface of the greater wing of the sphenoid (*small solid arrow*) and the posterolateral wall of the maxillary sinus (*open arrow*).

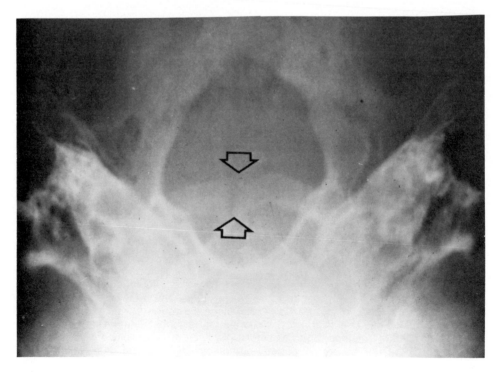

Fig. 1.14 The *open arrows* indicate the posterior arch of C_1 projecting through the foramen magnum.

posed upon the lateral margin of the foramen magnum and extend laterally toward the squamosal portion of the temporal bone. The air cells of the petrous pyramid and the mastoid process (*c*) are found at the junction of the pyramid and the squamosal portion of the temporal bone.

Both the lambdoidal (Fig. 1.13*e*) and the coronal (*d*) sutures are visible in this examination. The coronal suture has a wide arc, while that of the lambdoidal suture is short. Wormian bones are frequently found in the lambdoidal suture. The sagittal suture (*g*) is visible at the midline.

Grooves for the bilateral transverse sinuses (Fig. 1.13*h*) and the sigmoid sinuses (*i*) are commonly identifiable. The sphenomaxillary fissure (*s*) is formed by the sphenomaxillary surface of the greater wing of the sphenoid (*small solid arrow*) and the posterolateral wall of the maxillary sinus (*open arrow*). The neck of the mandible is indicated by (*f*).

The roentgen study of the skull of infants and children requires the same projections as described earlier. However, there are distinct differences in the appearance of the skull of infants and young children as compared to the adult skull. The most obvious difference is the disproportion between the bones of the calvarium with respect to those of the face. At birth, the cranium is normally much larger than the face.

During infancy, the anterior and posterior fontanelles are open and radiographically visible. The anterior fontanelle generally closes during the 2nd year and the posterior fontanelle by the 2nd month. Normally, all of the major suture lines are open. Minor sutures, such as the metopic suture (Fig. 1.15) and the innominate synchondrosis (Fig. 1.16), may be visible during infancy.

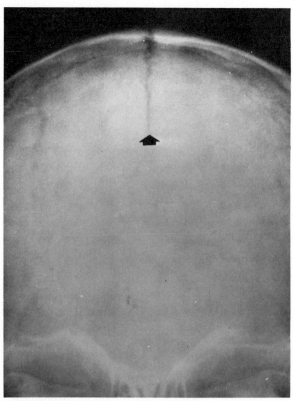

Fig. 1.15 The *arrow* indicates the metopic suture of the frontal bone.

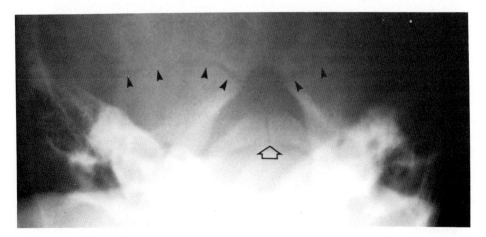

Fig. 1.16 The innominate synchrondosis (*arrowheads*) extend from the posterolateral margin of the foramen magnum into the occipital bone. The *open arrow* indicates the ununited posterior arch of the atlas vertebra.

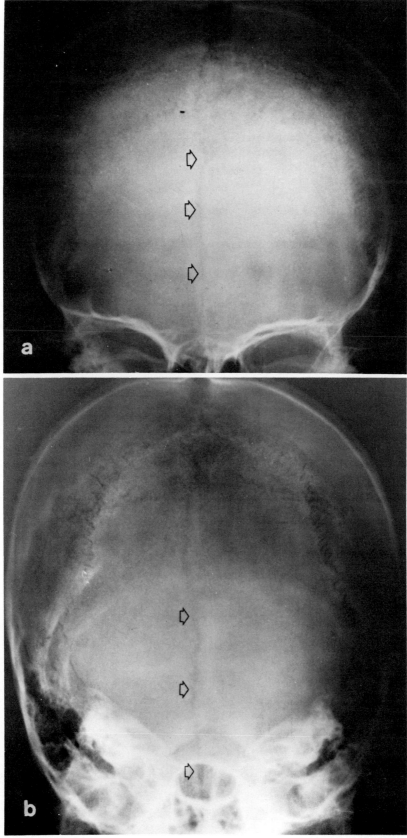

Fig. 1.17 The *arrows* indicate the persistent metopic suture as seen in the posteroanterior **(a)** and the occipital **(b)** projections of a normal adult skull. This normal variant should be distinguishable from a linear fracture by virtue of uniform width, faintly sclerotic margins, and irregular course.

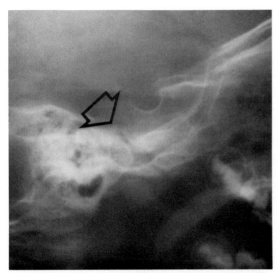

Fig. 1.18 The *arrow* identifies the spheno-occipital synchrondrosis. This normal structure, which occurs in the clivus, may persist until the age of 16–18 years as a radiolucent defect with sclerotic margins. The synchondrosis should not be mistaken for a fracture of the floor of the middle cranial fossa.

The metopic suture extends anteriorly from the anterior fontanelle a variable distance along the midline of the frontal bone. The bilateral innominate synchondrosis sutures are represented by curvilinear radiolucent lines of variable length that extend laterally from the posterolateral margins of the foramen magnum. While these sutures usually fuse and become obliterated during childhood, the metopic suture may persist as a normal variant into adulthood (Fig. 1.17). These normal structures should not be mistaken for linear, nondepressed fracture lines.

The spheno-occipital synchondrosis (Fig. 1.18) appears as an obliquely vertical radiolucent defect with sclerotic margins in the clivus at the junction of the sphenoid and occipital bones. This temporary joint may persist until the age of 16–18 years.

Lack of fusion of the planum sphenoidale with the chiasmatic sulcus ["the unfused planum sphenoidale" (12)] (Fig. 1.19) is a rare developmental variant that can simulate a basilar skull fracture. The radiographic characteristics of the unfused planum sphenoidale include a superior position of the anterior portion of the osseous discontinuity and the sclerotic margins of the sharply oblique separation. Fractures in the region of the planum sphenoidale (Fig. 1.20) may be distinguished from the developmentally unfused planum by the vertical fracture line, the sharp irregular, nonsclerotic margins of the fragments, the inferior position of the anterior fragment and the commonly associated pneumocephalus.

As seen in the radiographs of the normal adolescent and adult skull, the cranial sutures (Fig. 1.12, *solid*

arrows) are serrated, have sclerotic margins, and frequently contain Wormian bones. The location of the major sutures is constant in children and adults. A knowledge of their location and radiographic appearance helps distinguish sutures from fracture lines. The squamosal suture, as seen in the frontal projections (Fig. 1.2 and 1.3) is the suture most frequently mistaken for a fracture. This suture, which is obliquely oriented with respect to the lateral wall of the cranium, is seen end-on in frontal projections and casts an obliquely vertical radiolucent defect in the region of the floor of the temporal fossa, thus resembling a fracture line. The regular, slightly sclerotic margins and the fact that the suture is a paired structure establishes its true identity.

Radiographic Manifestations of Trauma

Computed tomography (CT) provides direct evidence of intracranial trauma and is, therefore, the radiographic diagnostic examination of choice when there is clinical indication for the roentgen examination of the skull following trauma. CT is not only appropriate in the patient with head trauma but is also indicated in the evaluation of seizure, "stroke," and intracranial inflammation.

Computed tomography demonstrates many of the effects of intracranial trauma better than any other

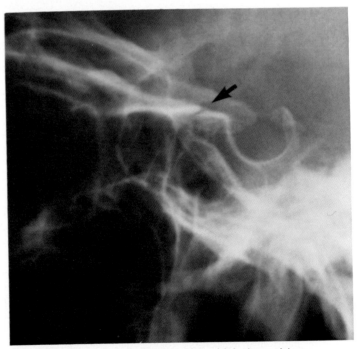

Fig. 1.19 The unfused planum sphenoidale (*arrow*) is a normal developmental variant. The superior portion of the anterior portion, the direction of inclination of the defect, and its smooth, parallel, densely sclerotic margins are characteristic of this variant.

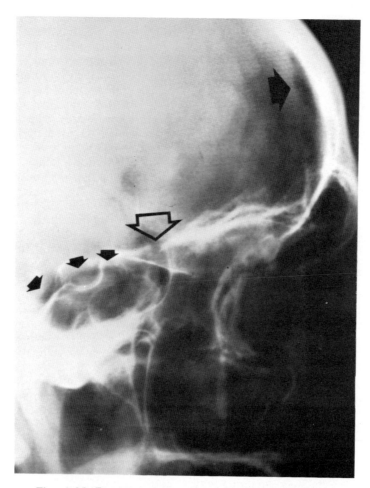

Fig. 1.20 Fracture of the planum sphenoidale (*open arrow*). The fracture line is vertically situated, its margins are sharply irregular, and the anterior fragment is on the same plane as the posterior fragment. These features, together with the pneumocephalus (*solid arrows*) distinguish the fracture from developmental lack of fusion of the planum (Fig. 1.19).

imaging method. A positive CT scan, with or without the demonstration of a fracture on plain skull radiographs, provides the definitive diagnosis of epidural hematoma, a surgical emergency, and subdural hematoma. Intracerebral hemorrhage, even when occurring beneath an overlying peripheral intracranial hematoma, may be recognized only by CT. The evaluation of depressed skull fractures and the associated cerebral edema or hemorrhage is best demonstrated by CT (13). As early as 1975, Feindel reported that CT scanning was indicated in patients with complex head injuries for the localization and evaluation of superficial hematomas and epidural and subdural hematomas, as well as for the determination of the extent of hemorrhage, contusion, and edema (11). A study of 5000 CT brain scans performed at the Swed-

ish Medical Center (Denver, Colorado) has concluded that CT scanning is the radiographic examination of choice early in the evaluation of patients with head trauma (8). Because CT is so effective in demonstrating all types of intracranial hemorrhage, it has largely eliminated the need for cerebral angiography in the evaluation of the patient with head trauma (10).

Fractures of the base of the skull are notoriously difficult to recognize by routine radiographic procedures including rectilinear tomography. Basilar skull fractures are best demonstrated, and, indeed, may only be demonstrated, by CT. Such fractures are commonly associated with major complications (14).

Throughout the literature is the constant reminder that the more severe the injury, the more likely the CT scan is to demonstrate an intracranial abnormality. However, the reverse does not necessarily follow. That is to say, the absence of a demonstrable skull fracture or neurologic sign by no means excludes the possibility of significant intracranial injury. This feature of acute head trauma is reflected in the recent report of Zimmerman et al. (9), indicating that there is no correlation between the presence or absence of a skull fracture and the presence of an intracranial abnormality and that 50% of pediatric patients with diffuse cerebral edema may be conscious at the time of admission to the emergency department. Therefore, the indication for CT scanning in the patient with acute head trauma must be established on an individualized basis.

Thirty of 109 children, ranging in age from 3 months to 17 years, were found to have subarachnoid hemorrhage on the basis of CT scans performed following acute head trauma. Only 15 of the 30 patients with subarachnoid hemorrhage had skull fractures. While there was no specific correlation between the presence or absence of skull fracture and the subarachnoid hemorrhage, the subarachnoid hemorrhage occurred in 87% of the more severely injured patients (15).

General cerebral swelling is the most common finding in the pediatric patient with severe head trauma (9). The edema occurs in the immediate post-trauma period. Patients with CT demonstration of cerebral swelling have a variable clinical presentation in the immediate post-trauma period. They may be unconscious immediately following trauma or they may deteriorate rapidly to unconsciousness after a lucent interval lasting from minutes to hours. Up to 50% of the patients who die from head injury are conscious on admission (9).

Based upon the large body of medical literature describing the unique advantages of CT scanning in the evaluation of patients with head and face trauma and because of the combination of noninvasiveness and the high degree of accuracy in the detection of intracranial complications of acute head trauma, CT is the radiographic procedure of choice in all cases of severe head trauma (9) and, today, constitutes "usual and customary" care of patients with acute head trauma.

The plain film study of the skull can neither establish nor exclude the presence of intracranial hemorrhage or edema directly. A fracture line which crosses a vascular groove in the inner table of the skull should certainly prompt the consideration of an epidural hematoma. Any depressed fracture should be considered to be associated with intracranial hemorrhage, cerebral edema, or both, and therapeutic measures indicated by the clinical findings should be instituted. Shift of calcified midline structures, i.e., the pineal, habenular commissure, or cerebral falx, following

head trauma should be considered indicative of intracranial hemorrhage until proven otherwise.

Unfortunately, calcification of the pineal gland, habenula or the cerebral falx occurs in only a small percentage of children and young adults, and it is in this age group that the incidence of cranial trauma is highest. The incidence of calcification of the pineal gland increases with age and is present in about 60% of all adult skulls (16).

Echoencephalography provides accurate localization of the midline structures. The important disadvantage of the ultrasound study is the limited information that it provides and the fact that failure to record either a midline shift or a hematoma does not exclude the presence of such a lesion.

While the roentgen and ultrasound studies are complimentary, even together they constitute an inadequate definitive diagnostic evaluation of the patient with head trauma.

Vascular injuries that result from head trauma may produce extracerebral, (epidural and subdural hematoma and subarachnoid hemorrhage), intracerebral, or intraventricular hemorrhage. Epidural hematoma is an extradural accumulation of blood which is most commonly associated with a fracture, causing a tear of one of the divisions of the middle meningeal artery (Fig. 1.21a) or vein or one of the dural sinuses. Although there is a high incidence of skull fracture with epidural hematoma (17), this lesion may occur without a fracture being demonstrable either radiographically or at surgery (18). Low-lying temporoparietal fractures may tear the middle meningeal artery or vein. Fractures involving the vertex may tear the superior sagittal sinus, and those that cross the lateral dural sinuses or the torcular Herophili (Fig. 1.21b) may result in epidural hematoma of the posterior cranial fossa. Thus, the location of skull fractures with respect to vascular grooves is important.

Epidural hematoma produces a characteristic biconvex area of high attenuation (increased density) immediately adjacent to the inner table of the skull (Fig. 1.22) which demonstrates increased attenuation with enhancement. Bergstrom et al. (19) and others have demonstrated that there is a rather uniform and constant decrease in the attenuation value of both epidural and subdural hematomas during the 1st month post-trauma.

Subdural hematoma is the accumulation of blood in the space between the dura and the cerebral cortex. Bleeding originates from severe contusion or laceration of the brain substance (20). This lesion is almost always related to trauma and frequently occurs without an associated skull fracture. The usual acute subdural clot is the result of hemorrhage caused by motion of the brain within its covering structures tearing connecting veins. This type of intracranial

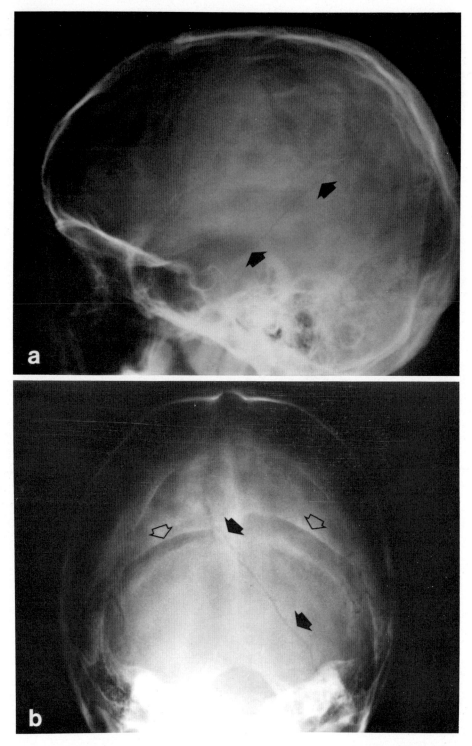

Fig. 1.21 (a) Linear, nondepressed fracture of parietal bone (*arrows*) which crosses the course of the posterior division of the middle meningeal artery and which caused the epidural hematoma seen in Figure 1.22. **(b)** Nondepressed linear fracture (*solid arrows*) crossing the torcular Herophili. The *open arrows* indicate the grooves for the transverse sinuses.

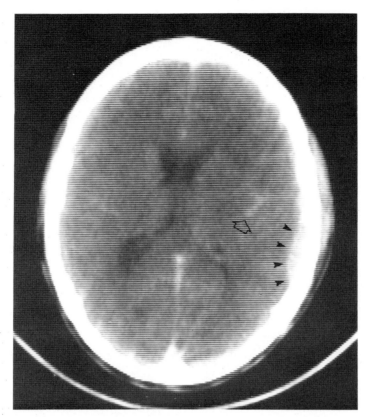

Fig. 1.22 Epidural hematoma (*arrowheads*) associated with nondepressed fracture seen in Figure 1.21**a**. Intracerebral hemorrhage is present in the parietal lobe (*open arrow*). The left lateral ventricle is compressed by the "mass effect" of the extracerebral injuries and tissue response.

motion is common and is caused by forces insufficient to produce skull fracture.

On CT, the typical acute subdural hematoma characteristically produces a peripheral biconcave (crescentric) zone of increased density (high attenuation) which parallels the concavity of the calvarium (Fig. 1.23). Because the acute subdural hemorrhage is free to fill the subdural space, the subdural hematoma is usually more extensive than the epidural hematoma. The subdural hematoma may extend into, or be confined to, the interhemispheric fissure. Bilateral subdural hematomas may be overlooked simply because of the bilaterality. Large epi- or subdural hematomas may exert a mass effect upon the ventricular system or displace the midline structures.

As noted above, subacute and chronic subdural hematomas have diminished density and, depending upon their age, may even be isodense. The presence of an isodense chronic subdural hematoma may be established on the basis of faint increase in density on a delayed scan made following enhancement. Secondary signs such as mass effect upon the ventricular system, displacement of midline structures, or unilateral effacement of cortical sulci suggest the presence of an isodense chronic subdural hematoma. In the absence of any of these CT signs, cerebral angiography should be considered and is the definitive diagnostic study. A radionuclide scan may be helpful in evaluating a possible isodense subarachnoid hematoma.

Acute or recurrent hemorrhage into a chronic or subacute subdural hematoma results in a different CT appearance. With the patient recumbent, the fresh blood will produce a zone of increased density in the dependent portion of the hematoma. The supernatent serum, or mixture of serum and cerebrospinal fluid (CSF), which entered the hematoma by osmosis, produces the zone of low attenuation (lucency). The resultant interface is usually sharply defined.

Subarachnoid hemorrhage is the accumulation of blood in the subarachnoid space caused by a contusion or laceration of the brain. Hematomas do not form in this space.

Cephalhematoma results from the organization of

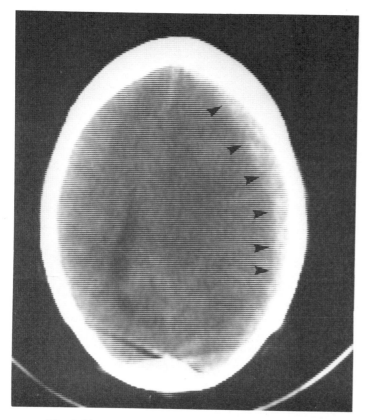

Fig. 1.23 Subdural hemorrhage (*arrowheads*). The crescentric density parallel to the inner table of the calvarium is the characteristic configuration of a subdural hematoma. The associated massive left cerebral edema has resulted in diminished attenuation of the parietal lobe and has completely obliterated the left lateral ventricle and displaced the midline structures to the right ("mass effect").

a subperiosteal hemorrhage secondary to head injury. It may or may not be associated with fracture of the underlying bone. Cephalhematoma is not an acute lesion; however, it is germaine to this discussion because of the presence of mass and calcification of its margins. Early, the calcification appears as a thin, shell-like density arising from the underlying bone (Figs 1.24 and 1.25). Ultimately, the entire hematoma calcifies and merges with the outer table of the skull. In the sagittal roentgenogram, this results in an area of increased thickness of the calvarium. In the lateral projection, a focal area of increased thickness of the calvarium. In the lateral projection, a focal area of increased density is visible.

Because multiple projections are needed to identify and localize some skull fractures (Figs. 1.26 and 1.27), every reasonable effort should be made to obtain a

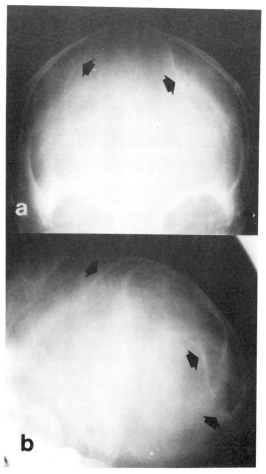

Fig. 1.25 (a, b) Calcification at the margins of bilateral parietal cephalhematomas.

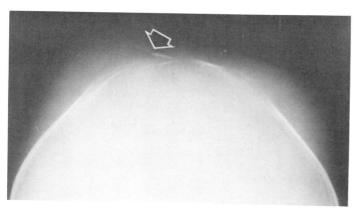

Fig. 1.24 Bilateral cephalhematomas. Calcification (*arrow*) is developing in the medial wall of the right cephalhematoma.

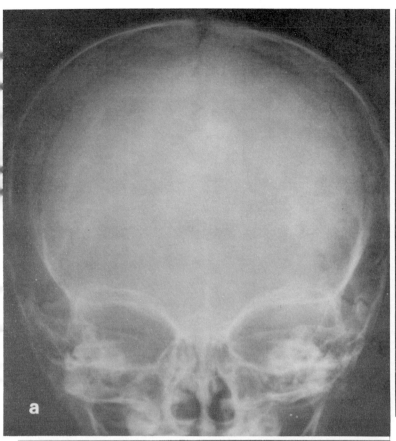

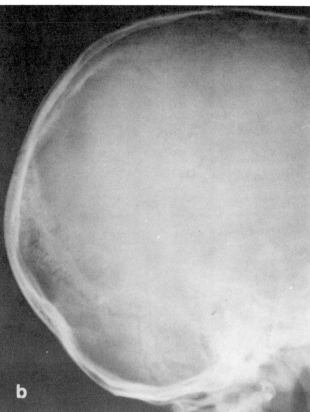

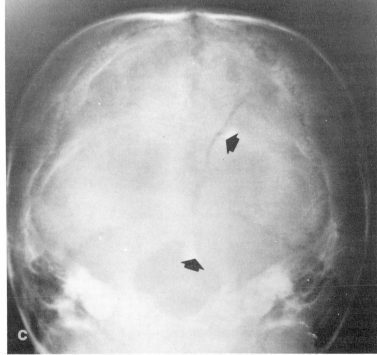

Fig. 1.26 Posteroanterior **(a)** and lateral **(b)** roentgenograms of the skull fail to reveal the fracture (*arrows*) involving the occipital bone, which is seen only in the occipital view **(c)**.

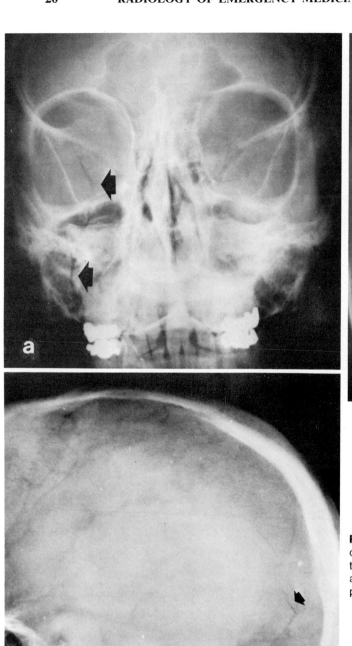

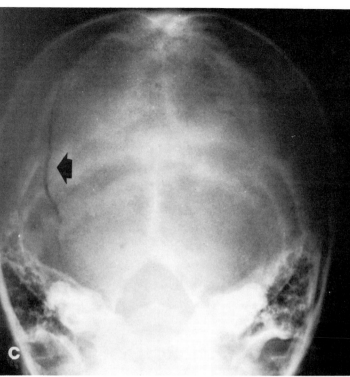

Fig. 1.27 The need for obtaining a complete roentgen examination of the skull is illustrated by this case. This fracture in the right side of the occipital bone (*arrows*) is poorly seen in the anteroposterior (a) and lateral **(b)** radiographs, but is clearly delineated in the occipital projection **(c)**.

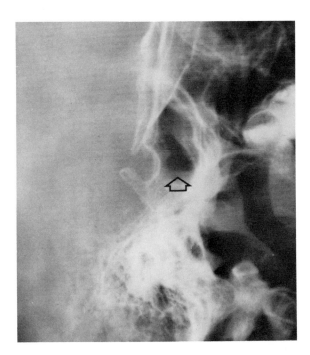

Fig. 1.28 Air-fluid level (*arrow*) in the sphenoidal sinus seen on the brow-up lateral roentgenogram of the skull. This indicates the presence of a fracture involving the sphenoidal bone, i.e., the base of the skull.

complete roentgen study of the skull at the time of initial examination.

Skull fractures are defined as closed or open, and these further classified as depressed or nondepressed (linear). Closed fractures are those in which there is no associated break in the overlying soft tissues. An open fracture is one in which communication does exist between the meninges and the outside air through the fracture defect and which is therefore associated with a high incidence of meningitis. Open fractures also include those which involve paranasal sinuses because, even though the skin may be intact, the fracture disrupts the mucous membrane of the sinus and permits contamination of meninges by air and mucous from the sinus. Open fractures of the middle cranial fossa extend into the sphenoid sinus. Middle fossa fractures are difficult to visualize and the presence of an air-fluid level within the sphenoidal sinus on the horizontal beam brow-up lateral radiograph (Fig 1.28) may be the only roentgen evidence of the existence of such a fracture.

Fractures involving only the anterior wall of the frontal sinus, even if the fragments are depressed, are not open fractures. Because the posterior wall remains intact (Fig. 1.29) there is no communication between the sinus cavity and the meninges and meningitis is not a complication.

Leakage of CSF is a specific sign of an open fracture of the skull. Open fractures of the frontal bone may involve both walls of the frontal sinus directly (Fig. 1.30) or may extend through the cribriform plate into the ethmoidal sinuses. The latter is the commonest cause of CSF rhinorrhea. Fracture of the petrous portion of the temporal bone involving the middle ear is the most common cause of CSF otorrhea (21).

Linear fractures are distinguishable from suture lines on the basis of the characteristics of their margins, their location, and unilaterality (Figs. 1.31 and 1.32).

The margins of nondepressed fractures are smooth and more sharply defined than the margins of either vascular markings (Fig. 1.33) or suture lines (Fig. 1.34).

Overlapping margins of depressed fragments produce an irregular band of increased density (Figs. 1.35 and 1.36).

The fragments of depressed fractures involving the frontal and parietal bossae may appear to be more severely depressed on the routine radiographs of the skull than is actually the case.

Tangential radiographs made with the skull rotated so that the fractured area is parallel to the central x-ray beam will afford an accurate assessment of the degree of depression (Figs. 1.37 and 1.38).

Comminuted, nondepressed fractures resulting from the impact of a low velocity blunt object have a rather characteristic, stellate pattern of fracture lines. This type of injury produces an inward bending of the tables of the calvarium, resulting in a peripheral circular fracture line and several additional linear fracture lines which radiate in spoke-like fashion from the peripheral fracture to the central point of maximum impact (Fig. 1.39).

Nontraumatic Lesions

Hair dressings (pomades) (Fig. 1.40) and wrinkles or folds of the scalp may produce opaque shadows that resemble intracranial calcification or nondepressed fracture lines.

Dermoids (epidermoids) are benign tumors that arise in the diploe. Radiographically, the dermoid produces a radiolucent defect with a rather sharply defined, faintly sclerotic margin (Fig. 1.41). It may contain a tiny calcific nidus. When the lesion arises in the diploe, it expands both tables of the skull and produces a palpable mass.

Primary and secondary neoplasms may involve the cranium. Multiple myeloma (Fig. 1.42) is the generalized primary malignant neoplasm that involves the cranium most commonly. Localized primary malignant tumors of the skull are infrequent. Metastatic lesions of the cranium are usually osteolytic (Fig. 1.43).

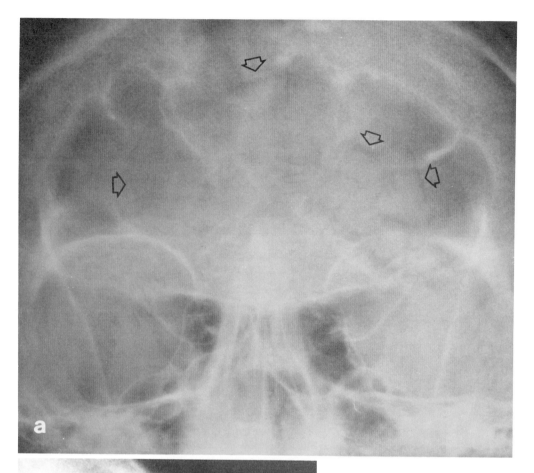

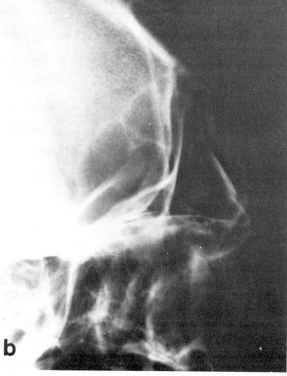

Fig. 1.29 This patient sustained a comminuted, depressed fracture of the anterior wall of the frontal sinus only (a). In the lateral radiograph (b) the posterior wall of the frontal sinus is seen to be intact. This, therefore, is not an open fracture.

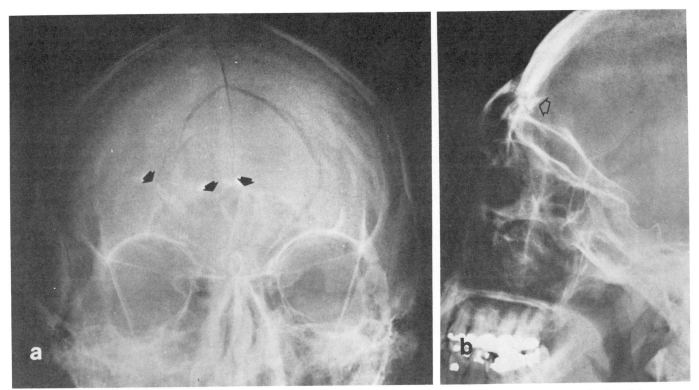

Fig. 1.30 Comminuted fracture of the frontal bone extending into the frontal sinus **(a)**. In the lateral projection **(b)**, a depressed fragment involving the posterior wall of the frontal sinus is indicated by the *open arrow*. This fracture, therefore, is an open fracture.

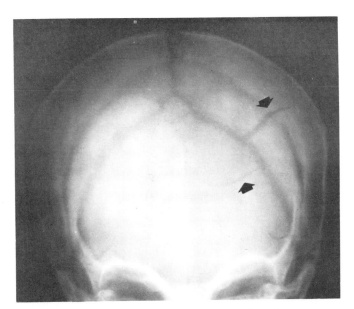

Fig. 1.31 In this posteroanterior projection, the *arrows* indicate the linear fracture line. The radiographic characteristics of the fracture line and its unilaterality should enable its distinction from the normal suture lines.

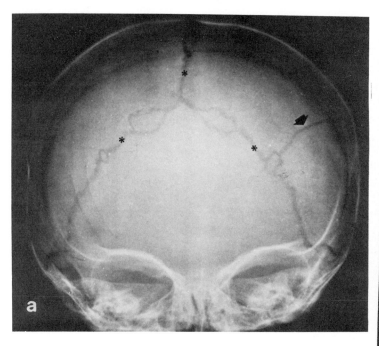

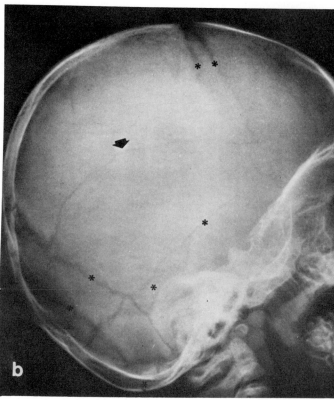

Fig. 1.32 (a, b) The radiographic differences between suture lines (*) in an older child and a fracture line (*arrows*) are well demonstrated by this illustration.

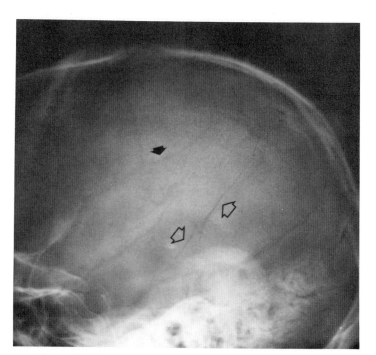

Fig. 1.33 The distinguishing features of a vascular marking (*solid arrow*) and a linear fracture (*open arrows*) are exemplified in this illustration.

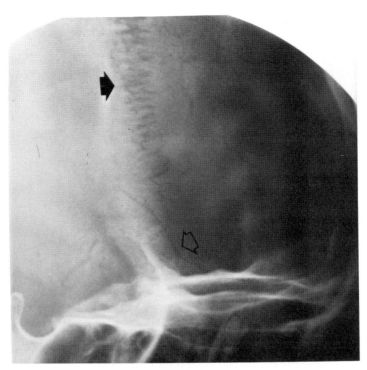

Fig. 1.34 The radiographic characteristics of the coronal suture (*solid arrow*) and a fracture line (*open arrow*) are evident in this lateral roentgenogram of the skull.

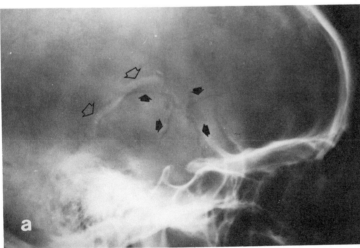

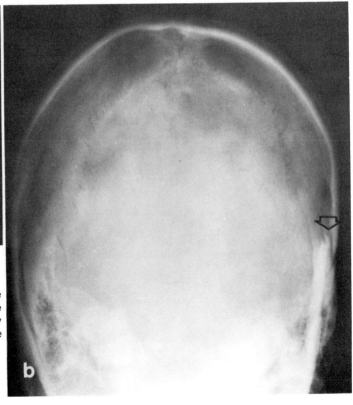

Fig. 1.35 (a, b) This patient sustained a blow to the left side of the head by a blunt instrument, resulting in a stellate fracture. The curvilinear band of increased density (*open arrows*) is caused by overlapping depressed fragments. The linear fracture lines are indicated by the *solid arrows*.

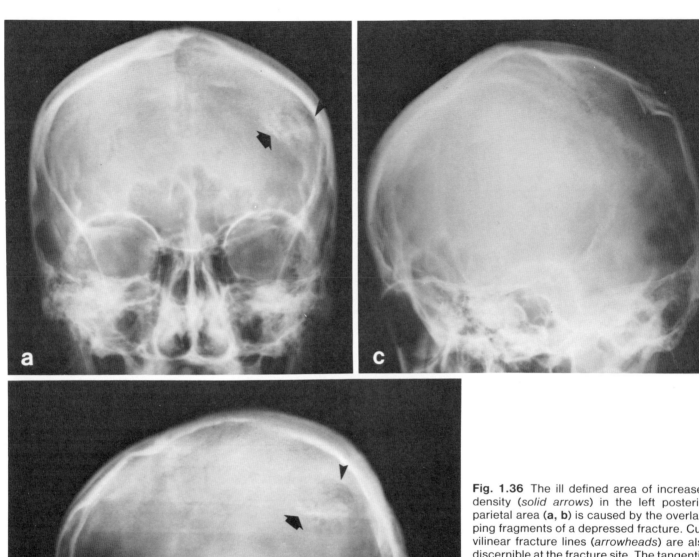

Fig. 1.36 The ill defined area of increased density (*solid arrows*) in the left posterior parietal area (**a, b**) is caused by the overlapping fragments of a depressed fracture. Curvilinear fracture lines (*arrowheads*) are also discernible at the fracture site. The tangential projection (**c**) confirms and establishes the magnitude of the depression.

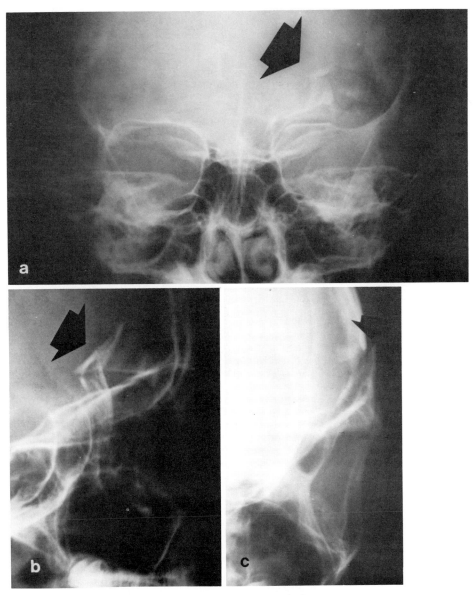

Fig. 1.37 In the routine anteroposterior
(**a**) and lateral (**b**) radiograph of the skull,
the fragments of the left frontal bone fracture appear to be severely depressed.
However, in the radiograph made with the
skull rotated and the central beam parallel
to the involved arc of the skull (**c**) the
degree of depression of the fragments is
accurately demonstrated.

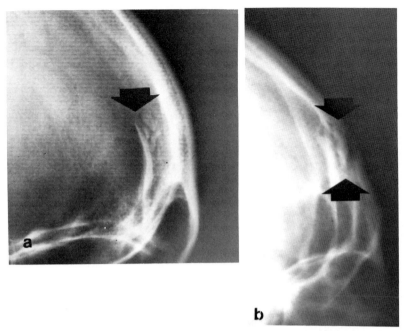

Fig. 1.38 In the lateral radiograph of the skull **(a)**, the fracture of the frontal eminence (*arrow*) appears to be severely depressed. The degree of actual depression of the fragment is more accurately depicted in the radiograph obtained with the skull rotated so that the involved arc of the frontal bossa is tangential to the central x-ray beam **(b)**.

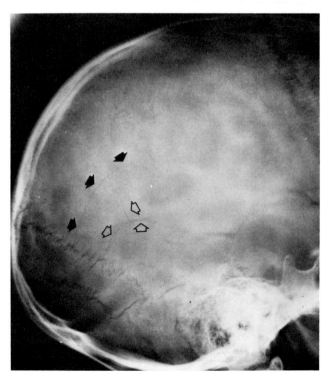

Fig. 1.39 Stellate fracture of the parietal bone. The peripheral circular fracture line is indicated by the *solid arrows*. The radiating linear fracture lines are indicated by the *open arrows*.

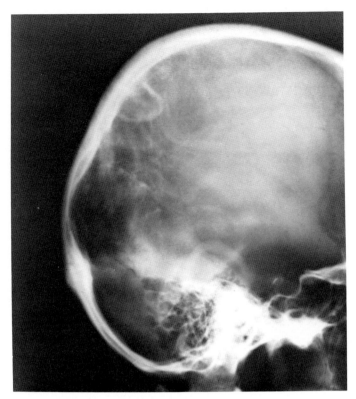

Fig. 1.40 The curvilinear densities overlying the posterior pariteal region are caused by braids which were dressed with hair pomade.

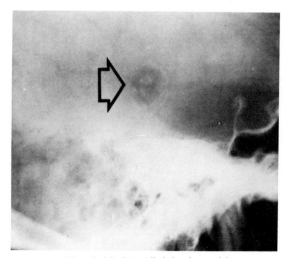

Fig. 1.41 Intradiploic dermoid.

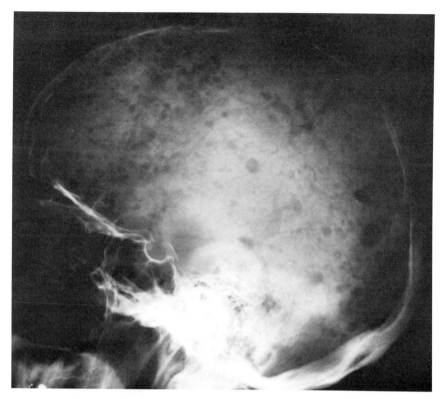

Fig. 1.42 Multiple myeloma.

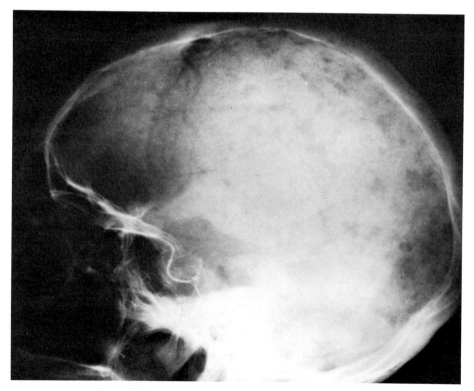

Fig. 1.43 Indistinctly marginated lytic metastatic lesions.

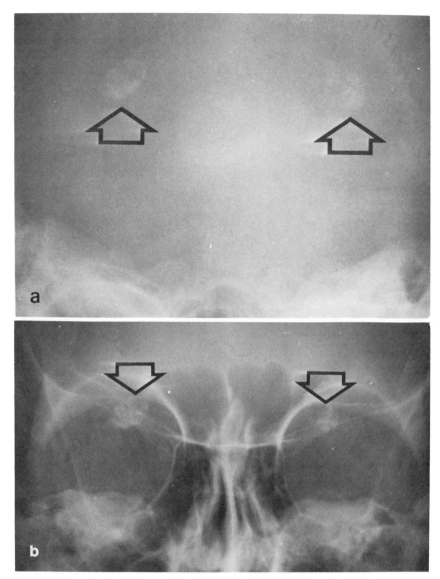

Fig. 1.44 (a, b) Calcified choroid plexuses of the lateral ventricles.

Tondreau (22) has classified intracranial calcifications as physiologic, pathologic non-neoplastic, and neoplastic. Physiologic calcifications commonly develop in normal intracranial structures such as the pineal, habenula, choroid plexus, dura, falx, tentorium, and Pacchionian bodies without a known pathologic etiology.

The incidence of pineal calcification has been previously noted. The habenula is reported to calcify in 47% of adults. Plaque-like calcification of the cerebral falx is common. The significance of calcification of these structures lies in the diagnostic usefulness of their radiologic localization. Displacement from the midline indicates the presence of a lesion on the side opposite the direction of displacement. The commonest causes for midline displacement are intracranial hemorrhage and cerebral neoplasms. It must be noted that small localized or thin diffuse intracranial hemorrhage or small cerebral neoplasms may exist without causing displacement of the midline structures. Therefore, the absence of lateral displacement of calcified midline structures does not exclude the possible presence of intracranial bleeding or tumor.

Calcification of the choroid plexuses of the lateral ventricles (Fig. 1.44) occurs in approximately 11% of patients (23). The radiographic significance of these

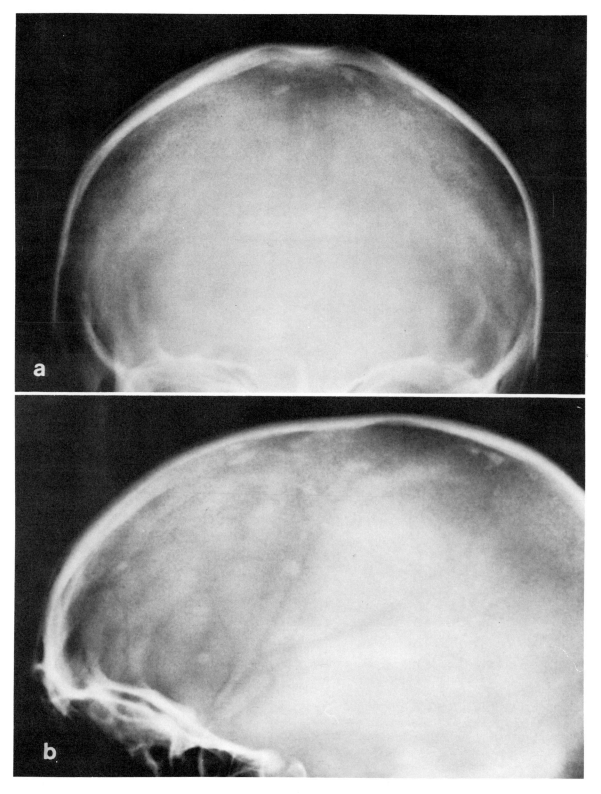

Fig. 1.45 (a, b) Pacchionian granulations.

calcifications rests primarily with their identification and the realization that they are not pathologic calcifications. Rarely, choroid calcifications may be displaced by a strategically situated brain tumor.

Pacchionian bodies (arachnoid granulations) function in the elimination of cerebrospinal fluids. These structures, which are located in depressions of the inner table of the skull at the vertex in the parietal and frontal areas, occasionally become calcified (6) (Fig. 1.45).

Of the pathologic, non-neoplastic calcifications, those of vascular origin are of interest in emergency medicine. Calcification of the wall of the siphon of the internal carotid arteries (Fig. 1.46) occurs in approximately 4–10% of skull roentgenograms from the sixth to the eighth decade (24). This calcification has no clinical significance. Particularly, its presence should not be equated with arteriosclerotic narrowing of cerebral arteries.

Calcification of the wall of an intracranial aneurysm is rare. Sub- or epidural hematomas are not calcified during the immediate post-traumatic phase. Chronic subdural hematoma may calcify in a shell-like distribution that resembles calcified pleural plaques.

Intracranial calcification caused by inflammatory disease is rare and is usually associated with uncommon conditions.

Calcification occurs in 15% of all intracranial neoplasms [see Gilbertson, cited in Camp (25)]. The oligodendroglioma and astrocytoma are the tumors that calcify most frequently.

Computed tomography is the diagnostic procedure of choice in the evaluation of the patient with acute,

nontraumatic onset of localizing or generalized intracranial signs and symptoms (26–29). CT can promptly and reliably detect intracranial vascular, neoplastic, inflammatory, and obstructive lesions and is able to distinguish between the common infarction and the uncommon intraparenchymal hemorrhage. Campbell et al (30), reported that 63% of all CT scans performed on patients with acute hemiparesis had positive (abnormal) CT scans. Fifty-nine percent of scans performed in the first 24 hours postictus were abnormal, while 66% of late (7–10 days postictus) CT scans were abnormal. It is important to be aware that in approximately 20% of Campbell's series, the initial CT scan was negative and that the second scan, performed 7–10 days later, was abnormal. Therefore, it is not reasonable to rely on an initial negative CT scan when the patient has definite intracranial symptoms. Additionally, 5% of all cerebral infarcts were isodense and could only be identified on the enhanced study. Peri-infarction edema developed in approximately 25% of patients, either initially or during the first 25 days following the ictus.

Computed tomography is not indicated in children with febrile or petit mal seizures but is indicated in other seizures, particularly the initial event, occurring in children and adults in order to detect remedial organic lesions (31).

Computed tomography is probably not indicated in the evaluation of children with chronic seizure disorders. Bachman et al. (32) have observed that in 70% of children with chronic seizure disorders, the CT scan was normal and only 2% of those with organic abnormalities had surgically correctable lesions.

Computed tomography is usually not indicated in

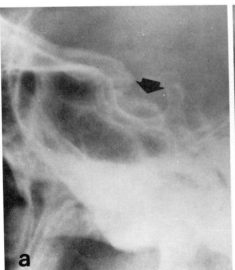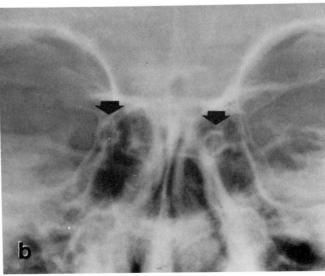

Fig. 1.46 Calcification of the siphon of the internal carotid artery superimposed upon the hypophyseal fossa **(a)** and projecting through the ethmoidal sinuses in the frontal projection **(b)**.

the study of the patient clinically suspected of cerebritis or encephalitis. However, when the diagnosis cannot be definitely established, when the differential diagnosis includes spontaneous subarachnoid hemorrhage, or when lumbar puncture cannot be performed, CT can be helpful in demonstrating the signs of diffuse cerebral edema, i.e., generalized compression of the ventricular system and effacement of the cerebral sulci, and by recording the absence of intracranial bleed or neoplasia.

Radionuclide brain scan is usually normal during the 1st week following a cerebrovascular occlusion, is considered inferior to CT in the detection of cerebral or intraventricular hemorrhage, and is of limited value in the detection of acute, post-traumatic sub- or epidural hematomas unless dynamic studies are performed (27, 30).

References

1. ALKER GJ, OH YS, LESLIE EV, LEHOTY J, PANARO VA, ESCHNER EG: Postmortem radiology of head and neck injuries in fatal traffic accidents. *Radiology* 114:611, 1975.
2. DAVIS D, BOHLMAN H, WALKER AE, FISHER R, ROBINSON R: The pathological findings in fatal craniospinal injuries. *J Neurosurg* 34:603, 1971.
3. BELL RS, LOOP JW: The utility and futility of radiologic skull examination for trauma. *N Engl J Med* 284:236, 1971.
4. PHILLIPS LA: A study of the effect of high yield criteria for emergency room skull radiography. HEW/Public Health Service/Bureau of Radiologic Health (FDA 78-8069), 1978.
5. DESMET AA, FRYBACK DG, THORNBURY JR: A second look at the utility of radiographic skull examination for trauma. *AJR* 132:95, 1979.
6. PENDERGRASS EP, SHEAFFER JP, HODES PJ: *The Head and Neck in Roentgen Diagnosis*, ed. 2. Charles C. Thomas, Springfield, Ill., 1956.
7. HARWOOD-NASH DC: Craniocerebral trauma in children. *Curr Probl Radiol* 3:3, 1973.
8. SEIBERT CE, SWANSON WR, DEBIASE J: *Computed Tomography and Head Trauma.* Swedish Medical Center, Denver, Colorado, 1976.
9. ZIMMERMAN RA, BILANIUK LT, BRUCE D, DOLINSKAS C, OBRIST W, KUHL D: Computed tomography of pediatric head trauma: Acute general cerebral swelling. *Radiology* 26:403, 1978.
10. FORBES GS, SHEEDY PF, PIEPGRAS DG, HOUSER OW: Computed tomography in the evaluation of subdural hematoma. *Radiology* 126:143, 1978.
11. FEINDEL W: Head and body scanning by computed tomography. *Can Med Assoc J* 113:273, 1975.
12. SMITH TR, KIER EL: The unfused planum sphenoidale: Differentiation from fracture. *Radiology* 98:305, 1971.
13. DAVES KR, TAVERAS JM, ROBERSON GH, ACKERMAN RH, DREISBACH JN: Computed tomography in head trauma. *Semin Roentgenol* 12:53, 1977.
14. CLAUSSEN CD, LOHCAMP FW, KRASTEL A: Computed tomography of trauma involving the brain and facial skull. *J Comput Assist Tomogr* 1:472, 1977.
15. DOLINSKAS CA, ZIMMERMAN RA, BILANIUK LT: A sign of subarachnoid bleeding on cranial computed tomographs of pediatric head trauma patients. *Radiology* 126:409, 1978.
16. PAUL LW, JUHL JH: *Essentials of Roentgen Interpretation*, ed. 2. Harper & Row, New York, 1965.
17. FERRIS EJ, SHAPIRO JH: Radiologic aspects of head trauma. *Mod Med* 38:104, 1970.
18. LAKE PA, PITTS FW: Recent experience with epidural hematomas. *J Trauma* 11:397, 1971.
19. BERGSTROM M, ERICSON K, LEVANDER B, SVENDSEN P: Computed tomography of cranial subdural and epidural hematomas: Variations of attenuation related to time and clinical events such as rebleeding. *J Comput Assist Tomogr* 1:449, 1977.
20. TORRES H: Acute head injuries. *Am Fam Physician* 2:88, 1970.
21. MILLER RH: CSF rhinorrhea and otorrhea. *Clin Neurosurg* 19:263, 1972.
22. TONDREAU RL: Intracranial calcification. Presented as Refresher Course, Radiology Society of North America, 1954.
23. CHILDE AE: Calcification of choroid plexus and its displacement by expanding intracranial lesions. *AJR* 45:523, 1941.
24. CAMP JD: Pathologic non-neoplastic intracranial calcification. *JAMA* 137:1023, 1948.
25. CAMP JD: Significance of intracranial calcification in roentgenologic diagnosis of intracranial neoplasms. *Radiology* 55:659, 1950.
26. BAKER HL, JR, HOUSER OW, CAMPBELL JK, ET AL: Computerized tomography of the head. *JAMA* 233:1304, 1975.
27. CHRISTIE JH, MORI H, GO RT, CORNELL SH, SCHAPIRO RL: Computed tomography and radionuclide studies in the diagnosis of intracranial disease. *AJR* 127:171, 1976.
28. TAVERAS JM, WOOD EH: *Diagnostic Neuroradiology*, ed. 2, p. 857, Williams & Wilkins, Baltimore, 1976.
29. NORMAN D, KOROBKIN M, NEWTON TH (Eds): *Computed Tomography.* C. V. Mosby, St. Louis, Mo., 1977.
30. CAMPBELL JK, HOUSER OW, STEVENS JC, WAHNER HW, BAKER HL, JR, FOLGER WN: Computed tomography and radionuclide imaging in the evaluation of ischemic stroke. *Radiology* 126:695, 1978.
31. NAIDICH TP, SOLOMON S, LEEDS NE: Computerized tomography in neurological evaluations. *JAMA* 240:565, 1978.
32. BACHMAN DS, HODGES FJ, III, FREEMAN JM: Computerized axial tomography in chronic seizure disorders of childhood. *Pediatrics* 58:828, 1976.

chapter two

Face

General Considerations

Although the face and skull represent distinct anatomic regions, they share bony components and frequently share in common injuries. For purposes of discussion, however, the face will be considered to include the eyes, nose, cheeks, and jaws. The bones comprising the face include the frontal, lacrimal, ethmoidal, sphenoidal, temporal, zygomatic, palatine, nasal, maxillary, and mandible.

The roentgen examination of the face demands precise positioning and optimal radiographic technique in order to accurately identify the normal structures and pathologic processes that involve them. The skeletal components are complex and compact. Many of the facial bones are thin and curved and their margins are not sharply demarcated. Superimposition of the bones of the face and some of the normal structures of the skull add to the difficulty of interpretation.

The roentgen diagnosis of facial fractures depends upon disruption of the normal configuration of individual facial bones and obscuration, or obliteration, of normally radiolucent spaces within the face such as the paranasal sinuses and the orbits.

Individualized oblique and tangential views, which must be personally supervised by the radiologist, are so commonly needed in the evaluation of facial trauma that their use is almost routine. Laminograms are frequently essential in delineating the extent and characteristics of abnormalities of the face.

The roentgen examination of the face of infants and children does not delineate the skeletal structures as distinctly as in adults because of their size and the relative lack of contrast between the facial bones and the soft tissues. The latter results from underdevelopment and poor aeration of the paranasal air spaces of the face. The nasal bones, particularly, are small and faintly ossified and may be impossible to examine

radiographically. Fortunately, facial fractures in children are uncommon and usually do not occur until after the facial skeleton is well developed.

Radiographic Examination

The routine radiographic examination of the face includes two projections made at different angles in the frontal position and the Waters', lateral, horizontal beam brow-up lateral, and extended base (Towne) views. The justification for two similar radiographs made in the frontal position is to provide different perspectives of the complex skeletal components of the face.

Radiographic Anatomy

The frontal projection may be made with the patient erect, prone, or supine. The frontal examination of the face made in the prone position with the nose and the chin resting on the radiographic table and the central beam centered on the meatocanthal line is seen in Figure 2.1. In this projection, the anatomy of the orbits (with the exception of the inferior orbital rim) and the retro-orbital skeletal structures are clearly delineated because the petrous pyramids are superimposed upon the maxillary antra. With minor further extension of the neck so that the nose is elevated and only the chin rests on the radiographic table, the petrous pyramids are projected more inferiorly revealing the inferior orbital rim in addition to the other orbital and retro-orbital skeletal structures (Fig. 2.2).

The prone frontal projection of the face made with the nose and forehead resting on the radiographic table and the central beam centered on the meatocanthal line is illustrated by Figures 2.3 and 2.4.

The Waters' projection (Fig. 2.5) is designed to

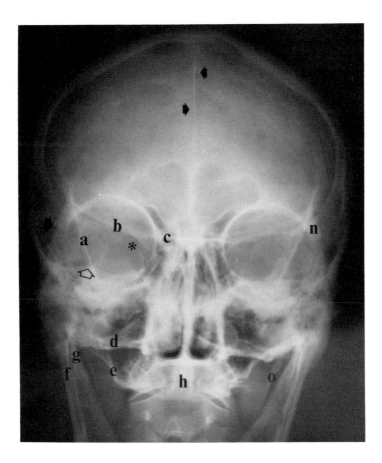

Fig. 2.1 This anteroposterior radiograph of the face is made with the patient prone with the tip of the nose and the chin resting upon the radiographic table. In this position, the petrous pyramids are projected through the maxillary sinuses rather than the orbits, resulting in unobstructed visualization of the orbital walls and roof. The superior orbital fissure is indicated by the asterisk (*), the zygomaticofrontal suture by the *solid arrow*, and the arcuate eminence by the *open arrow*. The lateral margin of the greater wing of the sphenoid bone which comprises the floor of the temporal fossa is indicated by *a*, the lesser wing of the sphenoid by *b*, the cribriform plate by *c*, the occipital bone projecting through the maxillary sinus by *d*, and the lateral wall of the maxillary sinus by *e*. The coronoid process of the mandible is indicated by *g* and the neck of the mandible by *f*. *h* indicates the odontoid process. The styloid process of the temporal bone is indicated by *o*. *n* represents the zygomatic process of the frontal bone. The *small arrows* in the midline of the skull indicate the cerebral falx, which is seen on end.

demonstrate the margins of the orbits, including the region of the zygomaticofrontal suture, the malar eminence, and at least the temporal process of the zygoma forming the anterior portion of the zygomatic arch, if not the entire arch, as well as the margins of the frontal and maxillary sinuses. The nasal bones and the vomer (the nasal septum) are seen end-on. The greater sphenoidal wing, as it constitutes the floor of the temporal fossa, produces the thin, linear density which extends obliquely from above downward and is projected inside the orbit, just medial to the lateral orbital wall.

The roentgen appearance of the zygomaticofrontal suture ranges from smooth complete fusion to total absence of bony union (Fig. 2.6). The latter appearance can be distinguished from a fracture on the basis of the similarity of each suture, the smooth sclerosis of the contiguous margins of the suture and the parallelism of the medial and lateral walls of each process forming the suture.

Occasionally air between the lids (Fig. 2.6a) or trapped beneath the upper lid (Fig. 2.6d) will produce

curvilinear lucent shadows which should not be confused for orbital emphysema, a sign of a medial orbital wall fracture (Fig. 2.32).

While the Waters' projection is usually obtained with the patient prone, a very similar and completely diagnostic demonstration of the skeletal anatomy of the face can be obtained in the supine position, i.e., the "reversed" Waters' projection (Fig. 2.7), when the patient's condition precludes the prone examination.

Rectilinear tomography made in the Waters' position (Fig. 2.8) may be required to establish the diagnosis of a blow-out fracture of the orbit and is the only method of determining the extent of the floor fracture and the possible presence of a medial wall fracture.

Further hyperextension of the neck and positioning of the skull with the point of the chin resting upon the x-ray table provides an "extended" Waters' view (Fig. 2.9).

It is difficult to discern the anatomy of the face, in the lateral projection, because of the superimposition of complex, paired structures, the effect of even minor

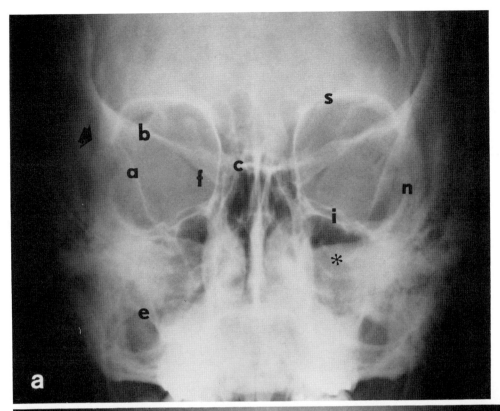

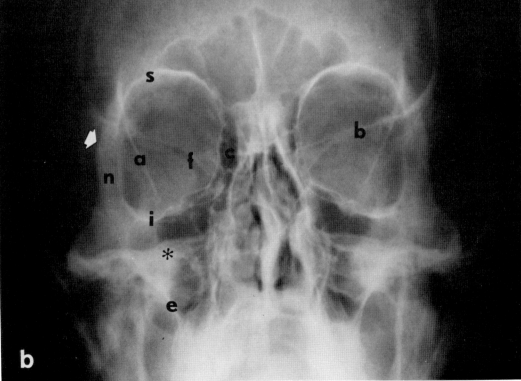

Fig. 2.2 This frontal projection of the face, which may be made either prone (**a**) or supine (**b**), clearly delineates all of the orbital and periorbital skeletal anatomy. The petrous pyramids (*) are entirely superimposed upon the maxillary antra. The *solid arrows* indicate the location of the fused zygomaticofrontal suture. The greater wing of the sphenoid, which constitutes the floor of the temporal fossa, is indicated by *a*, the lesser sphenoidal wing by *b*, the cribriform plate by *c*, and the anterolateral wall of the maxillary antrum by *e*. *s* is the superior, *n* the lateral, and *i* the inferior orbital rim. The superior orbital fissure is indicated by *f*.

37

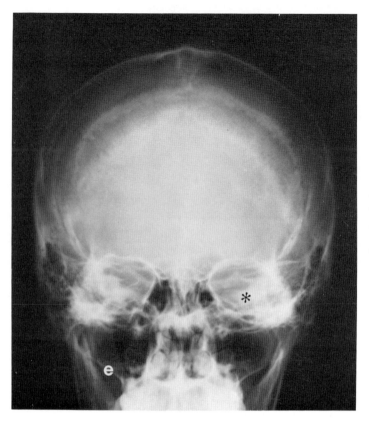

Fig. 2.3 Frontal projection of the face (and skull) made in the prone position with the nose and forehead resting on the radiographic table and the central x-ray beam centered parallel to the meatocanthal line. In this projection, the petrous pyramids (*) are superimposed upon the orbits obscuring the majority of the orbital skeletal anatomy. However, in this projection, the anterolateral margins of the maxillary antra (e) are optimally demonstrated.

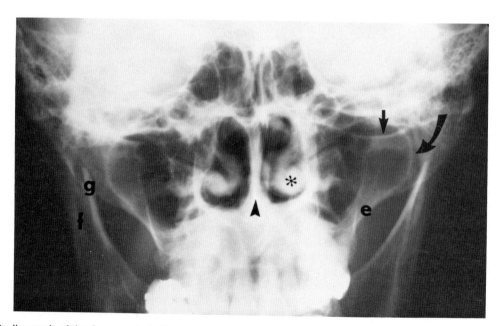

Fig. 2.4 Radiograph of the face made in the position described in Figure 2.3. The *stemmed arrow* indicates the inferior orbital rim, the *curved arrow* the lateral wall of the antrum, and e its anterolateral wall. The coronoid process of the mandible is indicated by g and the ascending ramus by f. The *arrowhead* indicates the nasal septum and the *asterisk* the inferior nasal turbinates.

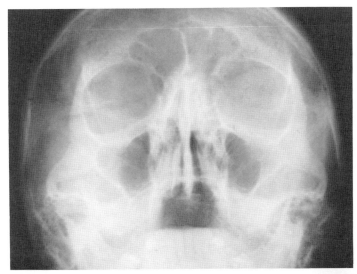

Fig. 2.5 Normal Waters' projection of the face.

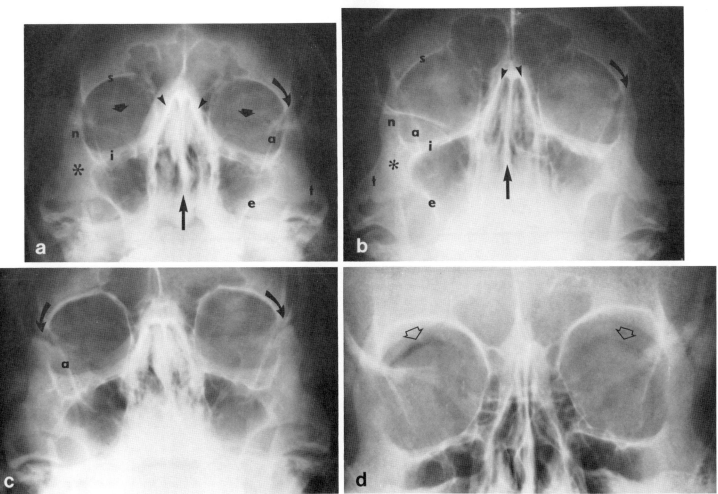

Fig. 2.6 Waters' projection of the face. In all examples *a* represents the greater sphenoidal wing comprising the floor of the temporal fossa, *e* the anterolateral wall of the maxillary antrum, *s* the superior orbital rim, *n* the lateral wall of the orbit, and *i* the inferior orbital rim. The asterisk (*) indicates the body of the zygoma (the malar eminence) and *t* the temporal process of the zygoma extending posteriorly to form the zygomatic arch. The *stemmed arrows* indicate the vomer (the nasal septum) and the *arrowheads* the nasal bones seen end-on. Air between the closed eyelids produces the thin curvilinear lucencies (*solid arrows*) transversely situated within the orbits (**a**). Air trapped *beneath* the upper eyelids may produce gently inferiorly concave lucent shadows (**d**, *open arrows*), which should not be mistaken for orbital emphysema. The *curved arrows* indicate the location of the solidly fused (**a, b**) and the completely open (**c**) zygomaticofrontal sutures.

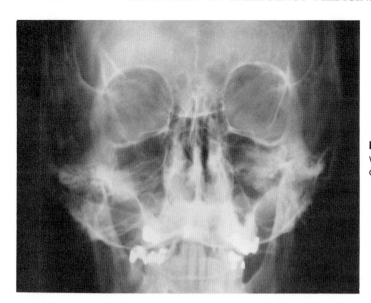

Fig. 2.7 Normal "reversed" Waters' projection obtained with the patient supine, the neck extended, and the central x-ray beam parallel to the meatocanthal line.

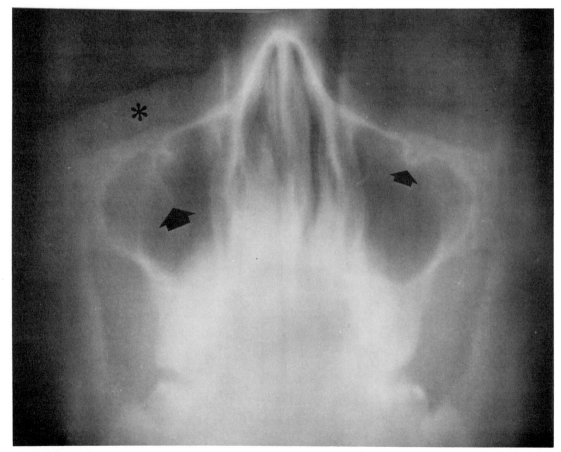

Fig. 2.8 Laminogram of the face made in the Waters' projection. The asterisk (*) indicates the soft tissue swelling over the right malar eminence. The *large solid arrow* in the right maxillary sinus indicates a normal bony septum. The *small solid arrow* in the left maxillary sinus indicates the infraorbital foramen.

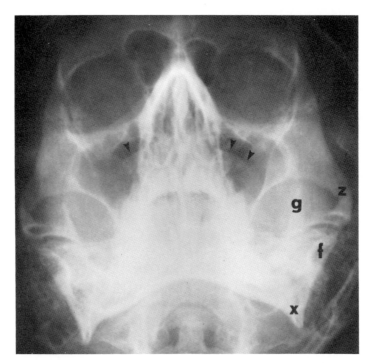

Fig. 2.9 Extended Waters' projection. The smooth, sharply defined, symmetrical soft tissue densities superimposed upon each maxillary antrum (*arrowheads*) represent the soft tissues of the upper lip. *f* is the ascending ramus, *g* the coronoid process, and *x* the angle of the mandible. *z* is the zygomatic arch.

imprecisions in positioning, and the effect of the divergent x-ray beam. However, a properly positioned lateral radiograph of the face obtained with optimum radiographic technique provides invaluable information about the sphenoid sinus, the naso-oropharynx, and the maxillary sinus including, particularly, its posterior wall and the pterygomaxillary (sphenomaxillary) fissure (Fig. 2.10). Fracture of the margins of the pterygomaxillary fissure is an integral part of the more extensive facial fractures, occurs frequently in less severe face injuries, and is associated with retropharyngeal hematoma which may compromise or occlude the nasopharyngeal airway (Fig. 2.11). Benign (hypertrophied adenoidal tissue) (Fig. 2.12)

and malignant (craniopharyngioma) masses may impair the nasopharyngeal air space. It is critically important, then, in the evaluation of the lateral radiograph of the face, to pay particular attention to the pterygomaxillary fissure and the naso-oropharynx.

The technical factors required to obtain a diagnostic roentgenogram of the face result in gross overexposure of the nose, thereby rendering this examination of little value in the diagnosis of nasal fractures.

The horizontal beam brow-up lateral roentgenogram is an important part of the radiographic examination of the injured face. The presence of a fluid level in the maxillary sinus of a patient with facial trauma is indicative of a fracture involving this sinus.

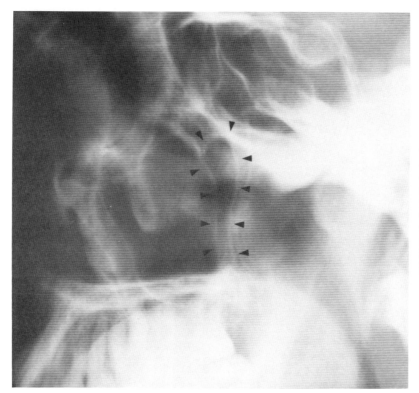

Fig. 2.10 Lateral radiograph of a normal face demonstrating the pterygomaxillary fissure (*arrowheads*) which contains the terminal portions of the maxillary artery and vein and the extensive pterygoid venous plexus. The posterior wall of the maxillary antrum constitutes the anterior margin of the fissure and the anterior cortical surface of the pterygoid process, its posterior margin. The pharyngeal aponeurosis and the superior constrictor muscle arise from the posterior edge of the medial pterygoid plate and extend posteriorly to form the posterior wall of the nasopharynx (see also Figs. 2.37 and 2.38).

Fig. 2.11 Horizontal beam (brow-up) lateral radiograph of the face of a patient with a complex zygomaticomaxillary fracture. The *arrowheads* indicate the size of the retropharyngeal hematoma which has completely obliterated the nasopharyngeal airway. The *open arrow* indicates the air-fluid level within the involved maxillary antrum.

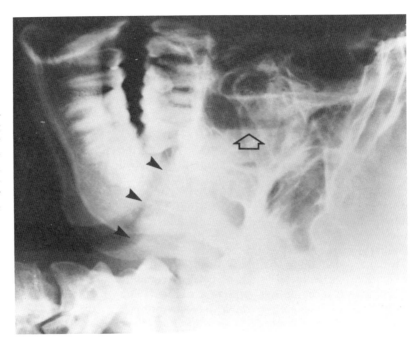

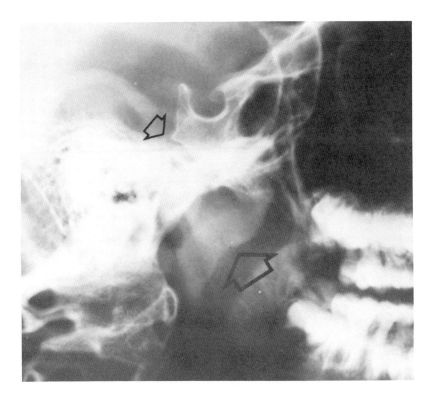

Fig. 2.12 The smoothly lobulated, sharply defined soft tissue mass in the nasopharynx (*large arrow*) represents adenoidal tissue. The *small arrow* indicates the normal spheno-occipital synchondrosis.

The fluid level may be the most obvious roentgen sign of a fracture of the face (Fig. 2.11) or a fracture of the skull that extends into the face (Fig. 2.13).

The lateral aspect of the anterior wall of the maxillary sinus, the malar eminence of the zygomatic bone, and the zygomatic arches are clearly delineated in the submentovertical (base) view (Fig. 2.14). The usual technique for obtaining the Hirtz view is modified by decreasing the radiographic factors so that the zygomatic arches, which are thin narrow structures, are visible on the roentgenogram.

The routine radiographic examination of the nose is simple and rewarding. Posteroanterior (Fig. 2.15) and Waters' (Fig. 2.16) views provide different frontal projections of the nasal bone. The lateral projection (Fig. 2.17) must be made with "soft tissue" technique because of the thinness of the nasal bones. This projection must also include the anterior nasal spine of the maxillae. The axial view of the nasal bones (Fig. 2.18) is obtained with an occlusal film held between the teeth and the x-ray tube directed caudad so that the central beam passes tangentially with respect to the nasal bones. Because of the variation in prominence of the nose and forehead, it may not always be possible to project the nasal bones free of the forehead. However, when it is possible, the axial view will permit identification of fractures not recognized on other projections and accurately reflects the magnitude of displacement of fragments.

The paranasal sinuses, while included in the routine radiographs of the face, are not sufficiently seen to permit definitive evaluation on these examinations. For this reason, special views of the sinuses must be specifically requested when the symptoms suggest an abnormality involving these structures. When the paranasal sinuses are examined for nontraumatic indications, the radiographs should be obtained with the patient sitting. If the patient's condition prevents the examination being made while erect, an adequate study can be made with the patient recumbent, provided that a horizontal beam brow-up lateral roentgenogram of the face is included to record a possible fluid level in the maxillary, sphenoidal, or frontal sinuses.

Radiographic examination of the middle ear requires the use of positions devised specifically to demonstrate the anatomy of this region. Because of the complexity of the middle and inner ears, a basic

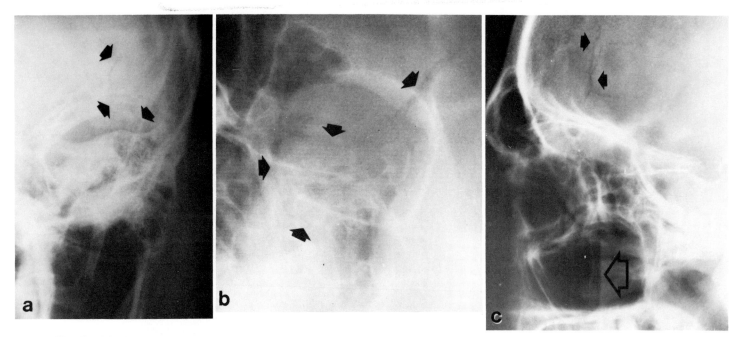

Fig. 2.13 In the frontal projection of the face (**a**), a fracture line is barely perceptible in the lateral aspect of the frontal bone extending into the roof of the orbit (*arrows*). In the Waters' projection (**b**), however, the fracture line is seen to involve the medial aspect of the orbit and extend into the maxillary sinus (*arrows*). The fluid level in the maxillary sinus seen in the horizontal beam lateral roentgenogram (**c**) is the most obvious roentgen sign of this subtle fracture.

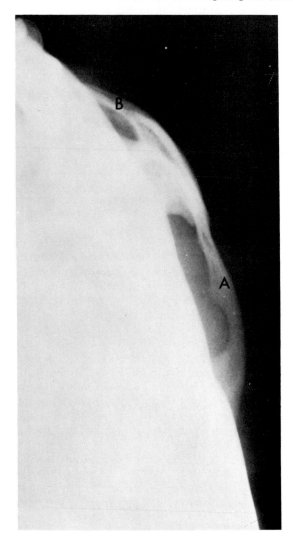

Fig. 2.14 Submentovertical projection demonstrating the zygomatic arch (*A*) and the anterior wall of the maxillary antrum (*B*).

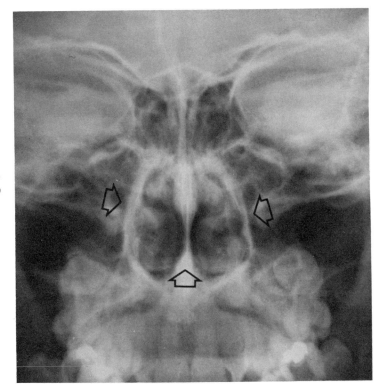

Fig. 2.15 Posteroanterior projection of the face. The *arrows* indicate the nasal process of the maxilla (lateral) and the nasal septum (midline).

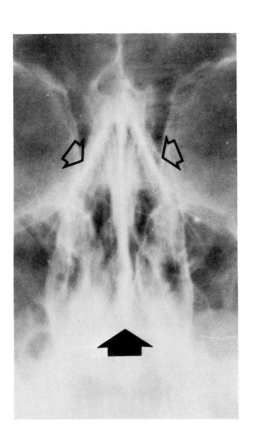

Fig. 2.16 Frontal projection of the nose made in the Waters' projection. The *open arrows* indicate the nasal bones and the *solid arrow* the nasal septum.

radiographic study should include examinations made in different planes along the sagittal axis, a lateral view, and a view designed to demonstrate the epitympanic recess. Fractures involving this area are best demonstrated by rectilinear or polydirectional tomography.

The mandible is routinely examined by means of anteroposterior (Fig. 2.19), true lateral, each oblique (Fig. 2.20), and extended Towne (Fig. 2.21) views and also, when indicated, a radiograph of the mandibular symphysis obtained with an occlusal film placed between the teeth and the x-ray tube centered on the submental region (Fig. 2.22). Special projections designed to examine the neck and condyle of the mandible include oblique views, positioned in such a way that the ascending ramus of the mandible is projected into the zygomatic fossa (Fig. 2.23), and lateral projections of the temporomandibular joints made with the mouth closed (Fig. 2.24a) and open (Fig. 2.24b). Frequently, a lateral laminogram of the temporomandibular joint is required to adequately evaluate the ascending ramus, neck, and condyle of the mandible.

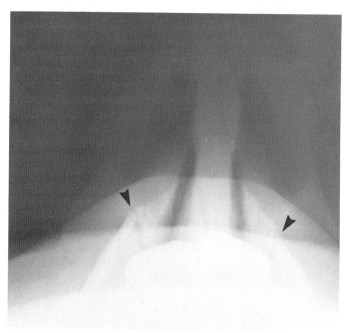

Fig. 2.17 Lateral radiograph of the normal nose. The *solid arrow* indicates the nasomaxillary suture. The anterior nasal spine of the maxilla is indicated by the *open arrow*.

Fig. 2.18 Axial view of the nasal bones. The *arrowheads* indicate the nasomaxillary sutures.

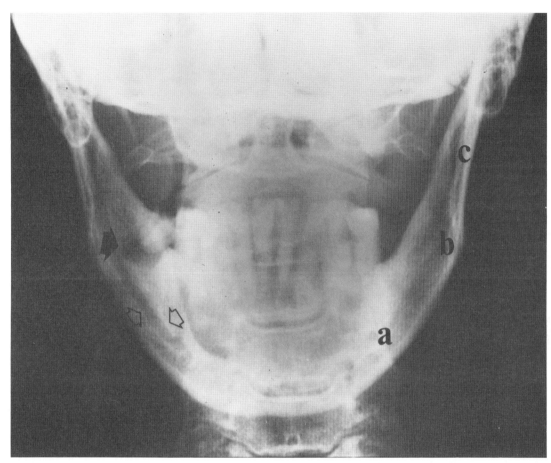

Fig. 2.19 Anteroposterior view of the mandible. *a*, horizontal ramus; *b*, angle; *c*, ascending ramus. The *open arrows* indicate the mandibular canal. In this projection, the mandibular symphysis is obscured by the superimposed density of the cervical spine, the coronoid processes are superimposed upon the proximal portion of the ascending ramus and the neck of the mandible, and the coronoid and condylar processes of the mandible are obscured by the mastoid process and the occipital bone. The *solid arrow* indicates a large periapical abscess about a retained root fragment.

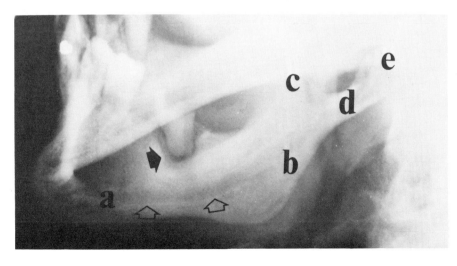

Fig. 2.20 Oblique view of the mandible. *a*, horizontal ramus; *b*, ascending ramus; *c*, coronoid process; *d*, neck; *e*, condyle. The *open arrows* indicate the mandibular groove. The *solid arrow* indicates a large periapical abscess.

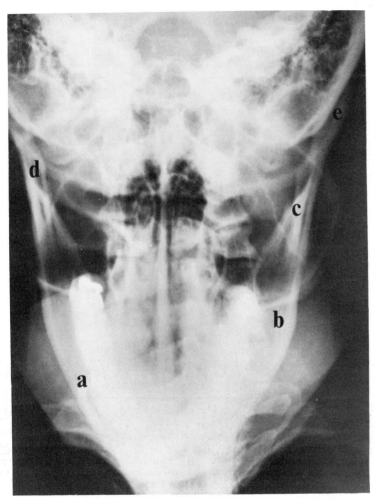

Fig. 2.21 Extended Towne view designed to demonstrate the proximal portions of the mandible. *a*, horizontal ramus; *b*, angle; *c*, coronoid process; *d*, neck; *e*, condyle.

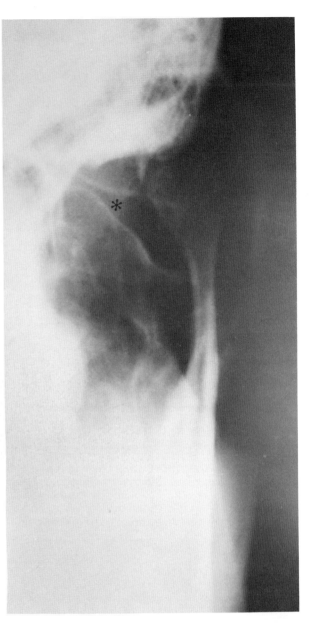

Fig. 2.23 Rotated oblique view designed to project the neck and condyle of the mandible through the temporal fossa. This view also provides an excellent demonstration of the sphenomaxillary fissure (*).

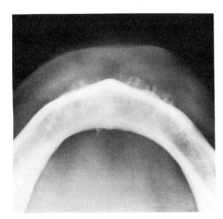

Fig. 2.22 "Occlusal" view of the symphysis of the mandible.

Radiographic Manifestations of Trauma

Soft tissue swelling about the eye and malar eminence can be seen radiographically as a homogeneous, ill defined density superimposed upon the maxillary antrum (Fig. 2.25), which projects above the orbital floor in the Waters' view (Fig. 2.8).

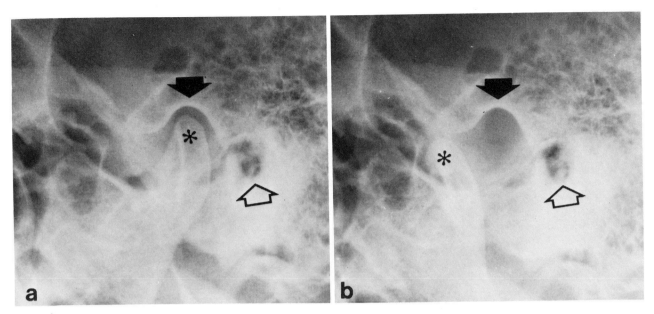

Fig. 2.24 Lateral examination of the temporomandibular joint with the mouth closed (**a**) and open (**b**). The asterisk (*) indicates the mandibular condyle, the *solid arrows* the mandibular fossa, and the *open arrows* the external auditory meatus.

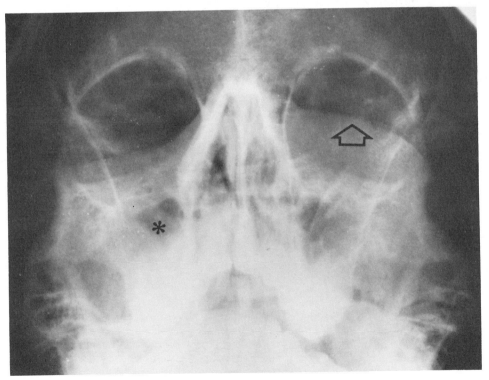

Fig. 2.25 This patient was struck over the *left* malar eminence. The *arrow* indicates soft tissue swelling of the cheek and lower eyelid. The right side of the face was not injured. Opacification of the right maxillary sinus (*) is due to a pre-existent, nontraumatic process.

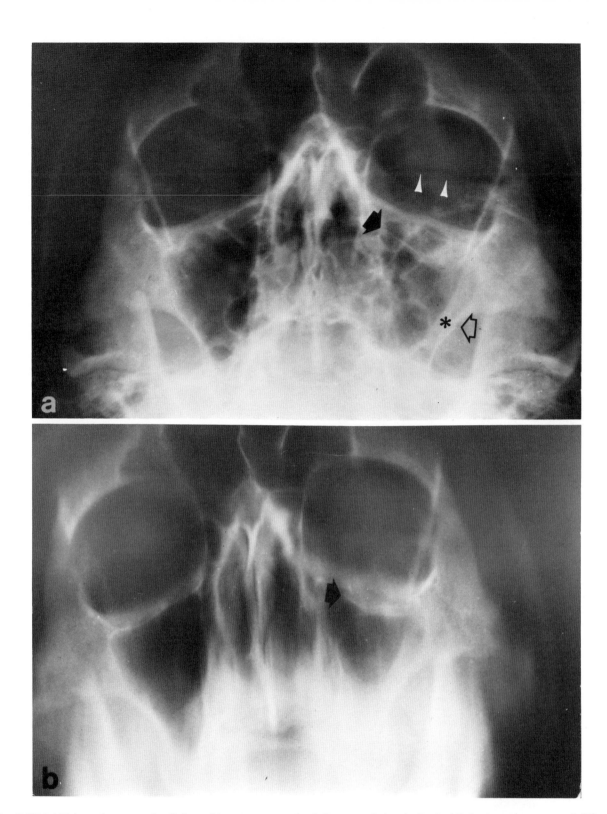

Fig. 2.26 (a) This patient sustained direct blunt trauma to the left eye and cheek. Periorbital edema has caused diffuse increased density of the left orbit and has made the palpebral fissure visible as a horizontally situated radiolucent line (*arrowheads*). Soft tissue swelling of the cheek has resulted in diffuse haziness of the left maxillary sinus. In addition, however, a sharply defined homogeneous soft tissue density is seen parallel to the anterolateral wall of the left maxillary sinus (*). This represents submucosal hemorrhage. The *open arrow* indicates a fracture in the anterolateral wall of the sinus. The *solid arrow* indicates the depressed fragment of a ''blow-out'' fracture of the left orbital floor. **(b)** Laminogram made in the Waters' projection. The *solid arrow* indicates the depressed blow-out fracture fragments.

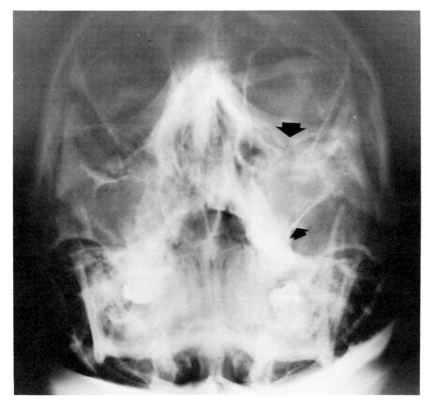

Fig. 2.27 This patient sustained severe, extensive facial trauma with multiple fractures of all of the bones of the face. The *arrows* indicate fractures in the left maxillary sinus. Uniform opacification of each maxillary sinus is the result of free hemorrhage into the sinus cavities.

The radiographic distinction between the increased density of the maxillary antrum, caused by superimposed soft tissue swelling, and that within the antrum, resulting from hemorrhage or pre-existing inflammatory disease, is difficult. However, as seen in Figures 2.8 and 2.25, the density produced by soft tissue swelling of the cheek is rather faint and is homogeneously distributed over the area of the right maxillary sinus. The walls of the antrum are intact. The typical, sharply defined, soft tissue density caused by submucosal hemorrhage resulting from fracture of the maxillary sinus is seen in Figure 2.26. When severe trauma of the face results in marked opacification of the maxillary sinus by free hemorrhage (Fig. 2.27), the presence of fracture lines or fragments and an air-fluid level within the antrum aid in the distinction between traumatic soft tissue changes and those caused by pre-existent, nontraumatic disease (Fig. 2.25).

Fractures of the face include the blow-out fracture of the orbit, those involving the zygoma and the midface (Le Fort).

The blow-out (1) of the orbit is caused by a blow striking the orbital rim in which the force is dissipated through the orbital contents, resulting in a fracture, usually of the orbital floor, and herniation of periorbital tissues into the subjacent maxillary antrum. In approximately 50% of patients, there will be a fracture of the medial wall, either alone or concomitant with the floor fracture, as evidenced by the presence of orbital emphysema (2). The blow-out fracture of the

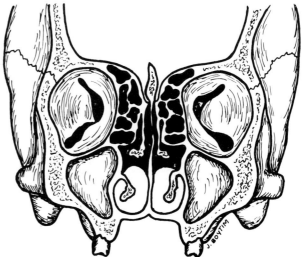

Fig. 2.28 Schematic representation of the structural support provided to the medial orbital wall by the ethmoid air cells. This support, theoretically, explains the reason that the blow-out fracture involves the thinner medial wall less often than the thicker orbital floor.

orbital floor is, by definition (3–9), limited to the floor and does not involve the inferior orbital rim. Although the medial orbital wall is thinner than the floor, it gains structural support from the adjacent ethmoidal air cells (Fig. 2.28). The medial orbital wall, therefore, being stronger than the thicker orbital floor, is less susceptible to fracture than is the floor.

Clinical signs of the blow-out fracture include enopthalmos, diplopia, and limited upward and outward gaze. The latter is secondary to entrapment of the inferior rectus and oblique muscles, or their sling, in the fracture defect. Medial wall fractures are characterized by the passage of air through the fracture defect into the involved orbit. The air gains access to the orbit only when the intranostril pressure is increased such as occurs with nose blowing. The passage of air into the orbit produces a pathognomonic "bubbling" sensation in the involved orbit. Because the air is typically superior and posterior to the globe, it

cannot be detected by palpation. Air within the orbit is referred to as orbital emphysema (2, 10).

Because the eyelids are usually swollen shut, the clinical signs of the blow-out fracture are of limited practical value. Since the orbital floor fracture does not involve the inferior orbital rim, palpation of the inferior rim will be negative. Therefore, recognition of the blow-out fracture depends upon a high index of suspicion and the radiographic examination.

The plain film signs of a blow-out fracture include the presence of a globular soft tissue mass projecting from the floor of the orbit into the superior portion of the maxillary antrum (Fig. 2.29) or the presence of a fracture fragment in the superior portion of the sinus (Fig. 2.30). The thin linear density of the depressed floor fragment has a characteristic attitude extending obliquely downward from medial to lateral. Thus, the fracture fragment is distinguishable from the normal, but inconsistent, maxillary sinus septum which is oriented in the opposite direction (Fig. 2.31).

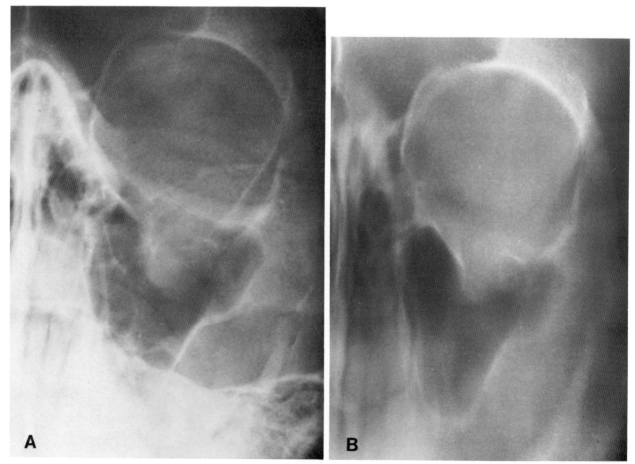

Fig. 2.29 Blow-out fracture of the floor of the left orbit. **(a)** Routine Waters' projection demonstrating a soft tissue mass extending into the maxillary sinus from the floor of the orbit. **(b)** Laminogram made in the Waters' projection demonstrates the soft tissue mass to better advantage. The depressed fracture fragment is represented by the obliquely situated, thin linear density.

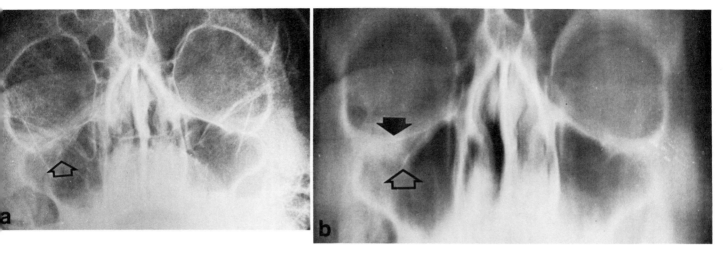

Fig. 2.30 (a) The *arrow* points to the thin, obliquely situated linear density in the superior portion of the right maxillary sinus which represents the depressed orbital floor fragment. Note the soft tissue swelling superimposed upon the right orbit. The depressed floor fragment (*open arrow*) is seen to better advantage in the laminogram made in the Waters' projection **(b)**. The *solid arrow* indicates the intact inferior orbital rim.

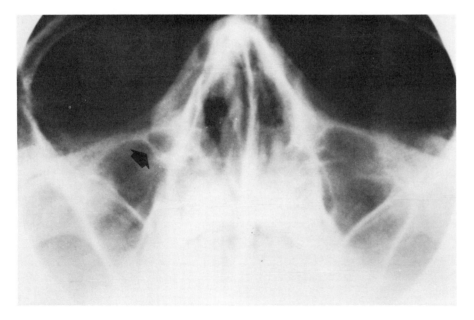

Fig. 2.31 The *arrow* indicates a normal, but inconsistently present, maxillary sinus septum. The septum is thicker than the depressed blow-out fracture fragments seen in other illustrations and its angle of obliquity is exactly opposite that of the blow-out fragment. These characteristics help distinguish the normal structure from a blow-out fragment.

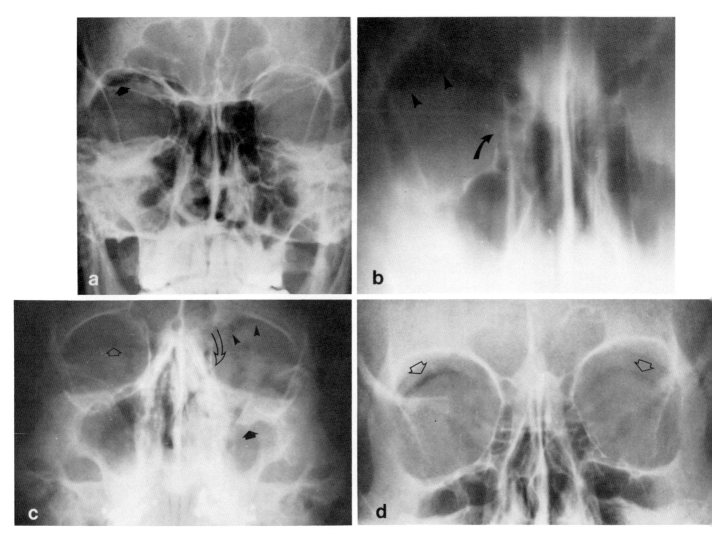

Fig. 2.32 Orbital emphysema secondary to medial wall blow-out fracture. In the frontal projection (**a**), the radiolucency in the superior aspect of the right orbit (*arrow*) represents air within the soft tissues superior to the globe. The medial wall fracture is not seen in this plain radiograph but is demonstrated (*curved arrow*) in the tomogram made in Waters' position (**b**). The superolateral surface of the globe (*arrowheads*), outlined by air in the periorbital tissues, is also seen in the tomogram. Orbital emphysema delineates the superomedial aspect of the left orbit (*arrowheads*) of a different patient in (**c**) who sustained a blow-out fracture of both the floor (*solid arrow*) and medial wall (*curved arrow*). Compare the appearance of the orbital emphysema (left eye) with the transverse lucency in the midthird of the right orbit (*open arrow*), which represents air in the palpebral fissure. The irregular curvilinear lucencies (*open arrows*) in the superior portion of the orbits of this patient who experienced no facial trauma represent air trapped beneath each upper lid (**d**).

Orbital emphysema, indicative of a medial orbital wall fracture, appears as a curvilinear lucency in the superior aspect of the orbit (Fig. 2.32). The sharply defined concave inferior aspect of the air collection outlines the superior arc of the eyeball. The characteristic appearance of orbital emphysema, with its sharply concave inferior margin representing the superior arc of the eyeball, should distinguish this pathologic air collection from the lucency caused by air physiologically located between the eyelids (Fig. 2.32c) and trapped beneath the upper lids (Fig. 2.32d).

Rectilinear or polydirectional tomography should be employed freely in the evaluation of suspected blow-out fractures, particularly when the plain films are equivocal or when a medial wall fracture is suspected.

Pseudo blow-out fracture (11) describes the situation in which there is blunt trauma to the orbit and equivocal signs of a blow-out fracture and in which both the plain radiographs and the tomograms suggest a soft tissue mass arising from the roof of the maxillary antrum but fail to demonstrate an orbital floor fracture. In this unusual circumstance, computed tomography of the face in routine and coronal sections will define the etiology of the changes seen on routine projections.

Fractures of the zygoma include the isolated fracture of the zygomatic arch and the more extensive zygomaticomaxillary injuries. The isolated fracture of the arch is the result of a direct blow causing various degrees of comminution and depression of the fragments. The fracture is not well demonstrated in the frontal (including the Waters') projections of the face, but is clearly visualized on the submentovertical view (Figs. 2.33 and 2.34). This fracture usually has no clinical significance other than the skeletal injury.

Before discussing malar fractures, it is important to review the anatomy of the malar bone (zygoma). Figures 2.35 and 2.36 depict the extensive articulation of the zygoma with the frontal, maxillary, and temporal bones. The body of the zygoma is dense, heavy boned and rarely fractured. Instead, the fractures typically occur in the weaker processes and at sites of articulation. Because of the anatomy of the zygoma and because fractures of the zygoma invariably (excepting the isolated arch fracture) involve the maxilla as well, these injuries are more accurately described as zygomaticomaxillary (12, 13) rather than malar

(14), zygomatic, or tripod fractures. The term tripod is particularly inappropriate because it infers that these fractures involve only the zygomatic arch and the lateral wall and inferior rim of the orbit, while completely ignoring the clinically important maxillary component of the lesion.

Zygomaticomaxillary fractures are usually the result of a direct blow to the malar eminence. Clinically, edema and ecchymosis involve the cheek and lower eyelid to varying degrees. The separate fragment is usually depressed, resulting in flattening of the malar eminence. This feature may be obscured by the soft tissue swelling. Other symptoms may include limitation of jaw movement or dental malocclusion, unilateral epistaxis, paresthesia of the distribution of the infraorbital nerve, unequal pupils, diplopia, limited upward and outward gaze, and difficulty in swallowing.

Pathologically, zygomaticomaxillary fractures include fractures of the lateral wall of the orbit (or separation of the zygomaticofrontal suture), the floor and inferior rim of the orbit, the anterior, lateral and posterior walls of the maxillary antrum, and the zygomatic arch. These lesions are classified as simple (nondisplaced) or complex (displaced). The latter are

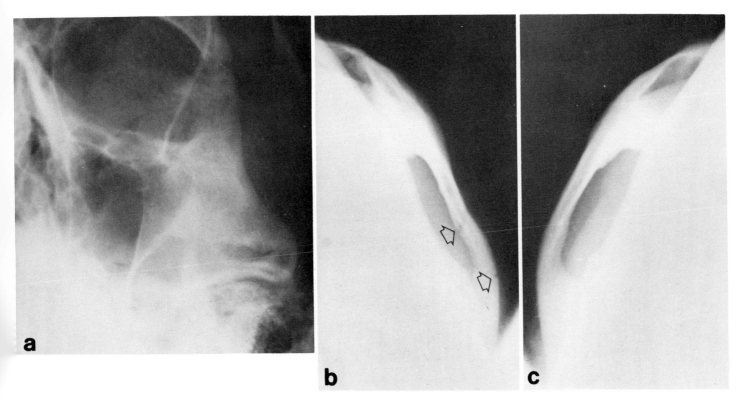

Fig. 2.33 This patient sustained direct trauma to the left zygomatic arch. In the frontal projection (**a**), a fracture line is barely perceptible in the temporal process of the zygoma. The comminuted fracture and depression of the fragments (*arrows*) are well demonstrated in the submentovertical view (**b**). The uninvolved right zygomatic arch (**c**) is shown for comparison.

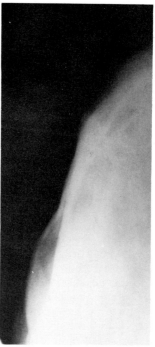

Fig. 2.34 Marked depression of a comminuted fracture of the right zygomatic arch.

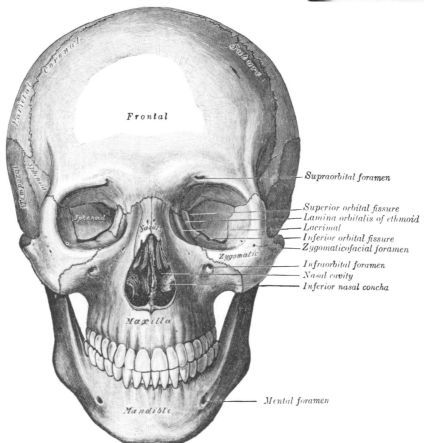

Fig. 2.35 Skull and face from the front. Note the relationship of the zygomatic to frontal, maxillary and temporal bones. (Reprinted with permission from C. M. Goss (Ed.): *Gray's Anatomy*, ed. 29. Lea & Febiger, Philadelphia, 1973.)

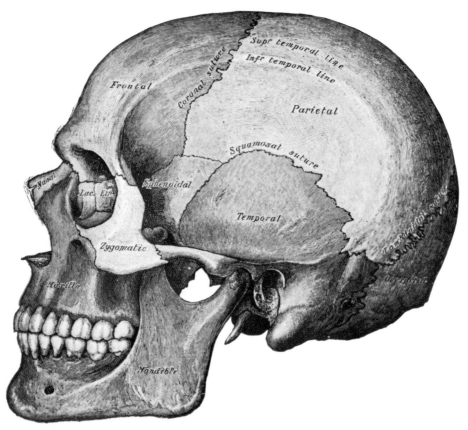

Fig. 2.36 Relationship of the zygomatic to the frontal, maxillary, and temporal bones in side view. (Reprinted with permission from C. M. Goss (Ed.): *Gray's Anatomy*, ed. 29. Lea & Febiger, Philadelphia, 1973.)

usually associated with a fracture of the pterygoid process of the sphenoid bone (15). Fractures of this magnitude commonly disrupt the vessels situated in the pterygomaxillary (pterygopalatine) fossa (Fig. 2.10). The resultant hemorrhage follows the fascial plane of the superior constrictor muscle, which arises from the medial pterygoid plate (Figs. 2.37 and 2.38), posteriorly into the posterior phyaryngeal wall, forming a retropharyngeal hematoma which can occlude the nasopharyngeal airway.

Radiographically, the simple zygomaticomaxillary fracture (Figs. 2.39–2.41) is characterized by non- or minimally depressed fractures at the sites previously described and clouding of the involved maxillary antrum. When present, free blood in the maxillary sinus produces an air-fluid level within the antrum. Demonstration of the air-fluid interface requires frontal or lateral radiographs made in either the erect posture (Fig. 2.42) or, when the patient's condition requires the roentgen examination to be made in the recumbent position, the horizontal beam lateral projection.

That component of the zygomaticomaxillary (and

Le Fort) fractures which involves the posterior wall(s) of the maxillary antrum may be seen on the lateral radiograph of the face but is best demonstrated on the extended Towne view (Fig. 2.43).

Simple zygomaticomaxillary fractures, although only minimally displaced, may be associated with fractures of other bones of the face or adjacent bones of the calvarium. The possibility of such other concomitant injury, which may be subtle, should be considered in all patients with facial trauma (Fig. 2.44).

The distribution of fractures of complex zygomaticomaxillary injuries is identical to that described in the discussion of simple zygomaticomaxillary injuries, except that the displacement of the fractures is greater in complex injuries (Fig. 2.45). Impairment or complete obstruction of the nasopharyngeal airway is common in complex zygomaticomaxillary fractures. This clinically significant aspect of the injury is difficult to recognize or appreciate by physical examination but will be readily apparent in a properly exposed lateral radiograph of the face (Fig. 2.11).

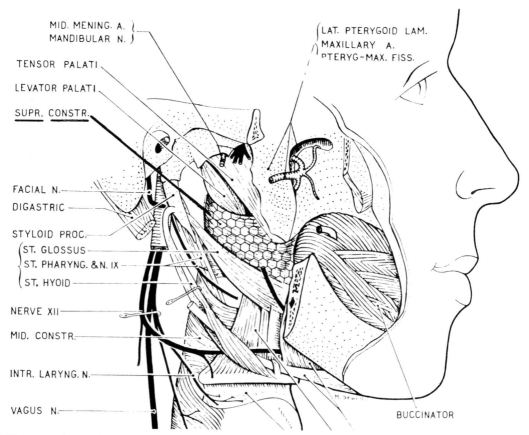

Fig. 2.37 Pharyngeal muscles seen from the side, indicating the relationship of the superior constrictor (*shaded*) to pterygoid bone and posterior pharyngeal wall. (Reprinted with permission from J. E. Anderson (Ed.): *Grant's Atlas of Anatomy*, ed. 7. Williams & Wilkins, Baltimore, 1978.)

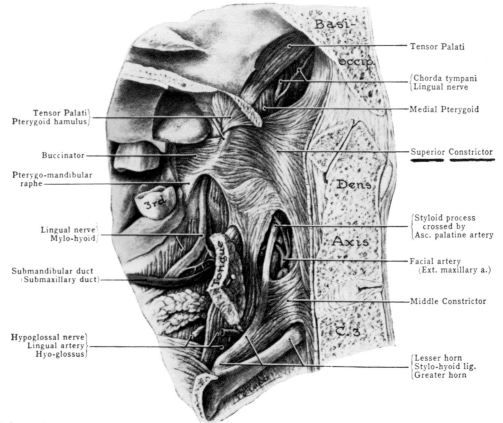

Fig. 2.38 Constrictor muscles seen from within. (Reprinted with permission from J. E. Anderson (Ed.): *Grant's Atlas of Anatomy*, ed. 7. Williams & Wilkins, Baltimore, 1978.)

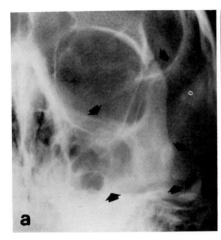

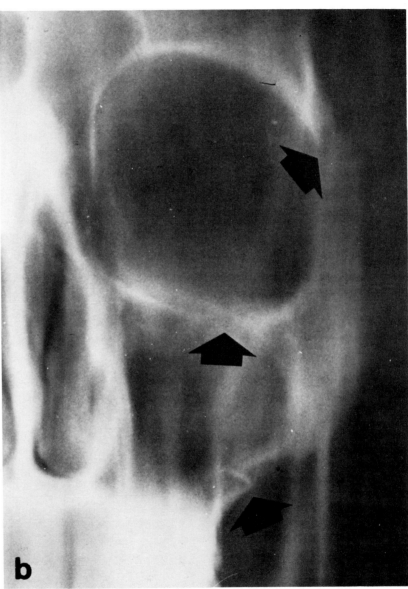

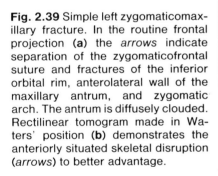

Fig. 2.39 Simple left zygomaticomaxillary fracture. In the routine frontal projection (a) the *arrows* indicate separation of the zygomaticofrontal suture and fractures of the inferior orbital rim, anterolateral wall of the maxillary antrum, and zygomatic arch. The antrum is diffusely clouded. Rectilinear tomogram made in Waters' position (b) demonstrates the anteriorly situated skeletal disruption (*arrows*) to better advantage.

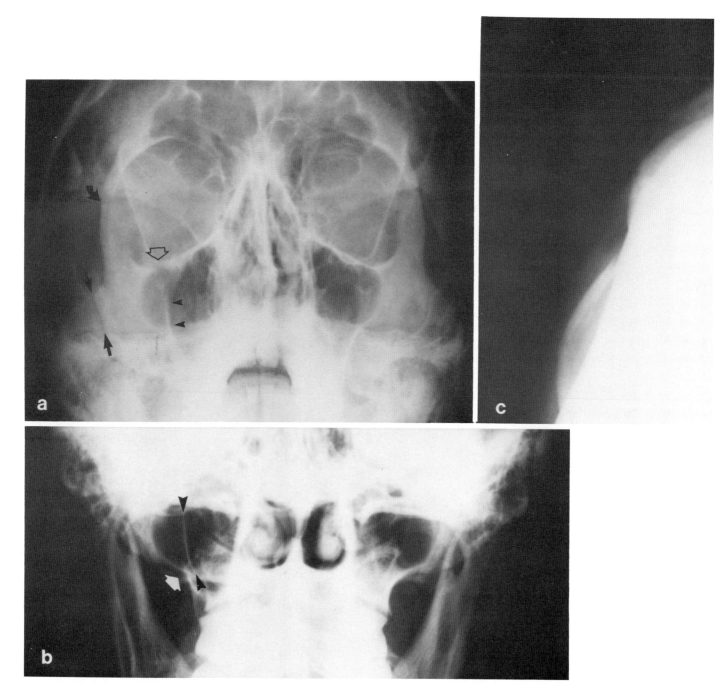

Fig. 2.40 Simple right zygomaticomaxillary fracture. The Waters' projection (**a**) discloses clouding of the right maxillary antrum, a vertically situated displaced fragment of the anterior wall of the antrum (*arrowheads*), a minimally displaced fracture of the inferior orbital rim (*open arrow*), and a vertical fracture line in the anterior portion of the zygomatic arch (*stemmed arrow*). The zygomaticofrontal suture is separated and slightly widened. Its components remain normally aligned (*curved arrow*). The frontal projection (**b**) reveals the depressed fracture of the anterolateral wall of the antrum (*white arrow*) and the vertical, displaced fracture of the anterior wall of the antrum (*arrowheads*). The depressed fracture of the anterior portion of the zygomatic arch is well seen in the submentovertical projection (**c**).

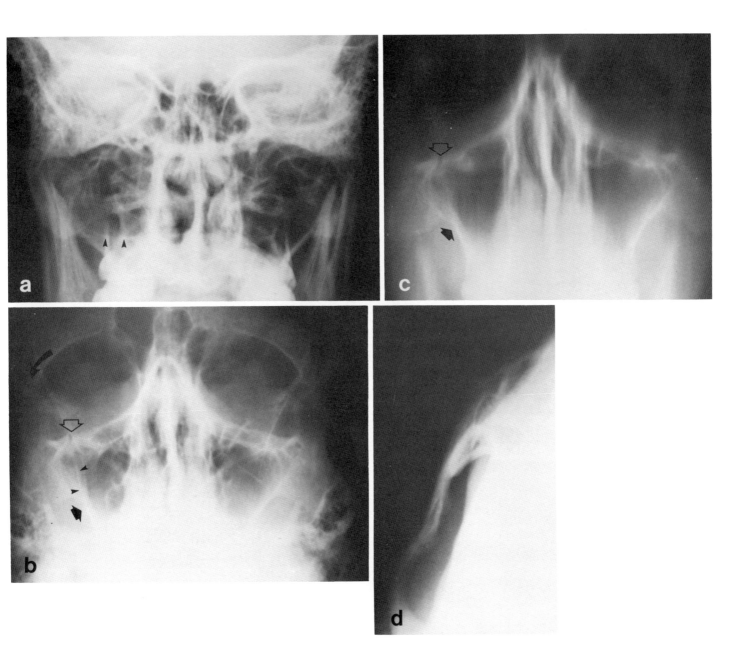

Fig. 2.41 Simple right zygomaticomaxillary fracture. In the frontal projection of the face (**a**) made in erect position, the only suggestion of skeletal injury is faint, diffuse opacification of the right maxillary antrum and a small air-fluid interface in its floor (*arrowheads*). In the Waters' projection (**b**), a slightly depressed fracture of the anterolateral wall of the antrum (*solid arrow*), a displaced, vertical fracture of the anterior wall of the antrum (*arrowheads*), a fracture of the inferior orbital rim (*open arrow*), and separation of the zygomaticofrontal suture (*curved arrow*) are evident. The fracture of the inferior orbital rim and of the anterolateral wall of the maxillary antrum are seen to better advantage in the rectilinear tomogram made in Waters' position (**c**). The submentovertical projection (**d**) clearly delineates the depressed fracture of the zygomatic arch.

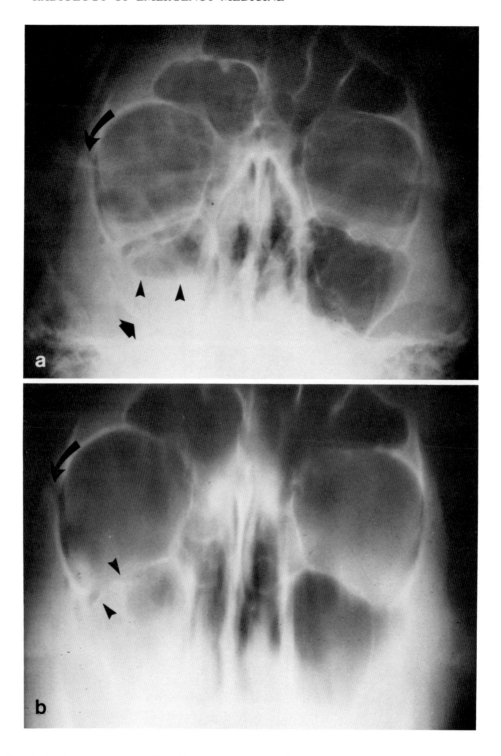

Fig. 2.42 Simple right zygomaticomaxillary fracture with an air-fluid interface in the right maxillary antrum. In the erect frontal projection of the face (**a**) an air-fluid level is evident in the right maxillary antrum (*arrowheads*). A fracture is evident in the anterolateral wall of the antrum (*solid arrow*), as is separation of the zygomaticofrontal suture (*curved arrow*). The tomogram made in Waters' position (**b**) confirms separation of the zygomaticofrontal suture (*curved arrow*) and identifies the comminuted, minimally displaced fracture of the floor of the right orbit (*arrowheads*).

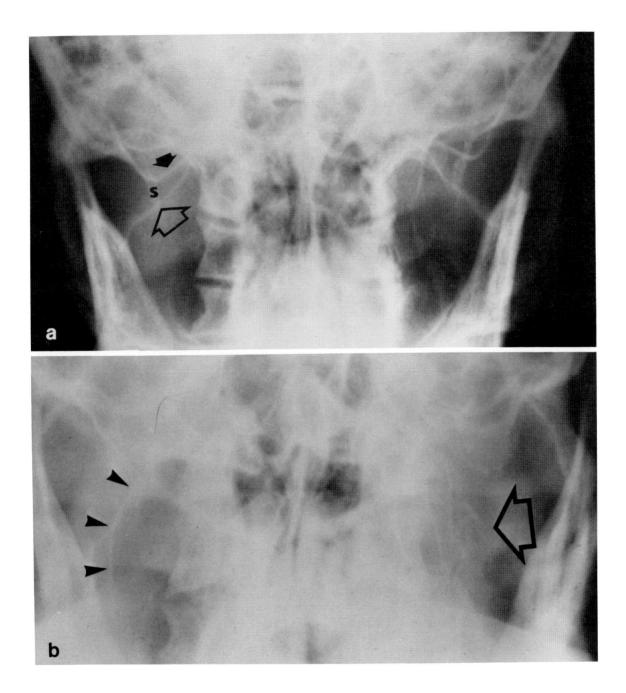

Fig. 2.43 In the normal extended Towne projection (**a**), the *open arrow* indicates the posterior wall of the maxillary antrum, *s* the sphenomaxillary fissure, and the *solid arrow* the sphenomaxillary surface of the greater wing of the sphenoid. A severely comminuted, depressed fracture involving the posterior wall of the left maxillary antrum (*open arrow*) of a patient with a zygomaticomaxillary fracture is seen in (**b**). The normal, intact posterior wall of the right antrum is indicated by the *arrowheads*.

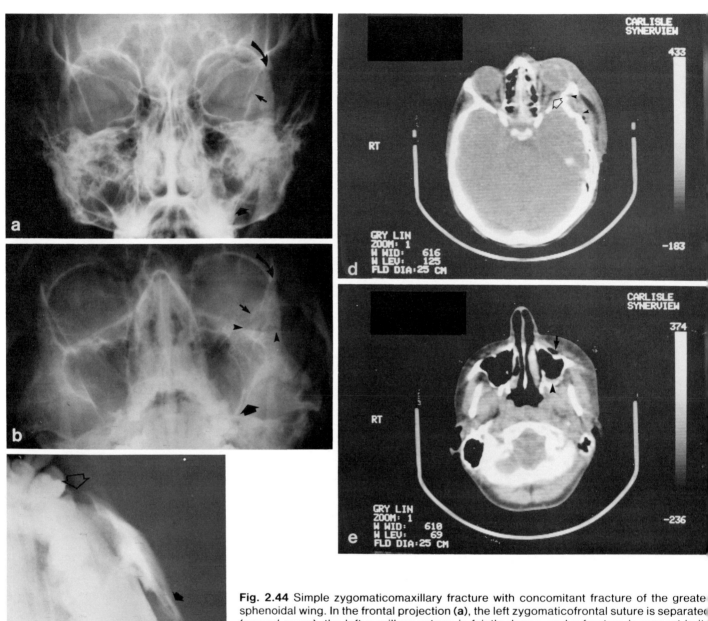

Fig. 2.44 Simple zygomaticomaxillary fracture with concomitant fracture of the greater sphenoidal wing. In the frontal projection (**a**), the left zygomaticofrontal suture is separated (*curved arrow*), the left maxillary antrum is faintly dense,·and a fracture is present in its anterolateral wall (*solid arrow*). In addition, and easily overlooked, is the fracture of the greater sphenoidal wing (*stemmed arrow*) as it passes obliquely projected through the orbit. The Waters' projection (**b**) demonstrates the separated zygomaticofrontal suture (*curved arrow*) and the fracture of the wall of the antrum (*large solid arrow*), confirms the comminuted fracture of the greater sphenoidal wing (*stemmed arrow*), and establishes a transverse fracture in the base of the frontal process of the zygoma (*arrowheads*). The submentovertical view (**c**) illustrates the fracture of the anterior wall of the left antrum (*open arrow*) and the minimally displaced fracture of the anterior portion of the zygomatic arch (*small solid arrows*). Computed tomograms (**d**, **e**) demonstrate proptosis of the left eye, displacement of the lateral rectus muscle (*open arrow*), and fractures of the lateral wall of the orbit; confirm the fracture of the greater sphenoidal wing (*arrowheads*, **d**); and confirm the depressed fracture of the anterior wall of the left maxillary antrum (*stemmed arrow*) and free fluid within the antrum (*arrowhead*, **e**).

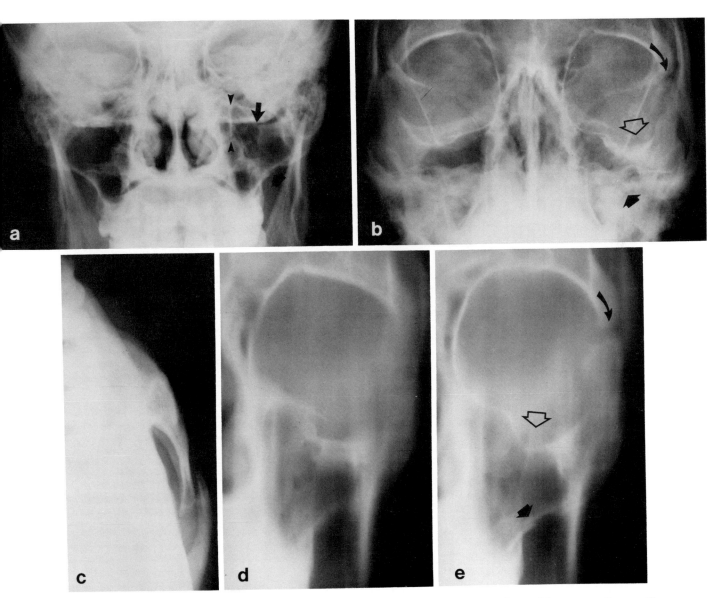

Fig. 2.45 Complex zygomaticomaxillary fracture. In the Caldwell projection (**a**), the signs of the zygomaticomaxillary fracture are very subtle. The left maxillary antrum is slightly, but definitely, clouded, its anterolateral wall is disrupted (*solid arrow*), a vertical fracture is present in its anterior wall (*arrowheads*), and a depressed fracture of the inferior orbital rim (*stemmed arrow*) is discernible through the superimposed density of the occiput. The anteroposterior projection (**b**) depicts the fracture-suture separation of the lateral orbital wall (*curved arrow*), a depressed fracture of the inferior orbital rim (*open arrow*), and the depressed fracture of the anterolateral wall of the antrum (*solid arrow*). The depressed, displaced fracture of the zygomatic arch is well demonstrated in the submentovertical view (**c**). The superficial rectilinear tomogram (**d**) clearly delineates the depressed fracture of the inferior orbital rim and the deeper tomogram (**e**) demonstrates the zygomaticofrontal suture separation (*curved arrow*), the depressed fracture of the orbital floor (*open arrow*), and the fracture of the anterolateral wall of the antrum (*solid arrow*).

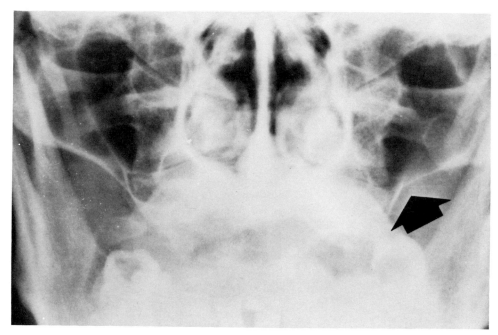

Fig. 2.46 Isolated, depressed fracture of the anterolateral wall of the maxillary sinus.

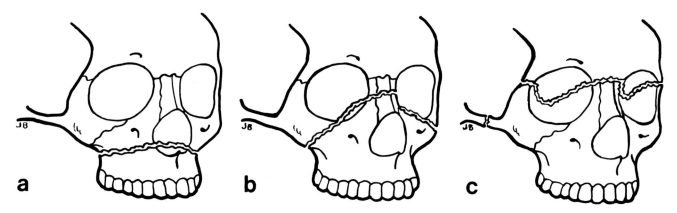

Fig. 2.47 Midfacial fractures according to the classification of Le Fort. **(a)** Le Fort I; **(b)** Le Fort II; **(c)** Le Fort III, craniofacial disjunction. (Modified from E.L. Ralston: *Handbook of Fractures.* C. V. Mosby, St. Louis, Mo., 1967).

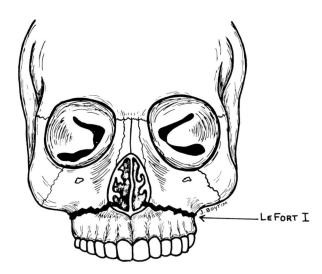

Fig. 2.48 Schematic representation of the Le Fort I fracture.

Midface fractures include fractures of the maxillary alveolar process, isolated fractures of the maxillary antrum, and the Le Fort fractures.

Fracture of the maxillary alveolar process is a transverse fracture limited to the alveolar process, most commonly in the incisor area, which may extend across the tips of the maxillary teeth. This fracture is readily apparent clinically and usually does not require radiographic examination to establish the diagnosis. Radiologic evaluation is indicated to determine the extent of the injury and the relationship of the dental apices to the fracture line. Roentgen evaluation requires the use of occlusal films since the alveolar process is usually not well seen in the standard projections of the face.

The isolated fracture of the maxillary antrum occurs uncommonly, is the result of direct trauma to the antrum inferior to the malar eminence, and is characterized, radiographically, by a fracture of its anterolateral wall with acute medial angulation at the fracture site (Fig. 2.46).

Approximately 25% of midface fractures are associated with cerebrospinal fluid (CSF) rhinorrhea secondary to fractures involving the cribriform plate (16). Le Fort II and III injuries constitute the majority of midface fractures associated with CSF rhinorrhea.

Le Fort fractures occur along the planes of structural weakness in the midface and are, by definition, bilateral and symmetrical injuries (Fig. 2.47) (17).

The Le Fort I fracture extends horizontally through each maxillary antrum and through each nostril above the level of the hard palate (Fig. 2.48). Consequently, fracture lines will be present in the anterolateral aspect of each antrum and the lateral wall of each nostril (medial wall of the maxillary antrum). The fractures extend through the antra circumferentially and can be identified in the anterior and posterior walls of the antra in lateral projection. Tomography is essential for the confirmation or detection of the minimally displaced fractures which are commonly obscured by superimposition of facial structures or antral hemorrhage. Free blood, commonly present in the maxillary antra, produces air-fluid levels in roentgenograms made with the horizontal beam. The pterygoid process is infrequently involved in the Le Fort I fracture (Fig. 2.49).

A pure Le Fort II fracture, as originally described, occurs infrequently because of the magnitude and direction of the causative force. Classically, the Le Fort II (pyramidal) fracture extends from the nasion bilaterally obliquely downward and laterally through the orbits and the maxillary antra medial to the body of the zygoma (Fig. 2.50). In the antra, the fracture extends posteriorly to involve the posterior wall and, commonly, the pterygoid processes. The Le Fort II fracture is, by definition, confined to the pyramidal distribution of the midface. It does *not* involve the lateral components of the face, i.e., the lateral orbital rims nor the zygomatic arches (Figs. 2.51–2.53).

Le Fort II fractures are commonly associated with a unilateral zygomaticomaxillary fracture (Fig. 2.54). In this instance, disruption of the lateral wall of the orbit and a fracture of the zygomatic arch on the right is present in addition to the pyramidal distribution of the Le Fort II fracture.

The Le Fort III fracture (craniofacial dysjunction), in distinction from the Le Fort II fracture, *does* involve the lateral walls of the orbits and the zygomatic arches (Fig. 2.55). The fracture lines extend from the nasion laterally, through the orbits to their lateral walls, as well as to the zygomatic arches. The fracture lines also extend through the roof and posterior wall of the antra and usually involve the pterygoid processes. Because the force required to produce a Le Fort III fracture is so severe and because the force is dissipated throughout the entire midface, the Le Fort III injury typically includes fractures in the Le Fort II distribution as well (Fig. 2.56). A pure Le Fort III fracture is rarely encountered clinically.

Le Fort III injuries are usually distracted or displaced and their radiographic demonstration is not difficult. However, rectilinear, polydirectional, or computed tomography is indicated, whenever the patient's condition will permit, to define the complete extent of the injury or to identify fractures not evident on the plain radiographs (Fig. 2.57).

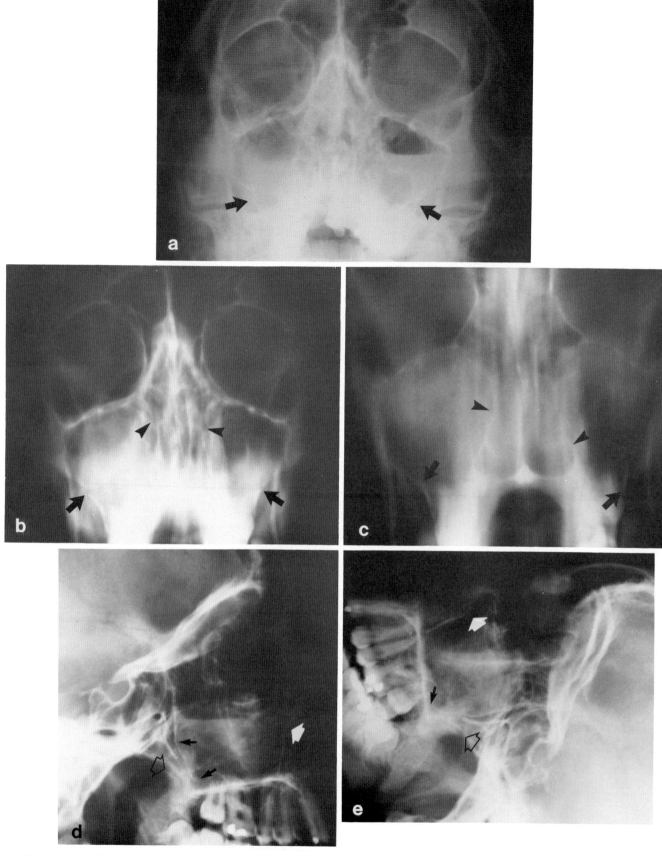

Fig. 2.49 Le Fort I fracture. Bilateral maxillary antral air-fluid levels are evident in the erect frontal radiograph (**a**). Minimally displaced fractures of the anterolateral wall of each antrum (*arrows*) are faintly perceptible through the density of the fluid within the antra. Tomograms made in frontal projection demonstrate the minimally displaced fractures of the antral walls (**b, c,** *arrows*) and of the lateral walls of the nostrils (**c,** *arrowheads*). Erect (**d**) and supine (**e**) horizontal beam lateral radiographs of the face demonstrate antral air-fluid levels, fractures of the anterior (*white arrows*) and posterior (*stemmed arrows*) antral walls and of the pterygoid process (*open arrows*).

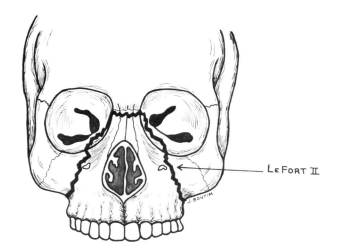

Fig. 2.50 Schematic representation of the Le Fort II (pyramidal) fracture.

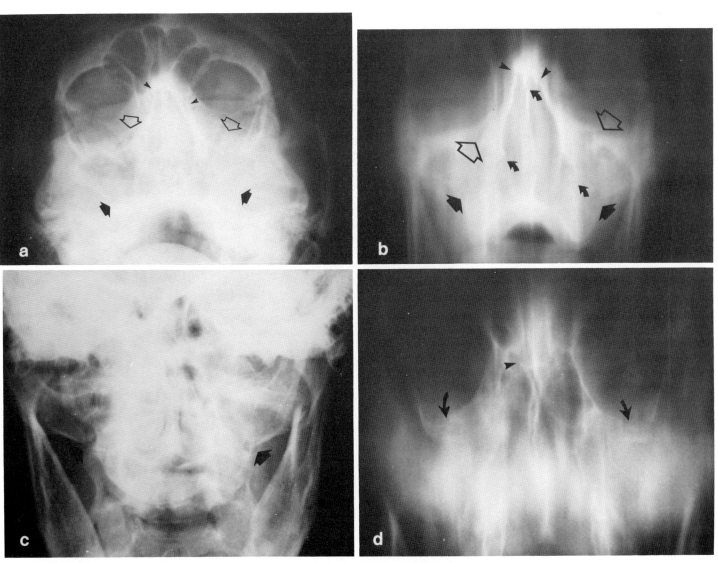

Fig. 2.51 Le Fort II fracture. In the erect Waters' projection (**a**), the most obvious roentgen signs are opacification of the left antrum and an air-fluid level in the right. Fractures are present in the anterolateral walls of each maxillary antrum (*solid arrows*) and fractures exist in the inferior rim of each orbit (*open arrows*) and each nasal bone (*arrowheads*). Note that the lateral orbital walls and zygomatic arches are intact. The tomogram made in Waters' position (**b**) demonstrates the fracture of the nasion (*arrowheads*), the inferior orbital rims (*open arrows*), and the lateral walls of the antra (*solid arrows*) to better advantage. Fractures of the nasal septum and medial wall of the antra (*curved arrows*) are also established. The maxillary antral fractures (*solid arrows*) are clearly seen in the frontal radiograph of the face (**c**). Each antrum is homogeneously opacified by blood. The more posterior tomogram (**d**) confirms the fractures of the orbital floor (*curved arrows*) and establishes fractures in the region of the nasion (*arrowhead*).

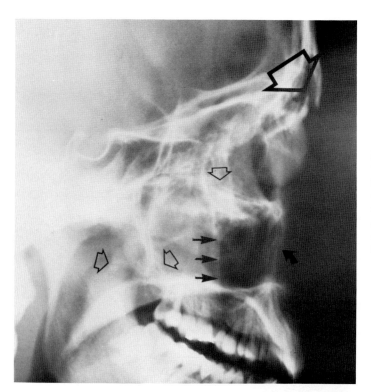

Fig. 2.52 Lateral radiograph of a patient with a Le Fort II fracture. The *large open arrow* indicates the displaced nasion fracture; the *small open arrows*, fractures of the orbital floor, the posterior wall of the antrum, and the tip of the lateral plate of the pterygoid process; the *curved arrow*, fractures of the anterior walls of the antra; and the *stemmed arrows*, the antral air-fluid level (radiograph made with patient supine and with a horizontal beam).

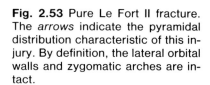

Fig. 2.53 Pure Le Fort II fracture. The *arrows* indicate the pyramidal distribution characteristic of this injury. By definition, the lateral orbital walls and zygomatic arches are intact.

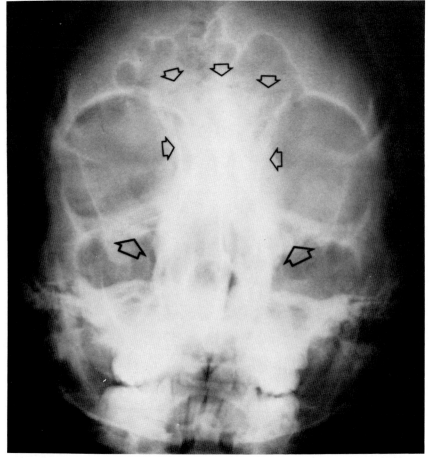

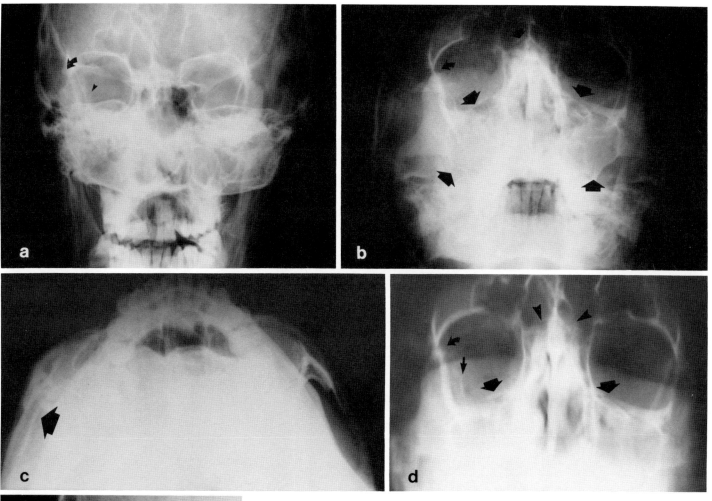

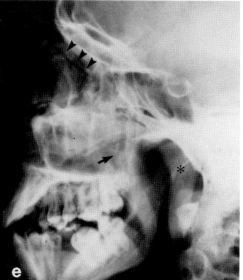

Fig. 2.54 Le Fort II fracture with simple right zygomaticomaxillary fracture. In the frontal projection (**a**), the displaced separation of the zygomaticofrontal suture is clearly demonstrated (*curved arrow*). Fracture of the lateral wall of the right orbit is further indicated by disruption of the greater wing of the sphenoid (*arrowhead*). Homogeneous opacification of the maxillary antra suggests the presence of free blood and, by inference, antral fractures. The appearance of the left zygomaticofrontal suture suggests either separation or fracture. However, the oblique density of the greater sphenoidal wing is intact and the medial cortices of the frontal and zygomatic processes are aligned. These observations militate against disruption of the suture. The Waters' projection (**b**) establishes the diagnosis of a Le Fort II fracture with an associated right zygomaticomaxillary fracture. The Le Fort II fractures (nasion, inferior orbital rims, and maxillary antra) are indicated by the *solid arrows*. The ethmoidal and maxillary sinuses are homogeneously and completely opacified by blood within their cavities. The right zygomaticofrontal suture is clearly disrupted (*curved arrow*). While the zygomatic arch fracture is not visible in either the frontal (**a**) or the Waters' (**b**) projection, it is seen (*solid arrow*) in the submentovertical view (**c**). The tomogram made in Waters' position (**d**) demonstrates fractures in the superior ethmoid sinuses (*arrowheads*) and confirms the fractures of the inferior orbital rims (*solid arrows*), the right greater sphenoidal wing (*stemmed arrow*) and separation of the right zygomaticomaxillary suture (*curved arrow*). The nasion fracture of the Le Fort injury (*arrowheads*) and of a posterior antral wall (*stemmed arrow*) and the retropharyngeal hematoma (*) are demonstrated in the lateral radiograph of the face (**e**).

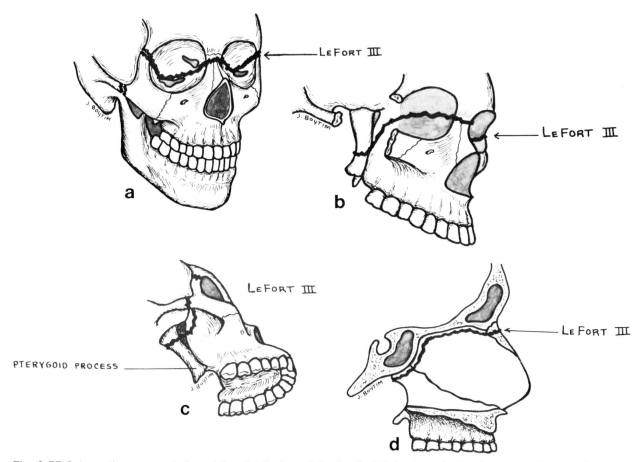

Fig. 2.55 Schematic representation of the distribution of the Le Fort III fracture. In (**b**), the zygomatic arch has been omitted to show the fracture line involving the orbit, the maxillary antrum, and the pterygoid process.

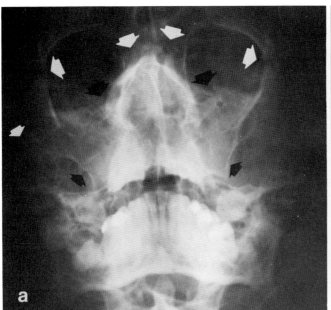

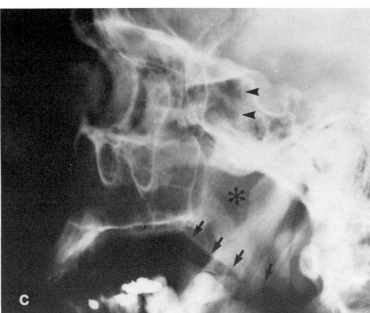

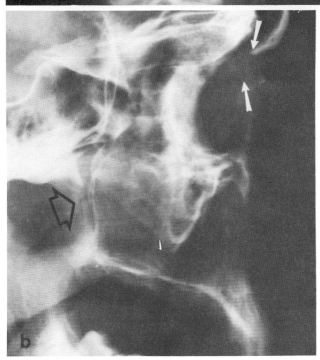

Fig. 2.56 Typical Le Fort III fracture with extension into the Le Fort II distribution. In the Waters' projection (**a**), the *white arrows* indicate the nasion fracture and fractures of the lateral orbital walls and the zygomatic arches (Le Fort III distribution). The *black arrows* indicate the fractures in the pyramidal distribution of a Le Fort II injury. Distraction of the nasion fragments (*stemmed arrow*) and fractures of the posterior wall of the antrum and the pterygoid process (*open arrow*) are evident in the lateral radiograph of the face (**b**). In the horizontal beam, brow-up lateral radiograph (**c**), the mottled lucencies of free air are evident in the region of the ethmoid sinuses and along the floor of the anterior cranial fossa; an air-fluid level is present in the sphenoidal sinus (*arrowheads*), indicating a concomitant fracture of the floor of the middle cranial fossa; and a large soft tissue mass (*) completely obliterating the nasopharyngeal airway and seriously compromising the oropharyngeal airway (*stemmed arrows*) represents a retropharyngeal hematoma secondary to the facial fracture.

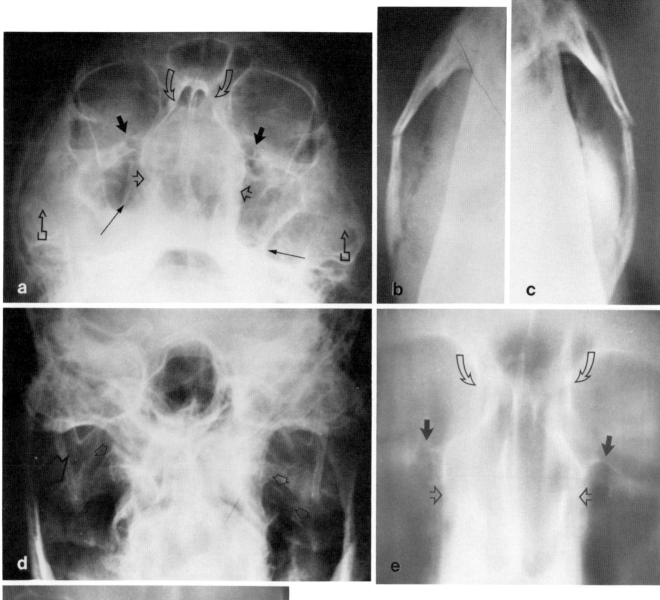

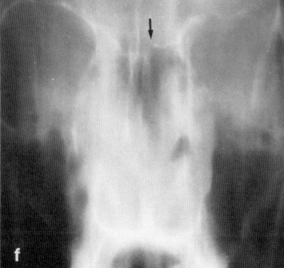

Fig. 2.57 Minimally displaced Le Fort III fracture. In the Waters' projection (**a**), the *open curved arrows* indicate the nasion fracture. The zygomatic arch fractures are indicated by the *box stemmed arrows*. Separation of the zygomaticofrontal sutures was not recognizable in this plane. Fractures in the pyramidal distribution are indicated by the *solid, open,* and *stemmed arrows.* The zygomatic arch fractures and subjacent subcutaneous emphysema were clearly demonstrated in the submentovertical radiograph (**b, c**). The extended Towne projection (**d**) records complete comminution of the posterior wall of each maxillary antrum. Only a few separate fragments are visible (*arrows*) in the region of the posterior antral walls. Rectilinear tomography demonstrated fractures in the medial walls of the orbits and antra (**e**) and in the cribriform plate (**f**).

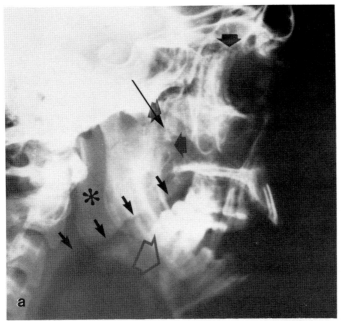

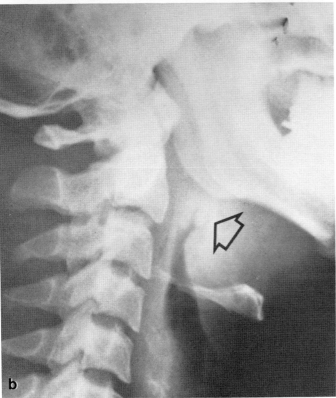

Fig. 2.58 Obstructing retropharyngeal hematoma in a patient with extensive facial trauma. The initial lateral radiograph of the face (**a**) demonstrated a large retropharyngeal mass (*) completely obstructing the nasopharynx and severely compromising (*stemmed arrows*) the oral airway. The *solid arrows* indicate some of the fractures of a Le Fort III injury and the *open arrow* a displaced fracture of the mandible. A tracheostomy was performed and shortly postoperatively a lateral radiograph of the pharynx (**b**) demonstrated complete obstruction of the upper airway (*open arrow*) by the retropharyngeal hematoma.

The most clinically significant feature of the Le Fort III injury is the retropharyngeal hematoma because it is life-threatening. The extensive soft tissue damage of the face, the obvious presence of blood in the nasal and oral cavities, and the frequently coexistent remote injuries, all typically present in patients with Le Fort III fractures, all require the attending physician's attention. The extensive damage to the face and the nasal and/or oral hemorrhage are usually considered to be the sole, or principal, etiology of airway obstruction. Not only is the development of a retropharyngeal hematoma masked by other more apparent clinical problems, but its detection by physical examination is extremely difficult. Therefore, the diagnosis of an obstructing retropharyngeal hematoma depends upon an awareness of the association of the hematoma with complex zygomaticomaxillary and Le Fort fractures, a high index of suspicion, and the routine inclusion of a lateral radiograph of the pharynx (Fig. 2.58) in all patients with these injuries.

Nondisplaced fractures of the nasal bones may be difficult to identify, particularly if the fracture line parallels the suture lines between the nasal bone and the nasal process of the maxilla (Fig. 2.59). The axial projection of the nose is particularly helpful in establishing the presence of this fracture (see Fig. 2.18, p. 46).

Fracture of the anterior nasal spine of the maxilla may occur as an isolated lesion (Fig. 2.60) or, more commonly, in association with a nasal fracture (Fig. 2.61). The anterior nasal spine fracture is particularly painful and is frequently the source of "unexplained" pain and tenderness in the midline of the upper lip at its junction with the nose. The radiographic examination, therefore, must include the area of the anterior nasal spine, be of sufficient diagnostic quality to adequately demonstrate this small process, and be specifically studied for this fracture.

Severe nasal fractures are frequently associated with more significant facial injury which may be either clinically unsuspected or masked by the soft tissue swelling and ecchymosis about the nose and face. Figure 2.62 is an example of a comminuted, nondisplaced nasal fracture associated with a clinically unsuspected blow-out fracture of the right orbit.

The mandible is the most frequently fractured bone of the face (18). The single fracture without associated temporomandibular dislocation (Figs. 2.63–2.65) occurred in 68% of mandibular fractures reported by Ivy and Curtis (19). Because of its configuration, stress applied to the mandible producing one fracture will be transmitted to another portion of the mandible and may produce multiple fractures (Fig. 2.66) or dislocation at the temporomandibular joint. It is, therefore, imperative that the entire mandible be carefully studied to exclude the presence of a double fracture.

Dislocation of the mandible may occur with or without direct trauma. The condyles usually dislocate

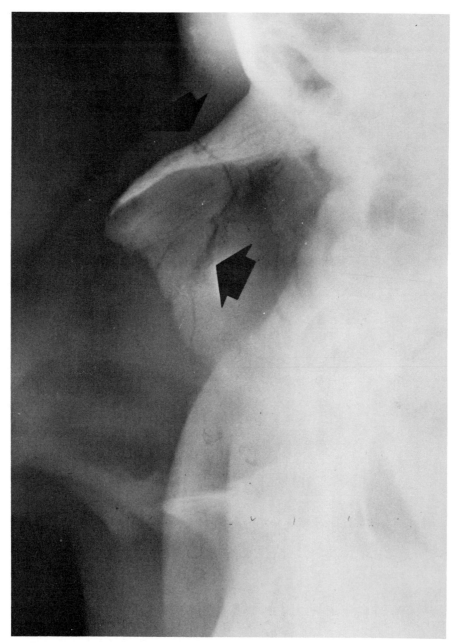

Fig. 2.59 The *arrows* indicate a nondisplaced, nondepressed fracture of the nasal bones. Note that the fracture line, even though resembling the nasomaxillary suture, does traverse the suture and that the fracture line is wider and its margins more irregular than the suture line. The anterior nasal spine of the maxilla is intact.

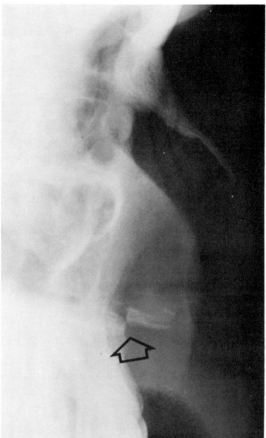

Fig. 2.60 Isolated, displaced fracture of the anterior nasal spine of the maxilla.

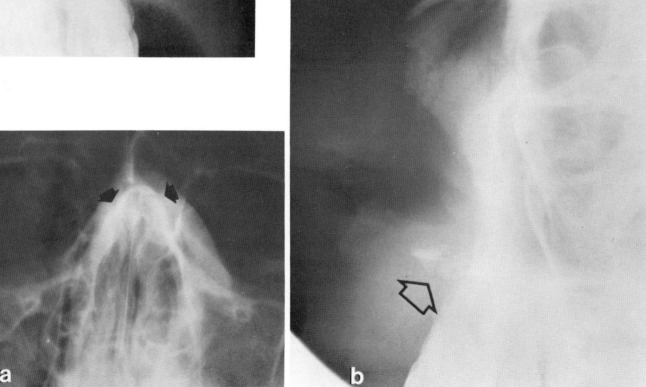

Fig. 2.61 Minimally displaced fractures of the tip of the nasal bones **(a)** associated with a comminuted fracture of the anterior nasal spine of the maxilla **(b)**.

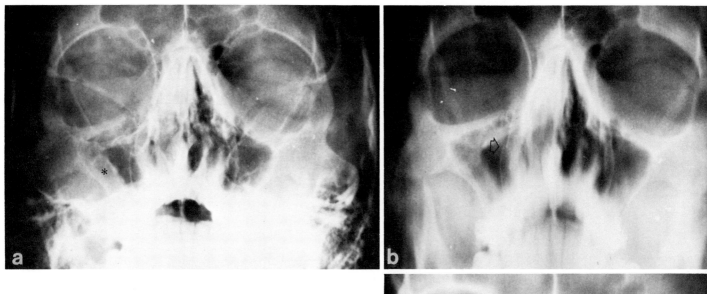

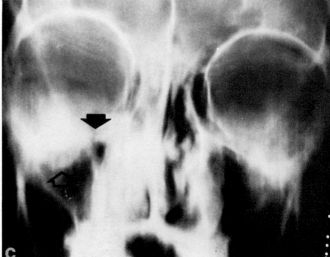

Fig. 2.62 Waters' projection **(a)** showing diffuse submucosal hemorrhage (*) in the right maxillary antrum and extensive soft tissue swelling of the right nostril. Clinically and radiographically, the patient had a displaced nasal fracture. The anterior tomogram **(b)** demonstrates a slightly displaced fracture of the nasal process of the right maxilla (*open arrow*). The most posterior tomogram **(c)** established a fracture in the medial aspect of the floor of the orbit (*solid arrow*) and orbital contents (*open arrow*) herniated into the subjacent maxillary antrum (a blow-out fracture).

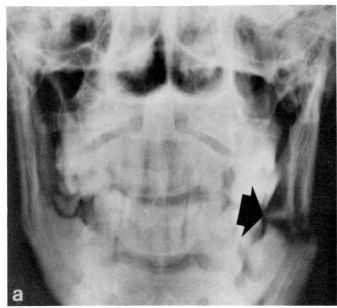

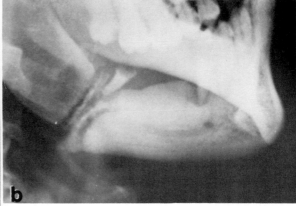

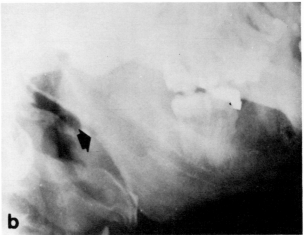

Fig. 2.63 (a) Single comminuted fracture through the angle of the mandible. The areas of rarefaction about the retained root fragment at the fracture site and the left canine tooth represent periapical abscesses **(b)**.

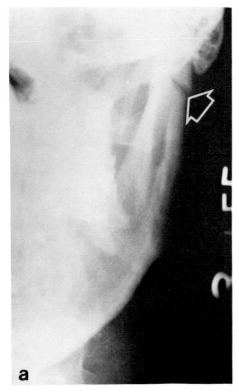

Fig. 2.64 (a, b) Single, minimally displaced fracture through the neck of the mandible on the left.

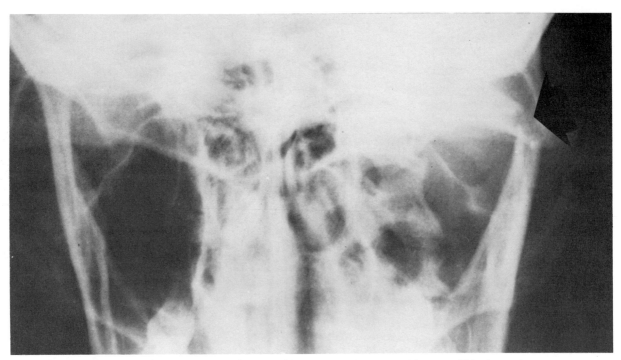

Fig. 2.65 Single, severely displaced fracture in the neck of the mandible (*arrow*).

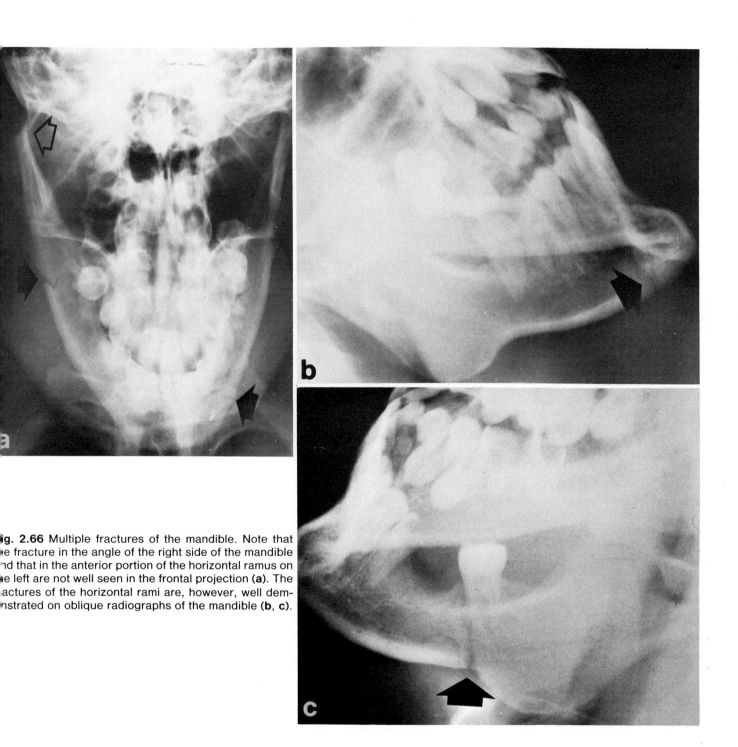

Fig. 2.66 Multiple fractures of the mandible. Note that the fracture in the angle of the right side of the mandible and that in the anterior portion of the horizontal ramus on the left are not well seen in the frontal projection (a). The fractures of the horizontal rami are, however, well demonstrated on oblique radiographs of the mandible (b, c).

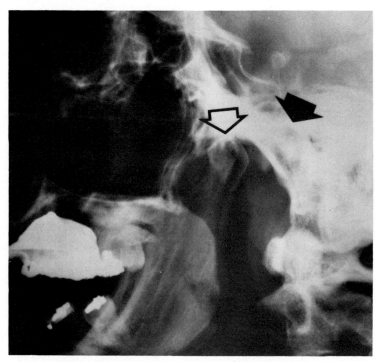

Fig. 2.67 Complete anterior dislocation of the temporomandibular joint. The location of the condyle is indicated by the *open arrow.* The position of the mandibular notch is indicated by the *solid arrow.*

anteriorly and superiorly out of the mandibular fossa to lie in front of the articular eminence (Fig. 2.67).

Mandibular fractures above the level of the notch may be difficult to identify radiographically, even when they are complete and displaced. Superimposed bones of the face or of the base of the skull frequently obscure the fracture line. Posteroanterior, anteroposterior, and Waters' projections (Fig. 2.68), individualized oblique projections made in the frontal position (Fig. 2.69), and lateral laminograms (Fig. 2.70) may be necessary to identify or confirm the presence of a fracture. If the patient's condition will permit, the base (Hirtz) view may provide an accurate delineation of the fragments (Fig. 2.71). If fracture lines occur in such a configuration that the body of the mandible constitutes a separate fragment, the unopposed action of the geniohyoid, the genioglossus, and the anterior belly of the digastric muscles may retract the separate fragments posteriorly. As a result, the tongue may be retracted posteriorly and may fill the oral and oropharyngeal cavities to such a degree that obstruction to the airway may occur (Fig. 2.72).

Posteriorly directed force applied to the body of the mandible and transmitted to the condylar processes may drive the condyles posteriorly and inferiorly out of the mandibular fossa against the anterior wall of the external auditory canal, producing a fracture of this portion of the temporal bone (Fig. 2.73) or a separation of the temporosphenoidal suture. Clinically, this injury is suggested by malocclusion, blood in the external auditory canal, or subcutaneous ecchymosis involving the anterior wall of the external auditory canal.

Nontraumatic Lesions

The smoothly sclerotic, gently irregular, parallel margins of the zygomaticotemporal suture (Fig. 2.74) should help distinguish this normal structure from an isolated fracture of the zygomatic arch.

Superimposition of the suture between the body and the greater cornua of the hyoid bone upon the mandible may simulate a fracture line (Fig. 2.75).

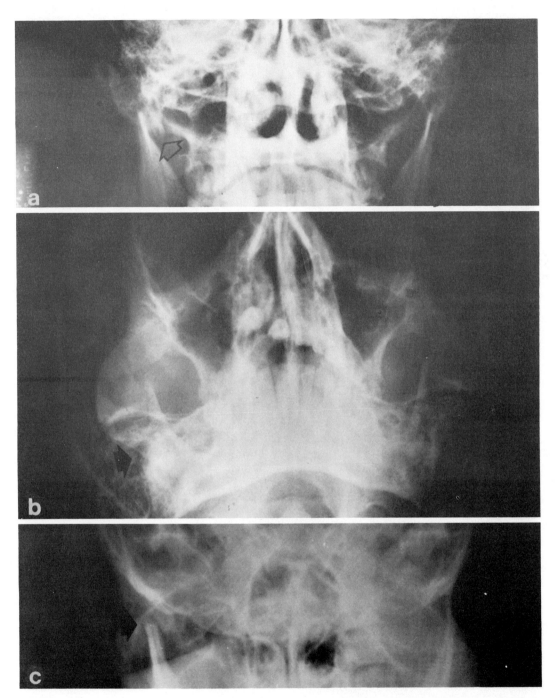

Fig. 2.68 Three frontal projections used to demonstrate fractures in the neck of the mandible. It is important to realize that these projections are useful to visualize a fracture at this site, since the fracture may not be recognizable on any one of the three. **(a)** Posteroanterior; **(b)** Waters'; **(c)** exaggerated base view.

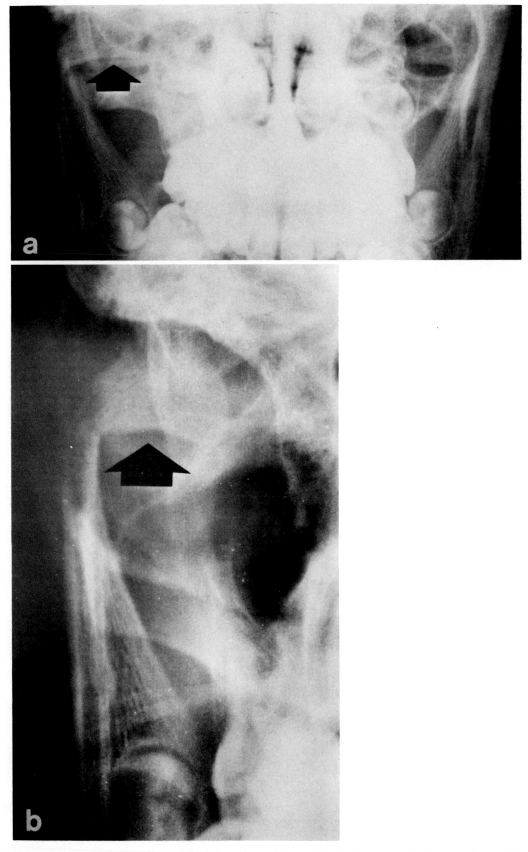

Fig. 2.69 Complete fracture in the neck of the mandible on the right (**a**). The proximal fragment (*arrow*) is angulated acutely medially resulting in dislocation at the temporomandibular joint. The fracture is obscured by superimposed densities of the bones of the face and the occiput. The same fracture is clearly demonstrated in the obliquely rotated frontal projection (**b**).

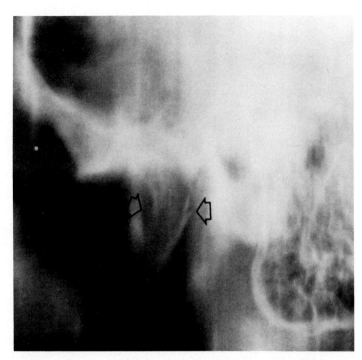

Fig. 2.70 Laminogram of the right temporomandibular joint made in lateral projection. The fracture line is indicated by the *arrows*.

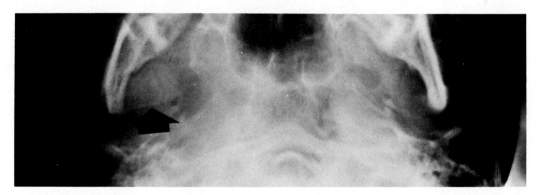

Fig. 2.71 Base view clearly demonstrating position of the proximal fragment of a fracture of the neck of the mandible.

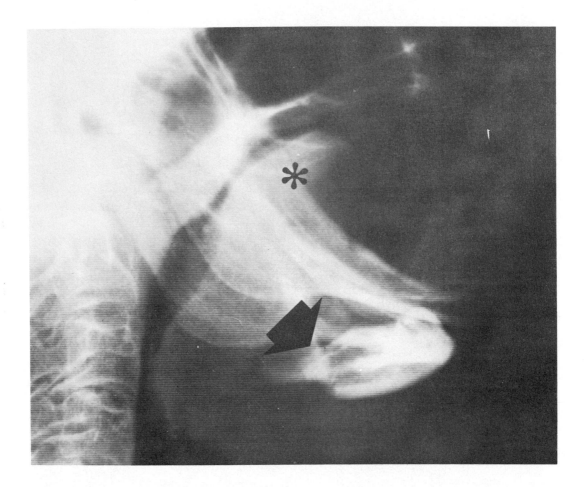

Fig. 2.72 Fracture of the anterior portion of each horizontal ramus of the mandible. The mandibular body and symphysis constitute a separate fragment (*arrow*). As a result of the proximal retraction of this fragment, the tongue (*) has also been retracted posteriorly obstructing the oral airway.

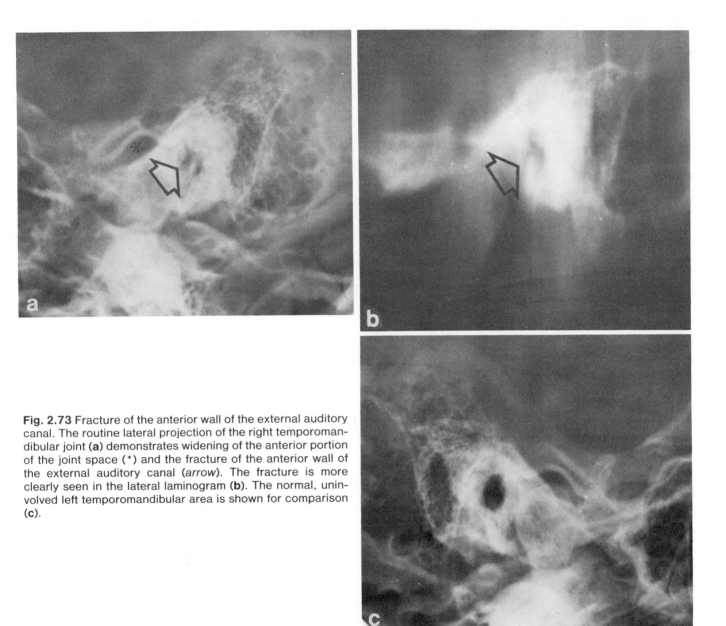

Fig. 2.73 Fracture of the anterior wall of the external auditory canal. The routine lateral projection of the right temporomandibular joint (**a**) demonstrates widening of the anterior portion of the joint space (*) and the fracture of the anterior wall of the external auditory canal (*arrow*). The fracture is more clearly seen in the lateral laminogram (**b**). The normal, uninvolved left temporomandibular area is shown for comparison (**c**).

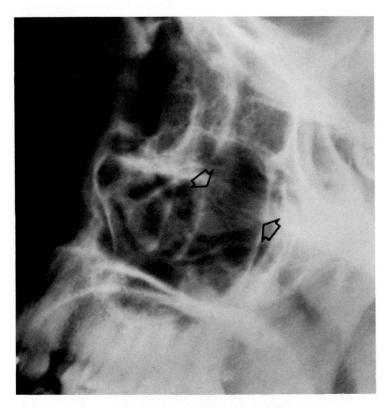

Fig. 2.74 The *arrows* indicate the zygomatico-temporal suture in the zygomatic arch. The sclerotic, sharply defined margins of the suture should help distinguish this normal structure from a fracture line.

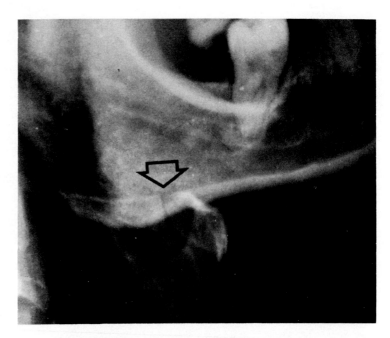

Fig. 2.75 The normal suture between the body and greater cornua of the hyoid bone (*arrow*) when superimposed upon the mandible could simulate a fracture line.

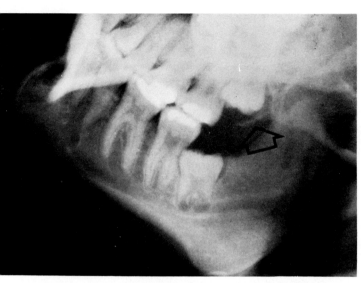

Fig. 2.76 The *arrow* points to a thin spicule of the alveolar bone partially covering the partially erupted maxillary third molar tooth. This is a normal finding and should not be misinterpreted as a fracture fragment, the wall of a lytic lesion, or a sequestrum.

The thin spicule of alveolar bone which normally overlies a partially erupted molar tooth (Fig. 2.76) may simulate a fracture, a sequestrum, or the wall of a lytic lesion.

Inflammation of the paranasal sinuses may involve one or all of the sinuses with faint haziness, discrete mucous membrane thickening (Fig. 2.77), or complete opacification.

Periapical abscess produces an area of bony destruction and resorption about the root of the involved tooth. The lamina dura is destroyed and the area of rarefaction extends into the adjacent alveolar bone (Fig. 2.63).

Polyps and retention cysts are common lesions of the maxillary sinus. Radiographically, these benign lesions produce a sharply defined, smooth, homogeneous soft tissue mass which usually arises from the floor of the sinus and projects into its cavity (Fig. 2.78).

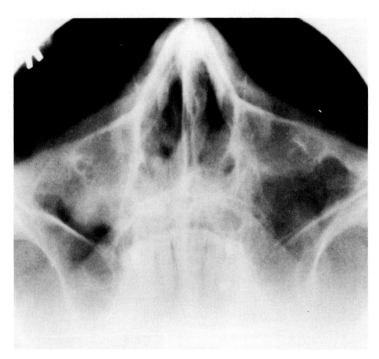

Fig. 2.77 Inflammatory mucous membrane thickening in the maxillary antra.

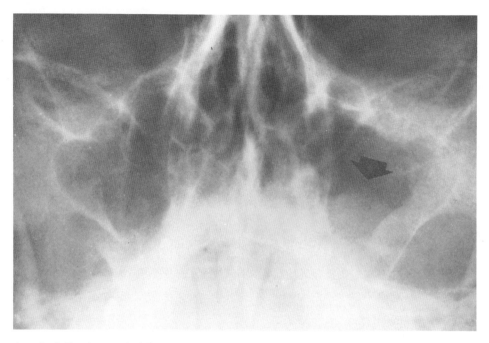

Fig. 2.78 The sharply defined, rounded, homogeneous soft tissue density in the floor of the left maxillary sinus (*arrow*) represents either a polyp or retention cyst. Note, also, the diffuse mucous membrane thickening within the left maxillary sinus.

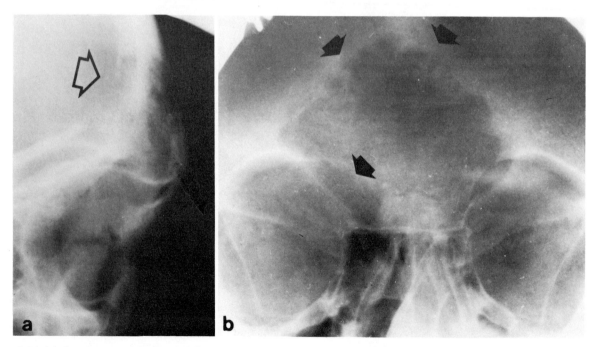

Fig. 2.79 (a) Carcinoma of the frontal sinus that has eroded through the posterior wall of the sinus. The large area of invasion and destruction of the frontal bone is evident. **(b)** The *arrows* indicate areas where the tumor has extended superiorly through the walls of the frontal sinuses and inferiorly through the wall of the right orbit.

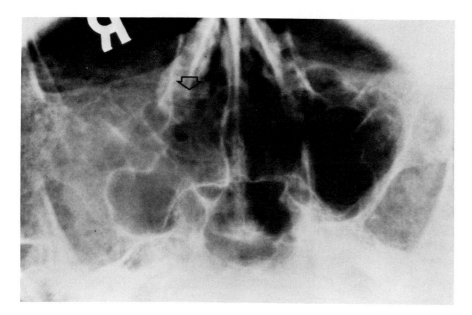

Fig. 2.80 The right maxillary sinus is irregularly opacified. The walls of the maxillary sinus are largely replaced by the soft tissue density. The medial wall, particularly (*arrow*), has been completely destroyed by the tumor which extends into the right nostril.

Fig. 2.81 Dentigerous cyst. The *arrows* indicate the clearly demarcated area of radiolucency which surrounds the unerupted third molar tooth. This benign cystic lesion, which results from degeneration of the enamel organ surrounding a developing crown, can produce marked enlargement of the jaw.

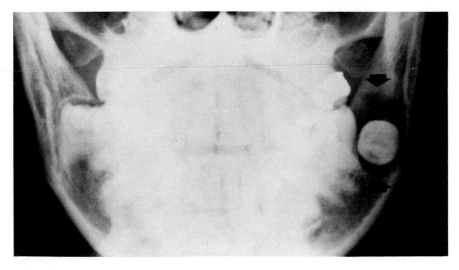

Malignant tumors of the paranasal sinuses may cause complete opacification of the involved sinus. Invasion of the bony walls of the sinus results in loss of its sharp cortical margin and mottled demineralization or destruction of the adjacent bone (Figs. 2.79 and 2.80).

Dentigerous cyst (Fig. 2.81) is the most common benign neoplasm of the mandible. Adamantinoma (Fig. 2.82) is a primary malignant tumor. This neoplasm, which involves the mandible more often than the maxilla, is characterized by a high incidence of local recurrence. Metastatic disease rarely involves the mandible but may do so either in the form of hematogenous foci or destruction of the walls of the mandibular canal by tumor involvement of the perineural lymphatic pathway.

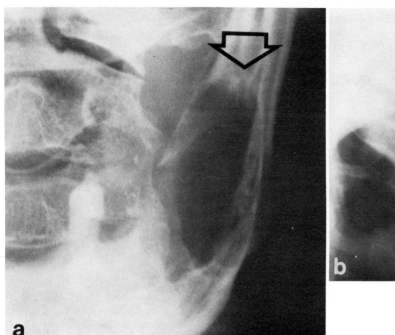
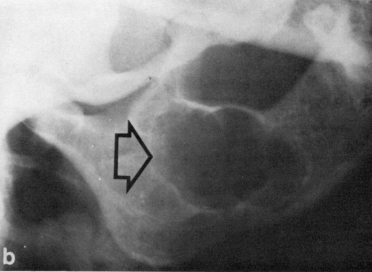

Fig. 2.82 (a, b) Adamantinoma of the mandible. Bony septa, cortical expansion, absence of new bone formation, sharply defined smooth wall, central location, and destruction of bone and dental roots are the usual roentgen characteristics of this tumor.

References

1. LEWIN JR, RHODES DR, Jr, PAVSEC EJ: The roentgeno-logic manifestations of fracture of the orbital floor (blow-out fractures). *AJR* 83:628, 1960.
2. LLOYD GAS: Orbital emphysema. *Br J Radiol* 39:933, 1966.
3. CRAMER LM, TOOZE FM, LERMAN S: Blow-out fracture of the orbit. *Br J Plast Surg* 18:171, 1965.
4. VIGARIO GD: Blow-out fracture of the orbit. *Br J Radiol* 39:939, 1966.
5. THORWARTH WT, BARDEN RP, GRAHAM TF: Recognition and management of fractures of the orbit. *AJR* 102:840, 1968.
6. ZIZMOR J, SMITH B, FASANO C, CONVERSE JM: Roentgen diagnosis of blow-out fractures of the orbit. *AJR* 87:1009, 1962.
7. POTTER GD: Radiological examination of the orbit. *CRC Crit Rev Radiol SCI* 2:145, 1971.
8. SMITH B, REGAN WF, Jr: Blow-out fracture of the orbit. *Am J Ophthalmol* 44:733, 1957.
9. CONVERSE JM, SMITH B, OBEAR MF, WOOD-SMITH D: Orbital blow-out fractures. *Plast Reconstr Surg* 39:20, 1967.
10. DODICK JM, GALIN MA, KWITKO M: Medial wall fractures of the orbit. *Can J Ophthalmol* 4:377, 1969.
11. EMERY AU, VON NOORDEN GK: Traumatic "pseudoprolapse" of orbital tissues into the maxillary antrum: A diagnostic pitfall. *Trans Am Acad Opthalmol Otolaryngol* 79:893, 1975.
12. VALVASSORI GE, HORD GE: Traumatic sinus disease. *Semin Roentgenol* 3:160, 1968.
13. ERMIND K: Transmaxillary approach in old and in fresh orbital fractures. In *Fractures of the Orbit,* edited by GM Bleeker and TK Lyle. Williams & Wilkins, Baltimore, 1970.
14. KNIGHT JS, NORTH JF: The classification of malar fractures. *Br J Plast Surg* 13:325, 1961.
15. UNGER JDeB, UNGER GF: Fractures of the pterygoid processes accompanying severe facial bone injury. *Radiology* 98:311, 1971.
16. GEORGIADE NG: The management of acute mid-facial-orbital injuries. *Clin Neurosurg* 19:301, 1971.
17. LeFORT R: Etude experimentale sur les fractures de la machoire superieure. *Rev de Chir* 23:208, 1901.
18. PENDERGRASS EP, SCHAEFFER JP, HODES PF: *The Head and Neck in Roentgen Diagnosis,* ed. 2. Charles C Thomas, Springfield, Ill., 1956.
19. IVY RH, CURTIS L: Fractures of the mandible: An analysis of 100 cases. *Dent Cosmos* 68:439, 1926.

chapter three

Spine

The majority of acute lesions of the spine are traumatic. "Spinal injury" conjures the image of a serious lesion which, at its worst, may be life-threatening and, at its best, may produce paralysis. The fact is that many injuries of the spine have no significance beyond the localized morbidity associated with the lesion itself. However, until the nature and extent of the spinal injury and its possible relationship to the spinal cord and nerve roots is accurately assessed, all patients who are unconscious or who have a history of significant injury to the spine should be considered as having a potentially serious lesion.

General Anatomic Considerations

Figure 3.1 illustrates the soft tissue anatomy of the spine. The anterior longitudinal ligament, a broad fibrous band extending from the anterior arch of the atlas to the sacrum, helps to maintain the relationship of the vertebral segments to each other. Fibers of this ligament, which extend cephalad from the anterior arch of the atlas to the basiocciput, constitute the anterior atlanto-occipital membrane.

A similar fibrous band, the posterior longitudinal ligament, is located in the vertebral canal along the posterior aspect of the vertebral bodies.

The interspinous, supraspinous, and intertransverse ligaments, as well as the various muscles of the spine, contribute to the stability of the spine and may be disrupted by acute trauma.

All of the vertebral segments except for the first cervical have a body as their main and largest component. The odontoid process of C_2 (Fig. 3.2), which lies posterior to the arch of C_1, is analogous to the body of the first cervical segment. The pedicles, which extend posteriorly from each side of the vertebral body, connect the body to the dense, heavy articular masses (pillar, lateral mass). Each articular mass has a superior and inferior articulating facet. The inferior and superior facets of contiguous vertebrae constitute an interfacetal (facetal, apophyseal, posterior) joint. The inferior facet of the segment above, anatomically, lies above and posterior to the superior facet of the segment below. The plane of inclination of the interfacetal joints varies throughout the spine, being approximately 35° in the cervical area and nearly vertical in the thoracic and lumbar areas. The laminae extend obliquely medially and posteriorly from the articular masses to fuse in the midline to form the spinous process. Together the pedicles, articular masses, and laminae form the posterior (neural) arch (Figs. 3.3–3.5).

Each vertebra has bilateral transverse processes which, in the cervical segments, contain a foramen for the passage of the vertebral artery. The vertebral bodies are separated and cushioned by fibrocartilaginous intervertebral disc material.

Because the problems of emergency medicine concerning the spine differ depending upon the area of the spine involved and because the radiographic examination is specific for the several parts of the spine, the segments of the spinal column will be considered individually.

CERVICAL SPINE

Radiographic Examination

The roentgen examination of the patient with acute cervical spine trauma is dictated by the condition of the patient.

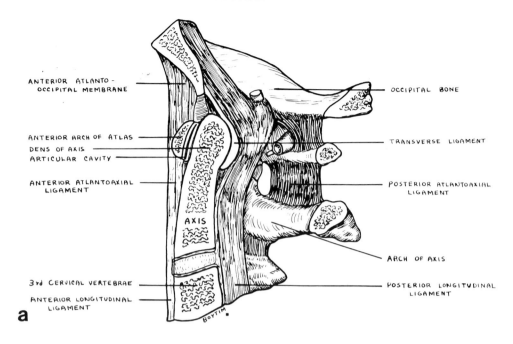

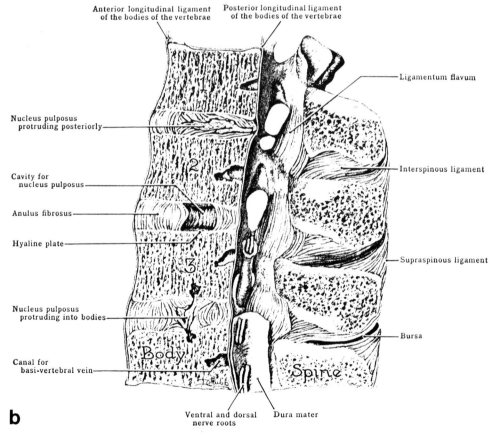

Fig. 3.1 Soft tissue anatomy in the upper cervical spine. Note the thickness and configuration of the anterior atlantoaxial ligament and the anterior longitudinal ligament through the upper cervical segments. The relationship of the odontoid process of C_2 to the anterior arch of C_1 and to the transverse atlantal ligament is well depicted in this sagittal section **(a)**. The extension of the anterior and posterior longitudinal ligaments into the lumbar area and the relationship of the interspinous ligament to the spinous processes is seen in **(b)**. (Reprinted with permission from J. E. Anderson (Ed.): *Grant's Atlas of Anatomy*, ed. 6. Williams & Wilkins, Baltimore, 1972.)

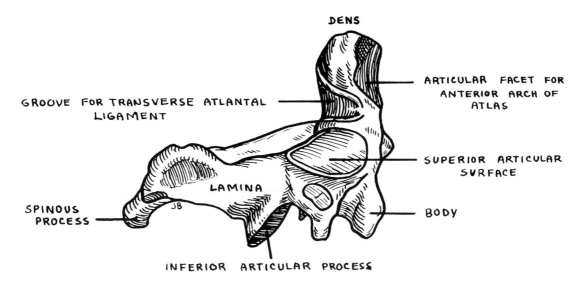

Fig. 3.2 The second cervical vertebra (axis or epistropheus) seen from the side. Note the presence of the groove for the transverse atlantal ligament in the posterior aspect of the base of the dens.

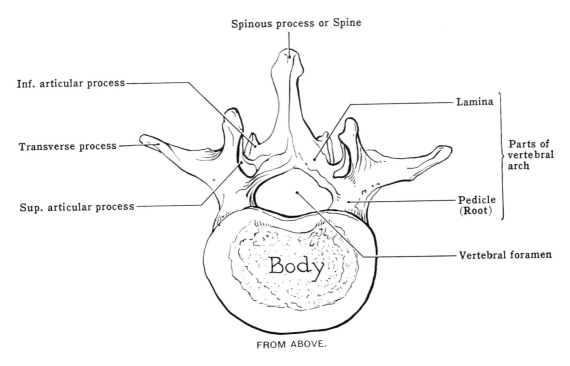

Fig. 3.3 A typical vertebra seen from above. The pedicles comprise the lateral walls of the neural canal. The laminae form the posterior aspect of the neural arch and fuse to form the base of the spinous process. (Reprinted with permission from J. E. Anderson (Ed.): *Grant's Atlas of Anatomy*, ed. 6. Williams & Wilkins, Baltimore, 1972.)

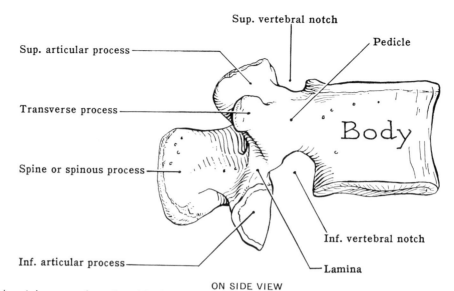

ON SIDE VIEW

Fig. 3.4 A typical vertebra seen from the side. Note the location of the paired superior and inferior articular processes (facets). (Reprinted with permission from J. E. Anderson (Ed.): *Grant's Atlas of Anatomy*, ed. 6. Williams & Wilkins, Baltimore, 1972.)

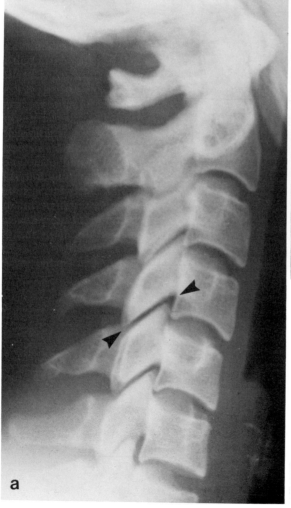

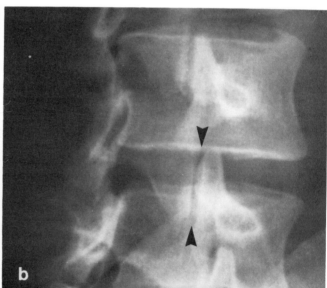

Fig. 3.5 The plane of the interfacetal joints of the cervical spine (**a**, *arrowheads*) is approximately 35° to the horizontal, while that of the facetal joints of the thoracic and lumbar spine (**b**) is essentially vertical.

The horizontal beam lateral radiograph of the cervical spine, obtained with the patient supine, is the single most important roentgen examination of the severely injured (unconsciousness, evidence of significant head or neck trauma, signs of cervical cord or root injury, multiple long bone fractures, "total body smash") patient. This examination should be made as soon as the patient's condition has been stabilized and, if possible, before nasogastric or endotracheal intubation (Fig. 3.6). When a diagnosis can be established from the horizontal beam lateral projection, no other views are indicated initially and more detailed roentgen examination may be delayed until the pa-

tient's condition will permit. If the horizontal beam lateral radiograph is not definitive, or if a fracture of the posterior neural arch is suspected, supine oblique projections (Fig. 3.7) (1) should be obtained. This projection permits diagnostic, although slightly distorted by magnification, evaluation of the posterolateral aspect of the vertebral bodies, the pedicles, articular masses, interfacetal joints, and laminae. Every reasonable effort consistent with the patient's condition should be made to completely visualize all seven cervical vertebrae (Fig. 3.8). If, for whatever reason, the lower cervical segments are obscured in lateral projection, a composite reconstruction of these verte-

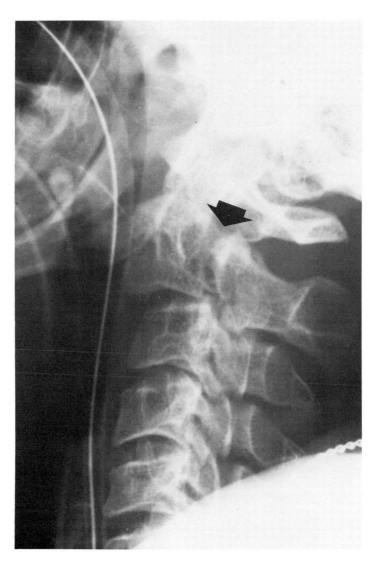

Fig. 3.6 Horizontal beam lateral radiograph of the cervical spine demonstrating a hangman's fracture of the axis (*arrow*). An endotracheal and a nasogastric tube are in place.

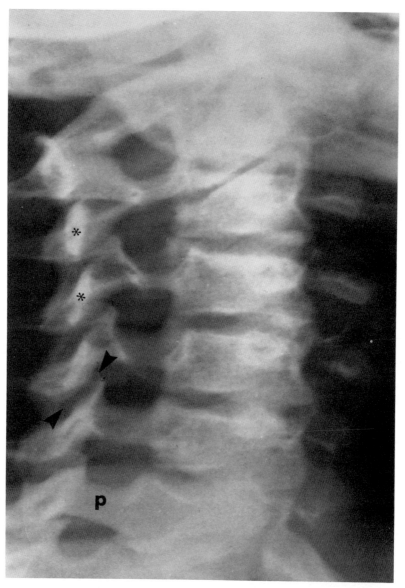

Fig. 3.7 Supine oblique radiograph of a normal adult cervical spine. The minor distortion and magnification, which is secondary to the short TFD and tube angulation, does not materially detract from the diagnostic qualities of this projection. *p* indicates the pedicle extending from the posterolateral aspect of the vertebral body to the articular mass. The *arrowheads* indicate an interfacetal joint space, and the *asterisks*, laminae, seen end-on. The alignment of the interfacetal joints and the laminae reflects the normal ''shingle'' relationship of the cervical articular masses.

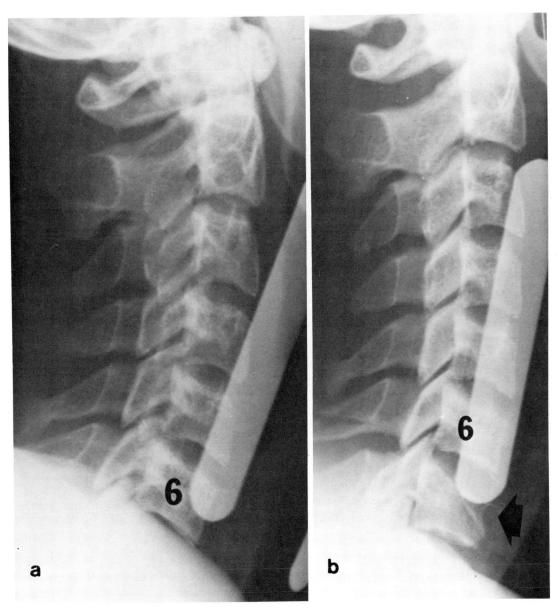

Fig. 3.8 This illustration emphasizes the inadequacy of a lateral roentgenogram of the cervical spine that fails to include the seventh vertebra. In the initial lateral projection **(a)**, the density of the shoulders completely obscured the fraction of C$_7$ **(b,** *arrow*).

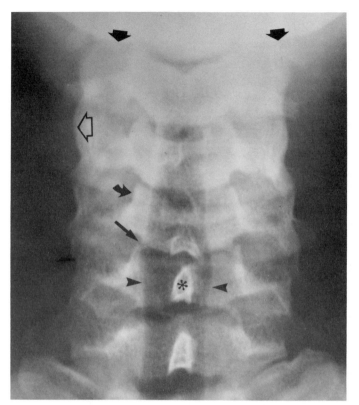

Fig. 3.9 Anteroposterior radiograph of the cervical spine. The atlantoaxial articulation is completely obscured by the superimposed density of the mandible and occiput (*solid arrows*). The major points of interest in this projection are the spinous processes, the tracheal air column, the joints of Luschka and the uncinate processes, and the lateral columns. The spinous processes (*) and the tracheal air column (*arrowheads*) are normally midline structures. The joints of Luschka (*stemmed arrow*), including the uncinate processes (*curved arrow*), should be symmetrically and vertically aligned at all levels. The lateral cortical margin (*open arrow*) of the lateral columns, which represents the lateral cortex of the anatomically superimposed articular masses, appears as a smooth, gently undulating, seemingly intact density. The lateral column itself normally appears as though it is a solid intact structure. Normally, the interfacetal joint spaces are not visible in this projection.

brae is possible from each supine oblique projection.

In the less severely injured patient, a definite sequence of radiographic projections must be followed. Depending upon the patient's condition, the examination can be made in either the erect or supine posture. If clinical signs of cervical cord or root damage are present, the cervical spine should be appropriately immobilized prior to the roentgen study. The lateral radiograph of the cervical spine should be obtained first because this projection provides the single most comprehensive evaluation of the cervical spine. (The visualization of all seven cervical segments in lateral projection is sufficiently important to warrant this emphasis by repetition.) The anteroposterior projection of the lower cervical segments (Fig. 3.9) and the "open-mouth" radiograph of the atlantoaxial articulation (Fig. 3.10) should be obtained next, followed by each oblique (Fig. 3.11) projection.

The studies enumerated above, i.e., the anteroposterior (including the open-mouth), the lateral, and each oblique projection, constitute the "basic" examination of the cervical spine. These projections must be evaluated prior to obtaining any additional views. If the basic study is equivocal, if the study suggests the possibility of an anterior subluxation (hyperflexion sprain), or if the history indicates a flexion injury, only then are lateral flexion (Fig. 3.12) and extension (Fig. 3.13) projections indicated. In the patient with acute cervical trauma, positioning for the lateral flexion and extension radiographs must be under the personal supervision of a physician. Rectilinear (Fig. 3.14) or polydirectional tomography should be used freely (2–4) to confirm or determine the true extent of fractures incompletely visualized on the plain radiographs. Computed tomography is invaluable in the detection of fractures and the displacement of fragments not otherwise radiographically visible (Fig. 3.15) (5–7). The pillar view (Fig. 3.16) (8–10), especially designed to visualize the articular masses en face, is indicated any time a fracture of the articular masses is suspected clinically or radiographically. The pillar view is obtained with the patient supine, the head rotated to one side, and the neck extended, if possible. The x-ray tube must be angled caudad 30–35° in order that the central beam passes parallel to the articulating facets of the lateral masses.

Radiographic Anatomy

The cervical spine normally includes the uppermost seven vertebral segments. In both children and adults, a smooth lordotic curve extends through the cervical

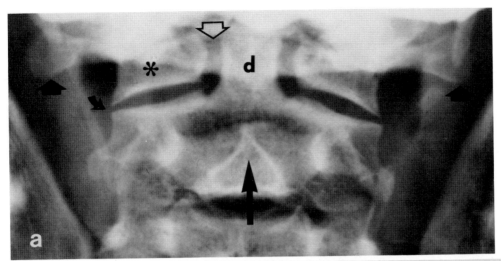

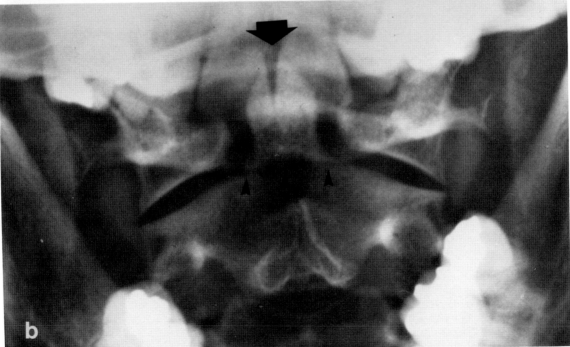

Fig. 3.10 Open-mouth projection of the normal upper cervical spine (atlantoaxial articulation, **(a)**. The dens (*d*) is centered between the lateral masses of C₁ (*) and the width of the lateral atlantodental intervals (ADT) (*open arrow*) is symmetrical. The lateral margins of the contiguous articulating facets of the atlas and the axis (the lateral atlantoaxial joints) are symmetrical (*curved arrow*). The bifid spinous process of the axis (*stemmed arrow*) is a midline structure. The transverse processes of the atlas (*solid arrows*) are symmetrical. **(b)** Normal open-mouth projection in which the lucency superimposed upon the dens (*solid arrow*) represents the interdental space between the maxillary central incisor teeth. The inferior, slightly convex, transverse lucency across the base of the dens (*arrowheads*) represents the Mach effect related to the inferior cortex of the posterior arch of C₁ superimposed upon the dens. These common artifacts should not be misinterpreted as fractures of the dens.

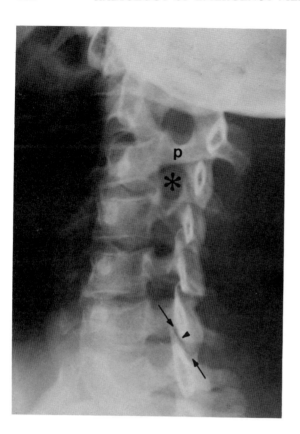

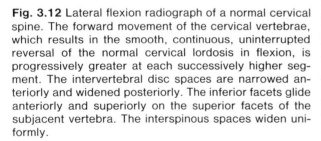

Fig. 3.11 The pedicles (*p*) and intervertebral foramina (*) are radiographically visible only in the oblique projection. This view also demonstrates the posterolateral aspect of the vertebral bodies, the normal relationship of the articular masses, and the anatomy of the interfacetal (facetal, apophyseal, posterior) joints (*stemmed arrows*). Notice that the inferior facet of the vertebra above (*arrowhead*) lies superior and posterior to the superior facet of the subjacent vertebra. In this respect, then, the inferior facet of the vertebra above actually constitutes the superior facet of the interfacetal joint.

Fig. 3.12 Lateral flexion radiograph of a normal cervical spine. The forward movement of the cervical vertebrae, which results in the smooth, continuous, uninterrupted reversal of the normal cervical lordosis in flexion, is progressively greater at each successively higher segment. The intervertebral disc spaces are narrowed anteriorly and widened posteriorly. The inferior facets glide anteriorly and superiorly on the superior facets of the subjacent vertebra. The interspinous spaces widen uniformly.

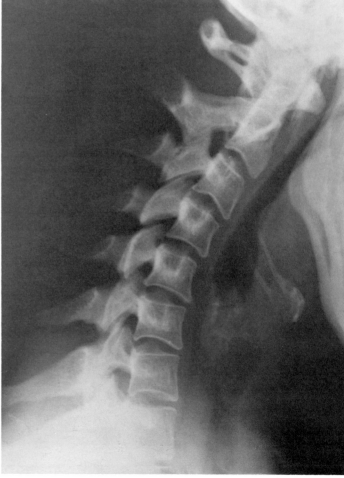

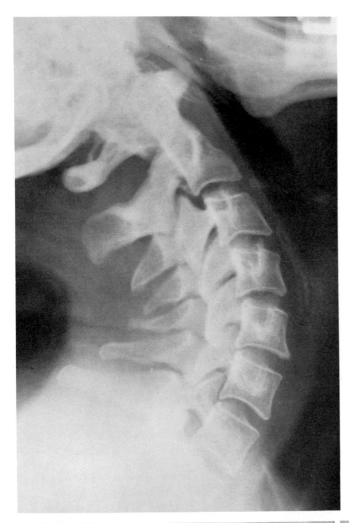

Fig. 3.13 Normal cervical spine seen in lateral hyperextension position. The normal cervical lordotic curve is uniformly and smoothly accentuated in this projection. There is minor widening of the anterior portion of the intervertebral spaces and minor narrowing posteriorly. In hyperextension, the inferior articulating facets glide posteriorly upon the adjacent superior articulating facets and interspinous spaces are narrowed as the result of convergence of the spinous processes from C_2–C_7.

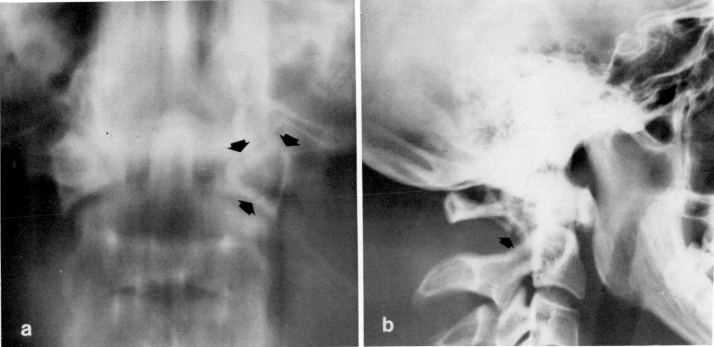

Fig. 3.14 Anteroposterior rectilinear tomogram **(a)** demonstrates a minimally displaced Jefferson bursting fracture and minimally displaced fractures of the left lateral mass of C_1 (*solid arrows*) which were not visible on the plain open-mouth projection. In the lateral radiograph **(b)**, the minimally displaced fractures of the posterior arch of the atlas are indicated by the *arrow*. The soft tissue mass extending from anterior to the body of C_2 to the clivus represents a retropharyngeal hematoma secondary to the atlas fracture.

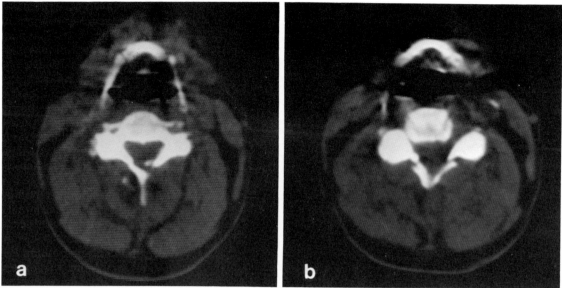

Fig. 3.15 Computed tomograph demonstrating bilateral laminar fractures, with displacement of fragments into the neural canal, which were not visible on plain films of the cervical spine.

area (Fig. 3.17). Obliteration of the lordotic curve is commonly thought to be indicative of muscle spasm and, therefore, a pathologic finding. However, the normal cervical lordosis may be straightened or reversed in 20% of asymptomatic patients in the neutral lateral position, and in 70%, the lordosis will be reversed if the neutral lateral radiograph is made in the "military" or "West Point," i.e., chin-on-the-chest, position (Fig. 3.18) (11). Reversal of the cervical lordosis may also be the result of muscle spasm. The

appearance of the spine is identical in either instance. The distinction rests with the clinical findings relative to the neck.

Alteration of the soft tissue anatomy of the cervical area constitutes a particularly valuable diagnostic clue to the recognition of highly significant, but subtle, musculoskeletal injuries. The prevertebral soft tissue shadow and the interspinous spaces must be studied before directing attention to the vertebral bodies and their appendages.

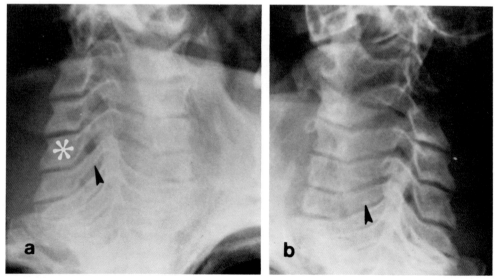

Fig. 3.16 The pillar view (**a, b**) is designed to visualize the articular masses (*) of the lower cervical segments en face. Portions of the laminae (*arrowheads*) may be recorded as well. Notice the normal variation in size and configuration of the articular masses in this patient with no known history of cervical spine trauma.

duces narrowing of the interspace between the lateral masses (vertical approximation) (Fig. 3.19b). The fundamental point here is that the asymmetry of the lateral masses of C_1 with respect to the dens or of the lateral masses of C_1 and C_2 may be normal findings and, in the absence of a history of trauma to the cervical spine, should not be equated with subluxation or dislocation of the atlantoaxial joint.

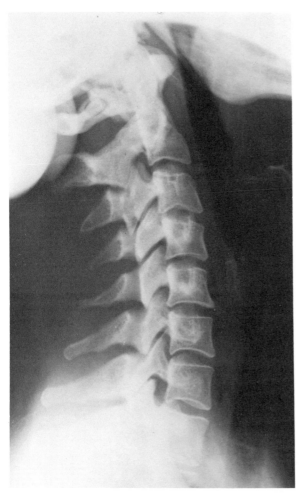

Fig. 3.17 Neutral lateral radiograph of a normal adult cervical spine demonstrating the smooth, normal continuous, cervical lordosis. The criteria of a true lateral projection, i.e., superimposition of the posterior cortex of the paired articular masses and of the interfacetal joint spaces, are clearly evident.

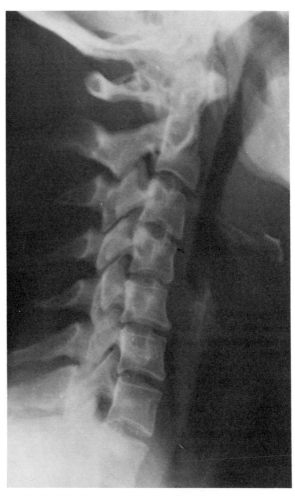

Fig. 3.18 This is the lateral projection of the cervical spine of an entirely asymptomatic patient who was asked to assume the "military" or "West Point" position, in which the chin is tucked sharply upon the neck. Compare the attitude of the angle of the horizontal ramus of the mandible in this illustration with that of Figure 3.17. The attitude of the mandible with respect to the cervical spine, in this illustration, is characteristic of the military position. The assumption of this position is the sole explanation for the reversal of the normal cervical lordotic curve and the concomitant widening of the interspinous spaces. This positional change in the alignment of the cervical vertebrae should not be misinterpreted as an indication of soft tissue damage.

The radiographic appearance of the normal adult cervical spine is seen in Figures 3.9–3.11 and 3.17. Evaluation of the atlantoaxial articulation in the open-mouth projection requires an understanding of the effect of physiologic motion at this level upon the relationship of the atlas and axis.

The atlantoaxial joint permits flexion, extension, rotation, vertical approximation (11), and lateral bending (gliding) (12,13). Both rotation (Fig. 3.19) and lateral bending (lateral tilting of the head with respect to the cervical spine) (Fig. 3.20) physiologically produce asymmetry of the lateral masses of C_1 with respect to the dens as well as asymmetry between articulating surfaces of the lateral masses of C_1 and C_2. Additionally, extreme rotation of C_1 on C_2 pro-

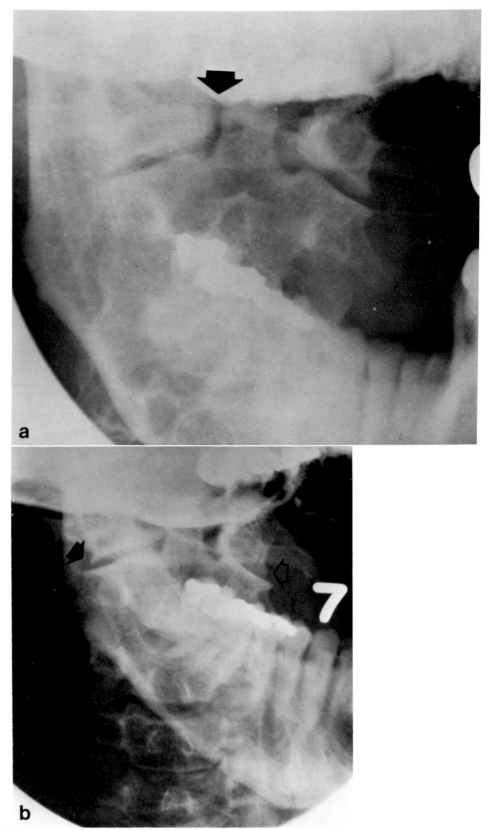

Fig. 3.19 (a) The normal atlantoaxial articulation demonstrating the effect of moderate rotation. The *arrow* indicates the asymmetry between the lateral masses of C_1 and the dens. In addition, note the apparent narrowing of the space between the lateral masses of C_1 and C_2 on the right. This, also, is physiologic and is caused by the anterior movement of the lateral mass of C_1 upon the lateral mass of C_2. In addition, the left lateral mass of C_1, which has rotated posteriorly, assumes a truncated configuration. **(b)** Normal cervical spine with maximum rotation of the head to the left. Note the marked degree of asymmetry of the right lateral mass of C_1 with respect to that of C_2 (*solid arrow*) and the asymmetry of the lateral masses of C_1 with respect to the dens. These relationships are physiologic. On the left side (*open arrow*) the appearance of the lateral masses suggests frank dislocation. In addition, the left lateral mass of C_1 has rotated posteriorly with respect to that of C_2, resulting in obliteration of the joint space. This has been called ''vertical approximation.''

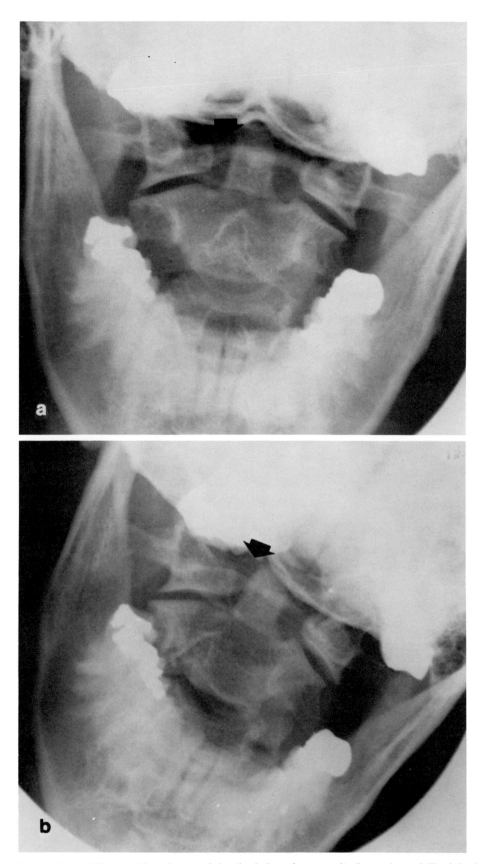

Fig. 3.20 The effect of lateral tilt upon the atlantoaxial articulation. As a result of pure lateral tilt of the head to the left, the atlas moves laterally, causing asymmetry of the articulating masses of C_1 with respect to C_2. Consequently, the dens is eccentrically located with respect to the lateral masses of C_1 and the space between the right lateral mass of C_1 and the dens (the right lateral atlantodental interval, *arrow*) is narrower than on the left **(a)**. With greater lateral tilt, the changes described in **(a)** are accentuated and, in addition, the spinous process of C_2 is displaced to the right of the midline, indicating rotation of C_2 to the left. It is important to realize that all of these changes are the result of a physiologic motion at the atlantoaxial level and that they do not indicate atlantoaxial subluxation or dislocation.

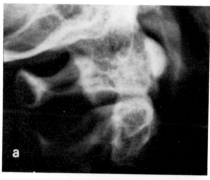

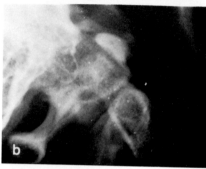

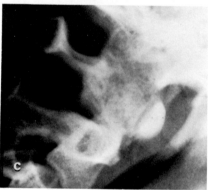

Fig. 3.21 The relationship between the anterior arch of C_1 and the dens of C_2 in the neutral lateral position is seen in **(a)**. Note the close proximity of the contiguous surfaces of the dens and the anterior arch of C_1. In hyperextension **(b)** and hyperflexion **(c)**, the relationship between the dens and the anterior arch of C_1 remains constant. This relationship is maintained by the extremely dense transverse atlantal ligament. Widening of the space between the contiguous surfaces of the dens and the anterior arch of C_1 greater than 3 mm indicates laxity or disruption of the transverse atlantal ligament.

Under normal physiologic conditions, lateral movement of the atlas on the axis of as much as 4 mm is possible. Less severe degrees of atlantoaxial asymmetry are not uncommon, appearing as a normal variant. Rotary scoliosis extending into the cervical spine, muscle spasm, torticollis, and laxity of the ligaments of the atlantoaxial articulation due to rheumatoid arthritis may all produce asymmetry of the lateral masses of C_1 with respect to the odontoid process. This knowledge, in conjunction with the results of extensive evaluation of the C_1–C_2 area in normal subjects, cadaver specimens, and in patients with cervical spine trauma but without fracture or dislocation, has led Hohl and Baker (14) to conclude that "the diagnosis of subluxation of the atlanto-axial joint or injury to the odontoid process cannot be made on the basis of unilateral displacement of the atlas with respect to the axis."

In the lateral projection, the anterior surface of the ring of C_1 is normally in the plane that would correspond to the extension of the smooth curve of the anterior surface of the cervical vertebral bodies projected in a cephalad direction from C_2. Approximately 15° of extension and flexion is possible at the C_1–C_2 level. Through this range of motion, the dens retains a very close relationship to the anterior arch of C_1 (Fig. 3.21). The relationship between the odontoid and the anterior arch of C_1 is maintained by the dense transverse atlantal ligament of C_2 which passes posterior to the dens (Fig. 3.22). Greater than 3 mm of separation of the dens from the anterior arch of C_1 or anterior displacement of the anterior arch of C_1 beyond the plane defined above suggests an abnormality of the transverse atlantal ligament of C_2 (15).

The lateral radiograph of the cervical spine (Fig. 3.23) is of more value in the evaluation of the acute processes of the cervical spine and neck than is the anteroposterior radiograph. The smooth, gentle lordotic curve of the cervical spine is seen in the neutral lateral position. In hyperflexion, the mid and upper cervical segments glide anteriorly upon the next inferior segment, reversing this curve. Normally, the amount of forward movement is progressively greater at each successively higher level, resulting in a smooth, continuous concavity throughout the cervical spine. The inferior articulating facets of the vertebrae glide anteriorly upon the superior articulating facets of the vertebra immediately beneath. Normally, the articulating facets remain in apposition and the apophyseal joints are not disrupted. The space between the spinous processes is slightly and uniformly widened in this projection (Fig. 3.12).

In the lateral radiograph made with the cervical spine extended, the lordotic curve is uniformly and smoothly accentuated, resulting in minor widening of the intervertebral spaces anteriorly and minor narrowing posteriorly. The inferior articulating facets glide

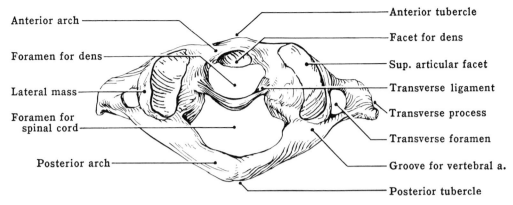

Fig. 3.22 The atlas seen from above demonstrating the relationship of the dens to the anterior arch of C₁ and the relationship of the transverse atlantal ligament to the posterior surface of the dens. (Reprinted with permission from J. E. Anderson (Ed.): *Grant's Atlas of Anatomy*, ed. 6. Williams & Wilkins, Baltimore, 1972.)

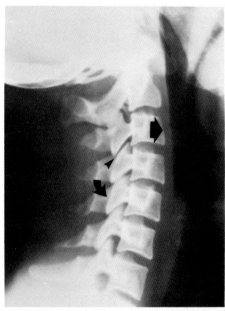

Fig. 3.23 Normal cervical spine in neutral lateral projection. The precise superimposition of the posterior cortical margins of the paired articular masses (*curved arrow*) and of the paired interfacetal joint spaces (*arrowhead*) are the criteria of a true lateral radiograph of the cervical spine. The height of the interspinous spaces is similar from C₂ through C₇. In adults, the width of the prevertebral soft tissue density (*solid arrow*) anterior to the body of C₃ normally should not exceed 4 mm.

posteriorly on the adjacent superior articulating facets and the space between the spinous processes is uniformly narrowed as the spinous processes converge (Fig. 3.13).

The soft tissue density anterior to the body of C₃ is sharply delineated by air in the hypopharynx. Normally, the thickness of these soft tissues rarely exceeds 4 mm in adults (Fig. 3.23). This is a reliable normal finding, and an increase in the width of the soft tissue shadow at this level should be considered abnormal and due to edema, hemorrhage, or abscess until proven otherwise.

The esophagus begins at the level of C₄, and from this level inferiorly the prevertebral soft tissue density is thicker than at the C₃ level. From the level of C₄ inferiorly, the prevertebral soft tissues are demarcated anteriorly by air normally present in the trachea. The thyroid and cricoid cartilages lie anterior to the bodies of C₄ and C₅. These structures can be identified by their irregular calcification (Fig. 3.24). In the frontal radiograph of the cervical spine (Fig. 3.25), the calcified lateral walls of the thyroid cartilage may be seen extending obliquely upward from medial to lateral.

The anterior margin of the hypopharyngeal air shadow represents the base of the tongue. The narrow, anteriorly thickened, horizontally situated bony density superimposed upon the prevertebral soft tissues, extending across the hypopharyngeal air shadow and the base of the tongue, is the hyoid bone. The major ossification centers are present at, or shortly after, birth. The greater cornua and the body may not unite until adulthood, thereby simulating a fracture of the hyoid (Fig. 3.26). Careful evaluation of the characteristics of the adjacent margins of the body and the greater cornua should enable one to distinguish between fracture and un-united ossification centers.

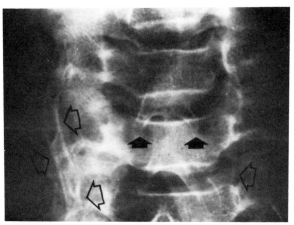

Fig. 3.25 In the frontal projection of the cervical spine, calcification in the lateral and medial surfaces of the walls of the thyroid cartilage may appear as thin, obliquely situated parallel linear calcifications superimposed upon the cervical vertebrae (*open arrows*). These normal densities should not be misinterpreted as foreign bodies. The *solid arrows* indicate a bifid spinous process.

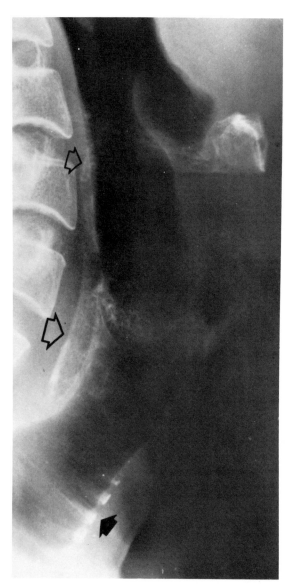

Fig. 3.24 The thyroid and cricoid cartilages can be seen in the routine lateral examination of the cervical spine. However, when the radiographic exposure factors are altered to "soft tissue" technique, these structures are well seen. Calcification in the thyroid cartilage (*open arrows*) is extremely variable both in amount and distribution. The characteristics of the calcifications have no clinical significance. The *solid arrow* represents calcified tracheal cartilage.

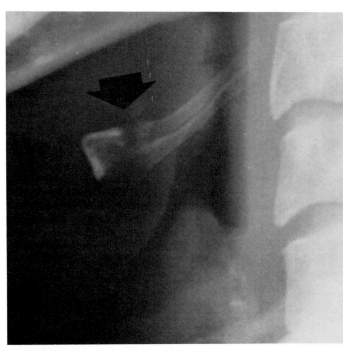

Fig. 3.26 The *arrow* indicates the normal epiphyseal line between the body and the major cornua of the hyoid bone. This structure is visible, normally, until adulthood and may persist as an ununited variant throughout life. The epiphyseal line may be mistaken for a fracture of the hyoid bone.

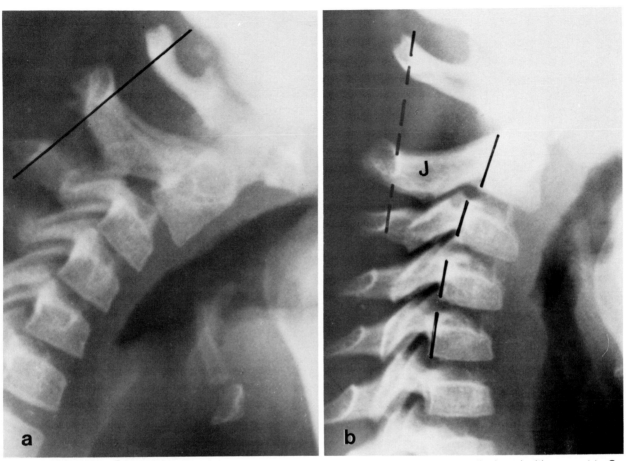

Fig. 3.27 Physiologic pseudosubluxation of C₂. In both **(a)** and **(b)**, the axis is anteriorly displaced with respect to C₃, simulating subluxation or dislocation. The fact that the posterior cortex of the neural arch of C₂ lies on the posterior cervical line (**a**, *solid line*; **b**, *broken line*) indicates that the forward translation of C₂ is physiologic.

In approximately 25% of children to the age of 8 years, the axis is anteriorly displaced with respect to C₃ (16). This relationship is physiologic and is attributed to normal laxity of the ligaments during this age group, the shallow plane of the articular facets at the C₂–C₃ level, and the fact that this level is the transition between the cervicocranium and the lower cervical spine. It has been established that if the posterior cortex of the neural canal of the axis lies on an imaginary line connecting the posterior cortex of the neural canal of C₁ and C₃ (the posterior spinal line), in neutral or flexion lateral radiographs, the anterior displacement of C₂ is physiologic (Fig. 3.27) (17,18). Should the body of C₂ be anteriorly displaced and the posterior cortex of its neural canal be posterior to the posterior spinal line, a bilateral pedicle fracture of the axis may be inferred.

Over 50% of the anterior arch of the atlas lies above the tip of the dens in approximately 20% of patients under the age of 8 years (Fig. 3.28) (16). This is due to the physiologic laxity of the soft tissues of the upper cervical spine at this age. This normal relationship should not be misinterpreted as atlantoaxial dislocation or subluxation.

The space between the posterior surface of the anterior arch of the atlas and the anterior surface of the dens (the anterior atlantodental interval), while remaining constant during flexion and extension in adults, is variable in infants and children. In flexion, the width of this space may physiologically reach 6 mm.

If great care is not taken in positioning the patient and in timing the radiographic exposure for the lateral examination of the neck in infants, the prevertebral soft tissues will buckle, simulating the appearance of a retropharyngeal mass. The pseudomass will disappear if the neck is hyperextended and the exposure timed to coincide with deep, forced inspiration such as occurs during crying (Fig. 3.29).

The end-plate epiphyses become radiographically visible between the 15th and 20th years and fuse to the vertebral bodies at approximately age 25. During

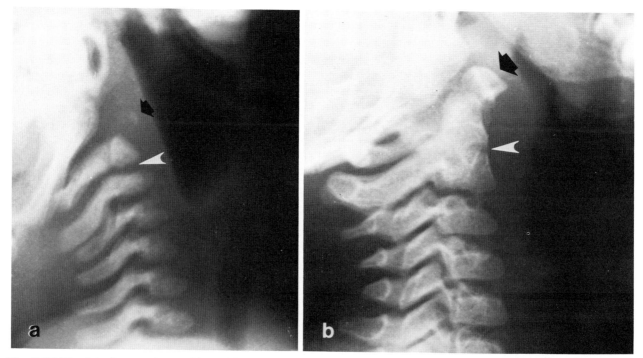

Fig. 3.28 Physiologic superior position of the anterior arch of the atlas (*arrows*) with respect to the tip of the dens in an infant **(a)** and in a child **(b)**. The horizontal radiolucent defect in the anterior portion of the body of the axis (*arrowhead*) represents the partially fused subchondral synchondrosis.

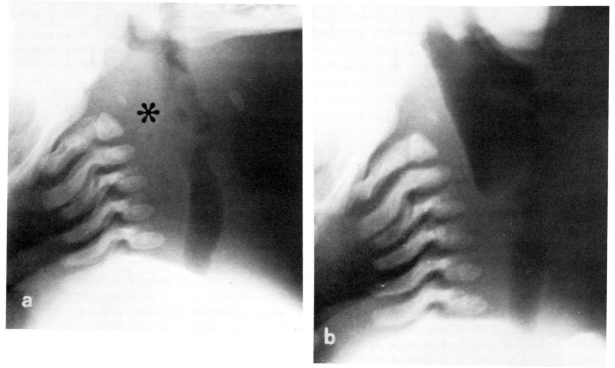

Fig. 3.29 These two lateral roentgenograms of a normal infant's neck were made within minutes of each other. In **(a)**, the exposure was made during expiration. The * indicates buckling of the normally loose mucosal and submucosal soft tissues of the hypopharynx and their simulation of a pharyngeal or retropharyngeal mass. Note that practically no air is seen in the hypopharynx. **(b)** was made with the neck hyperextended and the radiographic exposure timed to coincide with maximum inspiration. The apparent retropharyngeal mass seen in **(a)** has disappeared.

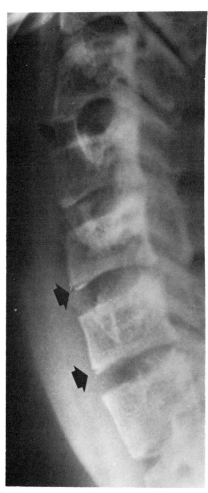

Fig. 3.30 The *arrows* indicate the normally present partially calcified end-plate epiphyses of several of the cervical vertebral bodies. These normal structures are radiographically visible between the 15th and 20th years and fuse by age 25. They should not be interpreted as avulsion fractures.

this interval, the un-united annular epiphyses may resemble avulsion fractures. Knowledge of the presence of these centers, the ages of their appearance and fusion, and the uniform appearance of all of the vertebral bodies identify these as normal structures (Fig. 3.30).

The anteroposterior examination of the cervical spine consists of the open-mouth projection of the atlantoaxial articulation (Fig. 3.10) and the anteroposterior view of the lower cervical segments. The roentgen anatomy of the atlantoaxial articulation and the radiographic appearance of the effects of physiologic motion at this level have been previously described and illustrated (Figs. 3.19 and 3.20).

The frontal projection of the lower cervical spine (Fig. 3.9) demonstrates the vertebral bodies and their end-plates, the joints of Luschka, and the spinous processes, which normally are located in the midline

of the spine. The lateral columns which lie lateral to the lateral margins of the vertebral bodies represent the superimposed articular masses. The smoothly undulating, seemingly continuous lateral margin of the lateral columns represents the lateral cortex of the superimposed articular masses. The interfacetal joint spaces are not visible in the frontal projection because of their oblique orientation to the x-ray beam. The tracheal air column produces a sharply demarcated lucency superimposed upon the midline of the mid and lower cervical vertebrae. The proximal ends of the margins of the air column converge symmetrically into the subglottic area.

The styloid process is a slender, cylindrical spur of bone that arises from the inferior aspect of the temporal bone. It may vary in length from 5 to 50 mm and, in the lateral radiograph of the neck, may be seen extending from the base of the middle cranial fossa toward the hyoid bone. The styloid process arises from two ossification centers which usually fuse by adulthood. These centers may, however, remain permanently ununited, thus simulating a fracture (Fig. 3.31).

The oblique projections (Fig. 3.11) are used to study the pedicles and the relationship of the articulating facets that comprise the apophyseal joints. Fractures of the posterior elements and dislocations of the apophyseal joints are demonstrated to best advantage in this projection.

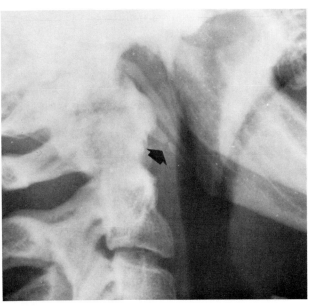

Fig. 3.31 The *arrow* points to a normal variant of the styloid process which, in this instance, arose from two ossification centers. The smooth, sharp density of the contiguous margins of the growth centers distinguish this variant from a fracture.

Radiographic Manifestations of Trauma

An understanding of the mechanisms and the pathophysiology of injury which lead to a classification of cervical spine injuries is essential to the interpretation of the roentgen manifestations of cervical spine trauma. The works of Beatson (19), King (20), Whitley and Forsyth (21), Holdsworth (22), and Fielding and Hawkins (23) provide the genesis for a classification of cervical spine injuries based upon the mechanism of injury (Table 3.1) and the degree of stability of the acute injury (Table 3.2). In order for a classification of cervical spine injuries to be practically useful, it must assume the pragmatic attitude that the injuries are caused by pure forces, i.e., flexion or extension, or by a combination of pure forces, i.e., flexion and rotation or extension and rotation. While such a classification may not be universally accepted, it does achieve validity through practical application and wide acceptance.

Flexion

Flexion injuries are those caused by pure, or dominant, flexion and include anterior subluxation (hyperflexion sprain), bilateral interfacetal dislocation, simple wedge fracture, "clay-shoveler's" fracture, and the flexion tear-drop fracture.

Anterior subluxation (hyperflexion sprain) (22,24) is the pathologic lesion caused by the least amount of flexion force capable of producing an organic lesion, less than 700 psi (25), and consists of disruption of the posterior ligament complex (22). It is a purely soft tissue injury characterized radiographically by an abrupt kyphotic angulation at the level of injury. As a result of anterior rotation or displacement of the involved vertebra, the interspinous space is inappropriately widened ("fanning"), the inferior facets of the involved vertebra move upward and forward with respect to the contiguous facets of the subjacent vertebra, and the disc space is widened posteriorly and narrowed anteriorly. The involved vertebra either rotates anteriorly, pivoting on the anterior-inferior corner of its body, or is displaced slightly anteriorly. The radiographic signs of anterior subluxation are accentuated in the lateral flexion radiograph and are reduced in extension (Figs. 3.32 and 3.33). Anterior subluxation is distinguished from straightening of the cervical lordosis secondary to positioning or muscle spasm by virtue of the localized kyphotic angulation in anterior subluxation and the diffuse straightening, or reversal, of the normal cervical lordosis caused by the military position or muscle spasm (Fig. 3.34).

Anterior subluxation, although innately stable, is associated with 20% delayed stability (Fig. 3.35) (26), an incidence greater than with any other cervical

Table 3.1
Cervical Spine Injuries: Mechanism of Injury

Flexion
1. Anterior subluxation
2. Bilateral interfacetal dislocation
3. Simple wedge fracture
4. Clay shoveler's fracture
5. Tear-drop fracture

Flexion-Rotation
1. Unilateral interfacetal dislocation

Extension-Rotation
1. Pillar fracture

Vertical Compression
1. Bursting fracture
   a. Jefferson of C_1
   b. Lower cervical vertebrae

Extension
1. Hyperextension dislocation
2. Extension tear-drop fracture
3. C_1 posterior neural arch fracture
4. Hangman's fracture
5. Hyperextension fracture-dislocation

Table 3.2
Cervical Spine Injuries: Degree of Stability

Stable
1. Anterior subluxation
2. Unilateral interfacetal dislocation
3. Simple wedge fracture
4. Bursting fracture
5. Fracture posterior arch, C_1
6. Pillar fracture
7. Clay shoveler's fracture

Unstable
1. Hyperextension dislocation
2. Bilateral interfacetal dislocation
3. Flexion tear-drop fracture
4. Extension tear-drop fracture (stable in flexion, unstable in extension)
5. Hangman's fracture
6. Jefferson bursting fracture
7. Hyperextension fracture-dislocation

spine injury. The frequency of delayed instability may be inherent in the healing of ligamentous injuries or may be related to failure to recognize the lesion and/or inappropriate initial treatment.

Bilateral interfacetal dislocation is essentially a pure soft tissue injury caused by hyperflexion. As a result of the severe hyperflexion, the posterior complex, the posterior longitudinal ligament, the intervertebral disc, and the anterior longitudinal ligament are completely torn. The inferior facets of the involved vertebra are dislocated upward and forward and come to lie in the intervertebral foramen anterior to the articular masses of the subjacent vertebra. The involved vertebra is anteriorly displaced a distance greater than

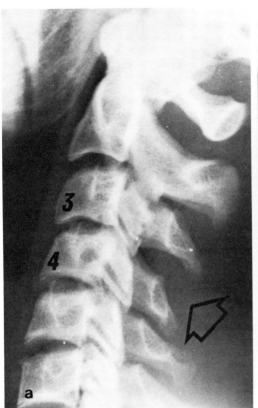

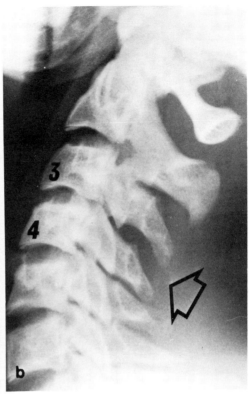

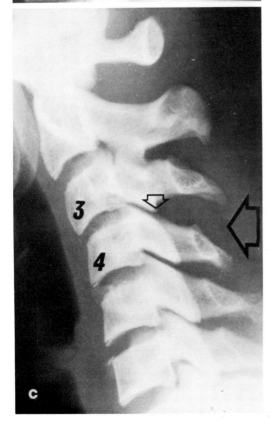

Fig. 3.32 (a) Minor anterior subluxation of C₃ on C₄ seen in the neutral lateral radiograph. The interspinous space (*arrow*) is abnormally widened, indicating a tear of the interspinous ligament at this level. **(b)** In hyperextended lateral position, the subluxation is reduced and the interspinous space appears normal. **(c)** In hyperflexion, the subluxation is exaggerated, the interfacetal joints become asymmetrical, and the interspinous space widened posteriorly.

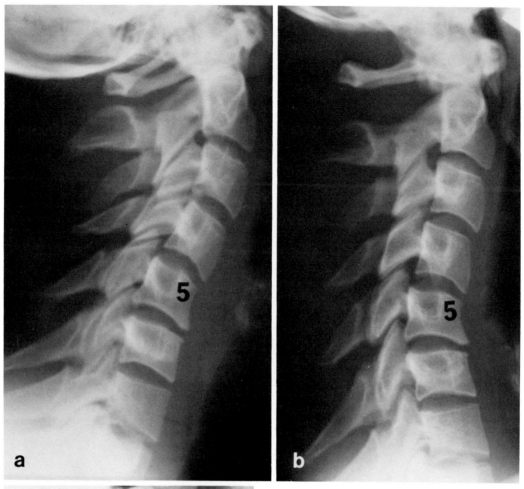

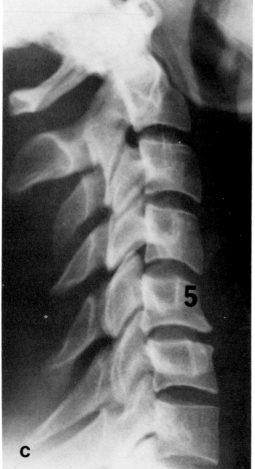

Fig. 3.33 Anterior subluxation of C_5 on C_6. In the neutral lateral projection **(a)**, there is an abrupt hyperkyphotic angulation of the cervical spine at the level of C_5. The interspinous space is widened, the inferior facets of C_5 are displaced upward and forward with respect to the superior facets of C_6, and the disc space is widened posteriorly and narrowed anteriorly. These changes are accentuated in flexion **(b)** and reduced in extension **(c)**.

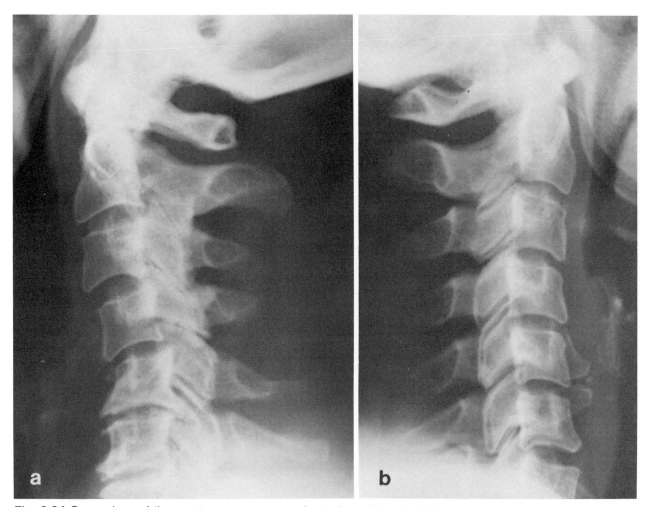

Fig. 3.34 Comparison of the roentgen appearance of anterior subluxation **(a)** with reversal of the cervical lordosis caused by the military position **(b)**. In **(a)**, anterior subluxation of C_4 on C_5 is indicated by an acute kyphotic angulation limited to the C_4–C_5 level, forward displacement of C_4 on C_5, anterior narrowing and posterior widening of the fourth disc space, upward and forward displacement of the inferior facets of C_4 on the superior facets of C_5, and widening of the fourth interspinous space. In contradistinction, the military position **(b)** has resulted in a smooth, continuous reversal of the cervical lordosis throughout the entire cervical region.

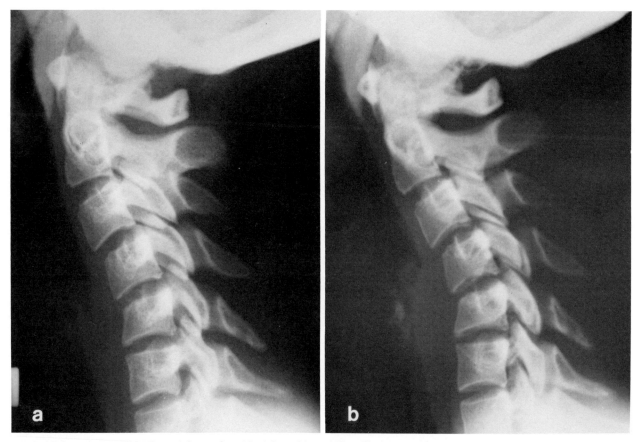

Fig. 3.35 Anterior subluxation of C₄ on C₅ with delayed instability. The neutral lateral radiograph obtained at the time of injury **(a)** demonstrates the roentgen signs of anterior subluxation of C₄ on C₅. The neutral lateral radiograph made 3 months later **(b)** reveals a greater degree of subluxation than was present on the initial examination.

50% of the anteroposterior diameter of a vertebral body. A tiny avulsion fracture fragment characteristically arises from one of the involved articular facets. The fragment may be seen radiographically and is invariably seen at the time of surgery or autopsy. The tiny fragment has little clinical significance relative to the extensive soft tissue injury (27). Because of the complete loss of ligamentous and skeletal integrity at the level of bilateral interfacetal dislocation, this lesion is initially unstable.

The simple wedge fracture (Fig. 3.36) is caused by mechanical compression of one vertebra between adjacent vertebrae during flexion. The simple wedge fracture is characterized by anterior loss of stature of the involved vertebral body and, usually, disruption of the anterior cortex, in lateral projection. In the anteroposterior radiograph, the involved vertebral body appears intact. This fracture is stable because the ligaments remain intact and the normal relationship of the interfacetal joints is maintained.

Clay-shoveler's fracture (Fig. 3.37) is an avulsion injury involving the spinous process of C₇, T₁, or C₆,

in that order of frequency. The fracture involves the spinous process itself, and the fracture line has a characteristic slightly obliquely horizontal orientation and location in the proximal portion of the spinous process. The fracture results from abrupt flexion of the head and neck against the tensed soft tissues of the posterior aspect of the neck. This fracture is stable.

The flexion tear-drop fracture (Fig. 3.38) is the most devastating of all cervical injuries. As described by Schneider and associates (28), the flexion tear-drop fracture is actually a fracture-dislocation of one of the cervical vertebrae caused by a massive flexion injury of the cervical spine. The injury is, by definition, associated with the acute anterior cervical cord syndrome of instant, complete quadriplegia and loss of pain, touch, and temperature sensations, but with retention of posterior column sensations of position, motion, and vibration. The cord damge is secondary to the severe hyperkyphotic angulation at the level of fracture-dislocation. Pathophysiologically, the lesion is characterized by complete disruption of all the soft tissues at the level of injury, including the posterior ligament complex, the posterior longitudinal ligament, the intervertebral disc, and the anterior longitudinal ligament, by subluxation or dislocation of the interfacetal joints, and by a typical fracture of the anterior-inferior corner of the involved vertebral body. Radiographically, the lesion derives its name from the characteristic triangle shaped, displaced fragment involving the anterior-inferior corner of the vertebral body. Other signs include the flexed attitude of the involved vertebra and those above it, acute kyphosis at the level of injury, prevertebral soft tissue swelling, and, posteriorly, signs of disruption of the posterior ligament complex (Fig. 3.38).

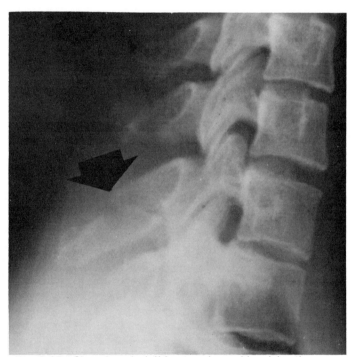

Fig. 3.37 ''Clay-shoveler's'' fracture (*arrow*) involving the spinous process of C$_7$.

Flexion-Rotation

Unilateral interfacetal dislocation (UID) (''locked'' vertebra) is the injury produced by simultaneous flexion and rotation. The dislocation occurs on the side opposite the direction of the rotation and consists of anterior dislocation of one articular mass (inferior facet) with respect to the contiguous subjacent articular mass. In the process, the posterior ligament complex is disrupted. The dislocated articular mass comes to rest in the intervertebral foramen, anterior to the subjacent articular mass. In this position, the dislocated articular mass is mechanically wedged in the

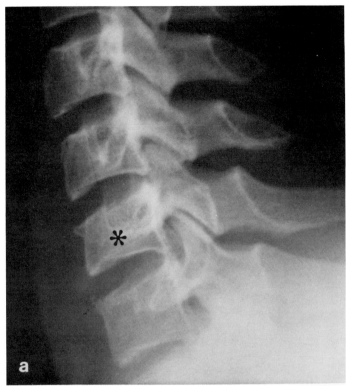

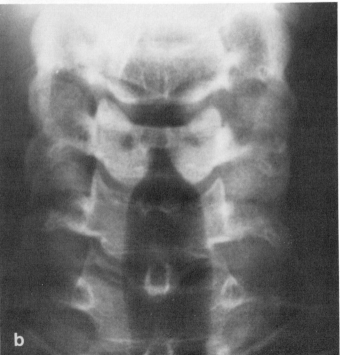

Fig. 3.36 Simple wedge fracture. In the lateral projection **(a)**, there is anterior loss of stature and disruption of the anterior cortex of the involved vertebral body (*). In the frontal projection **(b)**, the involved vertebral body appears intact and the fracture is not recognizable.

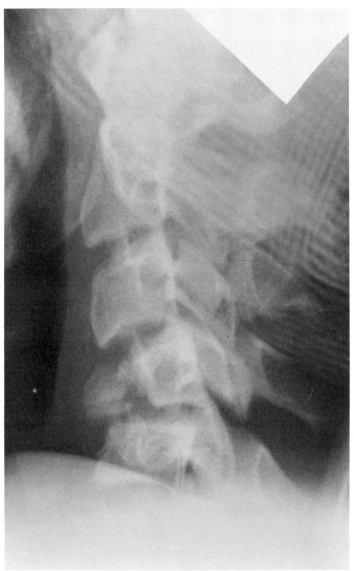

Fig. 3.38 Flexion tear-drop fracture.

foramen, hence the name "locked" vertebra. Therefore, UID is a stable lesion.

The roentgen signs of UID are the changes secondary to the rotation and flexion at and above the level of dislocation. In the anteroposterior radiograph the spinous processes at and above the level of dislocation are displaced from the midline to the side of the dislocation (the side opposite the direction of rotation). The lateral margin of the lateral column, on the same side, will appear disrupted at the level of dislocation (Fig. 3.39).

In the lateral projection the dislocated vertebra is anteriorly displaced with respect to the subjacent vertebra a distance less than one-half the anteroposterior diameter of a vertebral body. The rotational component of the injury is evidenced by the asymmetry of the articular masses at and above the dislocation. The posterior cortical margins of the articular masses on the side of the dislocation lie anterior to those on the opposite side. The interfacetal joint spaces on the side of dislocation become superimposed on the vertebral bodies and consequently, may be, difficult to identify. At the level of the dislocation, the dislocated articular mass is usually identifiable lying anterior to its contiguous subjacent articular mass. On the opposite side, the inferior facet of the articular mass is subluxed with respect to its contiguous facet; i.e., the inferior facet of the nondislocated articular mass is displaced upward and forward with respect to its contiguous facet, but it remains above and behind the facet below in the typical attitude seen in anterior subluxation.

Oblique projections are necessary to identify the side of the dislocation (Fig. 3.40a). On the opposite oblique view, the nondislocated articular mass will be in the subluxed, or "perched," attitude (Fig. 3.40b). If the positioning for the oblique projections does not display the interfacetal joints, the relationship of the laminae, seen end-on, accurately reflects the relationship of the articular masses and the facetal joints.

While UID is, by definition, a soft tissue injury, as with dislocations involving other joints, a small fracture may involve either component of the dislocated joint.

Fig. 3.39 Unilateral interfacetal dislocation of C_6 on C_7. In the frontal projection **(a)**, the spinous processes from C_6 upward are displaced to the left (*arrows*). Spina bifida occulta of C_7 and T_1 is an incidental finding. In the lateral radiograph **(b)**, C_6 is anteriorly displaced with respect to C_7. While the facetal dislocation cannot be specifically identified on this projection, the rotational component is evident by virtue of the lack of superimposition of the posterior cortices of the articular masses (*arrowheads*) above the level of dislocation. The left anterior oblique projection **(c)** demonstrates the anterior dislocation of the left lateral mass of C_6(*) with respect to that of C_7. The inferior articulating facet of C_6 (*arrowhead*) should normally lie above and behind the superior facet of C_7 (*open arrow*). In the right anterior oblique projection **(d)**, the articular mass (and lamina)(*) is subluxed with respect to the articular mass of C_7.

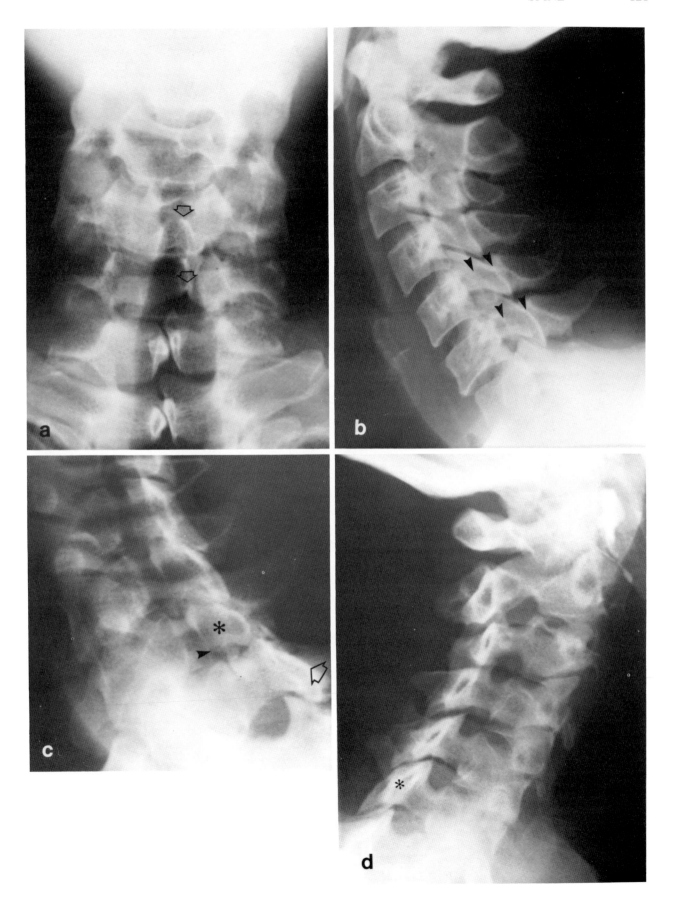

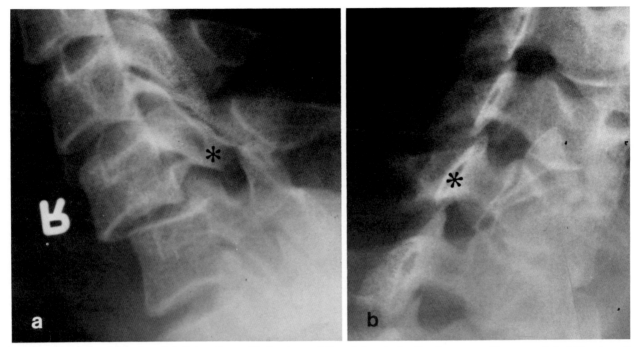

Fig. 3.40 Unilateral interfacetal dislocation with fracture of the dislocated articular mass. The amputated (fractured) mass (*) is dislocated into the intervertebral foramen anterior to the subjacent articular mass **(a)**. In the opposite oblique **(b)**, the subluxed articular mass (*) is "perched" upon the subjacent articular mass.

Extension-Rotation

Combined extension and rotation is the causative mechanism of the pillar fracture (10,11). The force is dissipated on a lower cervical articular mass on the side of the rotation. Radiographically (Fig. 3.41), the lateral margin of the lateral column is disrupted at the level of the fracture and a curvilinear lucent defect, which represents either the mass fracture or an interfacetal joint made visible by virtue of rotation of the mass fragments, is visible in the frontal projection. In the lateral radiograph, posterior displacement of the posterior mass fragment produces lack of superimposition of the posterior cortical margins of the articular masses only at the level of the mass fracture. This finding has been called the "double outline" sign (10). Oblique and pillar views are required to confirm the fracture. Rectilinear tomography may delineate the fracture more clearly. The diagnosis of an acute pillar fracture requires the demonstration of a fracture line in the involved articular mass. Simple asymmetry or variations in stature of articular masses is *not* sufficient evidence to warrant the diagnosis of an acute pillar fracture. Because the pillar fracture is limited to the articular mass, this lesion is considered stable.

Vertical Compression (Axial Loading)

Vertical compression injuries of the cervical spine are those resulting from a force delivered to the top of the skull at the precise instant that the cervical spine is straightened. This mechanism of injury is responsible for the "Jefferson bursting" fracture of the atlas and, in the lower cervical spine, the "burst" fracture.

The Jefferson bursting fracture (29,30) consists, by definition, of bilateral fractures of both the anterior and the posterior arch of the atlas. Radiographically (Fig. 3.42), the Jefferson fracture is characterized by bilateral lateral displacement of the articular masses of C_1. In the lateral projection (Fig. 3.43), the most striking roentgen sign is usually prevertebral soft tissue swelling which extends from anterior to the body of C_2 to the clivus.

In the lower cervical spine, vertical compression (axial loading) force produces the burst ("bursting," "compression," "dispersion") fracture. The pathophysiology of this fracture, as described by Roaf (31), begins with the intervertebral disc. The compressive force transmitted to the lower cervical spine is initially dissipated in the intervertebral disc, resulting in bulging of its annulus fibrosis. As the force persists and

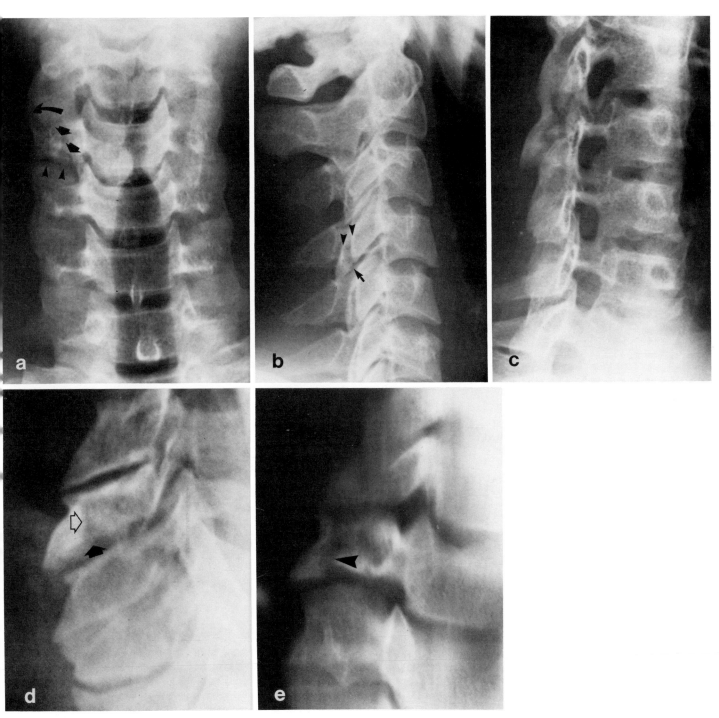

Fig. 3.41 Pillar fracture. In the frontal projection **(a)**, the lateral margin of the lateral column is disrupted (*curved arrow*), fracture lines (*solid arrows*) and the anterior margin of an interfacetal joint (*arrowheads*) are visible. The "double outline" sign (*arrowheads*)—inappropriate lack of superimposition of the posterior cortices of the articular masses at the level of the fracture—and a defect in the inferior facet of the involved pillar (*stemmed arrow*) are seen in the lateral radiograph **(b)**. The fracture line is clearly evident in the oblique projection **(c)**. In the pillar view **(d)**, the inferior facet is disrupted (*solid arrow*) and a fracture line is suggested (*open arrow*). Rectilinear tomography **(e)** confirms the presence of the pillar fracture (*arrowhead*).

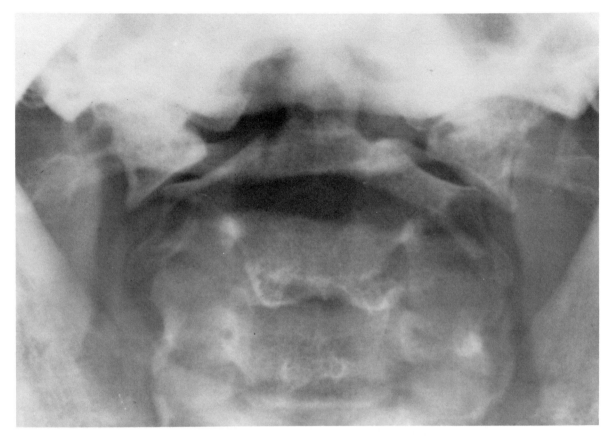

Fig. 3.42 The radiographic appearance of a "Jefferson bursting" fracture of C_1. Note that the lateral masses of C_1 are displaced laterally with respect to the superior articulating surface of the lateral masses of C_2. This degree of lateral displacement of the articular masses of the atlas is highly suggestive of disruption of the transverse atlantal ligament.

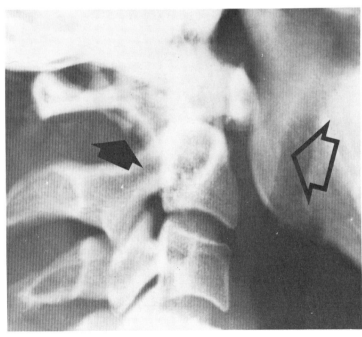

the annulus resists rupture, the liquid nucleus pulposus is forced through the inferior end-plate of the immediately superiorly adjacent vertebral body. Herniation of the nucleus pulposus causes an abrupt increase in pressure within the centrum of the body, which in turn is dissipated by exploding the vertebral body from within outward, resulting in the comminuted dispersion fracture which characterizes this injury. The posterior fragment of the vertebral body impinges upon or penetrates the ventral surface of the cord to varying degrees. Consequently, the presenting neurologic signs may vary from minor transient paresthesia (Fig. 3.44) to complete quadriplegia (Fig. 3.45). While some authorities consider the burst fracture to be simply a minor variant of the anterior teardrop fracture (25,32), most consider it to be a distinct entity because of the variability of cord involvement and the attitude of the cervical spine radiographically.

Fig. 3.43 Jefferson bursting fracture, lateral projection. The *solid arrow* indicates the minimally displaced posterior arch fractures. The prevertebral soft tissue swelling is indicated by the *open arrow*.

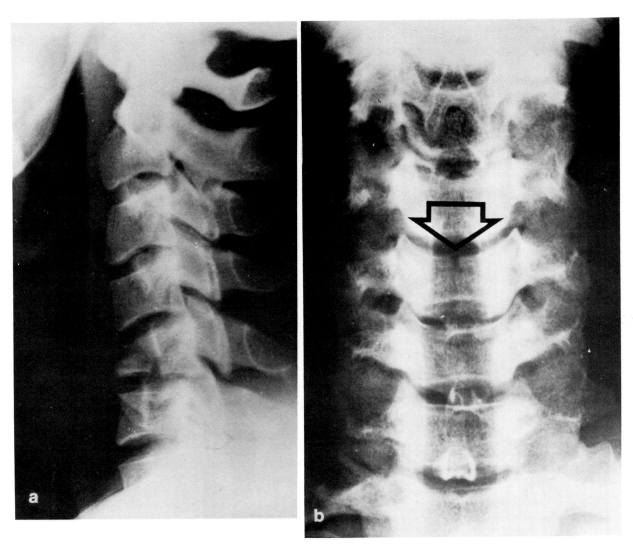

Fig. 3.44 "Burst" (bursting, compression, dispersion) fracture of C₅. In the lateral projection **(a)**, the cervical spine is straight. The comminuted fracture, with extension of a fracture line through the inferior end-plate and posterior displacement of the posterior fragment, is typical of this injury. The vertical fracture line in the center of the vertebral body (*open arrow*) is the characteristic roentgen sign of the "burst" fracture in frontal projection **(b)**. This patient experienced only temporary upper extremity paresthesias.

The characteristic appearance of the burst fracture is seen in Figure 3.44. A vertical fracture line extending through the midportion of the vertebral body, seen on the anteroposterior projection, distinguishes the burst fracture from the simple wedge fracture. In the lateral projection, the cervical spine is essentially straight. The involved vertebral body is comminuted and one of the fracture lines involves the inferior end-plate. The posterior inferior fragment is posteriorly displaced a variable distance. The posterior elements remain intact. For this reason, and because the annulus of the disc and the anterior longitudinal ligament are intact, the burst fracture is generally considered to be stable.

Hyperextension Injuries

The hyperextension dislocation is caused by a straight, posteriorly directed force striking the face or mandible, causing abrupt hyperextension of the head and cervical spine. The anterior longitudinal ligament is torn as the dislocated vertebra and those above it are displaced posteriorly. In addition, either there is a complete horizontal tear of the intervertebral disc or the inferior end-plate of the dislocated vertebra is separated from the disc. In either event, the posterior dislocation of the involved vertebra results in stripping of the posterior longitudinal ligament from the posterior cortex of the subjacent vertebra and acute an-

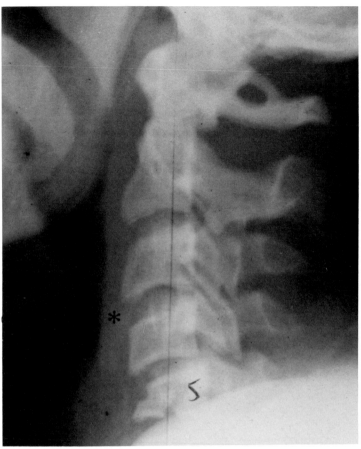

Fig. 3.45 Burst fracture of C₅ in a young man who became a quadriplegic at the instant of impact. Note that the attitude of the cervical spine is straight, the body of C₅ is comminuted and a fracture line extends through its inferior end-plate, and the posterior fragment is posteriorly displaced. The prevertebral soft tissue shadow (*) is abnormally widened secondary to hemorrhage and edema.

terior angulation of the spine. Consequently, the cervical cord is pinched between the posteriorly dislocated vertebral body and the anterior angulation of the lamina and the ligamentum flava. The neurologic signs range from transient paresthesia to complete quadriplegia, depending upon the degree of cord injury. As the causative force ceases, the head and dislocated vertebrae usually return to the normal anatomic position. This sequence of events has led to the description of the "quadriplegic patient with normal appearing cervical spine" (33,34). This misconception has been perpetuated in current literature (32,35).

Radiographically, hyperextension dislocation is characterized by essentially normal alignment of the cervical vertebrae and *diffuse prevertebral soft tissue*

swelling (Fig. 3.46). The latter sign, which represents hemorrhage and edema secondary to ligamentous disruption, and which is invariably present, should stimulate a high index of suspicion regarding a hyperextension dislocation. Rarely, a vacuum defect may be present within the torn intervertebral disc, or a thin, flat fracture fragment avulsed from the inferior end-plate may be present in the anterior aspect of the superior portion of the disc space.

Fracture of the posterior arch of the atlas (Fig. 3.47) is caused by compression of the posterior arch between the heavy occipital bone and spinous process of the axis. This fracture is stable.

The hyperextension tear-drop fracture (Fig. 3.48) is an avulsion fracture at the site of attachment of the anterior longitudinal ligament on the anterior inferior corner of the body of the axis. The separate fragment is characteristically triangular. This fracture occurs principally in association with osteoporosis and osteoarthritis of the cervical spine. It is considered unstable in extension because, in effect, the anterior longitudinal ligament is disrupted though stable in flexion, since the posterior elements and the posterior ligament complex are intact.

The hangman's fracture (traumatic spondylolisthesis) is a bilateral pedicle fracture limited, by definition, to the axis. It derives its name from its morphological similarity to the skeletal injuries associated with judicial hanging. The most common cause of hangman's fracture today is a high speed automobile accident involving abrupt deceleration in which the head and upper cervical vertebrae (cervicocranium) are thrown or forced into hyperextension, producing the bilateral pedicle fracture. When the force is expended, the head and cervicocranium assume an anterior position with respect to the lower cervical segments. Radiographically, the hangman's fracture (Fig. 3.49) is characterized by disruption of the pedicles and forward displacement of the cervicocranium with respect to the lower segments. While the cord may be severely damaged by this injury, the incidence and magnitude of cord injury is surprisingly low, because the anteroposterior diameter of the spinal canal is greatest at the axis and the bilateral pedicle fractures produce an "auto-decompression" of the cord. Prevertebral soft tissue swelling is common and may impede the hypopharyngeal airway (Fig. 3.50).

Hyperextension fracture-dislocation is caused by a continuous circular force impacting on the chin or low on the face and driving the head and neck into maximum extension. As the force continues in a circular fashion, it is dissipated upon the articular masses, resulting in severely comminuted fractures or, if there is a rotational component, interfacetal dislocation on one side. Because the skeletal integrity of the articular masses is disrupted by fracture or dislo-

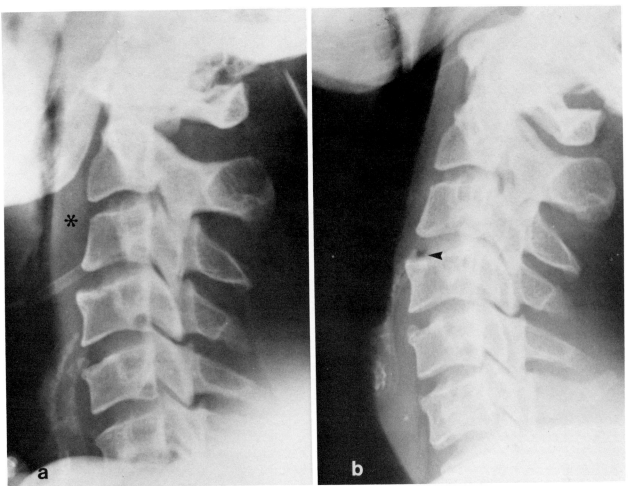

Fig. 3.46 Hyperextension dislocation. This injury has also been inaccurately described as ''the syndrome of paraplegia with normal appearing cervical spine.'' In the immediate postinjury, horizontal beam lateral radiograph **(a)**, although the vertebrae are intact and normally aligned, the prevertebral soft tissue shadow, from C_5 to the clivas, is distinctly abnormally thickened and ill defined, reflective of soft tissue hemorrhage and edema secondary to disruption of the anterior longitudinal ligament and the involved intervertebral disc. This finding, in a patient with cervical cord neurologic deficits and an injury to the face or forehead, is characteristic of hyperextension dislocation. In the radiograph obtained 7 days postinjury **(b)**, the prevertebral soft tissue swelling is obviously diminished and the ''vacuum'' defect (*arrowhead*) in the third interspace indicates the level of the dislocation.

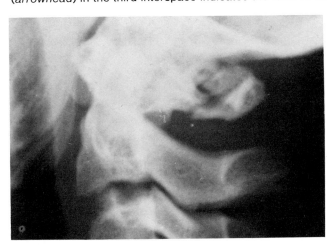

Fig. 3.47 Fracture of the posterior arch of the atlas.

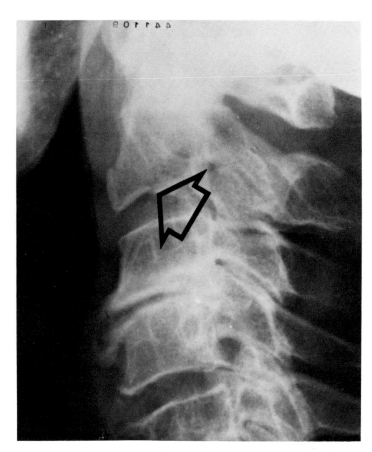

Fig. 3.48 Extension tear-drop fracture (*arrow*). This fracture, by definition, involves the anterior inferior corner of C_2. The triangular shape of the separate fragment, osteoporosis, and degenerative arthritis are all characteristic of this injury.

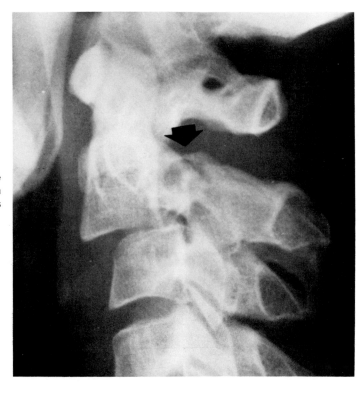

Fig. 3.49 Hangman's fracture. The arrow indicates the pedicle fractures. The axis and the entire cervicocranium are displaced *anteriorly*, even though the hangman's fracture is a hyperextension injury.

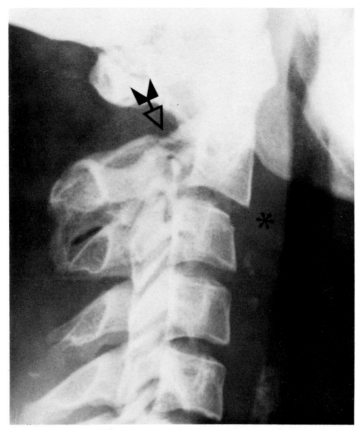

Fig. 3.50 Diffuse prevertebral soft tissue swelling (*) secondary to a hangman's fracture. The *arrow* indicates the pedicle fractures.

cation, the involved vertebra is displaced *anteriorly* by the continuous, circular hyperextension force. It is critically important to recognize the roentgen signs of an extension injury in order that inappropriate immobilization or management not be instituted.

The roentgen signs of hyperextension dislocation are illustrated in Figure 3.51. Because the skeletal injury involves the posterior elements, fracture lines or the cortical margins of rotated pillar fragments disrupt the lateral column and its lateral margin in the frontal projection. In lateral view, the intact body of the involved vertebra is *anteriorly* displaced and prevertebral soft tissue swelling is evident. The normal anatomy of the articular masses and the interfacetal joints is disorganized as a result of the skeletal injuries. Oblique and pillar views and tomography are all indispensable and identify the location and extent of the fracture, confirm the site of dislocation when present, and demonstrate fractures not demonstrated on plain radiographs.

Fracture of the dens may involve the tip (type I), the base (type II), or the superior portion of the body

of the atlas (type III). This lesion is not common, is difficult to diagnose, and carries a high incidence of fatality due to compression of the medulla. The most common site is at the junction of the base of the dens with the body of C$_2$ (Fig. 3.52). Obtaining adequate radiographic visualization of the dens is difficult because of superimposition of the maxillary incisor teeth or the occipital bone. A satisfactory radiograph is even more difficult to obtain when the patient has a fractured dens, has considerable discomfort or paralysis, and will not permit any motion of the head or the cervical spine. In lateral projection, the dens may be obscured by the lateral masses and transverse processes of C$_1$ and C$_2$ and, unless the fragments are displaced, the fracture line is likely to be missed. Prevertebral soft tissue swelling is always present. Laminographs of the C$_1$-C$_2$ area are of great assistance in visualizing the dens and the fracture line.

The dens ossifies from two major centers and from a secondary center at the tip. Failure of the major centers to unite with the body of the axis results in the dens constituting a separate "loose body" called the

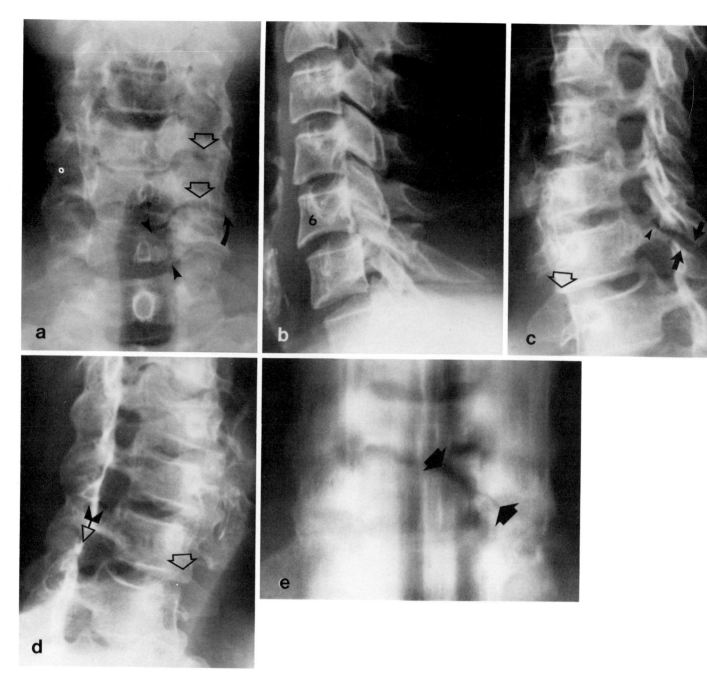

Fig. 3.51 Hyperextension fracture-dislocation of C_6 on C_7. In the frontal projection **(a)**, an oblique fracture is present in the left lamina of C_6 (*arrowheads*). The anterior margins of the left fifth and sixth interfacetal joints are visible (*open arrows*) and the lateral margin of the lateral column is disrupted (*curved arrow*). In the lateral radiograph **(b)**, the intact body of C_6 is anteriorly displaced. The anatomy of the posterior elements from C_5 through C_7 is disorganized. The lateral masses of C_6 and the adjacent facetal joints are distorted. Displaced fractures are present in the laminae and base of the spinous process of C_6. In the left **(c)** and right **(d)** anterior oblique projections, the fracture of the lateral mass (*stemmed arrows*) and forward displacement of C_6 (*open arrow*), and the partial dislocation (perched) of C_6 on C_7 (*winged arrow*) are evident, respectively. Rectilinear tomography **(e)** confirms the comminuted fracture involving the left larmina, articular mass, and pedicle of C_6 (*arrows*).

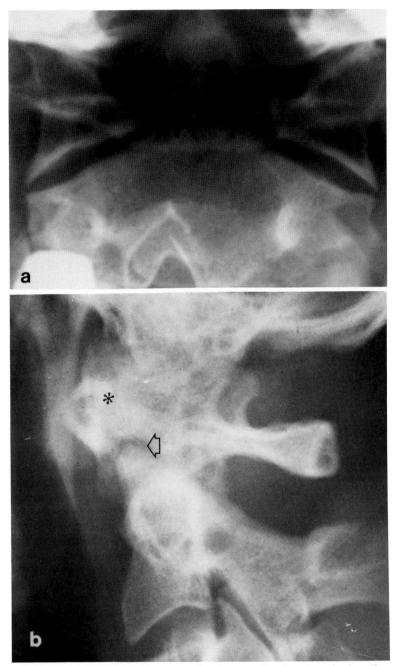

Fig. 3.52 Minimally displaced type II fracture of the dens. The fracture line involves the junction of the base of the dens and the body of the axis (*arrows*). The inferiorly convex density traversing the body of the axis (*arrowheads*) is the inferior margin of the posterior arch of the atlas and should not be mistaken for a fracture.

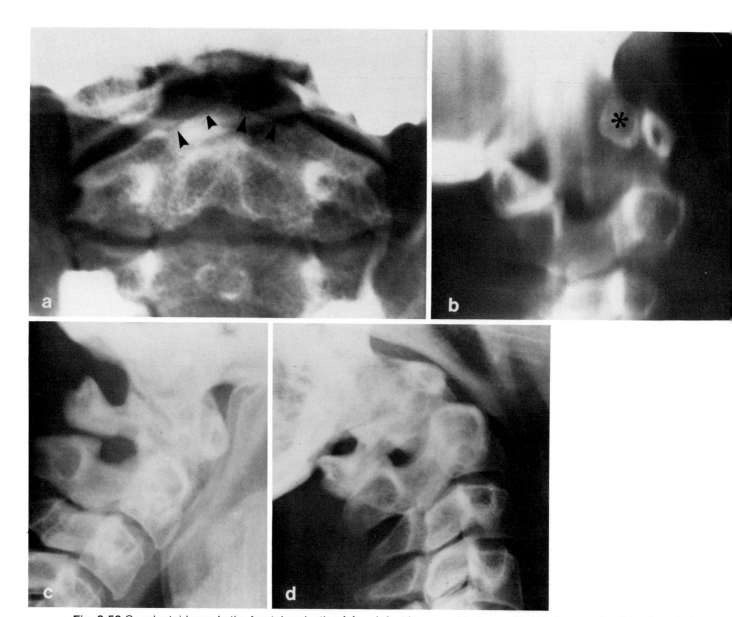

Fig. 3.53 Os odentoideum. In the frontal projection **(a)**, a defect is present between the inferior margin of the dens and the superior convex superior surface of the body of the axis (*arrowheads*). Lateral tomograms **(b)** confirm the presence of the rudimentary separate dens (*) posterior to the anterior arch of the atlas. Lateral flexion **(c)** and extension **(d)** radiographs delineate the range of abnormal motion of the os odentoideum and the atlas with respect to the body of the axis.

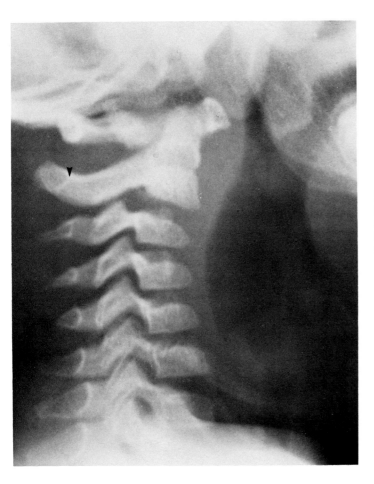

Fig. 3.54 Physiologic dislocation of C_2. In this neutral lateral radiograph of a child *without* history of cervical spine trauma, the posterior cortex of the neural canal of C_2 (*arrowhead*) lies posterior to the spinolaminar line (see also Fig. 3.27).

os odentoideum (Fig. 3.53). While the os odentoideum has traditionally been considered a developmental variant, Fielding et al. (36) have described the dens as a separate body following nonunion of a type II dens fracture. The clinical significance of this lesion rests in the abnormal range of motion (instability) between the os odentoideum and atlas and the body of the axis which constitutes a potential hazard to the upper cervical cord. The congenital, or acquired, os odentoideum can be distinguished from an acute type II dens fracture by the smooth, dense sclerotic margins of the contiguous surfaces of the os odentoideum and the axis and absence of prevertebral soft tissue swelling.

Physiologic anterior displacement of the axis on C_3 occurs in approximately 25% of children to the age of 8 years. Swischuk (17) has demonstrated that the posterior cortex of the neural canal of C_2 normally lies posterior to the posterior spinal line in neutral (Fig. 3.54) lateral radiograph and lies on or 1-2 mm anterior to the posterior spinal line in flexion. The posterior spinal line is an imaginary line extending from the posterior cortex of the spinal canal of C_1 to C_3.

Atlanto-occipital dislocation, which may be anterior (Fig. 3.55) or posterior (Fig. 3.56) and atlantoaxial

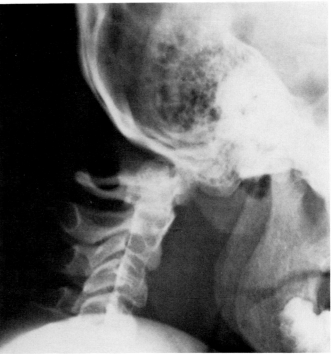

Fig. 3.55 Anterior atlanto-occipital dislocation.

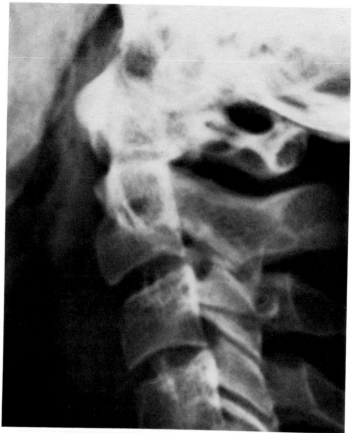

Fig. 3.56 Posterior atlanto-occipital dislocation.

rotatory dislocation, in which the atlas is rotated approximately 90° on the axis, are incompatible with life because of the associated cord damage.

Direct trauma to the larynx may result in fracture of the thyroid cartilage. If the cartilage is sufficiently calcified, the fracture line may be radiographically discernible. Laryngeal fracture is commonly associated with air in the soft tissues of the neck (Fig. 3.57).

Differential Diagnosis

Cervical Spine

Torticollis ("wry neck") is clinically manifest by lateral tilt and rotation of the head. Both lateral tilt and rotation are physiologic motions at the atlantoaxial articulation. The roentgen appearance of the atlantoaxial articulation in torticollis (Fig. 3.58), then, reflects the physiologic changes in the atlantoaxial relationship attributable to rotation and lateral tilt. In rotation, the articular mass of the atlas on the side opposite the direction of rotation moves anteriorly and assumes an oblique or eccentric attitude toward the central x-ray beam. Consequently, this articular

mass is increased in transverse diameter and the space between the mass and the dens is diminished. Contrarily, the opposite lateral mass moves posteriorly during rotation of the head and assumes a truncated configuration. The atlantodental interval on this side (the side of the direction of rotation) is either unchanged or is increased in width. Depending upon the magnitude of rotation, the lateral margins of the contiguous facets of the atlas and axis may not be superimposed. In lateral tilt, the atlas glides laterally with respect to the axis in the direction of the tilt. Consequently, the articular masses of the atlas are eccentric with respect to the dens so that the space between the mass and the dens is wider on the side in the direction of the tilt and narrower on the opposite side. The lateral margins of the inferior facets of the atlas are displaced in the direction of the tilt with respect to the contiguous superior facets of the axis. This asymmetry of the articular facets has been described as "unilateral" or "bilateral offset," and the alteration of the normal atlantoaxial relationship secondary to physiologic rotation and lateral tilt has been described as "rotational subluxation" and "physiologic dislocation" (37, 38). These terms, which connote a pathologic process, are misleading since neither

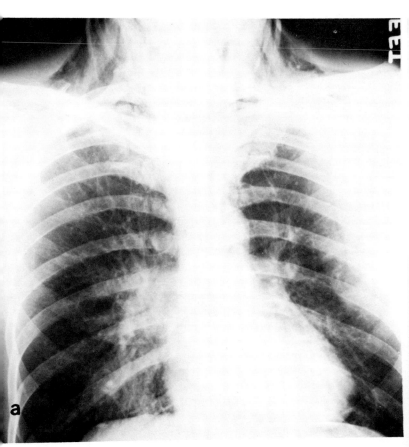

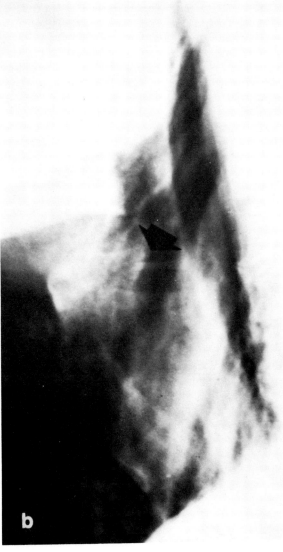

Fig. 3.57 (a) Fracture of the larynx with extensive subcutaneous emphysema of the neck. In the lateral radiograph of the neck **(b)**, the *arrow* indicates a concomitant fracture of the hyoid bone.

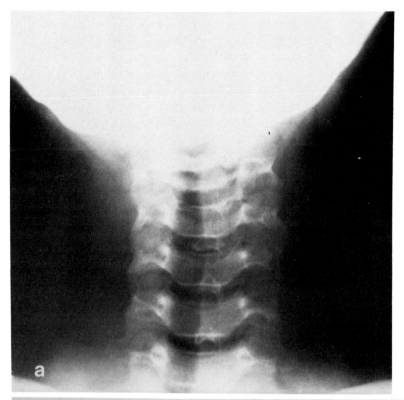

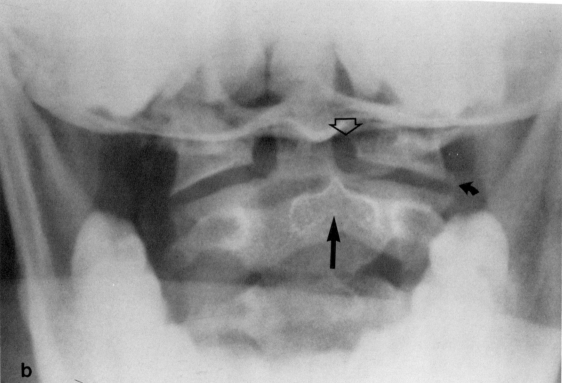

Fig. 3.58 Torticollis ("wry-neck"). The rotation and lateral tilt of the head to the right, with respect to the cervical spine, is obvious in the anteroposterior radiograph of the cervical spine **(a)**. The roentgen signs of atlantoaxial rotary displacement are evident in the open-mouth projection **(b)**. These include an increase in the transverse diameter of the left lateral mass of C_1, a decrease in the width of the left lateral atlantodental interval (*open arrow*), asymmetry of the lateral margins of the lateral atlantoaxial joints (*curved arrow*), and displacement of the spinous process of C_2 to the left (*stemmed arrow*).

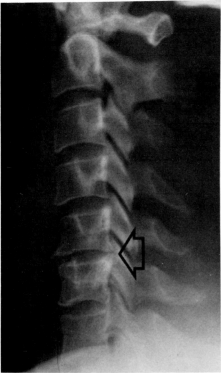

Fig. 3.59 Degenerative arthritis involving a single level of the cervical spine.

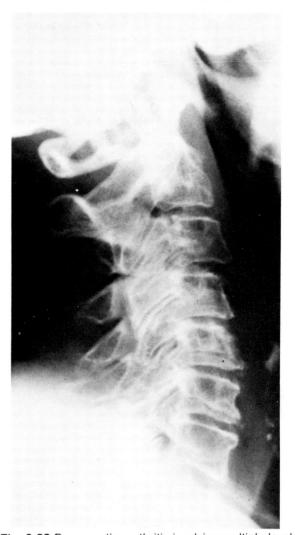

Fig. 3.60 Degenerative arthritis involving multiple levels of the cervical spine.

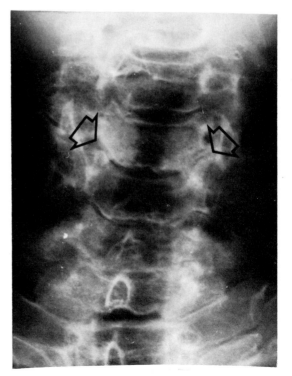

subluxation nor dislocation exists. "Atlantoaxial rotary displacement," advocated by Fielding and Hawkins (23), accurately describes the roentgen appearance of the atlantoaxial articulation in torticollis. In addition to the changes described above which occur during rotation and lateral tilt, the axis also *rotates* during, and in the direction of, lateral tilt. This is manifest radiographically by displacement of the bifid spinous process of the axis off the midline to the side opposite the direction of the tilt.

Degenerative arthritis may be localized to a single level of the cervical spine (Fig. 3.59) or may involve the entire cervical area (Fig. 3.60). Degenerative changes of the Luschka joints are seen in the frontal projection (Fig. 3.61). Narrowed intervertebral spaces, anterior and posteriorly projecting osteophytes, and degenerative changes of the interfacetal joints are best seen in lateral projection. Pain in the neck, shoulder, or upper extremity may be caused by cervical root compression secondary to osteophytic encroachment upon the intervertebral foramina. Oblique projections of the cervical spine are necessary to evaluate this cause of root pain (Fig. 3.62).

Primary or secondary malignant disease may involve the spine and may be the cause of symptoms

Fig. 3.61 Osteoarthritic changes of the Luschka joints consisting of narrowing of the joint spaces and the formation of reactive sclerosis and osteophyte formation.

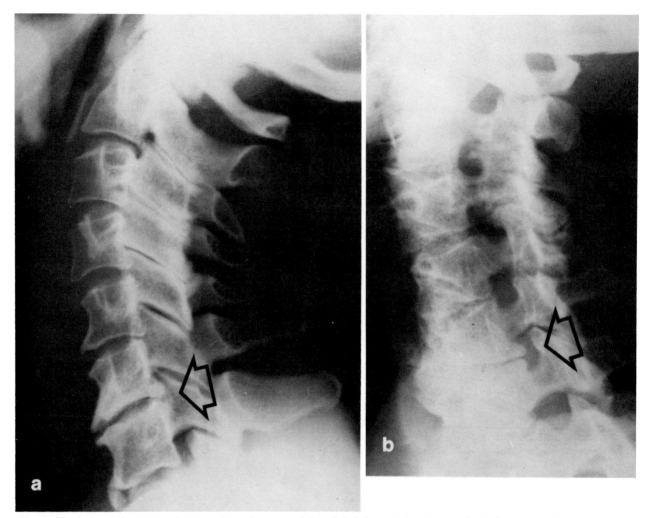

Fig. 3.62 Moderately severe degenerative changes of the sixth intervertebral space including narrowing of the space with sclerosis of its contiguous surfaces and anterior and posterior (*open arrow*) osteophytes **(a)**. In the oblique projection **(b)**, bony encroachment upon the left sixth intervertebral foramen (*open arrow*), which impinged upon the cervical root, is clearly evident.

referable to the particular area of involvement. Metastasis is more frequent than primary neoplasia and may be either osteolytic (Fig. 3.63) or osteoblastic. Pathologic fractures may occur (Fig. 3.64).

Increase in width of prevertebral soft tissue shadow may be caused by a retropharyngeal abscess (Fig. 3.65) or the presence of opaque (Fig. 3.66) or nonopaque (Fig. 3.67) foreign bodies in the prevertebral soft tissues.

THORACOLUMBAR SPINE

Radiographic Examination

The thoracic and lumbar portions of the spine are similar in many regards and it is therefore convenient to consider them together.

Routine radiographs of the thoracic spine consist of anteroposterior and lateral projections. The anteroposterior view is seen in Figure 3.68. While this projection is designed primarily to visualize the thoracic spine and adjacent soft tissues, it may also include portions of the shoulder girdles and the rib cage. Displaced rib fractures will usually be recorded on this projection, but nondisplaced or incomplete fractures in that arc of the ribs between the anterior and posterior axillary lines may not be demonstrated. Therefore, if rib fracture is suspected, either clinically or radiographically, oblique projections of the rib cage must be obtained.

It is very important to realize that the upper thoracic vertebrae cannot be visualized in routine lateral projections because of the superimposition of the shoulders (Fig. 3.69). Adequate radiographic evaluation of

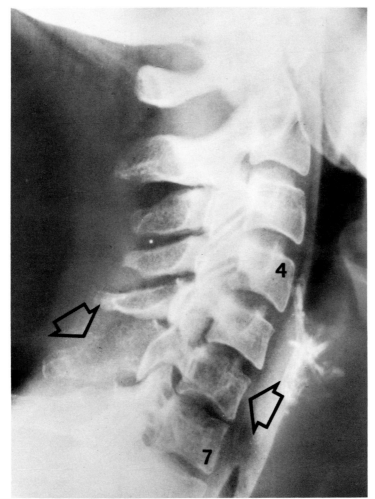

Fig. 3.63 Osteolytic metastatic disease of the cervical spine.

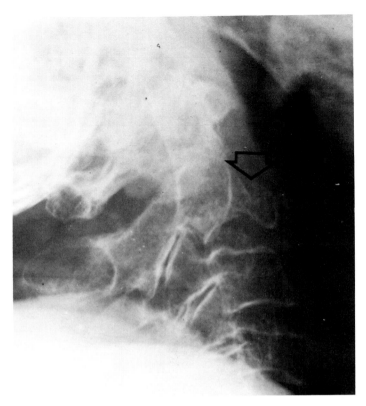

Fig. 3.64 Pathologic fractures caused by metastatic disease (*arrow*).

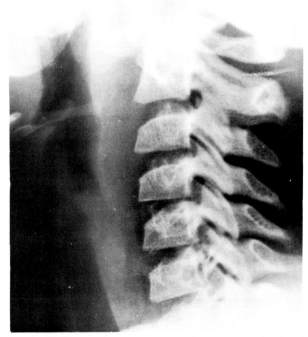

Fig. 3.65 Diffuse increase in width of prevertebral soft tissue swelling due to a retropharyngeal abscess.

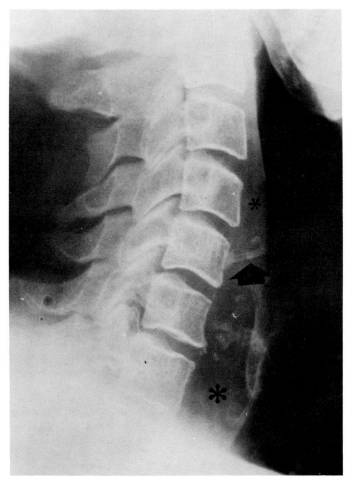

Fig. 3.66 Prevertebral soft tissue swelling (*) is secondary to the opaque foreign body (*arrow*).

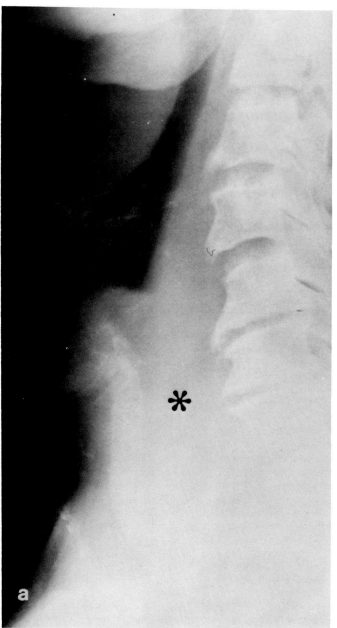

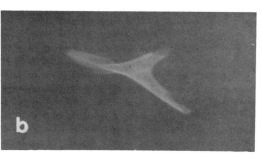

Fig. 3.67 (a) Marked prevertebral soft tissue swelling (*) is caused by a chicken bone lodged in the posterior wall of the cervical esophagus. (b) Radiograph of the extracted chicken bone which was completely obscured by the soft tissue density.

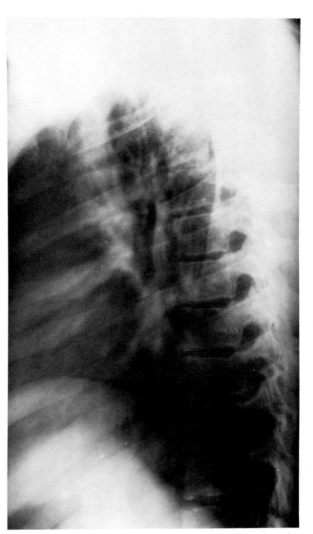

Fig. 3.69 Lateral radiograph of the normal thoracic spine. Note that the upper thoracic segments are obscured by the superimposed density of the shoulders.

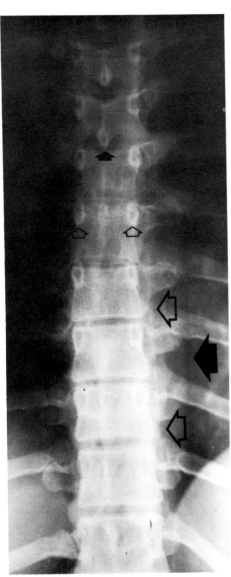

Fig. 3.68 Anteroposterior radiograph of the normal thoracic spine. The *small open arrows* indicate the pedicles and the *small solid arrow* a spinous process. The *large open arrows* indicate the paraspinous soft tissue shadow ("mediastinal stripe"), which is caused by the mediastinal pleural reflection of the left lung. The shadow of the lateral margin of the descending thoracic aorta can be seen extending obliquely downward lateral to the paraspinous stripe (*large solid arrow*).

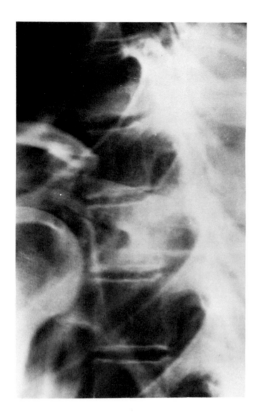

these segments of the spinal column requires the use of the Fletcher view, which is made with the patient obliqued from the true lateral position so that one shoulder lies anterior and the other posterior to the spine (Fig. 3.70). Therefore, the attending physician must indicate that the upper thoracic segments are to be examined radiographically in order that the appropriate view may be obtained initially.

The sensory distribution of the anterior primary divisions of the thoracic nerves is useful in clinically localizing the level of thoracic spine injury and, consequently, that area of the thoracic spine which requires critical roentgen evaluation. Thus, it is helpful to remember that the third, fourth, fifth, and sixth thoracic nerves supply the thoracic wall with the fourth dermatome coinciding with the nipple line. The lower seven supply the lower thoracic cage and the abdominal wall, with the 10th thoracic dermatome coinciding with the level of the umbilicus and the 11th with the inguinal area. The first and second thoracic nerves are distributed chiefly to the upper extremity, the axilla, and the axillary border of the scapula.

Fig. 3.70 Fletcher projection made with the patient in a slight degree of obliquity from the lateral position. Because the shoulders are now located anterior and posterior to the spine, the lower cervical and upper thoracic vertebral bodies are visible.

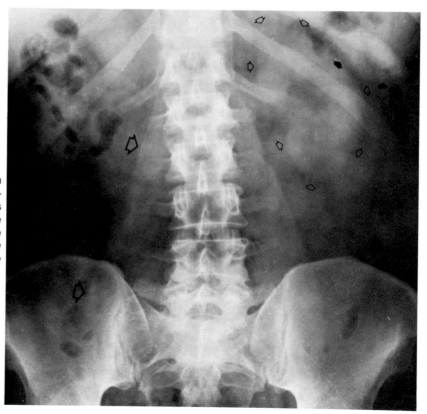

Fig. 3.71 Anteroposterior radiograph of a normal lumbar spine. This examination should include the lower ribs bilaterally as well as portions of the pelvis. The *small solid arrows* indicate the tip of the spleen; *the small open arrows*, the left kidney; and the *large arrows*, the psoas muscle.

fracture of the lumbar transverse processes. The resultant retroperitoneal hematoma obscures the soft tissue plane of the psoas shadow, thereby rendering it radiographically unidentifiable.

The lower thoracic segments must be included in the lateral radiograph of the lumbar spine (Fig. 3.72) for the same reasons discussed in reference to the frontal examination.

In positioning the patient for the routine lateral roentgenogram of the lumbar spine, the central x-ray beam is centered over the L_2-L_3 level. Because of the peripheral divergence of the x-ray beam, the lumbosacral space is depicted as being narrowed on this examination. For this reason, a special, coned down lateral "spot" projection has been devised in which the x-ray beam is centered between the surfaces of the lumbosacral space. When this study is properly executed, the width of the lumbosacral space may be accurately assessed (Fig. 3.73).

Positioning the patient for the lateral spot radiograph of the lumbosacral space requires the patient to be placed in the lateral position with the side against the table built up with sponges to assure that the lumbar spine is parallel to the table top. Thus, it is apparent that this amount of patient motion is contraindicated for a patient with an acute traumatic history and suspected lumbar fracture. It is therefore extremely important, and it is the responsibility of the referring physician, to indicate precisely the basis for and the type of radiographic examination desired of the lumbar spine.

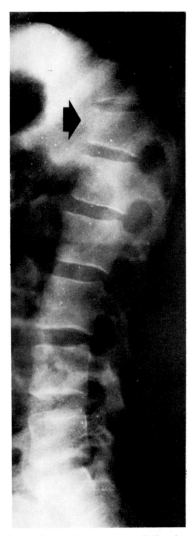

Fig. 3.72 Lateral roentgenogram of the lumbar spine. The lower thoracic segments must be included in this projection. Note the fracture of T_{12} (*arrow*). The lumbosacral intervertebral space is not well depicted in this view because of the divergence of the x-ray beam.

The anteroposterior examination of the lumbar spine should include the lower thoracic vertebrae, the lower ribs, and portions of the pelvis (Fig. 3.71). Because abnormalities of the lower thoracic spine, ribs, or pelvis may be obscured by signs and symptoms of lumbar pathology, those portions of these areas recorded in the frontal projection of the lumbar spine must be examined with particular care. Further, it is not sufficient to limit the study of this radiograph to the skeletal parts. In a properly positioned and exposed roentgenogram, the hepatic, splenic, renal, and psoas shadows will usually be visible to some degree. These must be evaluated, particularly in patients who have sustained trauma. Absence of the psoas shadow may be the most apparent finding in instances of

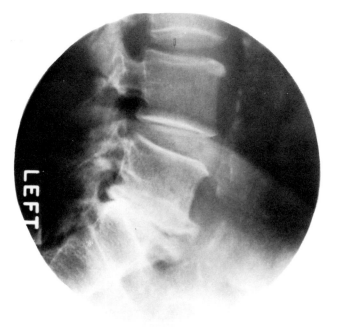

Fig. 3.73 Lateral "spot" radiograph of the lumbosacral space, which is involved with severe degenerative disease.

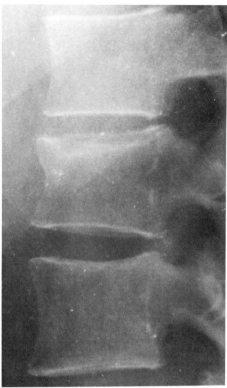

Fig. 3.74 Acute compression fracture of L₁. The superior end-plate is impacted into the centrum and the superior aspect of the anterior margin of the body is buckled. The vertebral body is "wedged" anteriorly in the characteristic configuration of a compression fracture.

To summarize, anteroposterior and lateral radiographs of the lumbar spine and pelvis are initially the only projections required to evaluate this area in a patient with an acute traumatic history. Under these circumstances, the lateral examination must be made using a horizontal beam with the patient supine in order to prevent unnecessary movement of the patient.

In the absence of a history of acute trauma, the routine radiographic study of the lumbosacral spine and pelvis should include the anteroposterior view of the lumbar spine and pelvis, a lateral radiograph of the lumbar spine, and the lateral spot projection of the lumbosacral space. Oblique views may be indicated for evaluation of the posterior elements, as determined from information obtained on the routine study or from clinical data.

Radiographic Anatomy

The thoracic spine consists of 12 vertebral segments. Normally, paired ribs articulate with each thoracic segment. Anomalously, the 12th pair of ribs may be hypoplastic or absent.

The paraspinous soft tissue shadow, which is present to the left of the thoracic column (Fig. 3.68), represents the mediastinal pleural reflection of the left lung and is commonly referred to as the "mediastinal stripe." Distortion of this normal soft tissue shadow is frequently the most obvious radiographic sign of early or subtle pathologic processes involving the vertebra or intervertebral disc.

The lumbar spine consists of the five vertebrae located between the 12th thoracic and 1st sacral segments. Because of the frequency of anomalies at the lumbosacral segments, and especially if the 12th ribs are absent, it may be difficult to specifically enumerate the lumbar segments. However, the transverse processes of L₄ are usually canted slightly in a cephalad direction in distinction to those of the remainder of the lumbar spine (Fig. 3.71). When this characteristic is present, it serves as a useful landmark in identifying the lumbar segments.

Radiographic Manifestations of Trauma

Compression fracture is the commonest traumatic lesion of the thoracic and lumbar spine. This injury is caused by acute flexion of the spine such as occurs in a fall from a height or by a heavy weight striking the shoulders. Depending upon the magnitude of the flexion force, the fracture may consist simply of buckling of the superior plate (Fig. 3.74), anterior wedging (Fig. 3.75), or loss of stature (Fig. 3.76) of a vertebral body. The mechanism of this injury, and its relationship to those patients who sustain calcaneal fractures in a fall from a height, is very important in the total evaluation of these patients. Frequently, the calcaneal fracture will produce such morbidity that the patient may not be conscious of back pain due to an associated thoracolumbar fracture. Under these conditions, the spine must be specifically evaluated clinically. If there is the least suspicion of spinal injury, radiographic examination of the appropriate level of the spine is mandatory.

Comminuted fracture (Fig. 3.77) of the thoracolumbar spine is much less common than the simple compression fracture. It is usually caused by a severe abrupt flexion force which drives one vertebral body or its adjacent intervertebral disc into the superior plate of the next lower body. Any degree of comminution may occur. Posterior fragments may be driven posteriorly, producing cord compression or injury. The intervertebral disc is always injured with this fracture and there is a high incidence of ligamentous injury about the apophyseal joints and the posterior elements. Pedicle fracture may occur.

The Chance fracture (39) typically involves an upper lumbar vertebra. It is the result of a shearing, flexion injury which produces an obliquely horizontal

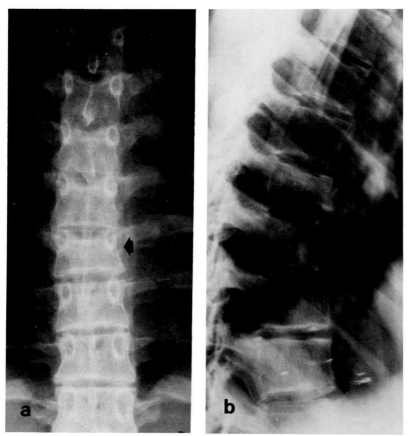

Fig. 3.75 This teenage patient sustained an acute compression fracture of one of the midthoracic vertebral bodies, with loss of stature and anterior wedging of the involved vertebral body (*solid arrow*). In the lateral projection **(b)**, the *open arrows* indicate ununited end-plate epiphyses. These should not be misinterpreted as avulsion fractures. In the frontal projection **(a)**, note the soft tissue density to the left of the involved thoracic segment. This mass represents the hematoma associated with the vertebral body fracture and is a reliable sign associated with primary osseous pathology.

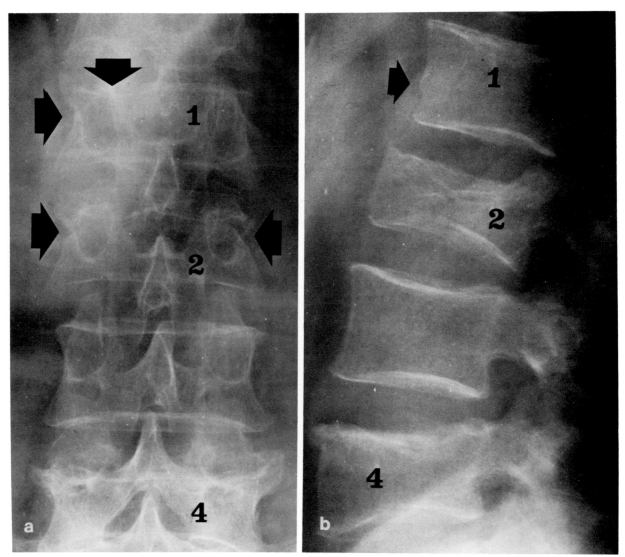

Fig. 3.76 (a, b) Acute compression fractures involve the bodies of L₁ and L₂. An old healed fracture involves the superior plate of the body of the fourth lumbar segment. Compare the radiographic characteristics. Note the absence of sclerosis of the fractures in the first and second segments in both frontal and lateral projections. The fracture lines are sharply defined and there is 50% loss of stature of the body of L₂.

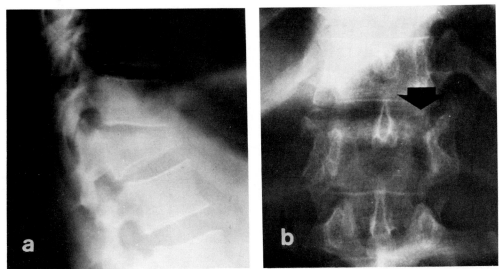

Fig. 3.77 Severely comminuted fracture of the body of L_1. The fragments are distracted and the body of T_{12} has been driven into the body of L_1. Note the posterior displacement of the posterior fragments with respect to the bodies of both T_{12} and L_2 (**a**). In the frontal projection (**b**), the *arrow* indicates a vertical fracture line through the left lateral portion of the vertebral body and separation of these fragments.

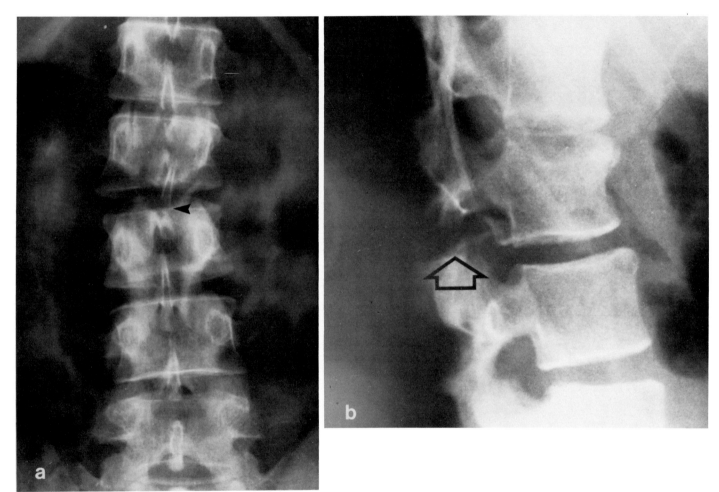

Fig. 3.78 Chance fracture of L₂. In the anteroposterior projection **(a)**, there is a scoliosis of the lumbar spine to the right. In the upper lumbar spine, the second vertebral body is eccentrically diminished in stature and the spinous process of L₂ is disrupted and angulated to the right (*arrowhead*). In lateral projection **(b)**, the horizontal fracture through the posterior elements is indicated by the *open arrow*. The body of L₂ is diminished in stature and wedged anteriorly, reflecting extension of the fracture through the vertebral body.

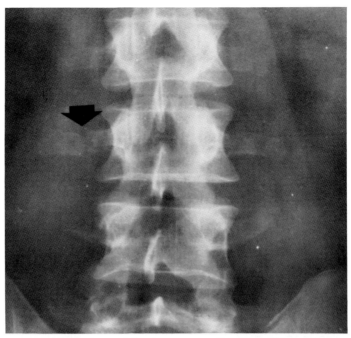

Fig. 3.79 The *arrow* indicates a vertically situated fracture across the base of the right transverse process of the third lumbar segment.

fracture of the spinous process, the pedicles, and the vertebral body. This lesion is typically associated with neurologic damage. The roentgen signs of a Chance fracture (Fig. 3.78) include loss of stature of the involved vertebral body, rotation of the segments at the level of injury, and either a fracture line or angulation of the spinous process of the involved segment in the frontal projection. In lateral projection, a horizontal fracture extends from the spinous process through the pedicles into the vertebral body.

Fracture-dislocation of the thoracolumbar spine is uncommon and is the result of a combination of flexion and rotary forces. The dislocation may be due either to displacement of one or both apophyseal joints or to fracture of the articular surfaces of these joints. In either event, there is marked ligamentous damage and injury to the disc and to the posterior longitudinal ligament. This type of injury is unstable and is frequently associated with either cord or nerve root involvement.

Fractures of the lumbar transverse processes occur frequently and are commonly overlooked radiographically. These fractures may be vertically situated across the base of the transverse process (Fig. 3.79) or they may consist simply of avulsion of the tip of the process (Fig. 3.80). The fragments may be slightly or markedly displaced. Because the psoas muscle arises in part from the lumbar transverse processes, the hematoma associated with transverse process fractures diffuses into the fascial plane adjacent to the muscle, thereby obliterating its radiographic identification (Fig. 3.81). The loss of this normal soft tissue finding may be the most prominent radiographic sign of lumbar transverse process fracture.

Nontraumatic Lesions

The radiographic study of the lumbosacral spine in patients suspected of acute herniation of the lumbosacral nucleus pulposus may be entirely negative or the involved space may be narrowed. With acute herniation, the contiguous surfaces of the space are usually devoid of degenerative changes. Muscle spasm may result in straightening of the normal lumbar lordotic curve.

Osteomyelitis of the vertebrae occurs infrequently. Gram-negative bacilli are the usual causative agents. Access to the vertebral column may occur via the vertebral veins of Batson, for example, following urinary tract instrumentation. These low virulence organisms produce narrowing of the disc space and destruction of the contiguous surfaces of the space without evoking reactive new bone formation. These changes are seen to best advantage in the lateral radiograph (Fig. 3.82).

In the frontal projection of the thoracic spine, the inflammatory process may produce a localized bulge of the paraspinous soft tissue shadow (the mediastinal

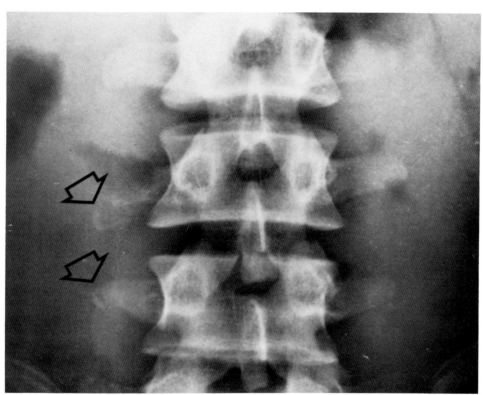

Fig. 3.80 Minimally displaced avulsion fracture of the tip of lumbar transverse processes.

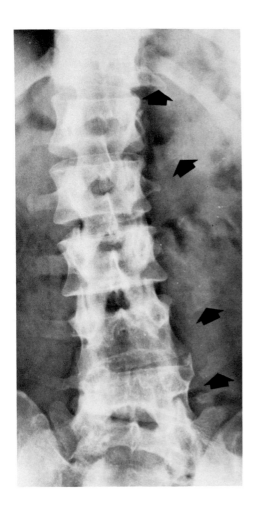

Fig. 3.81 The *arrows* indicate complete, displaced fractures of several lumbar transverse processes. The resultant retroperitoneal hematoma has caused obliteration of the psoas muscle shadow.

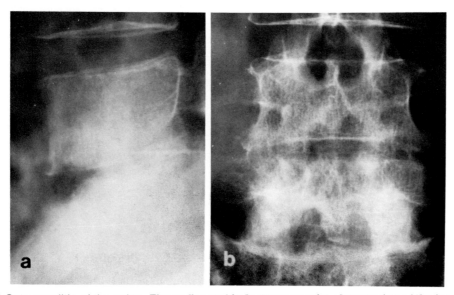

Fig. 3.82 (a, b) Osteomyelitis of the spine. The radiographic features consist of narrowing of the intervertebral space with destruction of the contiguous end-plate. Note the absence of reactive sclerosis.

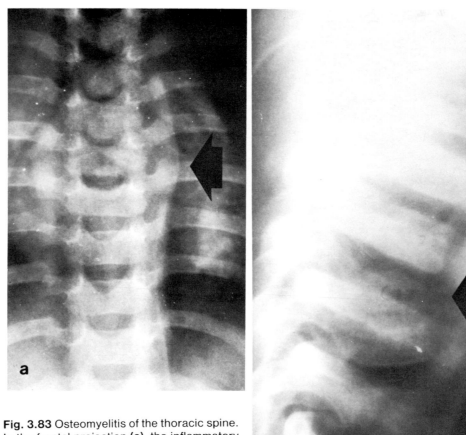

Fig. 3.83 Osteomyelitis of the thoracic spine. In the frontal projection **(a)**, the inflammatory reaction results in smooth, sharply defined lateral bulging of the mediastinal stripe (*arrow*). In the lateral projection **(b)**, the *arrow* indicates the lytic involvement of the vertebral body and loss of the subjacent intervertebral space.

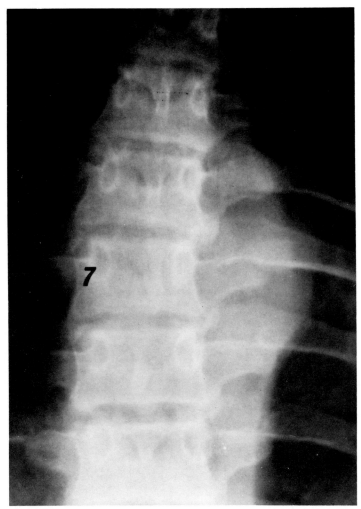

Fig. 3.84 The paraspinous soft tissue mass adjacent to the body of T7 was caused by Ewing's sarcoma of the seventh thoracic segment and the neck of the seventh rib.

stripe) at the level of involvement (Fig. 3.83). This soft tissue abnormality is not pathognomonic of infection but is an adjunctive radiographic sign of disease. A similar localized soft tissue mass may be caused by traumatic hematoma or primary neoplastic disease (Fig. 3.84).

In current practice, tuberculosis of the spine is much less common than osteomyelitis caused by gram-negative organisms. The radiographic appearance of tubercular osteomyelitis of the spine differs little from that caused by the coliform organisms.

In the elderly patient with diffuse demineralization of the spine secondary to osteoporosis, compression fractures with varying degrees of anterior wedging (Fig. 3.85) or buckling of the superior plate (Fig. 3.86) are common. It is frequently radiographically impossible to distinguish between old and acute fractures in patients of this age group. In the final analysis, this distinction must be made primarily on the basis of the history and physical examination of the patient.

Differential Diagnosis

While the major causes of acute symptoms referable to the spinal column are related to trauma, frequently soft tissue infection, intervertebral disc disease, preexistent congenital anomalies (Figs. 3.87 and 3.88), metabolic and primary or secondary neoplastic diseases may make radiographic interpretations difficult or may, themselves, cause some of the patient's clinical findings. Spina bifida occulta (Fig. 3.89) and anomalous growth centers of the transverse processes or rudimentary ribs may simulate fractures (Fig. 3.90). The ring epiphyses (Fig. 3.91) of the vertebral bodies, which have been previously described, may suggest an avulsion fracture.

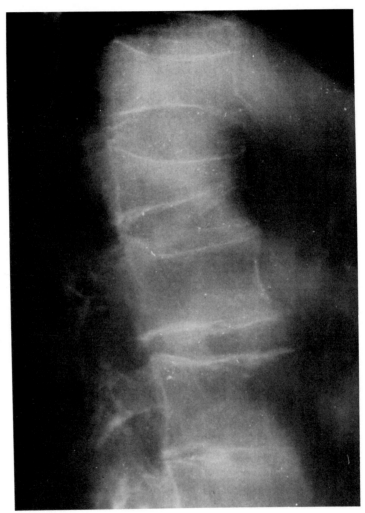

Fig. 3.85 Compression fracture secondary to senile osteoporosis.

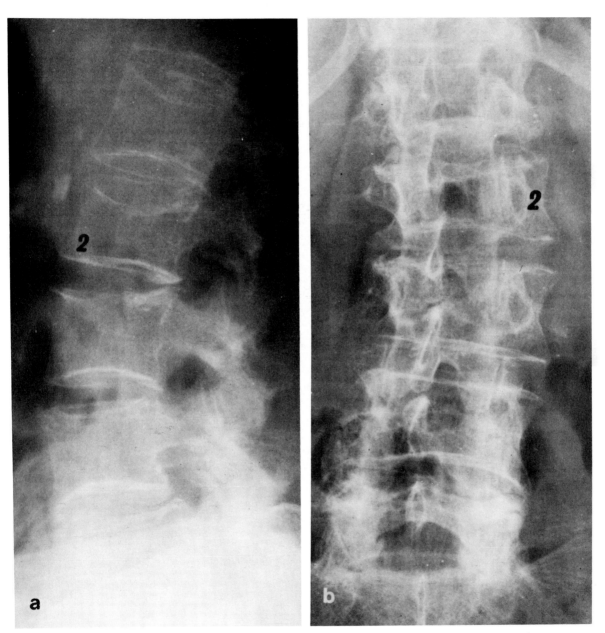

Fig. 3.86 (a, b) Buckling of the superior plate of L_2 in a patient with diffuse osteoporosis.

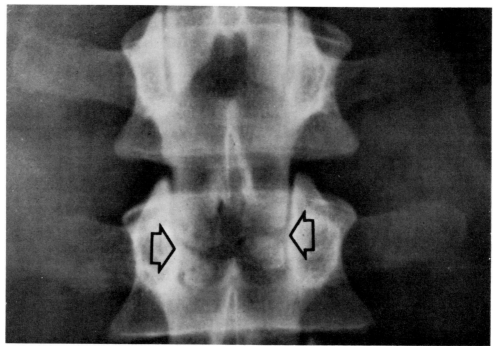

Fig. 3.87 The ununited secondary growth centers of the inferior articulating facets (*open arrows*) could be misinterpreted as representing acute fractures. The smooth, dense, sclerotic margins and the absence of a history of trauma indicate the true nature of this finding.

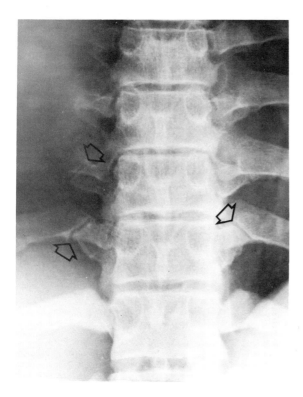

Fig. 3.88 Anomalous pseudoarthrosis between the transverse process and neck of the corresponding ribs. The radiographic characteristics of the contiguous surfaces of the transverse process and the rib should distinguish this variant from acute fracture.

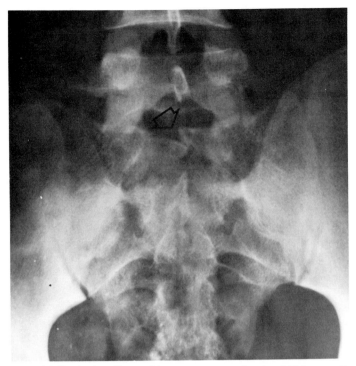

Fig. 3.89 Typical radiographic appearance of spina bifida occulta.

Fig. 3.90 The *open arrows* indicate rudimentary 12th ribs. This anomaly, particularly as it appears on the left, could be misinterpreted as a transverse process fracture. This type of variant commonly involves the 12th thoracic and first lumbar segments and should not be misinterpreted as a fracture.

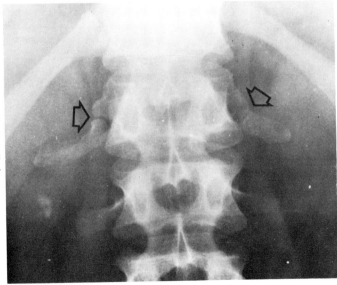

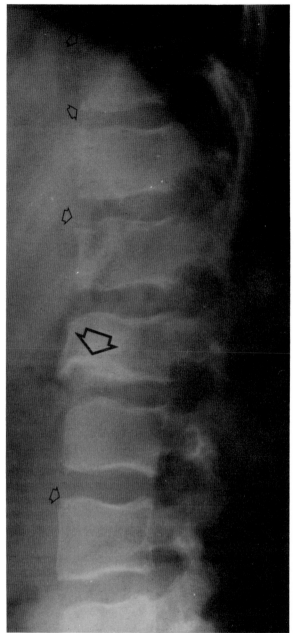

Fig. 3.91 The *small arrows* indicate ring epiphyses, which should not be mistaken for avulsion fragments. The *large arrow* indicates an area of healed juvenile osteochondritis.

Schmorl's nodule is a defect, usually in the superior surface of a vertebral body, caused by herniation of disc material through the end-plate. The herniation may occur at any portion of the end-plate not covered by the rim and may be single or multiple. The etiology of the herniation may be a single compressive trauma, repeated chronic stress, or degenerative disease. Radiographically, the Schmorl's nodule consists of one or more radiolucent defects which extend through the end-plate for a variable distance into the centrum. The margins of the defect are thin and irregularly sclerotic (Fig. 3.92). It is important to be aware that radiographically discernible Schmorl's nodules are generally considered to be asymptomatic (32).

Anomalies at the lumbosacral level are extremely common and, when anomalous alignment of the apophyseal joints at this level is included, may be encountered in as high as 50% of patients. The principal anomaly of the posterior element that is germane to this subject is spondylolysis. **This is a congenital developmental defect in the isthmus (pars interarticularis)** (Fig. 3.93) and may occur unilaterally or bilaterally at the same level or at multiple levels. This defect, which typically involves the fourth or fifth lumbar segments, may be suspected by a characteristic linear radiolucent defect on the frontal or lateral roentgenogram (Fig. 3.94). However, the oblique projection is required to confirm the presence of this defect.

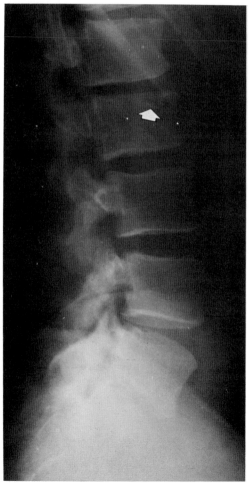

Fig. 3.92 Schmorl's nodule of the superior end-plate of L₂ (*arrow*).

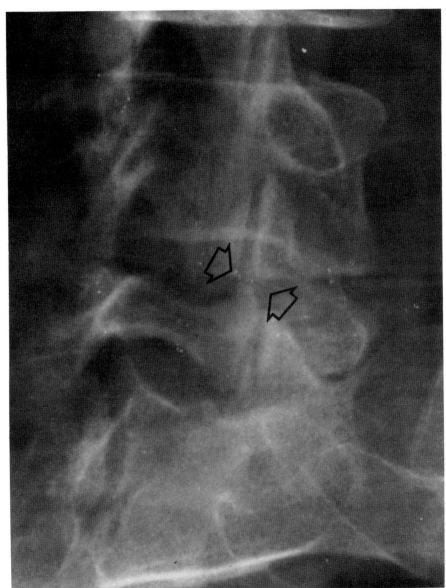

Fig. 3.93 The *arrows* indicate the lytic defect in the pars interarticularis. This is the defect of spondylolysis, and it is best demonstrated in the oblique projection.

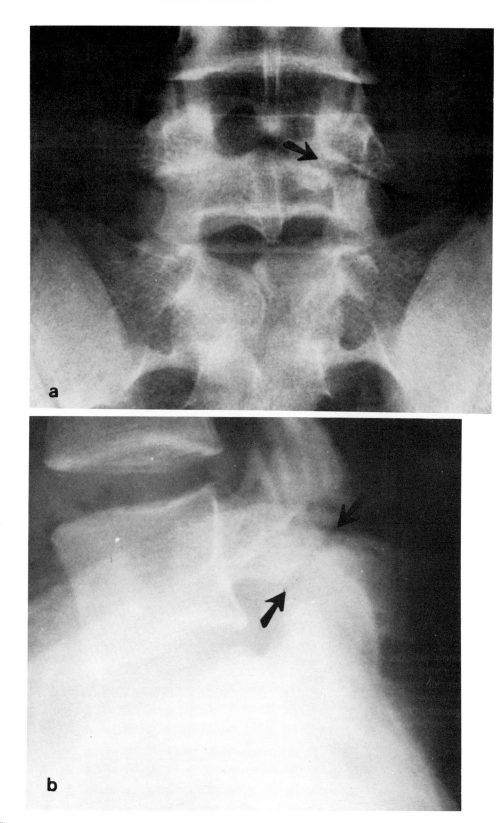

Fig. 3.94 The *arrows* indicate the appearance of the typical linear radiolucent defect in the frontal **(a)** and lateral **(b)** radiographs that are very suggestive of the presence of spondylolysis. This impression can only be confirmed by means of roentgenograms made in the oblique projection.

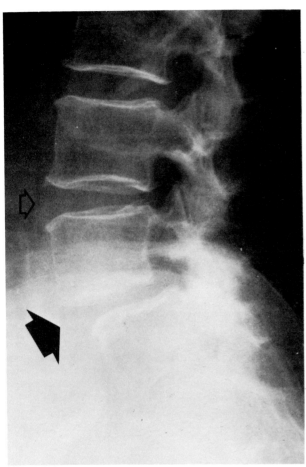

Fig. 3.95 Spondylolisthesis of L$_4$ on L$_5$ (*solid arrow*). *Open arrow* indicates soft tissue density of anteriorly bulging intervertebral disc.

When the defect is unilateral, there is no associated anterior slippage of one vertebral body upon the other. A bilateral spondylolysis may also exist without associated vertebral body displacement due to the stabilizing effect of the soft tissues.

When the pars interarticularis is disrupted bilaterally at the same level and the soft tissues are decompensated, the vertebral body may slip anteriorly with respect to the body below. This is spondylolisthesis (Fig. 3.95). While this anomaly is nearly always congenital or developmental, rare cases of traumatic spondylolisthesis have been reported (40, 41).

Transitional fifth lumbar or first sacral segments occur commonly and are characterized by pseudoarthrosis between the fifth lumbar and first sacral transverse processes or by the presence of a transverse, congenital defect in the normally fused sacral wing. "Sacralization" of the transverse process of L$_5$ may be unilateral or bilateral and is always associated with some degree of congenital narrowing of the corresponding intervertebral space. When the lumbosacral

space is congenitally absent or fused, the fourth lumbar interspace assumes the function of the lumbosacral space. In this role, it is subject to the same incidence of acute disc disease as the L$_5$-S$_1$ space.

"Limbus" vertebra refers to a thoracolumbar vertebra in which the anterior superior corner of the body constitutes a separate triangle shaped bony fragment (Fig. 3.96). The most common cause of the limbus vertebra is separation of the vertebral rim by extrusion of intervertebral disc material in an obliquely inferior course through the anterior aspect of the superior end-plate of the body. The etiology of the extruded disc material is a degenerative phenomenon secondary to repeated everyday stress (42).

The "separated vertebral edge" (limbus vertebra), which is the result of chronic, repeated stress, should be distinguishable from a fracture on the basis of its characteristic triangular shape, the dense, sclerotic margins of the separated rim and the contiguous surface of the vertebral body, and the uniform width of the lucent defect between the two (Fig. 3.96). Neither extension nor flexion fractures produce a separate triangular fragment of the anterior *superior* aspect of the vertebral body. The separate triangular fragment of the extension tear-drop fracture arises from the anterior *inferior* corner of the axis (Fig. 3.48). The separate fragments of the flexion tear-drop (Fig. 3.38) and the bursting fracture (Fig. 3.44) also characteristically involve the anterior *inferior* corner of the

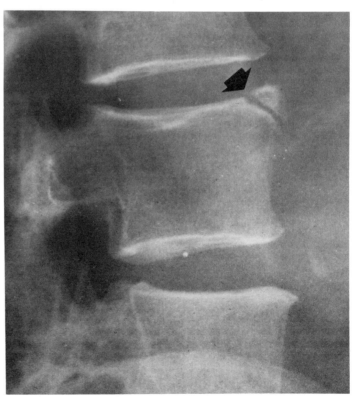

Fig. 3.96 Limbus vertebra.

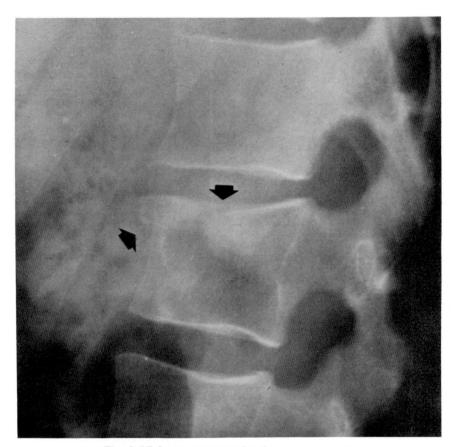

Fig. 3.97 Acute compression fracture (*arrows*).

body. Additionally, the contiguous surfaces of these fragments are neither densely sclerotic nor sharply defined and the lucent defect between the separate fragment and the vertebral body is not of uniform width, as in the instance of the vertebral edge separation. Acute compression fractures (Fig. 3.97), which frequently involve the superior end-plate and the superior aspect of the anterior cortex of the vertebral body, have a characteristic impacted, buckled appearance and should easily be distinguishable from the limbus vertebra.

References

1. HARRIS JH Jr: *The Radiology of Acute Cervical Spine Trauma.* Williams & Wilkins, Baltimore, 1978.
2. MILLER MD, GEHWEILER JA, MARTINEZ S, CHARLTON OP, DAFFNER RH: Significant new observations in cervical spine trauma. *AJR* 130:659, 1978.
3. MARAVILLA KR, COOPER PR, SKLAR FH: The influence of thin-section tomography on the treatment of cervical spine injuries. *Radiology* 127:131, 1978.
4. GARGANO FP, MEYER J, HONDEK PV, CHARYULU KKN: Transverse axial tomography of the cervical spine. *Radiology* 113:363, 1974.
5. KERSHNER MS, GOODMAN GA, PERLMUTTER GS: Computed tomography in the diagnosis of an atlas fracture. *AJR* 128:688, 1977.
6. COIN CG, PENNINK M, AHMAD WD, KERANEN VJ: Diving-type injury of the cervical spine: Contribution of computed tomography to management. *J Comput Assisted Tomography* 3:362, 1979.
7. TADMOR R, DAVIS KR, ROBERSON GH, NAW PFJ, TAVERAS JM: Computed tomographic evaluation of traumatic spinal injuries. *Radiology* 127:825, 1978.
8. WEIR DC: Roentgenographic signs of cervical injury. *Clin Orthop* 109:9, 1975.
9. ABEL MS: *Occult Traumatic Lesions of the Cervical Vertebrae.* Warren H. Green, St. Louis, Mo., 1971.
10. SMITH GR, BECKLEY DE, ABEL MS: Articular mass fracture: a neglected cause of post-traumatic pain? *Clin Radiol* 27:335, 1976.
11. WEIR DC: Roentgenographic signs of cervical injury. *Clin Orthop* 109:9, 1975.
12. HOHL M: Normal motions in the upper portion of the cervical spine. *J Bone Joint Surg* 46-A:1777, 1964.
13. FIELDING JW: Cineroentgenography of the normal cervical spine. *J Bone Joint Surg* 39-A:1280, 1957.
14. HOHL M, BAKER HR: The atlanto-axial joint. *J Bone Joint Surg* 46-A:1739, 1964.
15. McKEEVER FM: Atlanto-axoid instability. *Surg Clin North Am* 48:1935, 1968.
16. CATTELL HS, FILTZER DL: Pseudosubluxation and other normal variations of the cervical spine of children. *J Bone Joint Surg* 47-A:1295, 1965.
17. SWISCHUK LE: Anterior dislocation of C2 in children: Physiologic or pathologic. *Radiology* 122:759, 1977.
18. CAFFEY J: *Pediatric X-ray Diagnosis,* ed. 6. Yearbook Medical Publishers, Chicago, 1972.
19. BEATSON TR: Fractures and dislocations of the cervical spine. *J Bone Joint Surg* 45-B:21, 1963.
20. KING DM: Fractures and dislocations of the cervical portion of the spine. *Aust NZ J Surg* 37:57, 1967.
21. WHITLEY JE, FORSYTH HF: The classification of cervical spine injuries. *AJR* 83:633, 1960.
22. HOLDSWORTH F: Fractures, dislocations and fracture-dislocations of the spine. *J Bone Joint Surg* 52-A:1534, 1970.
23. FIELDING JW, HAWKINS RJ: Roentgenographic diagnosis of the injured neck. In *A.A.O.S. Instructional Course Lectures,* vol. XXV, chap. 7, p 149. C.V. Mosby, St. Louis, Mo., 1976.
24. BRAAKMAN R, PENNING L: The hyperflexion sprain of the cervical spine. *Radiol Clin Biol* 37:309, 1968.
25. SELECKI BR, WILLIAMS HB: *Injuries to the Cervical Spine and Cord in Man.* Australasian Medical Publishing Co., New South Wales, 1970.
26. CHESHIRE DJE: The stability of the cervical spine following the conservative treatment of fractures and fracture-dislocations. *Paraplegia* 7:193, 1969.
27. BEDBROOK GM: Stability of spinal fractures and fracture-dislocations. *Paraplegia* 9:23, 1971.
28. SCHNEIDER RC, KAHN EA: Chronic neurologic sequelae of acute trauma to the spine and spinal cord. Part I: The significance of the acute flexion or "tear-drop" fracture-dislocation of the cervical spine. *J Bone Joint Surg* 38-A:985, 1956.
29. JEFFERSON G: Fracture of the atlas vertebra. Report of four cases, and a review of those previously recorded. *Br J Surg* 7:407, 1920.
30. SHERK HH, NICHOLSON JT: Fractures of the atlas. *J Bone Joint Surg* 52-A:1017, 1970.
31. ROAF R: A study of the mechanics of spinal injuries. *J Bone Joint Surg* 42-B:810, 1960.
32. ROTHMAN RH, SIMEONE FA: *The Spine.* W.B. Saunders, Philadelphia, 1975.
33. TAYLOR AR, BLACKWOOD W: Paraplegia in hyperextension cervical injuries with normal radiographic appearance. *J Bone Joint Surg* 30-B:245, 1948.
34. TAYLOR AR: The mechanism of injury to the spinal cord in the neck without damage to the vertebral column. *J Bone Joint Surg* 33-B:543, 1951.
35. BEDBROOK, GM: Spinal injuries with tetraplegia and paraplegia. *J Bone Joint Surg* 61-B:267, 1979.
36. FIELDING JW, HENSINGER RN, HAWKINS RJ: Os Odontoideum. *J Bone Joint Surg* 62-A:376, 1980.
37. JACOBSON G, ALDER DC: An evaluation of lateral atlanto-axial displacement in injuries of the cervical spine. *Radiology* 61:355, 1961.
38. JACOBSON G, ALDER DC: Examination of the atlanto-axial joint following injury with particular emphasis on rotational subluxation. *AJR* 76:1081, 1956.
39. CHANCE CQ: Note on a type of flexion fracture of the spine. *Br J Radiol* 21:249, 1948.
40. SULLIVAN CR, BICKELL WH: The problem of traumatic spondylolysis. *Am J Surg* 100:698, 1960.
41. RUSSELL WJ, NAKATA H: Spondylolysis following trauma. *Radiology* 91:973, 1968.
42. SCHMORL G, JUNGHANNS H: *The Human Spine in Health and Disease.* Grune & Stratton, New York, 1971.

chapter four

Shoulder

General Considerations

Radiographically, the shoulder includes the distal end of the clavicle, the scapula, and the proximal end of the humerus. This definition has practical significance because the routine radiographic examination of the shoulder may not include the sternoclavicular joint and proximal end of the clavicle and does not include a complete radiographic examination of the scapula. Therefore, even though the scapula and clavicle will be discussed in this chapter, it must be understood that the radiographic studies designed to examine the calvicle and the scapula must be specifically requested.

Although the shoulder is a large, seemingly relatively simple joint, it must not be considered an uncomplicated structure radiographically. The anatomy of the shoulder and its relation to the trunk are the basis of serious radiographic diagnostic pitfalls peculiar to this joint.

Partial, or complete, acromioclavicular separation, fracture of the coracoid process, and direct posterior dislocation of the shoulder present special diagnostic problems, radiographically. If disruption of the acromioclavicular fibers is complete while the coracoclavicular ligament remains intact, separation of the acromioclavicular space may not occur unless this joint is stressed. Consequently, when an acromioclavicular separation is suspected, special views of the shoulder must be obtained with the patient erect and holding 15–20 pounds of weight in each hand. The radiographic examination of the uninjured shoulder serves as a normal baseline study for comparison with the similar examination obtained of the involved side. Fracture of the coracoid process of the scapula may only be established on the axillary projection of the shoulder.

Direct posterior dislocation of the shoulder may be extremely difficult to diagnose on routine anteroposterior roentgenograms of the shoulder. Superimposition of the humeral head upon the glenoid fossa or widening of the space between the humeral head and the glenoid fossa have each been described as signs of posterior dislocation of the shoulder. However, neither is sufficiently constant to be reliable and special views are necessary to establish this diagnosis.

Radiographic Examination

The routine radiographic examination of the shoulder is made in the anteroposterior position with the arm rotated both internally (Fig. 4.1) and externally (Fig. 4.2). When these projections are made in the usual position, neither provides a true frontal view of the glenohumeral joint space. The latter may be obtained by externally rotating the entire body so that the plane of the scapula parallels that of the cassette and by directing the central beam just medial to the articulating surface of the humeral head. The resulting radiograph (Fig. 4.3) provides a true measure of the glenohumeral space. These projections, which may be made with the patient either erect or supine, provide an adequate "survey" examination of the shoulder. However, as previously noted, they frequently do not provide definitive data relative to some of the traumatic lesions involving the shoulder.

Commonly, it will be necessary to obtain views of the shoulder made in planes other than the frontal projection. These may be either the transthoracic lateral (Cahoon) (Fig. 4.4) or the axillary view (Fig. 4.5). The Cahoon projection is easy for the patient, but positioning is critical in order to project the humeral head into the space between the posterior surface of the sternum and the anterior aspect of the

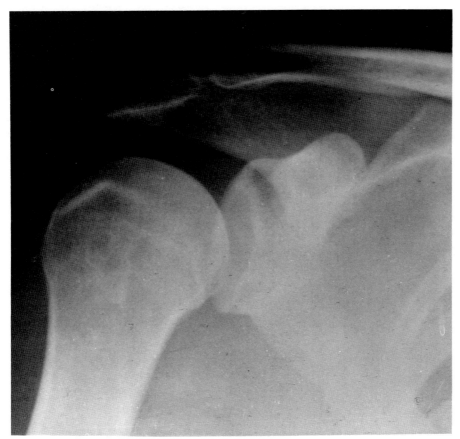

Fig. 4.1 Frontal radiograph of a normal adult shoulder in *internal* rotation. In this projection, neither tuberosity is seen in profile and the humeral head appears essentially round. The articulating surface of the humeral head is superimposed upon the posterior rim of the glenoid fossa, but is lateral to its anterior rim.

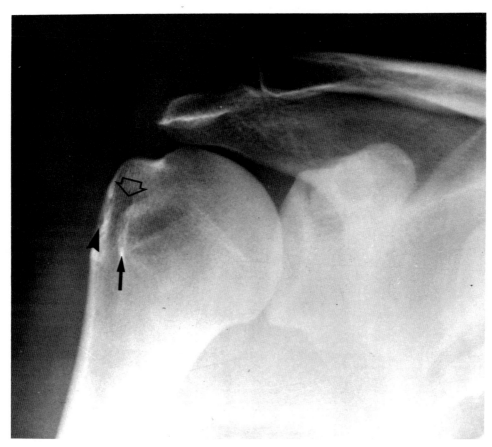

Fig. 4.2 Frontal radiograph of a normal adult shoulder in *external* rotation. The greater tuberosity (*arrowhead*) is seen in profile and the bicipital groove (*open arrow*) can be identified between it and the cortex of the lesser tuberosity (*stemmed arrow*). Note that the relationship of the humeral head to the glenoid fossa is similar to that seen in internal rotation (see Fig. 4.1).

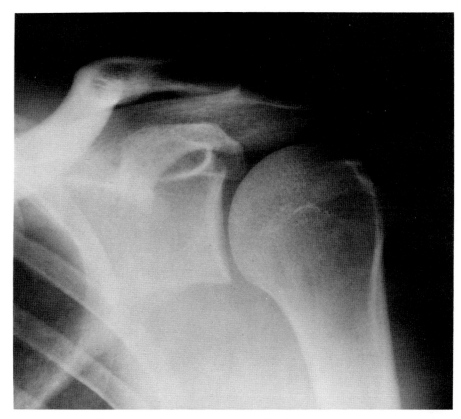

Fig. 4.3 True anteroposterior radiograph of the shoulder made with the patient externally rotated and the central x-ray beam directed just medial to the articulating surface of the humeral head. The purpose of this projection is to visualize the glenohumeral joint space *en face*.

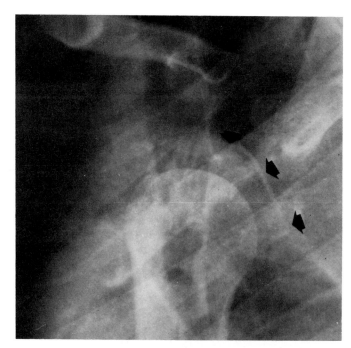

Fig. 4.4 Normal Cahoon projection of the shoulder. This view is also known as the transthoracic lateral or the "through-the-chest" lateral. The *arrows* indicate the glenoid fossa.

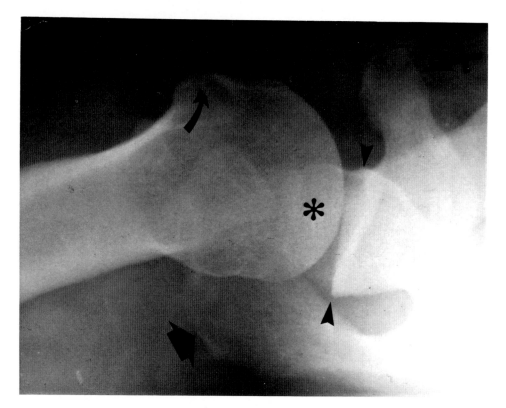

Fig. 4.5 Axillary projection of the right shoulder. The *stemmed arrow* indicates the coracoid process; the *arrowheads*, the glenoid fossa; the *solid arrow*, the acromium process; and the (*) the humeral head. In this view, the lesser tuberosity (*curved arrow*) is seen in profile and the glenohumeral relationship is seen in the coronal (caudocranial) plane.

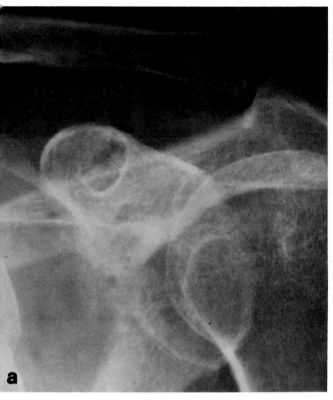
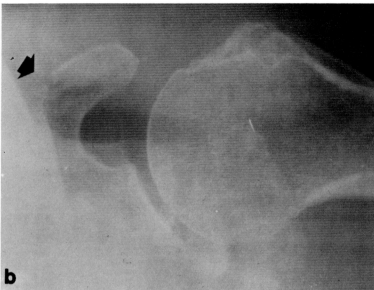

Fig. 4.6 The anteroposterior examination of the shoulder **(a)** is apparently negative. The axillary view **(b)** demonstrates a slightly displaced fracture (*arrow*) through the base of the coracoid process.

upper thoracic vertebral bodies. Even when optimum positioning is obtained, the glenoid fossa, being somewhat oblique to the central beam, is rarely well seen in this view.

The axillary view should be considered in the radiographic examination of the shoulder in all cases of trauma to the shoulder. Although frequently overlooked, the axillary view provides more information about the shoulder than any other single projection. It is the only view in which minimally displaced fractures of the coracoid process of the scapula (Fig. 4.6), cortical fractures of the anterior or posterior surfaces of the humeral head (Fig. 4.7), and direct posterior dislocation of the humerus can be demonstrated. The axillary view also demonstrates the direction of angulation of humeral neck fractures (Fig. 4.8).

Positioning for the axillary view is very simple and the demonstration of the anatomy of the shoulder is clear. The axillary view is best obtained in the supine position. Occasionally, because of severe pain in the shoulder, the patient cannot easily assume the supine position. Such a patient may be assisted in this by placing the x-ray table in the erect position with the foot step on the bottom end of the table. With the patient standing on the step, the table can be lowered

into the horizontal position and the patient comes into the supine posture without discomfort. When the patient is on a litter, the axillary view is easier to obtain than is the transthoracic lateral projection.

A few words of caution are necessary relative to the use of the axillary projection in the evaluation of the acute skeletal injury involving the shoulder. First, the axillary projection should be obtained only if the routine frontal projections are equivocal or do not permit a definitive roentgen diagnosis. Second, contrary to the positioning described for the axillary projection in standard textbooks, it is not necessary to extremely rotate nor abduct the arm 90° from the body to obtain a satisfactory axillary projection. Diagnostic transaxillary views (see Figs. 4.20, 4.22–4.24, and 4.27) can be obtained with only sufficient abduction of the arm (10–15°) to permit placing the x-ray tube between the hand and the hip with the central beam directed to the apex of the axilla. The cassette is placed above the shoulder in a plane perpendicular to the central ray. Finally, the radiologist must personally abduct the arm in order to assure maximum control and minimum movement during positioning. The purpose for these admonitions is to prevent any unnecessary motion of the injured shoulder during this diagnostic examination.

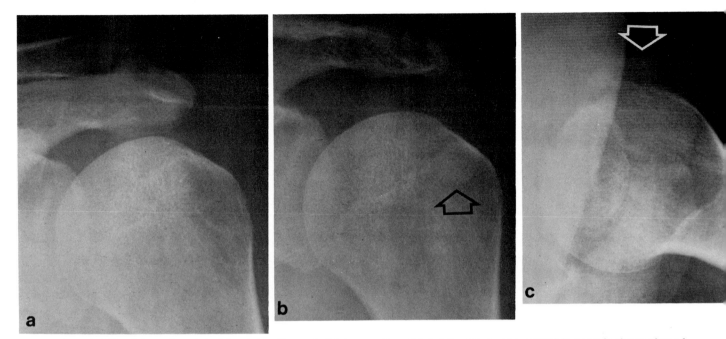

Fig. 4.7 The internally rotated frontal radiograph **(a)** is negative. A faint density (*open arrow*) is seen in the region of the greater tuberosity on the externally rotated examination **(b)**. The separate fracture fragment (*arrow*) is clearly seen in the axillary view **(c)**.

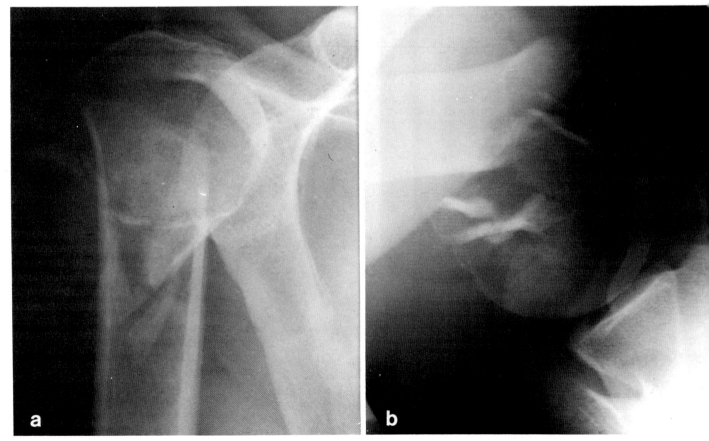

Fig. 4.8 Severely comminuted, displaced fracture of the surgical neck of the humerus **(a)**. The degree of displacement of the major fragments can only be appreciated in the axillary projection **(b)**.

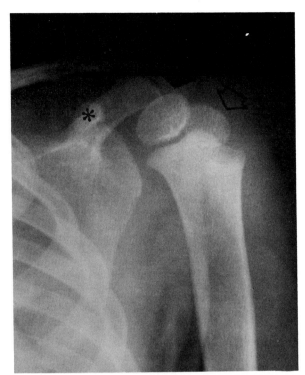

Fig. 4.9 Frontal projection of the normal shoulder of a child. The *arrows* indicate the ununited humeral head epiphyses and the asterisk (*) marks the coracoid process of the scapula.

Radiographic Anatomy

The radiographic appearance of the normal child's shoulder is seen in Figure 4.9.

Figure 4.10 illustrates the roentgen appearance of the normal adolescent shoulder. The apophysis of the coracoid process is clearly seen. The radiographic characteristics of an epiphyseal line, namely the dense sclerotic margin, variable width of the line, and its anatomic location, are illustrated at the surgical neck of the humerus. This figure also illustrates the effect of position upon the appearance of the epiphyseal line and indicates how an arc of the epiphyseal line may be projected in such a way as to resemble a fracture line.

The apophysis of the acromium process (Fig. 4.11) is a normal structure that can resemble an avulsion fracture fragment.

Radiographic Manifestations of Trauma

The diagnosis "acromioclavicular separation" refers to abnormal widening of the acromioclavicular joint, usually the result of a direct trauma to the point of the shoulder. This terminology completely ignores the significance of the coracoclavicular ligament in the support of the upper extremity and is misleading because there is no reference to coracoclavicular sep-

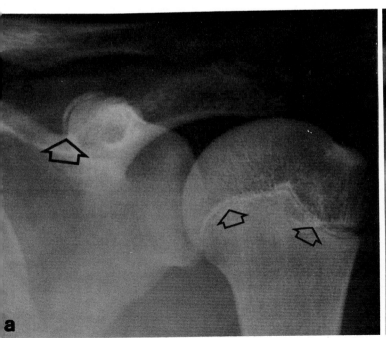

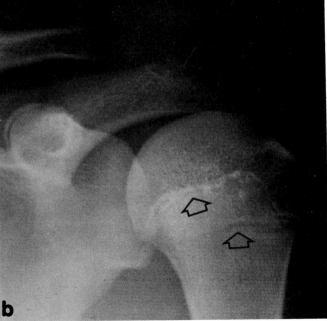

Fig. 4.10 Normal adolescent shoulder seen in two different frontal projections. In part **(a)**, the *large open arrow* indicates the apophysis of the coracoid process. The *smaller open arrows* indicate the proximal humeral epiphyseal line which, because the epiphyseal plate is precisely parallel to the central x-ray beam, produces a single radiographic shadow. In part **(b)**, the position of the humerus has been changed so that the plane of the epiphyseal plate is at an angle to the x-ray beam. Consequently, both the anterior arc of the epiphyseal plate (*superior arrow*) and the posterior arc (*inferior arrow*) produce separate radiographic images. Therefore, the inferior posterior arc of the epiphyseal plate should not be mistaken for a fracture line.

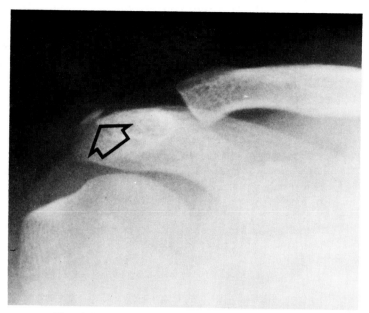

Fig. 4.11 The *arrow* indicates the secondary ossification center of the acromium process. This normal finding may be misinterpreted as an avulsion fracture. This apophysis usually appears at age 15 and unites about age 20.

aration, which is the most important soft tissue injury caused by this type of trauma. The normal ligamentous anatomy between the clavicle and the scapula is indicated in Figure 4.12. Radiographically, the location of the acromio- and coracoclavicular ligaments is seen in Figure 4.13.

Both the acromioclavicular and the coracoclavicular ligaments play a role in the radiographic appearance of the effects of a blow or fall upon the point of the shoulder. The acromioclavicular joint is enclosed by a thin capsule which is reinforced superiorly and inferiorly by acromioclavicular ligaments. The principal ligament between the clavicle and the scapula, however, is the coracoclavicular ligament which is thick, dense, and strong. The extent of the coracoclavicular separation has a direct bearing upon the degree of acromioclavicular separation.

Injuries of the acromioclavicular (and coracoclavicular) ligaments are classified as sprain (grade I), subluxation (grade II), and dislocation (grade III) (1).

When the force applied to the point of the shoulder is sufficient to disrupt both the relatively weak acromioclavicular ligament and the strong coracoclavicular ligament (grade III acromioclavicular dislocation), the scapula and its acromium are displaced downward and medially, resulting in both acromioclavicular and coracoclavicular separation (dislocation—grade III) (Fig. 4.14). Radiographically, complete ligamentous disruption is usually represented by widening of the acromioclavicular and coracoclavicular spaces in routine, erect, anteroposterior roentgenograms of the shoulder (Fig. 4.15).

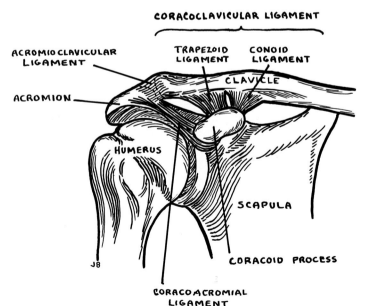

Fig. 4.12 Schematic representation of the normal ligamentous attachments between the acromium and the coracoid process of the scapula and the clavicle. (Modified from H.E. Conwell and F. C. Reynolds: *Key and Conwell's Management of Fractures, Dislocations and Sprains*, ed. 7. C. V. Mosby, St. Louis, Mo., 1961.)

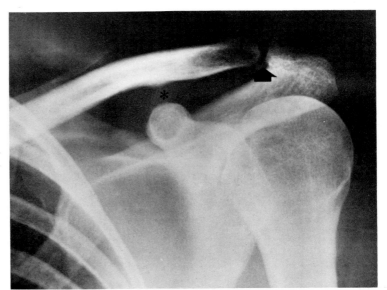

Fig. 4.13 Normal shoulder in the anteroposterior projection. The (*) indicates the location of the coracoclavicular ligament, and the *arrow* indicates the location of the acromioclavicular ligament.

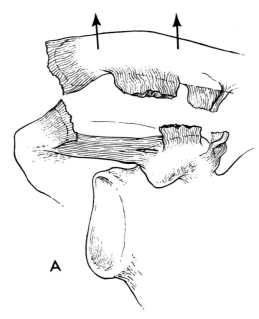

Fig. 4.14 Acromioclavicular separation. This line drawing depicts complete disruption of the acromioclavicular and the coracoclavicular ligaments. (Reprinted with permission from R. J. Schultz: *The Language of Fractures.* Williams & Wilkins, Baltimore, 1972.)

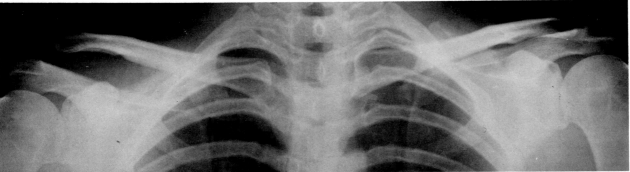

Fig. 4.15 The complete acromioclavicular and coracoclavicular separation is obvious in this frontal projection made with the patient erect, but without stressing the shoulder. Compare the changes on the right with the appearance of the normal left shoulder.

Partial or complete rupture of the acromioclavicular ligament may exist without disruption of the coracoclavicular ligament (subluxation—grade II) (Fig. 4.16), and the separation of the acromioclavicular joint may not be evident on routine radiographs of the shoulder. Therefore, when this condition is suspected, but not apparent on the routine radiograph, stress films are required. These examinations are made in the erect, anteroposterior position both with and without the patient holding 15- to 20-pound weights in each hand. The weight (sandbag) thus applied to the affected shoulder will stress the acromioclavicular and/or coracoclavicular ligaments, resulting in widening of these spaces (Fig. 4.17) thereby establishing the diagnosis. The sprain (grade I) consists of stretching or tearing of a few fibers of the acromioclavicular ligament. The acromioclavicular joint is stable and the coracoclavicular ligament is intact. This injury can only be detected by comparing stress views of the injured and uninjured shoulders. The roentgen sign of acromioclavicular sprain is minor widening of the acromioclavicular space.

The shoulder is the most frequent site of dislocation of any joint of the body, constituting approximately 50% of all dislocations (2). The explanation for this incidence reflects the configuration of the humeral head and the glenoid fossa, the relative size of each, the weakness of the shoulder capsule, and the fact that this major joint is frequently subject to injury.

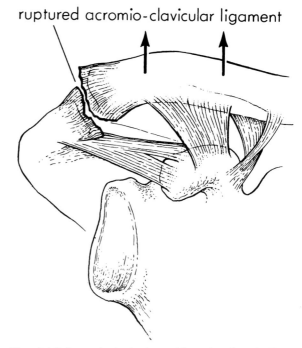

Fig. 4.16 Acromioclavicular subluxation (grade II separation). Note that only the acromioclavicular ligament is ruptured and that there is a slight separation of the acromioclavicular space. (Reprinted with permission from R. J. Schultz: *The Language of Fractures*. Williams & Wilkins, Baltimore, 1972.)

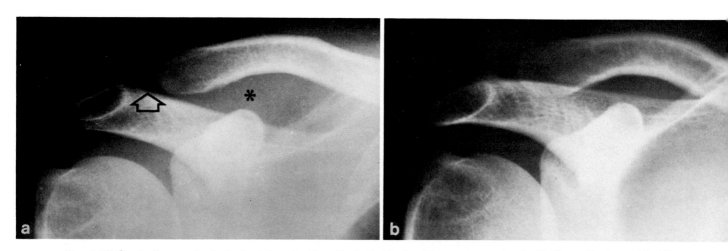

Fig. 4.17 Grade II acromioclavicular injury (subluxation). Each shoulder was examined with the patient erect holding a 15-pound sandbag in each hand. Part **(a)** is the acutely injured right shoulder. Part **(b)** is the uninjured left shoulder which has been reversed for ease of comparison. In part **(a)** the acromioclavicular space is widened (*open arrow*) and the inferior cortex of the distal end of the clavicle lies above the plane of the inferior cortex of the acromion. The asterisk (*) indicates the slightly widened coracoclavicular space, which probably represents simply stretching of this ligament.

Dislocations at the shoulder are, generally, clinically obvious. The indications for radiographic evaluation prior to reduction include establishing whether the humeral head lies anterior or posterior to the glenoid fossa and whether an associated fracture or loose body is present. Either the Cahoon or axillary projection is necessary to confirm the position of the head relative to the glenoid fossa, and one of these views is mandatory for a complete radiographic study of the shoulder.

Dislocations at the shoulder are classified on the basis of the final resting place of the humeral head with respect to the glenoid fossa and are designated, therefore, as anterior, inferior, posterior, and superior. Of these, the anterior dislocation, occurring most often as a subcoracoid dislocation (Fig. 4.18), is the most common. The inferior (subglenoid) dislocation is next in frequency. Posterior and superior dislocations are rare.

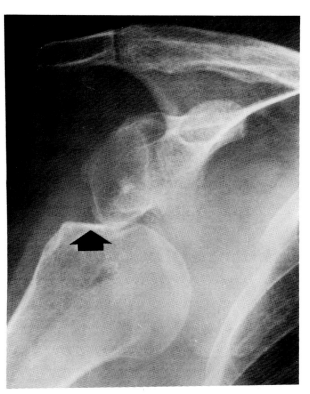

Fig. 4.19 Inferior (subglenoid) dislocation of the humerus with Hill-Sachs lesion. The *arrow* indicates the flattened segment of the greater tuberosity of the humerus caused by the impacted cortical fracture. This fracture, commonly associated with subglenoid dislocations, is the result of forceful impaction of the humeral head with the inferior rim of the glenoid fossa. The humeral lesion constitutes the Hill-Sachs lesion or "notch" defect.

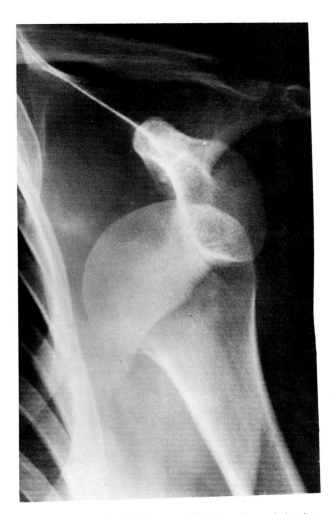

Fig. 4.18 Anterior (subcoracoid) dislocation of the humerus. There is no associated fracture.

Inferior dislocation of the humerus is frequently associated with a compression fracture of the humeral head, resulting in a flattened segment of the head referred to as the "notch" defect or "Hill-Sachs" (3) lesion (Fig. 4.19). This fracture is the result of forceful impingement of the superolateral aspect of the humeral head against the anterior or inferior rim of the glenoid fossa at the time of dislocation (Fig. 4.20).

One of the most common complications of glenohumeral dislocation is fracture of the anteroinferior rim of the glenoid fossa (Fig. 4.21) (4).

Luxatio erecta is an uncommon and extreme form of inferior dislocation of the shoulder. Luxatio erecta is the result of severe hyperabduction of the arm. In the process, the humeral head impinges upon the acromion process. The latter, acting as a fulcrum, forces the head anteriorly and inferiorly out of the glenoid fossa, where it becomes locked by the coracoid and acromion processes. Clinically, the arm is in a position of extreme abduction so that it is elevated parallel to the side of the head and the arm is typically

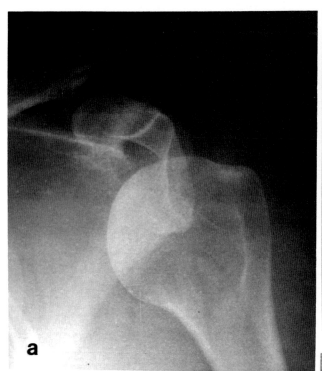

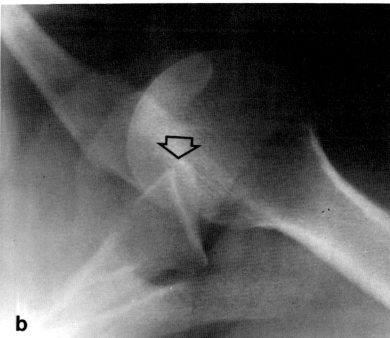

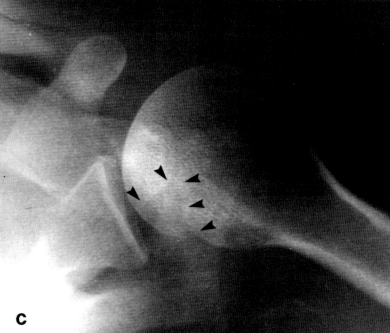

Fig. 4.20 Subcoracoid dislocation of the humerus illustrating the mechanism of the Hill-Sachs fracture. The anterior dislocation is obvious in **(a)**. The axillary projection **(b)** demonstrates the impaction of the humeral head upon the glenoid rim (*arrow*). The "notch" defect of the Hill-Sachs fracture (*arrowheads*), caused by impaction of the humeral head upon the glenoid rim, is clearly evident in the postreduction axillary projection **(c)**.

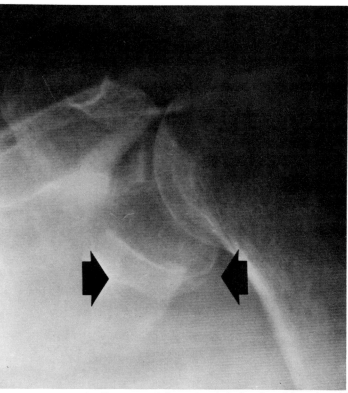

Fig. 4.21 Fracture of the anteroinferior rim of the glenoid fossa. The *arrows* indicate the displaced fragment.

held in a flexed position over the top of the skull. The radiographic appearance of luxatio erecta is seen in Figure 4.22. Figure 4.23 is an example of luxatio erecta associated with a comminuted fracture of the greater tuberosity.

Direct posterior dislocation of the shoulder is uncommon (4%) but constitutes a definite radiographic hazard because it is unrecognized in 40–50% of cases (3). This is because, in the frontal view, the roentgenogram is remarkably normal in appearance (Fig. 4.24). This radiographic fact, in conjunction with a history of trauma or recent convulsion, plus pain and limitation of motion, should make one suspect a posterior dislocation of the humerus. Two subtle changes have been described as being found in the anteroposterior projection of the posteriorly dislocated shoulder. The more common is the superimposition of the humeral head upon the glenoid fossa so that the articulating surface of the head seems to lie medial to the glenoid fossa. Secondly, Arndt and Sears (5) have described the "positive rim-sign" which consists of widening of the space between the articulating surface of the head and the anterior margin of the glenoid fossa. In their four cases of posterior dislocation, this distance measured 11 mm or more, as compared to

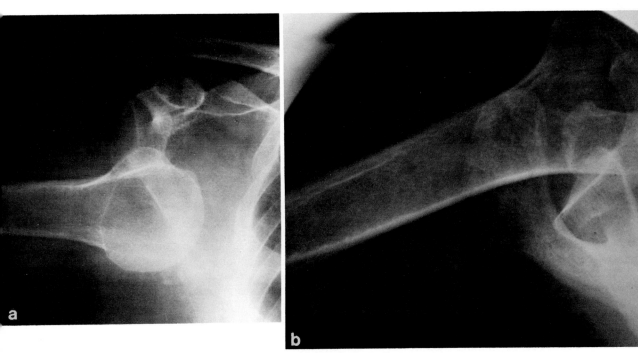

Fig. 4.22 Uncomplicated luxatio erecta in frontal (a) and axillary (b) projections. The abduction of the humerus characteristic of this injury is seen in the anteroposterior radiograph (a). Compare the attitude of the humerus in part (a) with that seen in subcoracoid (see Fig. 4.18) and subglenoid (see Fig. 4.19) dislocations.

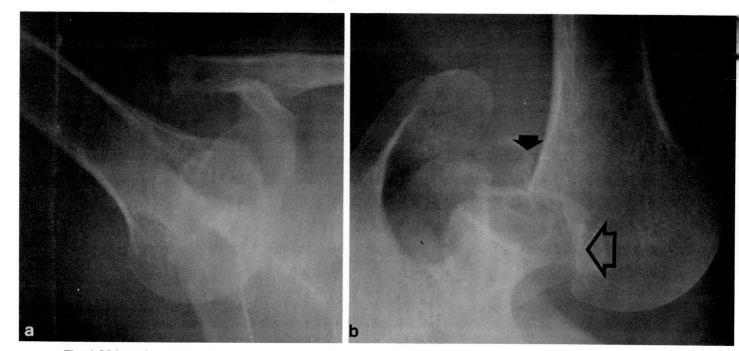

Fig. 4.23 Luxatio erecta with associated fracture of the greater tuberosity. The characteristic severe abduction of the arm is evident in the anteroposterior projection **(a)**. The associated fracture of the humeral head can be appreciated only in the axillary view **(b)**, where the *open arrow* represents the site of impaction and the *solid arrow* a displaced fracture fragment.

maximum normal separation of 6 mm. Figure 4.25 demonstrates this radiographic sign.

Posterior dislocation of the shoulder is typically associated with a fracture of the anteromedial aspect of the humeral head (6) caused by impaction of the head upon the posterior glenoid rim (Figs. 4.24 and 4.26). A curvilinear density superimposed upon the humeral head and roughly paralleling the articulating cortex of the head is caused by the depressed fragments and produces, in the frontal projection, what has been referred to as the "trough line" (7) (Figs. 4.24 and 4.26), which is an important sign of posterior fracture-dislocation of the shoulder.

Figure 4.26 is a rare case of bilateral fracture-posterior dislocation of the humeral head. In each an-

teroposterior roentgenogram, the fractures are obvious but the associated dislocation is not.

The posterior position of the humeral head can only be established by either a transthoracic lateral or an axillary view of the shoulder. While a transthoracic projection may be easier to obtain insofar as patient comfort is concerned, positioning is critical and the roentgenogram is commonly difficult to interpret because the glenoid fossa may not be well seen. The axial view, on the other hand, sharply depicts the posterior dislocation (Fig. 4.26) and may be obtained with only minimal inconvenience to the patient. Contrary to common opinion, an entirely satisfactory axillary projection of the shoulder may be obtained with only slight abduction of the arm.

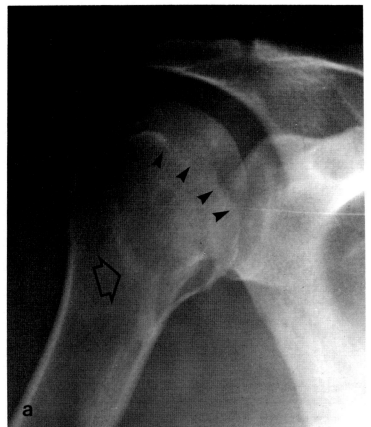

Fig. 4.24 Posterior fracture-dislocation of the shoulder. In the frontal projection **(a)**, important signs suggesting the correct diagnosis include the "light bulb" appearance of the proximal humerus, indicative of severe internal rotation which is characteristic of posterior dislocation, and the curvilinear cortical density of the depressed fracture fragments superimposed upon the humeral head (*arrowheads*) which produces the "trough line." The humeral head fracture is further indicated by the broad, dense band extending obliquely across the surgical neck (*open arrow*), which represents impacted and superimposed fracture fragments. In the axillary projection **(b)**, the posterior fracture-dislocation is clearly evident, as is the basis for the roentgen signs seen in the frontal projection. The superimposed fragments (*open arrow*) result in the broad, oblique density crossing the surgical neck and the cortical margin of the depressed fragments (*arrowhead*) produced the "trough line."

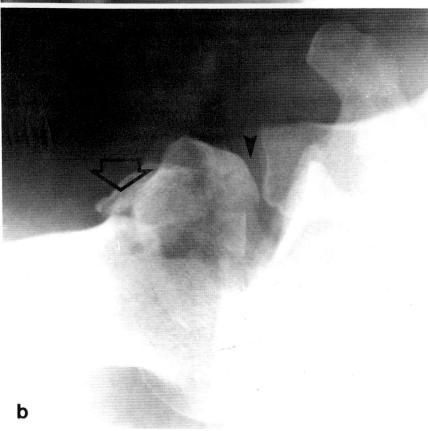

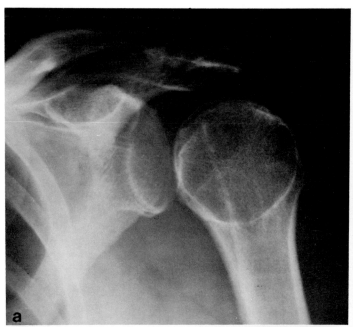

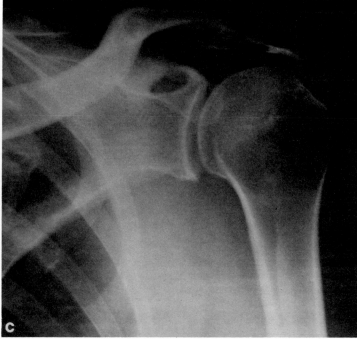

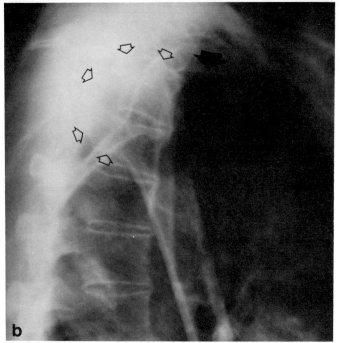

Fig. 4.25 Direct posterior dislocation of the humerus seen in frontal (a) and transthoracic lateral (b) projections. Part (c) is the frontal projection of the same patient's normal left shoulder, which has been reversed for ease of comparison. In the frontal projection of the dislocated shoulder (a), the relationship of the humeral head to the glenoid fossa and the acromion seems grossly normal. However, the space between the glenoid fossa and the adjacent cortical margin of the humeral head is abnormally wide (the positive rim sign) and, because of the severe internal rotation of the humerus, the superimposed cortex of the humeral head and neck are seen end-on, resulting in the "rifle barrel" or "light bulb" appearance of the head. In the Cahoon (transthoracic) projection (b), the proximal end of the humerus (*open arrows*) is posteriorly displaced with respect to the acromion process (*solid arrow*) and is abnormally superimposed upon the upper thoracic vertebrae.

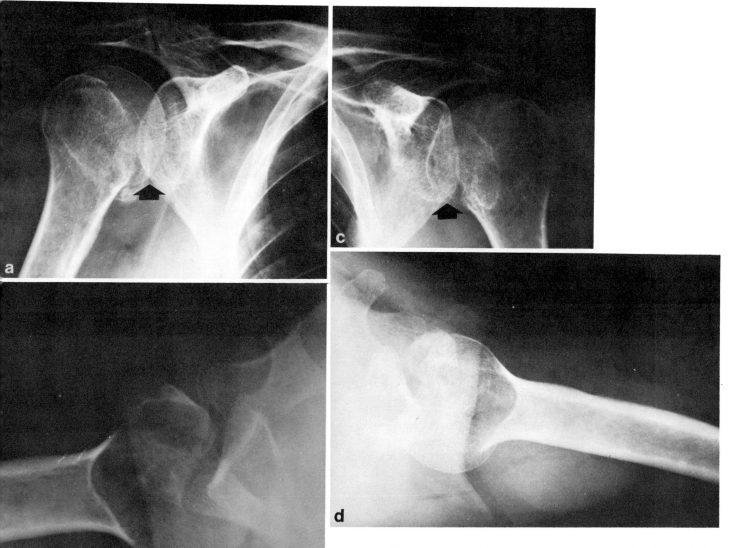

Fig. 4.26 Simultaneous, bilateral posterior fracture-dislocations of the shoulder. The significant radiographic signs, in the frontal projections **(a,c)**, are the ''trough line'' and narrowing **(a)** and obliteration **(c)** of the glenohumeral joint space (*arrows*). The posterior fracture-dislocations are clearly demonstrated in the axillary projections **(b,d)**.

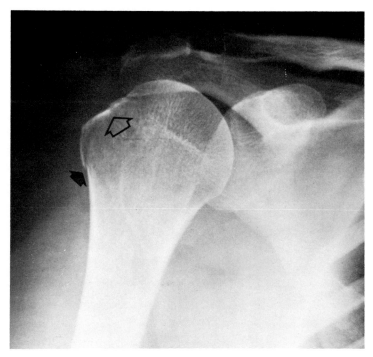

Fig. 4.27 Minimally displaced, impacted fracture of the greater tuberosity of the humerus. The *open arrow* indicates the flattened segment of the greater tuberosity. The *solid arrow* indicates the cortical fracture site.

Fractures of the proximal end of the humerus may involve the head, the greater tuberosity (Fig. 4.27) more frequently than the lesser, infrequently the anatomic neck (Fig. 4.28), and, commonly, the surgical neck (Figs. 4.29 and 4.30) and fracture-separation of the proximal humeral epiphysis (Fig. 4.31). The anatomic neck is the shallow groove or constriction just distal to the articular margin of the humeral head. The surgical neck is that constricted portion of the humerus situated distal to the level of the tuberosities and proximal to the insertion of the teres major and latissimus dorsi muscles. Neer (8) has prepared a current, detailed classification of proximal humeral fractures to which the reader is referred.

Minimally displaced fractures of the surgical neck occurring in patients in whom the proximal humeral epiphysis is not fused may not be recognized, the fracture line being misinterpreted to represent a segment of the epiphyseal line. However, a careful interpretation of the roentgenogram will reveal distinct differences between the characteristics of the fracture and the epiphyseal line (Fig. 4.32). The epiphyseal line can be recognized by its relatively constant location, the generally uniform width of the epiphyseal line throughout its extent, and its sclerotic margins.

The fracture, on the other hand, will be of varying width and its margins not sclerotic. The fragments may be distracted or impacted and overlapping of the fragments, or their cortical margins, may exist. Either the Cahoon or the axillary view is likely to show some degree of displacement of the fragments. Accurate comparison of the roentgen appearance of the injured shoulder with the contralateral normal shoulder may be necessary in order to accurately evaluate the proximal end of the humerus of the injured shoulder.

Nontraumatic Lesions

Nontraumatic conditions affecting the shoulder may produce acute, or severe, symptoms. One of the commonest of these is "bursitis," which may be inflammation of either a periarticular bursa or tendon. Frequently, periarticular soft tissue calcification associated with acute periarticular inflammation may resemble a thin cortical fracture fragment (Fig. 4.33). The roentgen characteristics of the calcific deposit and the absence of an acute traumatic history aid in establishing the true etiology of this soft tissue calcification.

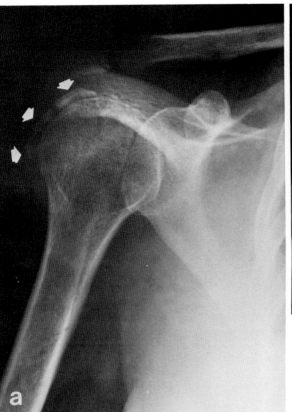

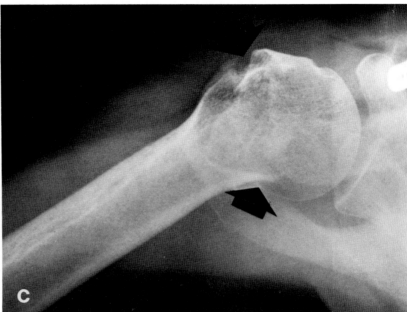

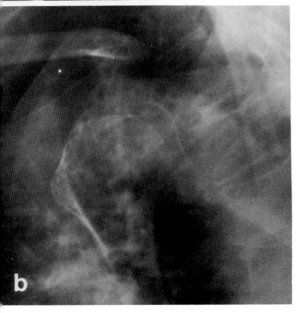

Fig. 4.28 Minimally displaced, impacted fracture of the anatomic neck of the humerus. In the internally rotated frontal projection **(a)**, thin cortical fragments (*arrows*) are present adjacent to the superolateral aspect of the humeral head. The anatomic neck fracture is not visible. None of the fractures are visible in the Cahoon ("through-the-chest") projection **(b)**. The axillary projection **(c)** demonstrates the slightly displaced, impacted anatomic neck fracture (*arrows*).

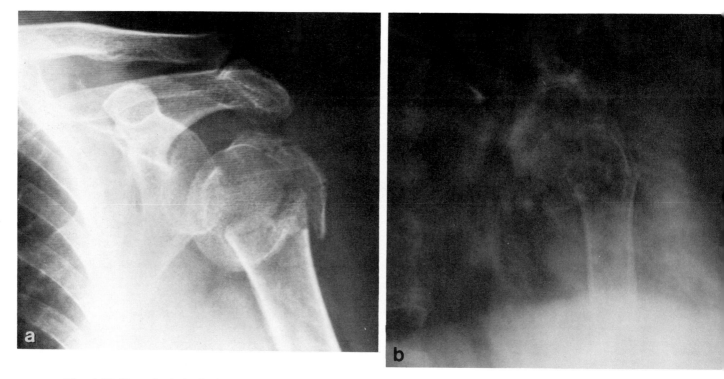

Fig. 4.29 Comminuted, displaced fracture of the surgical neck of the humerus seen in frontal **(a)** and Cahoon **(b)** projections.

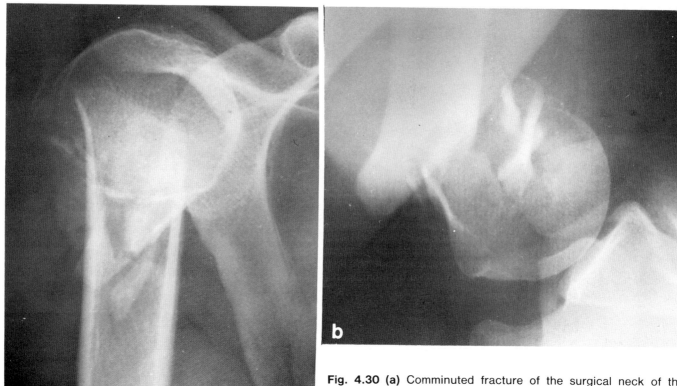

Fig. 4.30 (a) Comminuted fracture of the surgical neck of the rig humerus. The axillary view **(b)** shows the true extent of the displaceme of the major fragments.

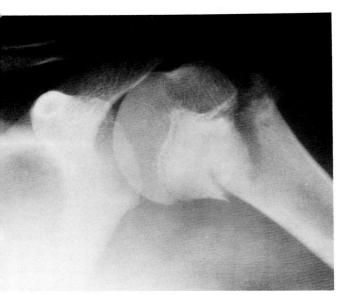

Fig. 4.31 Salter II epiphyseal injury of the proximal humerus.

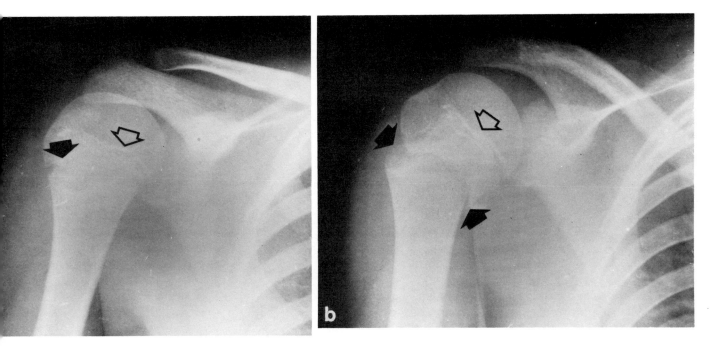

Fig. 4.32 Fracture of the proximal humeral metaphysis. In the internally rotated projection **(a)**, the fracture line (*solid arrow*) could be misinterpreted as the posterior arc of the epiphyseal line (*open arrow*). However, the externally rotated radiograph **(b)** clearly demonstrates the relationship between the epiphyseal line and the fracture line. Note the difference in the radiographic characteristics of the fracture line and epiphyseal line.

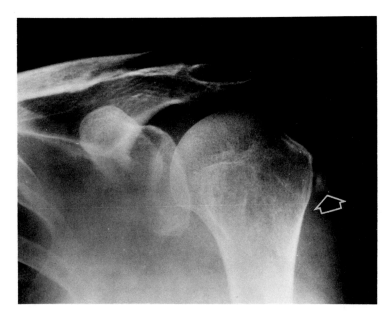

Fig. 4.33 Calcifying peritendinitis of the left shoulder. The soft tissue calcification indicated by the *solid arrow* simulates a thin cortical fragment seen "en face."

Pathologic fractures occurring in benign (Fig. 4.34) or malignant bone lesions may occur spontaneously or with minimal, commonly unrecognized trauma. These fractures may produce all the clinical signs and symptoms of an acute fracture of normal bone. Osteomyelitis of the humeral head (Fig. 4.35) and villonodular synovitis (Fig. 4.36) with involvement of the humeral head may produce a painful shoulder.

CLAVICLE

The radiographic examination of the clavicle consists of a straight anteroposterior projection and an anteroposterior projection with the central beam angled in a cephalad direction. Non- or minimally displaced fractures of the clavicle, poorly demonstrated in the straight frontal projection, will usually be seen in the angled view (Fig. 4.37). Occasionally, however, such a fracture may be difficult to recognize in each projection (Fig. 4.38). The presence of the fracture line on either examination, plus the physical findings, are sufficient to establish the diagnosis of a fracture.

Figure 4.39 demonstrates the typical deformity associated with mid-third clavicular fractures. The proximal fragment is displaced upward while the distal fragment is retracted inferiorly by the force of the pectoralis minor muscle and the weight of the upper extremity.

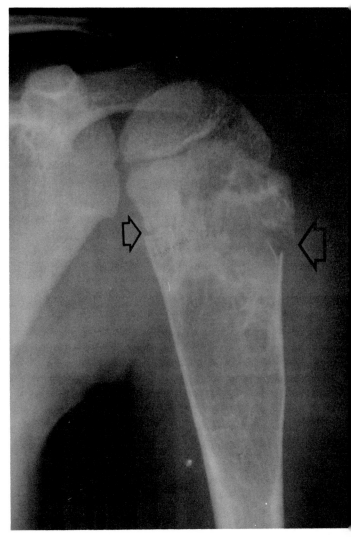

Fig. 4.34 Fracture through the wall of a benign lytic lesion in the proximal humeral metaphysis.

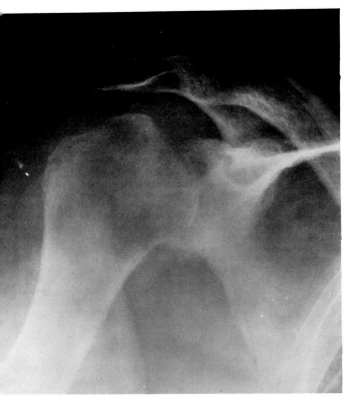

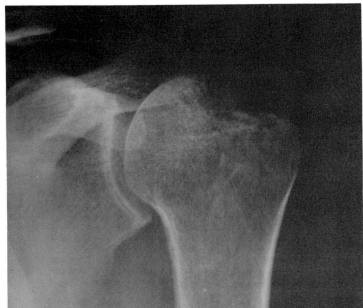

Fig. 4.35 Osteomyelitis of the humeral head. Note the irregular demineralization of the head and neck as well as destruction and erosion of the articulating surface of the head and glenoid fossa.

Fig. 4.36 Villonodular synovitis of the shoulder with erosion of the humeral head.

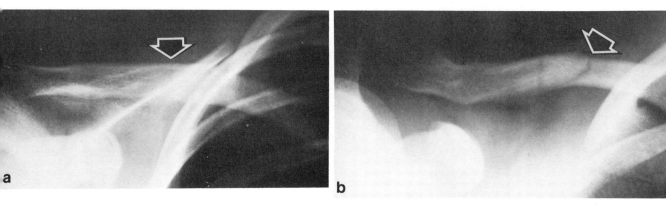

Fig. 4.37 The complete fracture in the mid-third of the right clavicle (*arrow*) can only be suspected in the straight anteroposterior projection (a). The presence of the fracture is clearly established, however, in the roentgenogram made with 15° cephalad angulation of the x-ray tube (b).

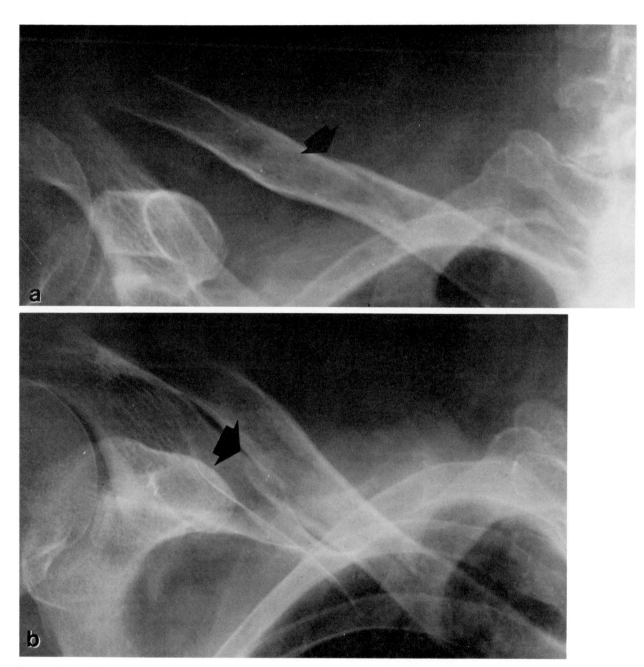

Fig. 4.38 (a,b) This subtle, minimally displaced fracture (*arrow*) in the mid-third of the clavicle is not well seen in either projection. However, the fact that portions of the fracture line can be seen in each projection indicates that it is a real finding.

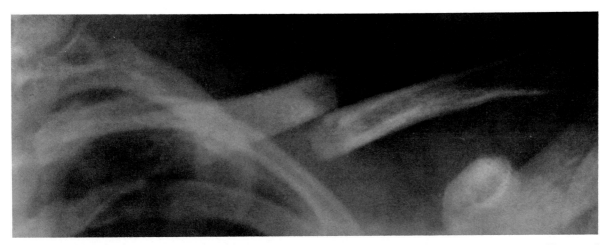

Fig. 4.39 Radiographic appearance of a typical, complete fracture in the mid-third of the clavicle. The proximal fragment usually overrides the distal fragment. The distal fragment is displaced inferiorly by the weight of the upper extremity and medially by the unopposed action of the muscular attachments from the clavicle to the anterior chest wall.

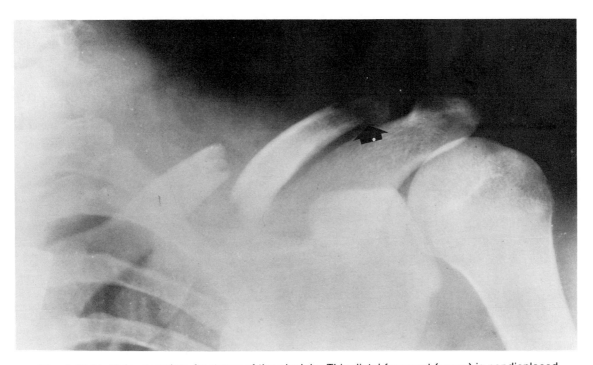

Fig. 4.40 Multiple, complete fractures of the clavicle. This distal fragment (*arrow*) is nondisplaced.

Outer third clavicular fractures are usually transverse and are usually nondisplaced (Fig. 4.40), the distal fragment being fixed by the acromioclavicular ligament and the proximal fragment by the coraco-clavicular ligament. If the distal end of the proximal fragment is elevated (Fig. 4.41), it indicates that the coracoclavicular ligament has been completely disrupted.

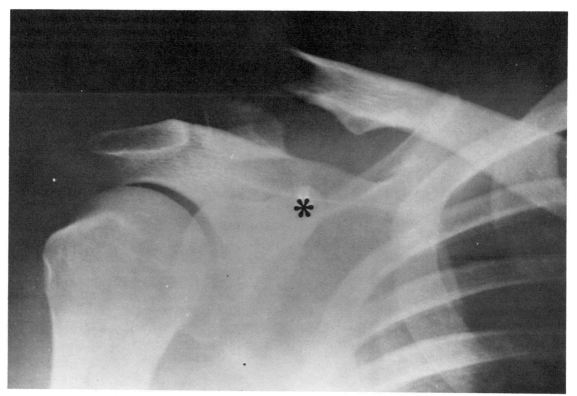

Fig. 4.41 Fracture of the lateral third of the clavicle resulting from severe force directed downward against the superolateral aspect of the shoulder. In this injury, the distal clavicular fragment retains its normal relationship to the acromium process and the acromioclavicular ligament is intact. The coracoclavicular ligament is disrupted, however, as evidenced by the increase in space between the coracoid process (*) and the clavicle.

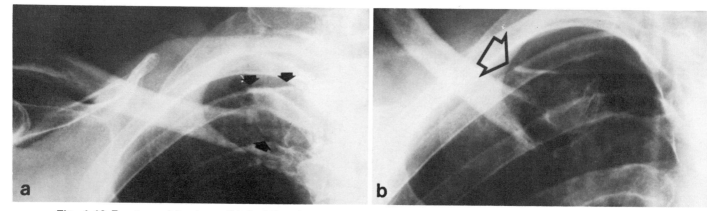

Fig. 4.42 Fracture of the inner third of the clavicle. Note that the fracture line is obscured by superimposed bony densities in both frontal (a) and oblique (b) projections.

Fractures of the inner third of the clavicle (Fig. 4.42) are uncommon and are particularly difficult to recognize because of the many superimposed bone shadows. Fractures close to the sternoclavicular joint may be demonstrable radiographically only by oblique views (Fig. 4.43) or by laminography. Computed tomography may be the most definitive procedure to diagnose subtle fractures, and dislocations, of the sternoclavicular joint. Because routine views of the clavicle may not demonstrate inner third fractures, and because special projections may be necessary to establish the diagnosis, it is critical that the clinical impression be transmitted to the radiologist in order that the appropriate views may be obtained.

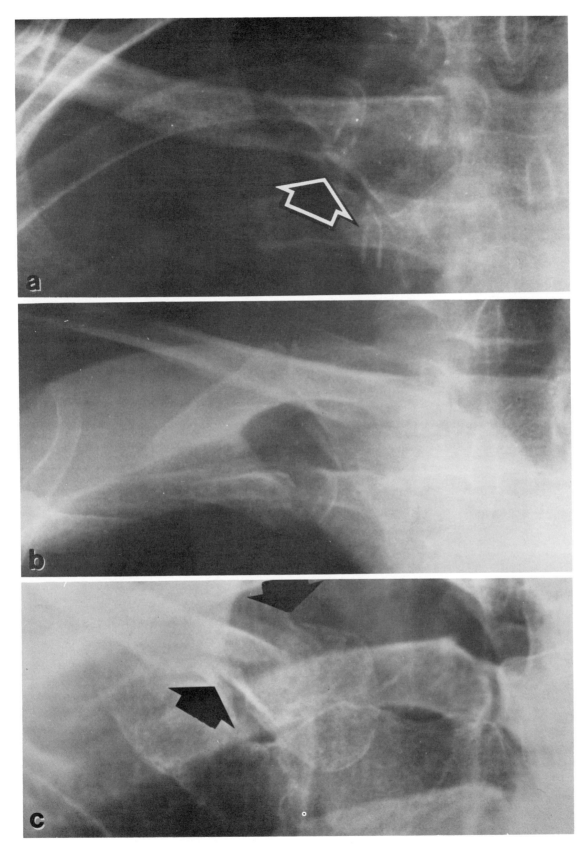

Fig. 4.43 Minimally displaced fracture of the inner third of the clavicle. Cortical irregularities (*arrow*) in the straight anteroposterior projection **(a)** merely suggest a fracture. The fracture is not visible in the roentgenogram made with the cephalically angled beam **(b)**. The fracture (*arrows*) is established only in the oblique projection **(c)**.

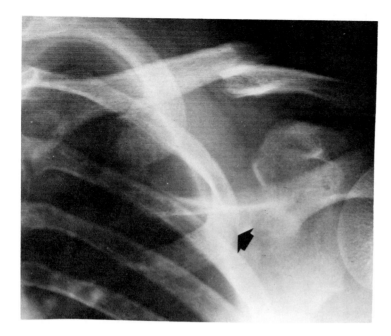

Fig. 4.44 The complete, displaced fracture in the mid-third of the clavicle is obvious. The associated, nondisplaced fracture in the second rib (*arrow*) is not readily apparent and could be overlooked.

Rib fractures may occur in association with fractures of the clavicle and may be masked, clinically, by the pain and deformity of the clavicular fracture. The physician must have a high index of suspicion for associated injury and must be satisfied that associated lesions have not been overlooked because of an obvious clavicular fracture (Fig. 4.44).

SCAPULA

Because the scapula is an integral part of the shoulder, many of the traumatic lesions affecting it, or the soft tissues related to it, have been previously discussed. In each of these instances, however, the scapula has not been the site of primary injury. This section deals with trauma affecting the scapula primarily.

The routine and special roentgen studies of the shoulder that have been previously described do not provide an adequate radiographic examination of the scapula. Therefore, when injury of the scapula is suspected, special scapular views must be obtained (4). These consist of anteroposterior (Fig. 4.45) and lateral (transcapular tangential, axial) (Fig. 4.46) projections.

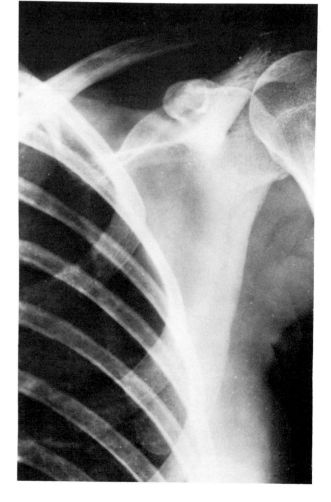

Fig. 4.45 Normal adult scapula seen in the frontal projection.

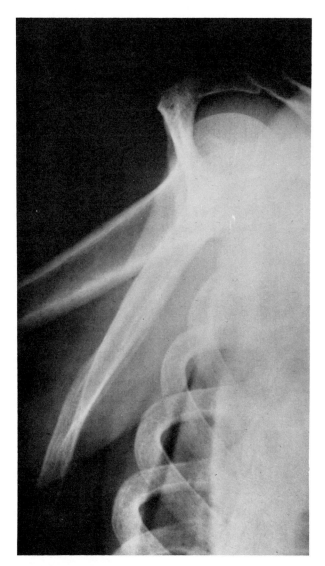

Fig. 4.46 Axial (tangential, lateral) projection of the normal adult scapula. Fractures occurring in the infraspinous portion of the scapula, which are frequently difficult to recognize in the anteroposterior projection of the scapula, are well seen in this view.

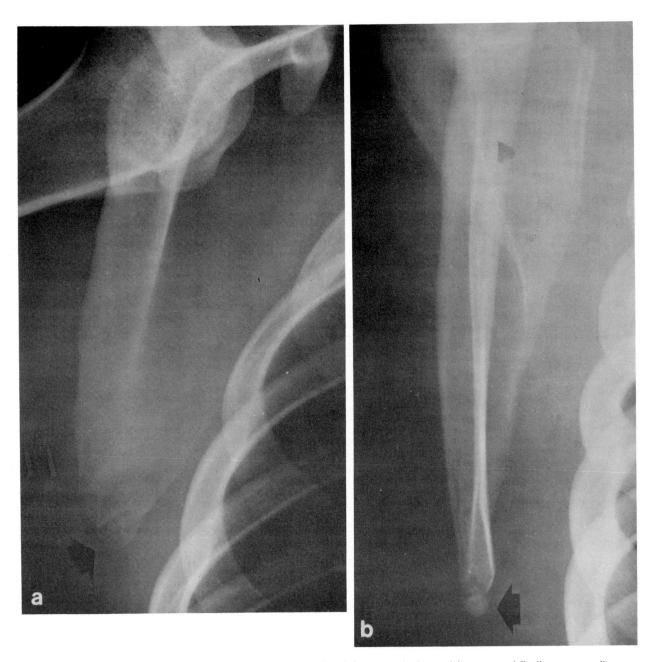

Fig. 4.47 (a, b) The ossification center at the inferior angle of the scapula (*arrow*) is a normal finding, generally seen between the ages of 15 and 25. It should not be misinterpreted as a fracture fragment. The location of the center and its smooth, sclerotic margins are characteristics that should help distinguish it from an acute fracture.

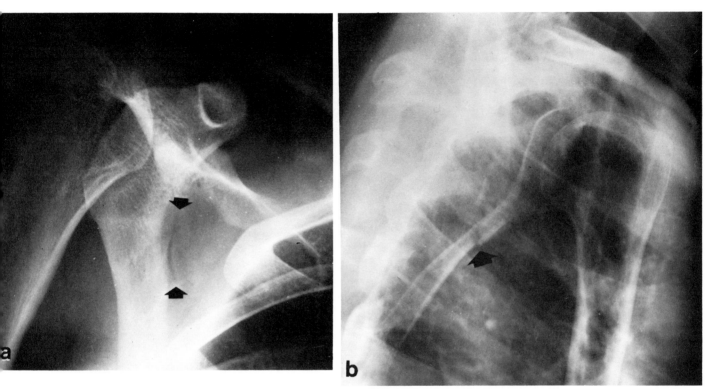

Fig. 4.48 The fracture line in the infraspinous portion of the scapula (*arrows*) is not well seen in the frontal projection (**a**); however, the fracture line is clearly identifiable in the lateral (Cahoon) view (**b**).

The secondary growth centers, their locations, and the radiographic characteristics of the epiphyseal lines must be considered when evaluating roentgenograms of the scapula of children and adolescents for fracture. The vertebral border ossifies from two centers, one in the middle and one at the inferior angle. The latter may not unite with the infraspinous portion of the scapula until age 25 years, and thus may simulate a fracture fragment. The typical radiographic appearance of this center is seen in Figure 4.47.

Fractures of the body of the scapula usually result from a direct, crushing-type injury (9). Fractures of the infraspinous portion, even when severely displaced, are notoriously difficult to identify in the anteroposterior view, but are clearly delineated in either the Cahoon (Fig. 4.48) or the axial view (Fig. 4.49).

Incomplete, nondisplaced fractures of the glenoid fossa may be difficult to identify on the plain roentgenograms of the shoulder but are usually clearly discernible on laminographic examinations (Fig. 4.50).

Fracture of the coracoid process is a rare injury (9–11), but probably occurs more frequently than has been reported. The reason for this is the fact that the coracoid process projects almost directly anteriorly in the routine frontal examinations of the shoulder. Consequently, the long axis of the coracoid process is essentially parallel to the central beam and, unless the coracoid fragments are grossly displaced, they are usually not visible on frontal examinations of the shoulder. Fractures of the coracoid process are clearly delineated in the axillary projection, however (Figs. 4.51 and 4.6).

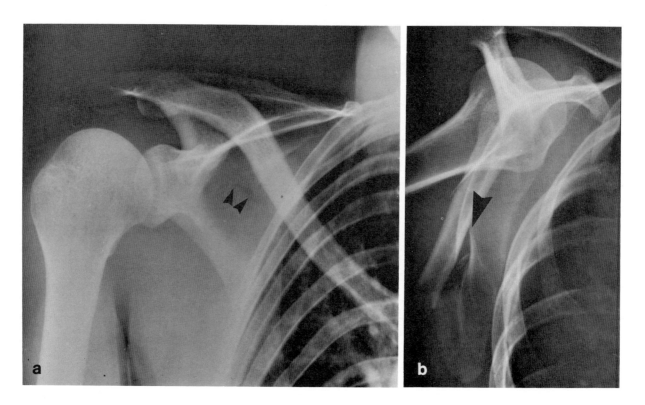

Fig. 4.49 The fracture line in the infraspinous portion of the scapula is barely perceptible in the frontal projection **(a)**. This fracture is represented by a vague radiolucent, slightly curvilinear, defect paralleling the sweep of the inferior margin of the clavicle (*arrowheads*). The axillary view **(b)**, however, clearly defines a comminuted, grossly displaced fracture.

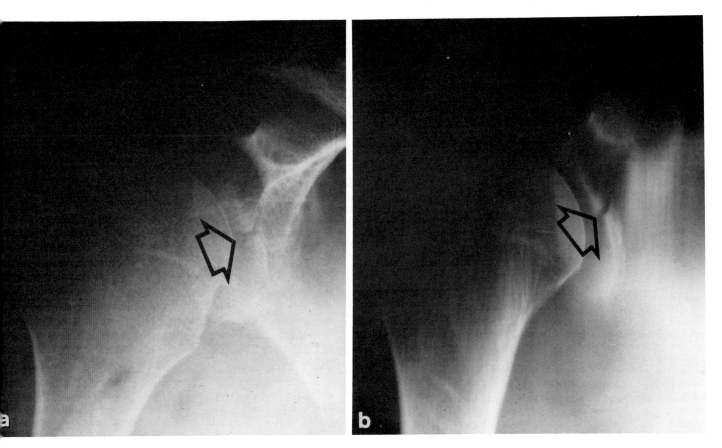

Fig. 4.50 The incomplete, nondisplaced fracture of the glenoid fossa, which is only vaguely seen on the routine roentgenogram **(a)**, is clearly delineated on the laminogram of the shoulder **(b)**.

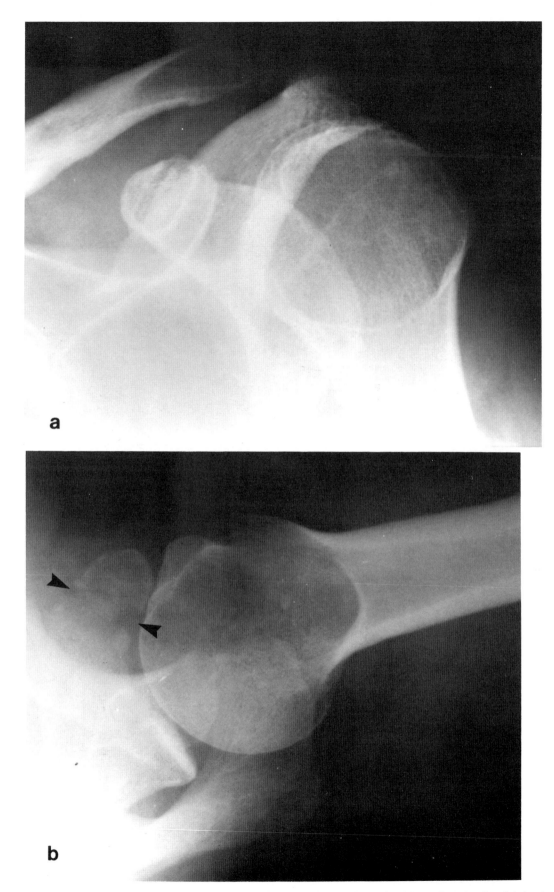

Fig. 4.51 Fracture of the coracoid process of the scapula. In the internally rotated frontal projection **(a)** the fracture is not discernible. In the axillary projection **(b)**, however, the transverse, slightly displaced and distracted fracture is clearly evident (*arrowheads*).

References

1. CAVE EF, BURKE JF, BOYD RJ: *Trauma Management.* Year Book Medical Publishers, Chicago, 1974.
2. CONWELL HE, REYNOLDS FC: *Key and Conwell's Management of Fractures, Dislocations and Sprains*, ed. 7. C.V. Mosby, St. Louis, Mo., 1961.
3. HILL HA, SACHS MD: The grooved defect of the humeral head: A frequently unrecognized complication of dislocations of the shoulder joint. *Radiology* 35:690, 1940.
4. PAVLOV H, FREIBERGER RH: Fractures and dislocations about the shoulder. *Semin Roentgenol* 13:85, 1978.
5. ARNDT JH, SEARS AD: Posterior dislocation of the shoulder. *AJR* 94:369, 1964.
6. FIGIEL SJ, FIGIEL LS, BARDENSTEIN MB, BLODGETT WH: Posterior dislocation of the shoulder. *Radiology* 87:737, 1966.
7. CISTERNINO SJ, ROGERS LF, STUFFLEBAM BD, KRUGLIK GD: The trough line: A radiographic sign of posterior shoulder dislocation. *AJR* 130:951, 1978.
8. NEER C: Displaced proximal humeral fractures. *J. Bone Joint Surg* 52-A:1077, 1970.
9. ROWE CR: Fractures of the scapula. *Surg Clin North Am* 43:1565, 1963.
10. IMATANI RJ: Fractures of the scapula: A review of 53 cases. *Trauma* 15:473, 1975.
11. FINDLAY RT: Fractures of the scapula and ribs. *Am J Surg* 38:489, 1937.

chapter five

Elbow

General Considerations

Precision in positioning the arm for the lateral radiograph of the elbow is of paramount importance, particularly in evaluating the position of the fragments of a supracondylar fracture. Minor degrees of obliquity or rotation in the lateral view will result in an examination that may be misleading because it may 1) obscure a minimally or nondisplaced fracture, 2) obscure positive olecranon fat pad signs, or 3) incorrectly reflect the alignment of the fragments.

The radiologist or the attending physician must be particularly critical of the lateral radiograph made immediately following the reduction of a supracondylar fracture. The acutely flexed position of the elbow and the posterior plaster splint which is commonly employed combine to make a true lateral roentgenogram difficult to obtain. An improperly positioned lateral radiograph made following reduction may lead to unnecessary attempts to reduce an already adequately reduced fracture. Conversely, the fragments may appear to be in satisfactory alignment when a correctly positioned lateral examination would show this to be untrue. Therefore, anything less than an optimum lateral radiograph of the elbow is unacceptable.

As in the radiographic examination of the other peripheral joints, the roentgenograms of the injured elbow may be equivocal because of the appearance of epiphyseal lines and epiphyses or because of the appearance of the normal soft tissue shadows about the elbow. In this instance, it is frequently helpful to obtain frontal and lateral radiographs of the opposite, uninvolved elbow for comparison purposes. In the interest of reducing unnecessary radiation exposure, it is no longer recommended that the opposite peripheral joint be examined *routinely*.

Radiographic Examination

The routine radiographic examination of the elbow includes anteroposterior, lateral, and each oblique projections. The anteroposterior and oblique views should be made with the arm extended as much as possible. In order to obtain a true lateral projection, the forearm should be flexed upon the arm 90° and should be positioned midway between pronation and supination with the thumb pointing upward.

Acute trauma to the elbow may prevent complete extension, thereby making it impossible to obtain a satisfactory examination in the frontal projection because, with the elbow flexed, the proximal radius and distal humerus become superimposed. Consequently, fractures of the radial head or distal humerus may be obscured and overlooked. When the elbow is partially flexed, it is possible to obtain a satisfactory frontal view of the proximal radius and ulna by placing the forearm on the radiographic table in the supine position and a satisfactory anteroposterior projection of the distal humerus with the arm resting upon the x-ray table. In each instance, the x-ray tube is angled 10° toward the joint.

Radiographic Anatomy

The radiographic appearance of the normal adult elbow in frontal and lateral projections is demonstrated in Figure 5.1. In the anteroposterior projection (Fig. 5.1a), note particularly the smooth, gentle, continuous concave sweep of the cortex from the neck to the head of the radius. Any disruption of this smooth arc is abnormal and, with the appropriate history and clinical findings, represents an acute fracture. The appearance of the normal radial neck cortex is particularly well demonstrated in anteroposterior (Fig. 5.2)

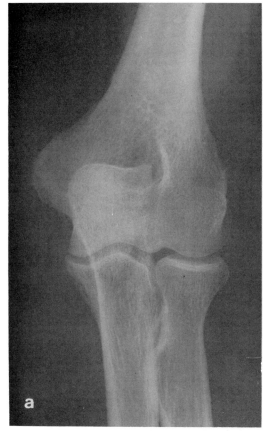

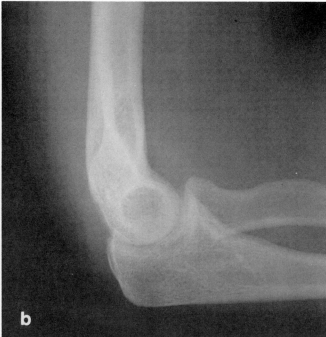

Fig. 5.1. Routine anteroposterior **(a)** and lateral **(b)** radiographs of a normal adult elbow. In the frontal projection, note the relationship between the articulating surface of the radius and the capitellum and the articulating surface of the coronoid process and the trochlea. Note, also, in the frontal projection, the normal smooth concave cortical sweep from the radial neck to the radial head. In the lateral projection **(b)**, note that the image of the coronoid process is superimposed upon the image of the radial head and that the soft tissue density about the elbow is homogeneous.

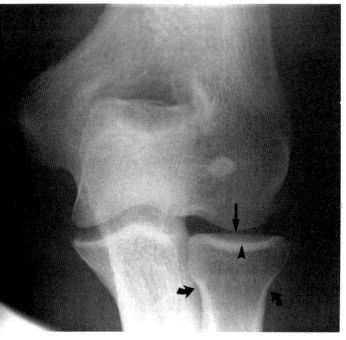

Fig. 5.2. Anteroposterior radiograph of a normal adult elbow. The radial neck cortical surface (*curved arrows*) is smoothly, gently, and continuously concave from the radial shaft to the base of the radial head. The concave proximal radial articulating surface produces a double cortical shadow in the frontal projection. The *stemmed arrow* indicates the rim and the *arrowhead* the concavity of the proximal radial articulating surface.

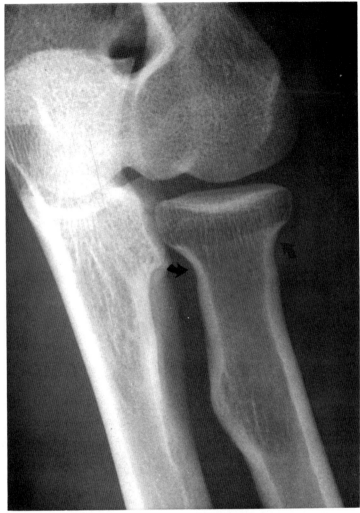

Fig. 5.3. Oblique radiograph of a normal adult elbow which demonstrates the normal concavity of the radial neck (*arrows*). (Compare with Fig. 5.28.) The radiolucency of the radial head is reflective of relatively thin cortex of the head.

and oblique (Fig. 5.3) projections. The cortex of the radial neck constitutes a smooth, continuous, graceful concave arc extending from the radial shaft to the base of the radial head. Any alteration of this configuration, including nothing more than a slight angulation, must be considered abnormal and, with a history of acute trauma, indicative of a radial neck fracture.

The concave surface of the radial head accounts for the double cortical margin normally seen in the frontal projection (Fig. 5.2).

In the lateral projection (Fig. 5.1b), the soft tissue density anterior and posterior to the distal humerus is usually homogeneous. Occasionally, however, the anterior distal humeral fat pad may normally be visible immediately adjacent to the cortex of the humerus.

The roentgen appearance of the normal elbow of an adolescent is seen in Figure 5.4.

The radiographic appearance of the normal child's elbow is seen in Figure 5.5. During this phase of development, only the capitellar epiphysis is ossified. A frequent misconception, based upon the appearance of the lateral projection of the elbow of young children, is that the capitellar epiphysis relates to the olecranon fossa of the ulna. The fact that the capitellum relates to the proximal end of the radius is clearly verified by the frontal projection (Fig. 5.5a).

Radiographic Manifestations of Trauma

Soft tissue changes are of singular diagnostic importance in trauma of the elbow and may often be the

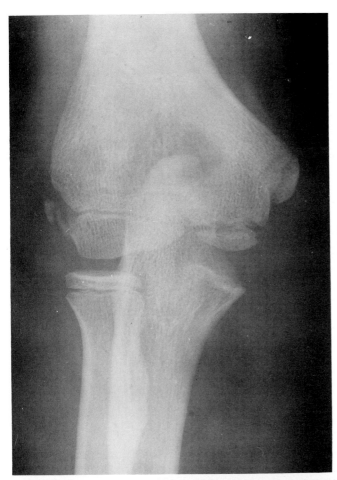

Fig. 5.4. Normal elbow of an adolescent patient showing epiphyseal and apophyseal lines that may simulate fracture lines.

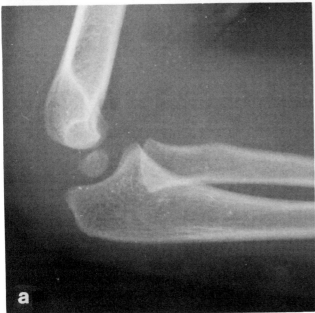

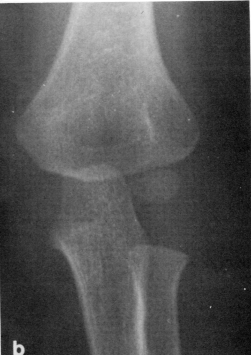

Fig. 5.5. Normal lateral projection of a 5-year-old patient (a). The apparent relationship between the capitellar epiphysis and the semilunar notch is a radiographic illusion since the capitellum actually relates to the radius (b).

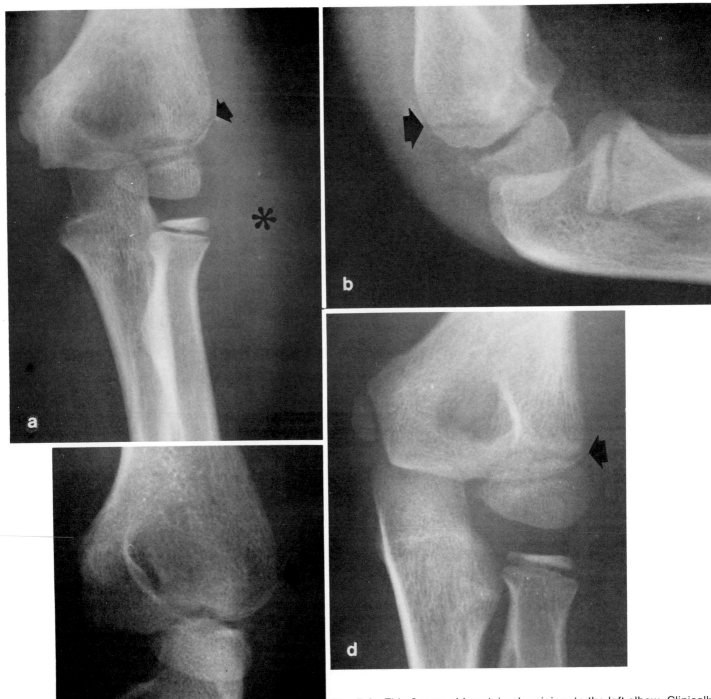

Fig. 5.6. This 8-year-old sustained an injury to the left elbow. Clinically, the elbow was swollen, painful, and tender. There was no limitation of motion. A subtle fracture is present in the lateral epicondylar metaphysis of the humerus. This fracture line is visible in all views but could be misinterpreted as an "epiphyseal line" or, in the anteroposterior (a) and oblique (c, d) views, as a relative radiolucency produced by superimposition of the capitellar epiphysis on the metaphysis. The soft tissue swelling along the lateral aspect of the elbow (*), the location of the fracture line in the lateral projection (b), and the capitellar epiphyseal subluxation clearly establish the true nature of this bony injury.

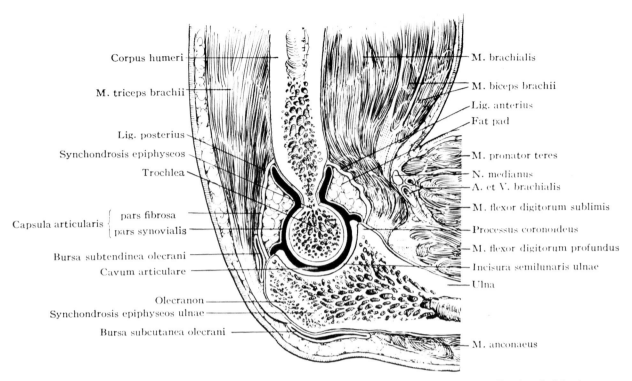

Corpus humeri

M. triceps brachii

Lig. posterius

Synchondrosis epiphyseos

Trochlea

Capsula articularis { pars fibrosa
pars synovialis

Bursa subtendinea olecrani

Cavum articulare

Olecranon

Synchondrosis epiphyseos ulnae

Bursa subcutanea olecrani

M. brachialis

M. biceps brachii

Lig. anterius

Fat pad

M. pronator teres

N. medianus

A. et V. brachialis

M. flexor digitorum sublimis

Processus coronoideus

M. flexor digitorum profundus

Incisura semilunaris ulnae

Ulna

M. anconaeus

Fig. 5.7. Sagittal section through the elbow showing the fat pad anterior and posterior to the distal end of the humerus lying outside the joint capsule. (Reprinted with permission from C.L. Callander: *Surgical Anatomy,* ed. 2. W. B. Saunders, Philadelphia, 1948.)

most obvious radiographic abnormality. Extracapsular soft tissue swelling may be diffuse, as in the instance of a supracondylar fracture (Fig. 5.6), or localized to the medial aspect of the elbow, such as with avulsion of the medial epicondylar apophysis (Fig. 5.13a).

The fat pad sign (1, 2) is an invaluable soft tissue finding in cases of intracapsular injury of the elbow. The anatomy about the distal end of the humerus is seen in Figure 5.7. Fat is present about the proximal part of the elbow joint capsule. Normally, the extrasynovial, intracapsular fat is "hidden" in the concavity of the olecranon and coronoid fossae and is usually not visible on the lateral radiograph of the normal elbow, except for a small amount which may be visible anterior to the coronoid fossa.

Injuries that produce intra-articular hemorrhage cause distention of the synovium. Concomitantly, the fat is forced out of the fossae, producing triangular-shaped radiolucent shadows anterior and posterior to the distal end of the humerus (Fig. 5.8), referred to as the "olecranon fat pad" sign. When present in a patient with a history of acute trauma to the elbow, the olecranon fat pad sign indicates the presence of an intra-articular hemorrhage, which in turn is almost

invariably (>90%) (3) associated with an intra-articular skeletal injury. When the olecranon fat pad sign was first described, it was thought to be specific for intra-articular hemorrhage (4). Subsequently, a positive fat pad sign has been observed in association with intra-articular fluid collections of nontraumatic origin (3).

Subluxation of the radial head in children usually occurs between the ages of 2 and 4 years and is a relatively common injury caused by forcible traction on the extended forearm. This injury usually occurs when the child is lifted by the hand or wrist with the upper extremity extended over the head. Clinically, the elbow is painful and the arm dangles at the side in the attitude of pronation. Supination is painful and restricted while flexion and extension are free. The diagnosis of subluxation of the radial head must be made on the basis of the clinical findings. Since the radial head epiphysis is not ossified at this age, subluxation of the radial head will not be visible radiographically (5). Therefore, radiographic examination of the elbow is not indicated when the clinical impression is subluxation of the radial head.

Dislocations of the elbow are reported to be second in frequency only to the shoulder dislocations (6). The

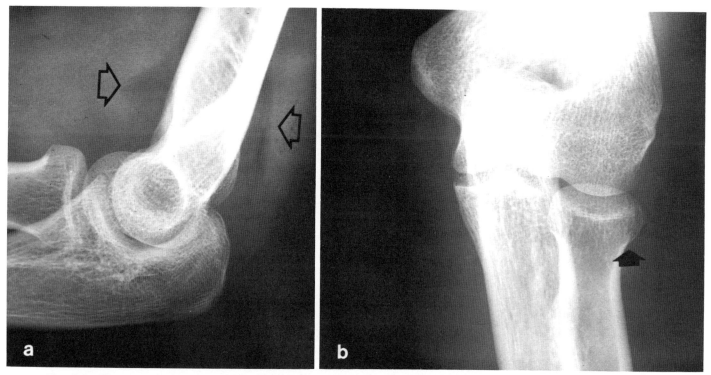

Fig. 5.8. The typical roentgen configuration and appearance of the anterior and posterior olecranon fat pad signs (*open arrows*) in the lateral radiograph **(a)**. This very prominent soft tissue finding signals the extremely subtle cortical disruption at the junction of the radial head and neck (*solid arrow*) seen in the frontal projection **(b)**.

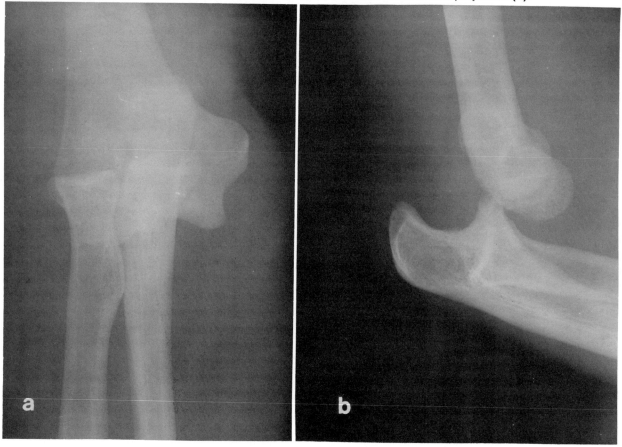

Fig. 5.9. (a, b) Complete posterior dislocation of the elbow.

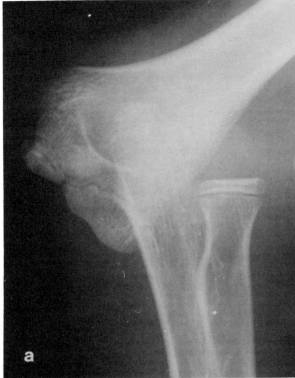

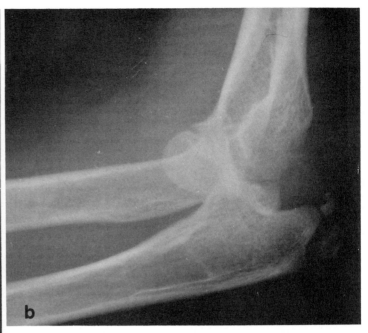

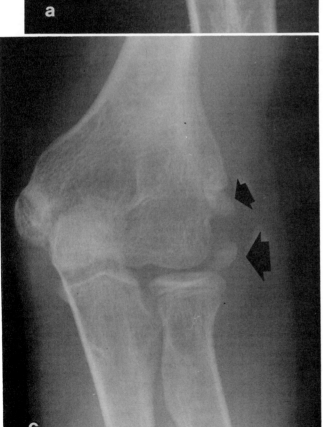

Fig. 5.10. Complete posterior dislocation of the elbow associated with separation of the medial epicondylar apophysis. In both the frontal (a) and lateral (b) projections, the dislocation is obvious, but there is no evidence of associated fracture or epiphyseal or apophyseal separation. Separation of the fractured medial epicondylar apophysis is evident only in the postreduction frontal projection (c).

commonest dislocation of the elbow consists of posterior displacement of the radius and ulna (Fig. 5.9).

Fractures or epiphyseal or apophyseal separations associated with a dislocation may not be discernible on the initial studies. Avulsion fractures of the coronoid process, subtle radial head fractures, and separations of the medial epicondylar apophysis may be recognized only on postreduction films. The pain of these injuries may be masked by the discomfort attributable to the dislocation itself. In order that such injuries be recognized as soon as possible, postreduction roentgenograms must be made routinely, preferably in multiple projections and prior to application of any immobilization device (Figs. 5.10 and 5.11).

Separation of the medial epicondylar apophysis is a common injury in adolescent children (Figs. 5.12 and 5.13). Because this lesion frequently involves the throwing arm of young baseball players, separation of the medial epicondylar apophysis is referred to as "little leaguer's elbow." The degree of separation may be so slight (Fig. 5.14) as to require comparison with the normal opposite elbow in order to establish the diagnosis. The usual appearance of the separation,

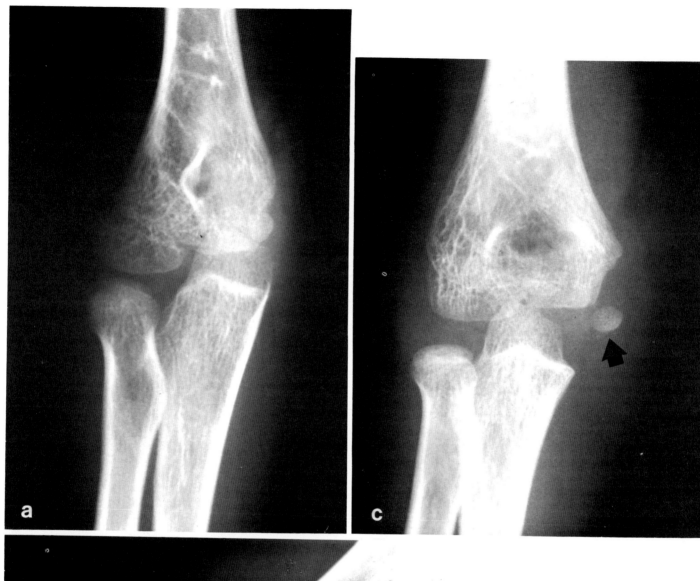

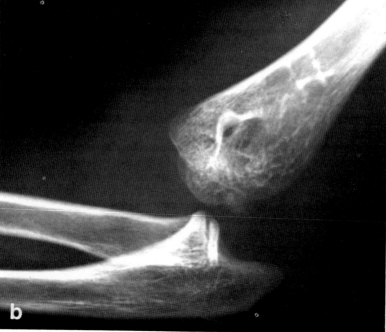

Fig. 5.11. Posterior dislocation of the elbow seen in frontal **(a)** and lateral **(b)** projections. There is no indication of the separated and displaced medial epicondylar apophysis (*arrow*) which is evident in the postreduction frontal radiograph **(c)** in either of the prereduction examinations.

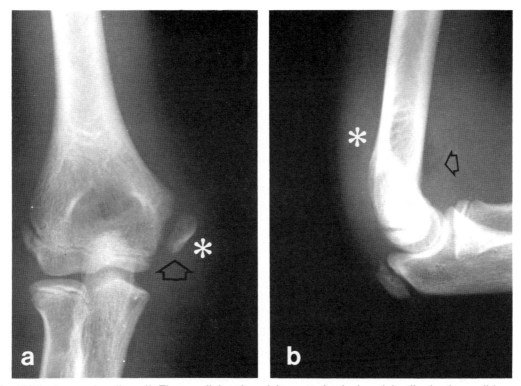

Fig. 5.12. "Little leaguer's elbow." The medial epicondylar apophysis is minimally (and possibly equivocally) separated (*open arrow*) in the anteroposterior radiograph of the elbow **(a)**. In the lateral projection **(b)**, the presence of the anterior olecranon fat pad sign (*open arrow*), indicating the presence of an intra-articular effusion (hemorrhage), provides strong supportive evidence that the apophysis is actually separated.

however, is seen in Figure 5.14. Depending upon the direction and magnitude of the force producing the separation, the medial epicondylar apophysis may be displaced anteriorly (Fig. 5.15), posteriorly (Fig. 5.16), or into the joint space between the trochlea and the coronoid process of the ulna (Fig. 5.17). In addition to the skeletal abnormality involving the medial apophysis, extracapsular soft tissue swelling is invariably present about the medial aspect of the elbow (Figs. 5.12–5.14). Because the medial epicondylar apophysis is an intracapsular structure, intra-articular hemorrhage secondary to its separation produces a positive olecranon fat pad sign (Fig. 5.12*b*).

Incomplete or minimally displaced supracondylar fractures of the humerus may be extremely difficult to recognize radiographically. The olecranon fat pad sign is usually the most obvious roentgen manifesta-

tion of this fracture and adds compelling significance to the subtle distal humeral abnormality (Figs. 5.18 and 5.19).

Displaced supracondylar fractures will be radiographically obvious in at least one projection (Fig. 5.20). The potential for vascular compromise (Fig. 5.21), culminating in Volkmann's contracture, exists in every displaced supracondylar fracture. As stressed previously, great care in positioning the elbow is required to ensure that pre- and postreduction roentgenograms accurately depict the alignment of the fragments of this fracture.

Although the fracture of the coronoid process of the ulna may occur as an isolated injury, it is usually associated with posterior dislocation or fracture-dislocation of the elbow (Fig. 5.22).

Radial head fractures may be classified as 1) linear,

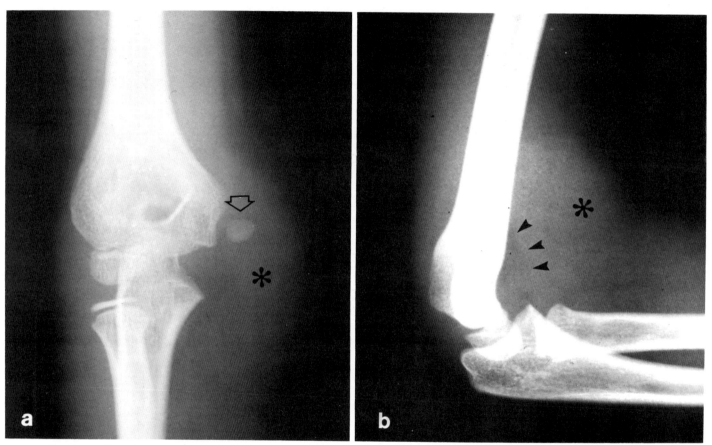

Fig. 5.13. Soft tissue swelling (*), localized to the medial aspect of the elbow, is the most striking roentgen sign of avulsion of the medial epicondylar apophysis (*open arrow*) in the frontal projection **(a)**. In the lateral radiograph **(b)**, diffuse soft tissue is present anteriorly (*) and the anterior olecranon fat pad sign (*arrowheads*), indicating an intra-articular hemorrhage, is evident.

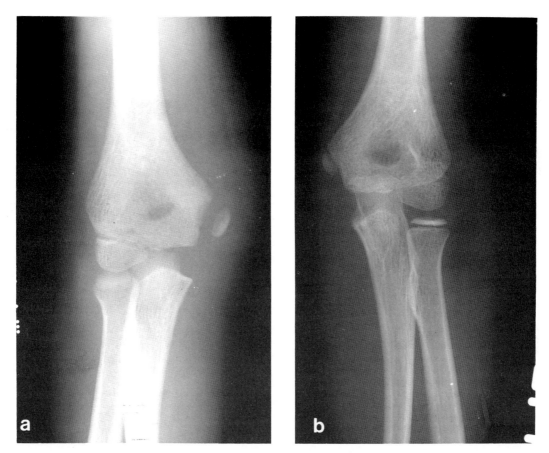

Fig. 5.14. This is the usual radiographic appearance of separation of the medial epicondylar apophysis as seen in frontal projection **(a)**. Note that the apophysis is clearly abnormally medially separated from the base of the adjacent metaphysis and that soft tissue swelling is present about the medial aspect of the elbow. The opposite elbow **(b)** is shown for comparison.

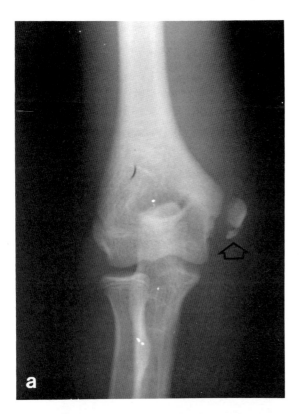

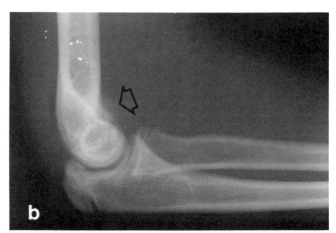

Fig. 5.15. Anterior displacement of the medial epicondylar apophysis (*open arrow*) is indicated in the lateral projection **(b)**. The fragmentation of the apophysis seen in the frontal projection **(a)** probably is developmental.

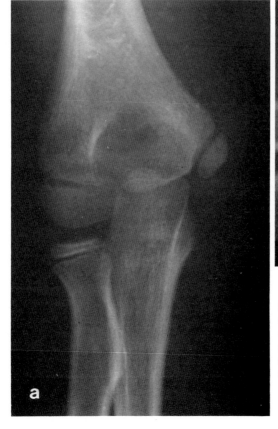

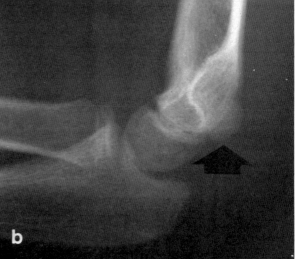

Fig. 5.16. Posterior displacement of the medial epicondylar apophysis. In the frontal projection **(a)**, the only clue of the bony abnormality is the soft tissue swelling about the medial portion of the elbow. The posterior displacement of the apophysis is indicated by the *solid arrow* in the lateral projection **(b)**.

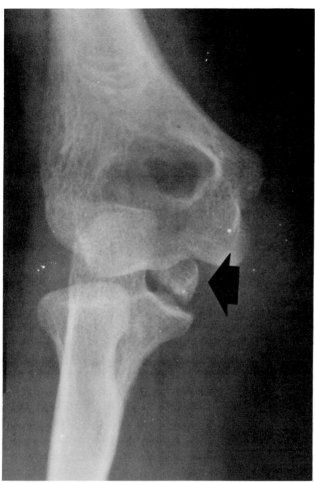

Fig. 5.17. Separation of the medial epicondylar apophysis associated with dislocation of the elbow. The radius and ulna are laterally dislocated with respect to the humerus. The *solid arrow* indicates the medial epicondylar apophysis which is severely displaced and which lies between the articulating surfaces of the trochlea and the coronoid process of the ulna. This degree of apophyseal displacement can only be found in association with dislocation of the elbow.

Fig. 5.18. In the lateral projection (a), the non-displaced supracondylar fracture line is indicated by the *solid arrow*. The *open arrow* emphasizes the olecranon fat pad sign which heralds the presence of significant intra-articular injury. The oblique projection (b) confirms the presence of the supracondylar fracture.

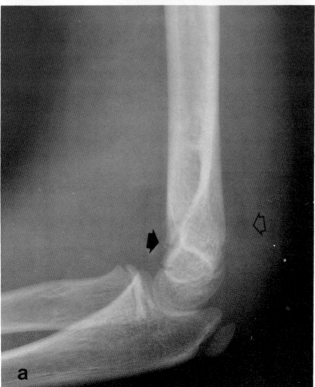

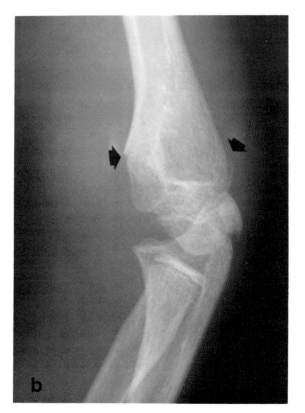

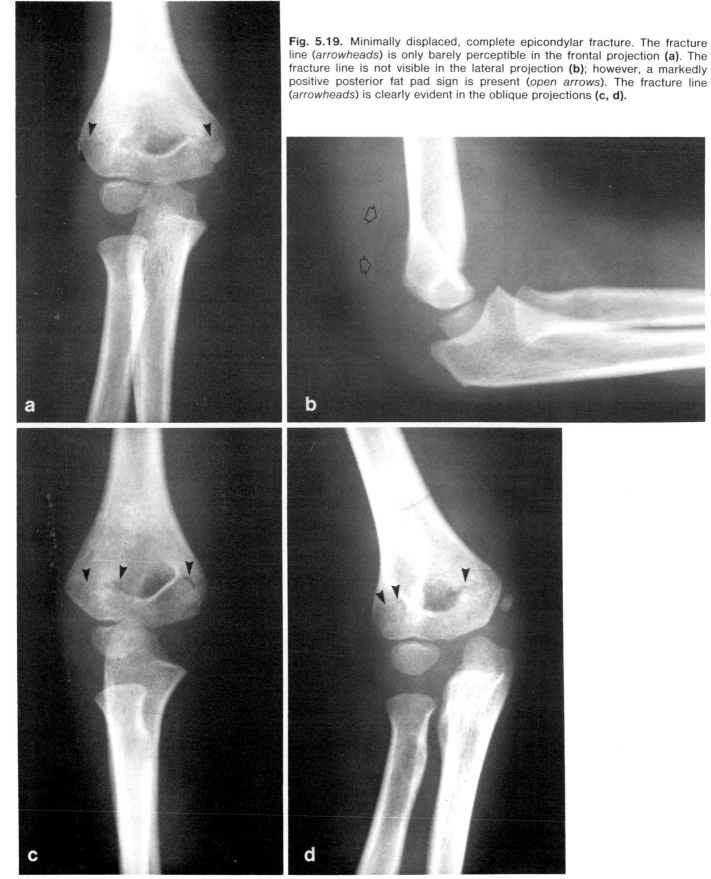

Fig. 5.19. Minimally displaced, complete epicondylar fracture. The fracture line (*arrowheads*) is only barely perceptible in the frontal projection **(a)**. The fracture line is not visible in the lateral projection **(b)**; however, a markedly positive posterior fat pad sign is present (*open arrows*). The fracture line (*arrowheads*) is clearly evident in the oblique projections **(c, d)**.

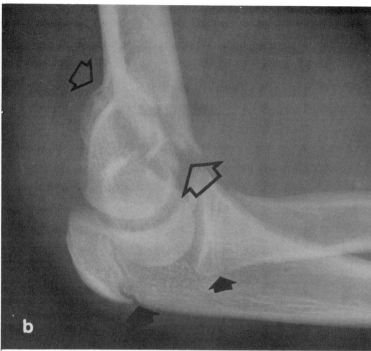

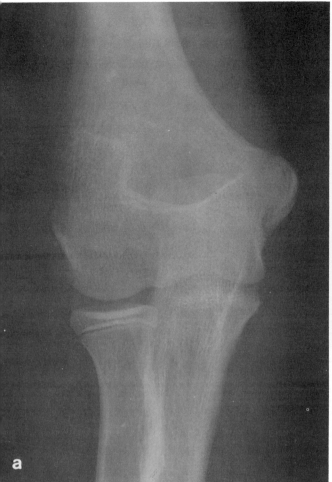

Fig. 5.20. The frontal projection **(a)** of the elbow of this patient gives little indication of the presence of a supracondylar fracture. The lateral projection **(b)** of the same patient clearly demonstrates the displaced supracondylar fracture (*open arrows*). The solid arrows indicate the proximal radial epiphysis and the olecranon apophyseal lines, which should not be mistaken for fracture lines.

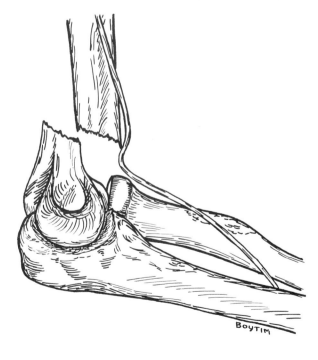

Fig. 5.21. Schematic representation of the effect of an unreduced supracondylar fracture upon the brachial artery.

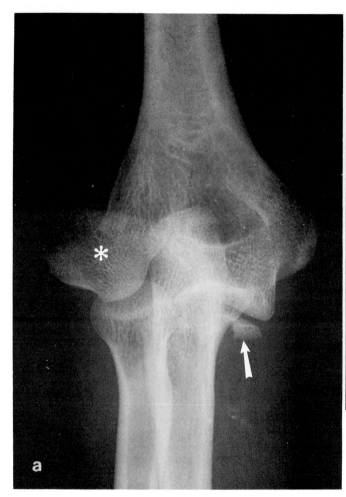

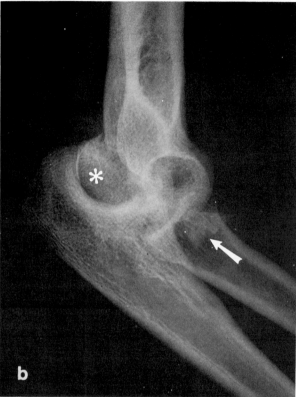

Fig. 5.22. This patient sustained a comminuted fracture-dislocation of the elbow. The capitellum (*) is displaced laterally and posteriorly. The small fragment (*arrow*) distal to the trochlea in the frontal view **(a)** and superimposed upon the radial head in the lateral projection **(b)** arises from the coronoid process of the ulna.

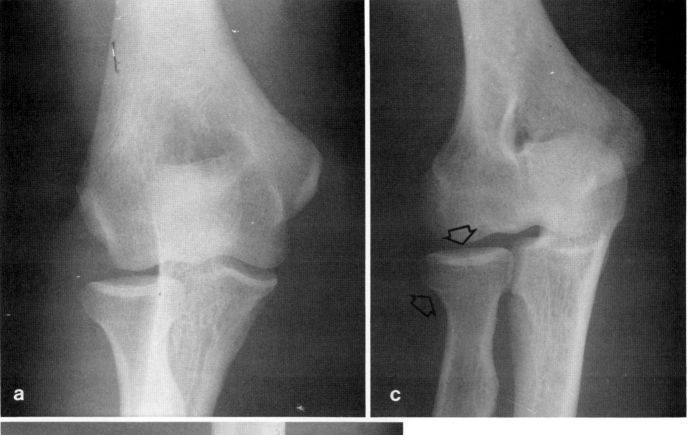

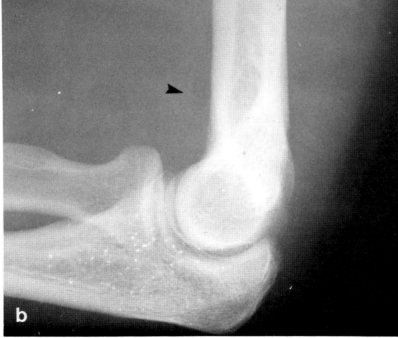

Fig. 5.23. Subtle, minimally depressed fracture of the radial head. The fracture is not visible in either the frontal **(a)** or lateral **(b)** projection. A very faint, abnormal anterior fat pad sign (*arrowhead*) is present in the lateral radiograph. The fracture line in the articulating surface of the radial head and the cortical impaction at the base of the head (*open arrows*) are evident only in the externally rotated oblique projection **(c)**. This patient emphasizes the importance of frontal, lateral, and oblique views in the evaluation of injuries of peripheral joints.

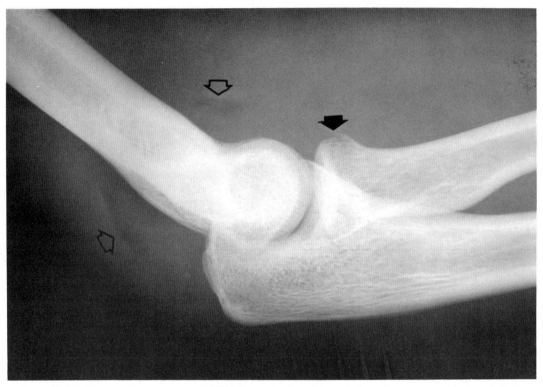

Fig. 5.24. Marginal fracture of the radial head (*solid arrow*). The fat pad signs (*open arrows*) signal the presence of the intra-articular fracture.

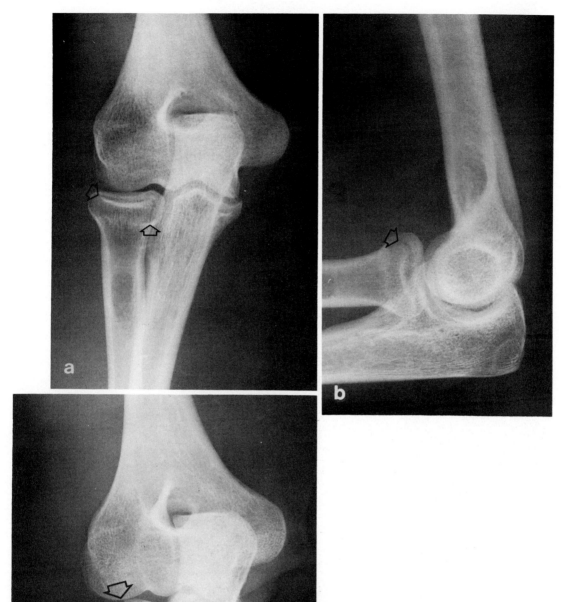

Fig. 5.25. (a–c) Depressed fracture of the radial head.

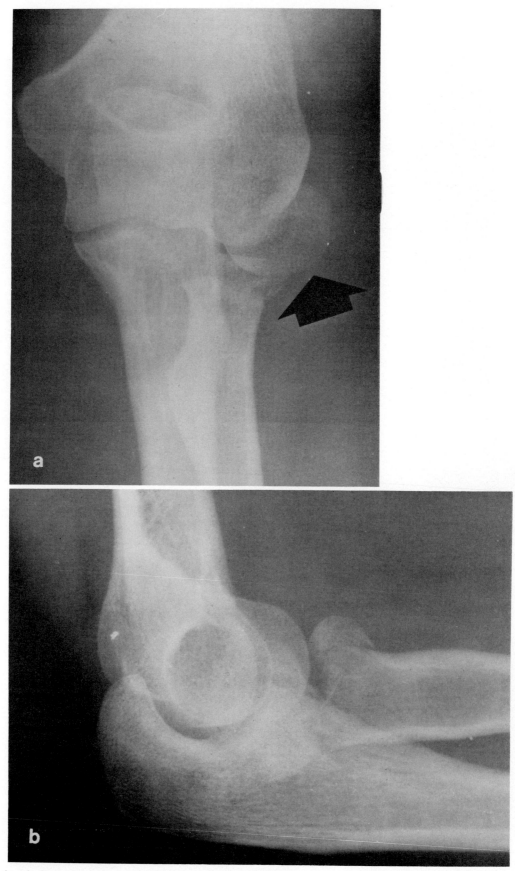

Fig 5.26. (a, b) Comminuted fracture of the radial head. The large proximal radial fragment lies free in the joint space (*solid arrow*).

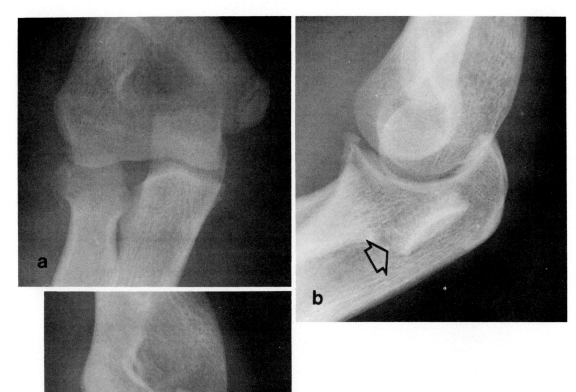

Fig. 5.27. (a–c) Displaced fracture of the radial neck.

nondisplaced (Fig. 5.23); 2) marginal (Figs. 5.8 and 5.24); 3) depressed (Fig. 5.25); and 4) comminuted (Fig. 5.26) (7).

Fractures of the radial neck are caused by the same mechanism that produces radial head fractures, namely, a fall on the outstretched hand with the forearm in supination. The force is transmitted along the radial shaft causing the radial head to impact upon the capitellum. The type of proximal radial fracture and the position of the fragments depends upon the magnitude and direction of the causative force. Consequently, radial head and neck fractures are considered together. Radial neck fractures may be displaced and obvious (Fig. 5.27) or minimally displaced and impacted. As such, the fracture may be very subtle and characterized only by disruption of the cortex and the presence of a faint, broad transverse

band of minimal increase in density at the junction of the head and neck (Fig. 5.28). The latter sign is caused by impaction of the trabeculae at the fracture site.

Fractures of the olecranon process result from a fall upon the forearm with the elbow flexed or from a fall directly upon the olecranon process itself. In the former instance, the distal end of the humerus acts as a fulcrum between the force of the fall upon the forearm and the force of the tensed triceps muscle. The fracture resulting from such an injury is usually transverse and usually not comminuted, and its fragments are usually only minimally separated (Fig. 5.29). Fractures resulting from a fall directly upon the olecranon process itself are usually comminuted and the fragments distracted (Fig. 5.30). When the fibrous covering of the olecranon process is torn in association with a fracture of this process, the fragments will be separated due to

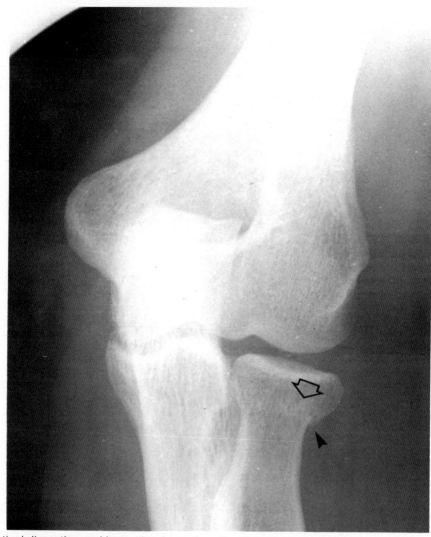

Fig. 5.28. The cortical disruption and impaction (*arrowhead*) and the faint transverse band of increased density (*open arrow*) caused by impacted trabeculae indicate the site of a subtle radial neck fracture.

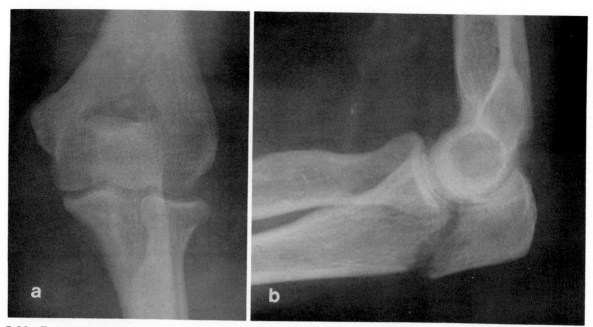

Fig. 5.29. Typical appearance of an olecranon process fracture caused by a fall upon the dorsum of the forearm. In the frontal projection **(a)**, the fracture is obscure because of the density of the superimposed distal end of the humerus and the oblique orientation of the fracture line with respect to the central x-ray beam. In the lateral projection **(b)**, the fracture is not comminuted and the fragments are only slightly distracted.

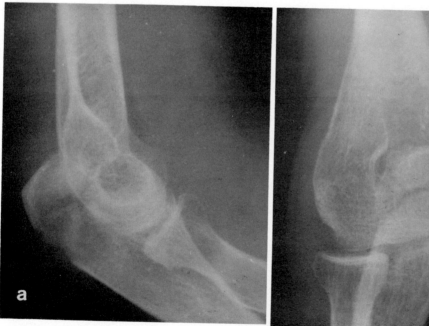

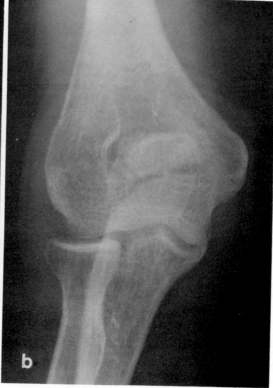

Fig. 5.30. (a, b) Comminuted, distracted fracture of the olecranon process.

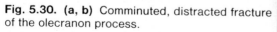

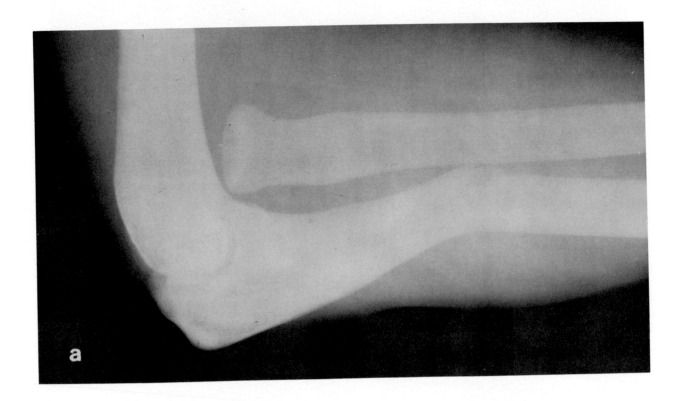

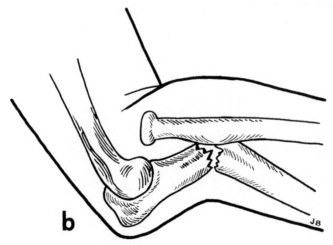

Fig. 5.31. (a, b) The Monteggia fracture consists of volar dislocation of the proximal end of the radius associated with a fracture in the proximal third of the ulna, with anterior angulation at the ulnar fracture site.

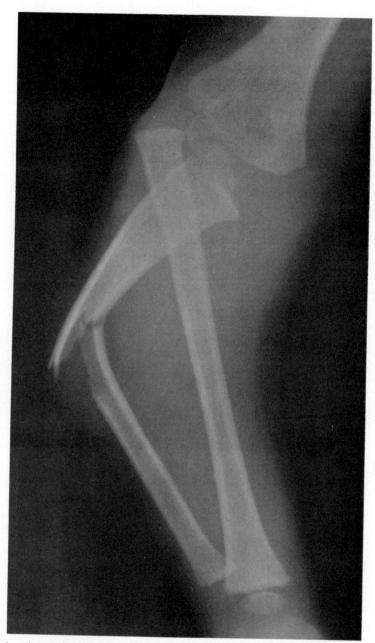

Fig. 5.32. This fracture has been described by Watson-Jones (8) as a "flexion" fracture of the Monteggia variety. It has also been referred to as a "reversed" Monteggia fracture. This injury is characterized by posterior dislocation of the proximal end of the radius and posterior angulation at the ulnar fracture site.

the unopposed pull of the triceps on the proximal fragment. If the fibrous covering is not disrupted, the fragments will be only minimally distracted.

The accessory ossification center (apophysis) of the olecranon process, which appears between 8 and 11 years and usually fuses by age 14 years, should not be mistaken for a fracture. The width of the apophyseal line and its parallel, smoothly undulating sclerotic margins (Figs. 5.12, 5.15, 5.18 and 5.20) together with

its characteristic location and inclination should all help distinguish this normal secondary ossification center from a fracture.

The Monteggia fracture (Fig. 5.31) consists of a fracture of the proximal portion of the ulna with volar angulation of the fragments associated with volar dislocation of the proximal radius. The injury is the result of force applied directly to the dorsum of the forearm or a forceful pronation injury of the forearm.

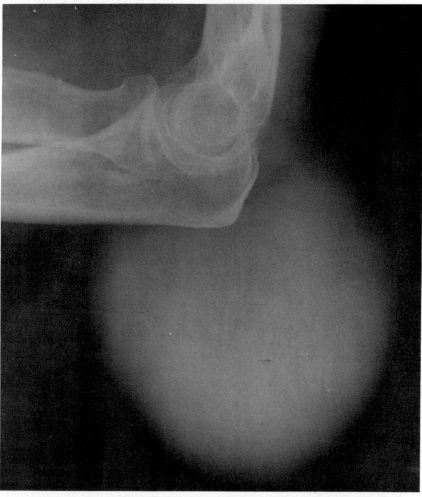

Fig. 5.33. The sharply defined, homogeneous soft tissue density arising from the posterior aspect of the elbow represents a posttraumatic fluid accumulation within the olecranon bursa.

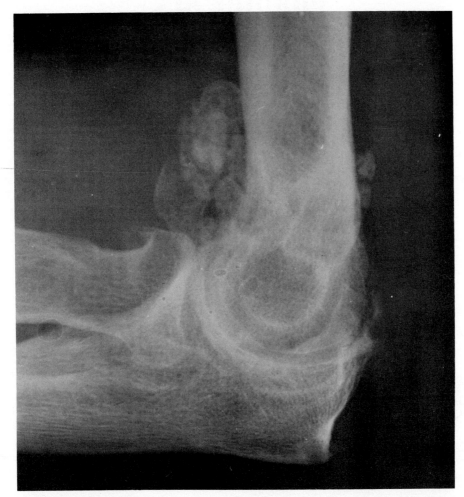

Fig. 5.34. The numerous loose bodies within the joint space are secondary to old trauma. The sharply defined sclerotic margins of the individual osteochondromata distinguish them from acute fracture fragments.

Volarly applied force to the proximal forearm is the cause of the "reversed" Monteggia fracture (Fig. 5.32), in which there is posterior angulation of the ulnar fragments and posterior dislocation of the proximal radius.

Differential Diagnosis

Direct trauma to the point of the elbow may result in accumulation of fluid within the olecranon bursa. Radiographically, this will appear as a homogeneous soft tissue density arising from the posterior aspect of the elbow (Fig. 5.33).

Osteochondromatosis of the elbow (Fig. 5.34) may produce acute clinical symptoms. There should be little difficulty in recognizing this entity radiographically.

References

1. BLEDSOE RE, IZENMARK JL: Displacement of fat pads in disease and injury at the elbow. *Radiology* 73:717, 1959.
2. NORELL HG: Roentgenologic visualization of the extracapsular fat: Its importance in the diagnosis of traumatic injuries of the elbow. *Acta Radiol* 42:205, 1954.
3. ROGERS LF: *Elbow Roentgenology of Fractures and Dislocations.* Grune & Stratton, New York, 1978.
4. NELSON SW: Some important diagnostic and technical fundamentals in the radiology of trauma. *Radiol Clin North Am* 4: 241, 1966.
5. DePALMA AF: *The Management of Fractures and Dislocations,* ed. 2. W. B. Saunders, Philadelphia, 1970.
6. CONWELL HE, REYNOLDS FC: *Key & Conwell's Management of Fractures, Dislocations and Sprains,* ed. 7. C. V. Mosby, St. Louis, Mo., 1961.
7. RALSTON EL: *Handbook of Fractures.* C. V. Mosby, St. Louis, Mo., 1967.
8. WATSON-JONES R: *Fractures and Joint Injuries,* ed. 4, vol. 1 (1952), vol. 2 (1955). Williams & Wilkins, Baltimore.

chapter six

Hand and Wrist

General Considerations

It is appropriate to emphasize that, although the hand and wrist are commonly considered as a single unit anatomically, radiographically, they are separate regions and the radiographic examination of the hand does not constitute an adequate study of the wrist nor vice versa. Further, there are special views of the hand and of the wrist that are peculiar to each and that have no application to the other. Therefore, it is mandatory that the attending physician determine as precisely as possible which part is to be studied radiographically and transmit this information accurately to the radiology department.

When it is clinically impossible to distinguish the precise area of involvement, limited radiographic examinations of both the hand and the wrist should be obtained. Appropriate additional views may be obtained subsequently as indicated.

During the adolescent period, when the epiphyses are undergoing fusion, the extreme variability in the radiographic appearance of the epiphyseal line may make interpretation of this shadow difficult. The type and location of the injury, the clinical findings, the radiographic appearance of the soft tissues, and the comparison of the roentgen characteristics of the injured and the uninvolved contralateral part should help in the radiographic evaluation of the injured part.

The soft tissue shadows, although commonly ignored, are valuable signs and may be the most prominent radiographic finding related to a significant, but subtle, bony abnormality. The value of careful appraisal of the soft tissue shadows cannot be overemphasized.

HAND

Radiographic Examination

Routine examination of the hand of patients of all ages consists of anteroposterior and oblique views made with the forearm in pronation (Fig. 6.1). In the oblique projection, it is necessary that the digits be spread sufficiently to prevent their superimposition upon each other.

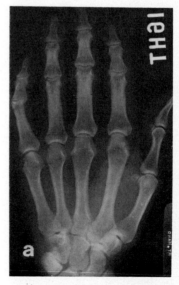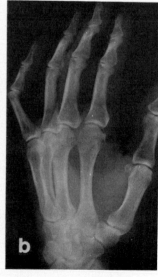

Fig. 6.1. The frontal **(a)** and prone oblique **(b)** projections constitute the routine radiographic examination of the hand. In the oblique projection, the digits must be separated to avoid superimposition.

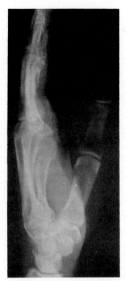

Fig. 6.2. The lateral projection of the hand has limited value because of the superimposition of all of the bones of the lateral four digits. This projection is, however, essential in the evaluation of the carpometacarpal area.

The lateral view of individual digits is extremely valuable and is readily obtained by flexing the uninvolved digits. The lateral projection of the hand (Fig. 6.2) is of limited value because of the superimposition of the metacarpals and the phalanges but is helpful in evaluating the carpometacarpal area.

The thumb requires special mention because none of the positions described above afford an anteroposterior view of this digit. The frontal view of the thumb is generally obtained with the forearm placed midway between pronation and supination and the thumb extended away from the volar surface of the hand (Fig. 6.3).

Special views of the hand include only the "reversed" oblique (Fig. 6.4), which is made with the forearm in supination, and the carpal tunnel view (Fig. 6.5). The latter is obtained with the forearm prone and the hand maximally extended at the wrist. The x-ray tube is angled 10° toward the elbow so that the central ray passes through the base of the hand. This projection has little application in the acutely injured patient but is used routinely in evaluation of the patient with a carpal tunnel syndrome.

The roentgen appearance of the growth centers is variable and occasionally may resemble an acute injury. An earlier dictum required a limited (frontal and lateral) examination of the contralateral, uninjured part to serve as the base line against which the injured part could be compared. The current generally accepted standard of practice is to *not* examine the opposite side *routinely.* Rather, the examination of the injured part should be studied and only if indetermi-

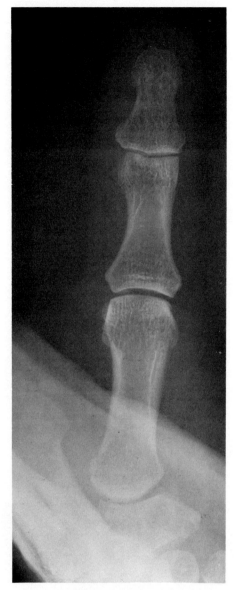

Fig. 6.3. Frontal projection of the thumb.

nate or equivocal should the opposite part be examined radiographically.

Radiographic Anatomy

The roentgen characteristics of the nutrient artery canals, the location of the epiphyses of the phalanges and metacarpals, the alignment and relationship of the carpal bones, and the radiocarpal angle constitute some of the practically important aspects of the radiographic anatomy of the hand and wrist.

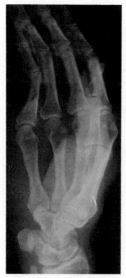

Fig. 6.4. "Reversed" oblique radiograph of the hand made in the supine oblique position.

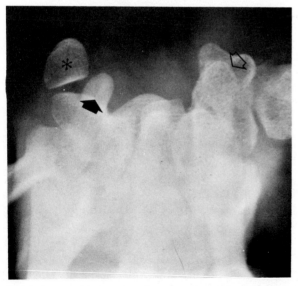

Fig. 6.5. Carpal tunnel view of the wrist. The *asterisk* (*) indicates the pisiform bone, the *solid arrow* the hook of the hamate, and the *open arrow* the tubercle of the navicular.

Nutrient artery canals (medullary foramen) (Fig. 6.6) are located near the middle of the phalangeal and metacarpal shafts and enter the bone from each side, passing obliquely distally. The margins of these normal vascular grooves are uniformly and smoothly sclerotic and parallel and converge distally. Nutrient artery canals are not constantly seen, radiographically. However, when present, their location, course, and roentgen characteristics should distinguish them from incomplete fracture lines.

The phalangeal and metacarpal epiphyses are not similarly located and, even among the metacarpals, the location of the growth centers is not uniform (Fig. 6.7). The phalangeal epiphyses are proximally situated. Those of the second, third, fourth, and fifth metacarpals are located distally and constitute the metacarpal head. The growth center of the first metacarpal is at its base. During the ages when the epiphyses are open and following their fusion, neither the epiphyseal line itself nor the thin linear sclerotic density that occasionally results from epiphyseal fusion should be mistaken for a fracture line. When fractures do include the epiphyseal portion of the bone, the difference in the radiographic characteristics between the fracture line and the epiphyseal line (Fig. 6.8) should permit identification of each.

The sesamoids are small, rounded bones imbedded in certain flexor tendons. Five sesamoid bones are commonly found in the hand. These include two lying volar to the first metacarpophalangeal joint (Fig. 6.9), one volar to the interphalangeal joint of the thumb, and one in the soft tissues anterior to the metacarpophalangeal joint of the index and little fingers. Sesamoid bones are characterized by dense, smooth cortical margins and a normal trabecular pattern.

The heads of the lateral four metacarpals constitute the knuckles of the closed fist. The force of a striking blow made with the fist is generally transmitted though the long axis of the metacarpals. When the direction and magnitude of forces is sufficient, a typical "Boxer's" fracture (Fig. 6.10) results. This fracture occurs at the metacarpal neck. The distal fracture is angulated volarly and may be canted slightly radially as well. The fifth metacarpal is most commonly involved, with the fourth being next in frequency.

Radiographic Manifestations of Trauma

Soft tissue swelling is an important, although frequently overlooked, aid to the roentgen detection of subtle skeletal injuries. Soft tissue swelling helps to direct attention to the bones of the area and adds significance to minor bony changes that might otherwise be overlooked (Figs. 6.11 and 6.12).

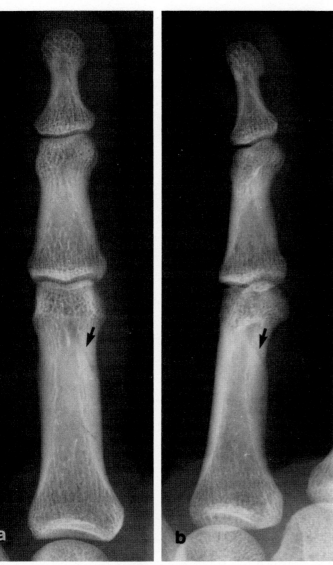

Fig. 6.6. The nutrient artery canal (medullary foramen) (*arrows*) in frontal **(a)** and oblique **(b)** projections.

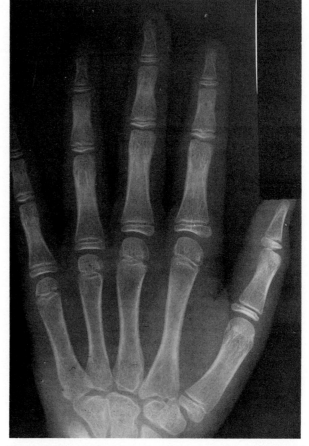

Fig. 6.7. Normal location of epiphyses of the hand. All of the phalangeal epiphyses are located at the proximal end. The metacarpal epiphyses, however, are all distally situated except for that of the first, which is proximal.

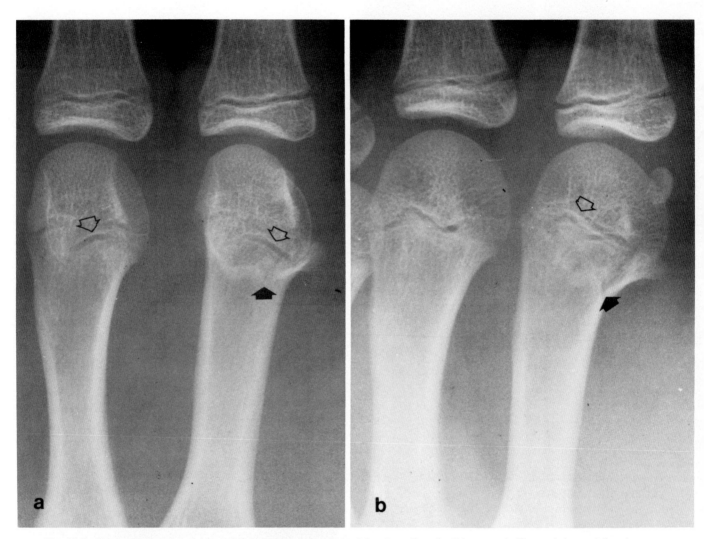

Fig. 6.8. Comparison of epiphyseal line (*open arrows*) and fracture line (*solid arrows*). The epiphyseal line is open (lucent) and its margins are sclerotic, parallel, and gently undulating. In contrast, the fracture line may be indicated by a broad band of increased density representing impaction of the fragments **(a)** or by an irregularly lucent defect with jagged, indistinct margins and cortical disruption **(b)**.

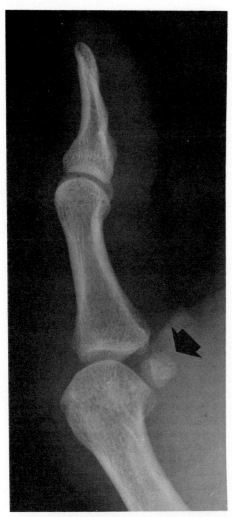

Fig. 6.9. The *arrow* indicates the sesamoids normally found at the first metacarpophalangeal joint.

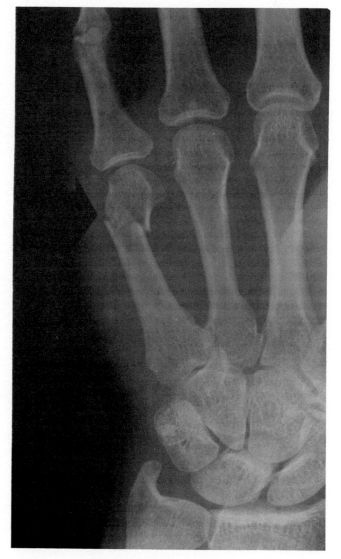

Fig. 6.10. ''Boxer's'' fracture.

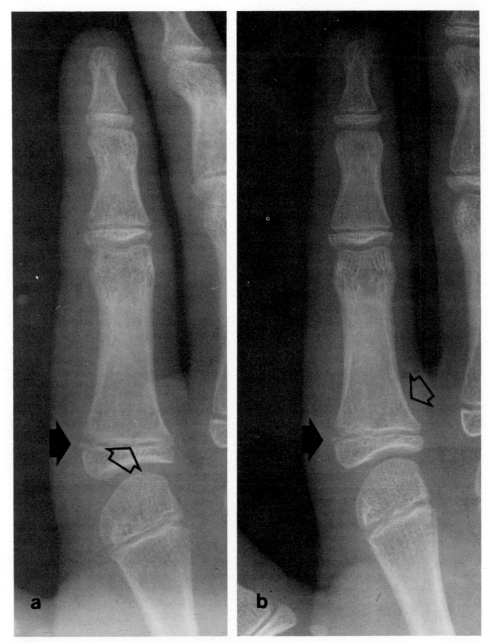

Fig. 6.11. Minimally displaced Salter II injury of the base of the proximal phalanx of the index finger. The oblique metaphyseal fracture line (*open arrows*) can be seen in both the oblique **(a)** and anteroposterior **(b)** radiographs. A tiny avulsion fragment arises from the radial aspect of the epiphyseal plate (*solid arrows*). The most striking roentgen sign of acute injury, however, is the diffuse soft tissue swelling of this digit. Note that the swelling is greatest at the metacarpophalangeal level.

cated in the periphery of the epiphyseal plate which may arise from either the metaphyseal or the epiphyseal margin of the plate (Fig. 6.16). Pathophysiologically, the Salter I injury consists of simply separation of the epiphysis from the metaphysis. Because the periosteum, which bridges the epiphyseal plate and attaches to the proximal margin of the epiphysis, remains intact, the epiphysis typically maintains its normal relationship to the metaphysis. Therefore, in the majority of instances, the Salter I epiphyseal injury cannot be established on the plain radiographs. It is only when the epiphyseal line is asymmetrically widened or a tiny avulsion fragment is seen within the periphery of the epiphyseal line that the diagnosis of a Salter I injury can be made radiographically.

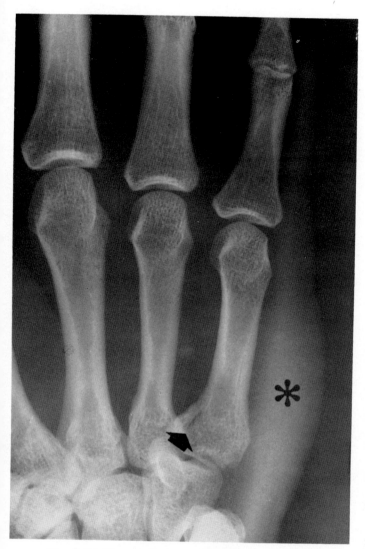

Fig. 6.12. The marked soft tissue swelling lateral to the base of the fifth metacarpal (*) calls attention to the subtle fracture in the base of this bone (*arrow*).

Interphalangeal and metacarpophalangeal dislocations (Figs. 6.13–6.15) are common injuries and usually result from a blow on the volar aspect of the digit forcing the base of the phalanx dorsally over the head of the next proximal bone. Postreduction radiographs should be obtained to exclude the presence of associated fracture or epiphyseal separation.

Epiphyseal injuries of the hand occur commonly. Figure 6.11 is an example of a Salter II injury. Although Salter's original definition of the Type I epiphyseal injury describes "complete separation of the epiphysis without any fracture through bone" (1), the definition has been expanded by common usage to include the presence of a tiny fracture fragment lo-

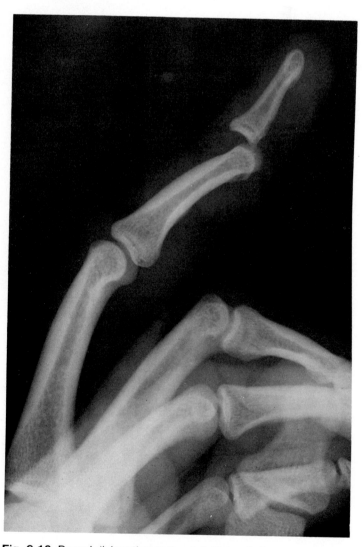

Fig. 6.13. Dorsal dislocation at the distal interphalangeal joint without associated fracture.

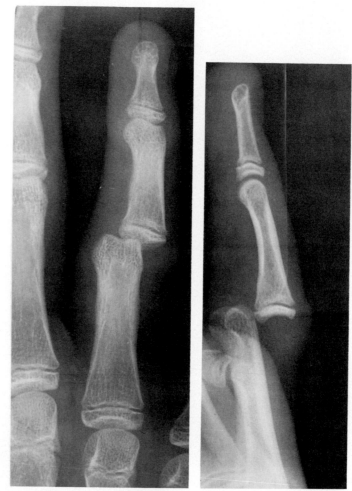

Fig. 6.14. Posterior dislocation at the proximal interphalangeal joint. There is no associated fracture. The epiphysis of the middle phalanx has maintained its normal relationship to the shaft.

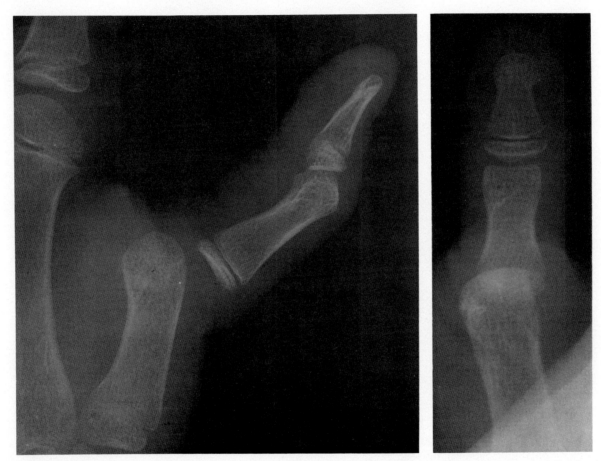

Fig. 6.15. Complete dorsal dislocation at the metacarpophalangeal joint of the thumb. There is no associated fracture nor epiphyseal separation.

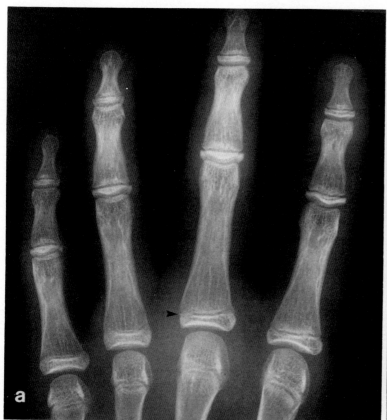

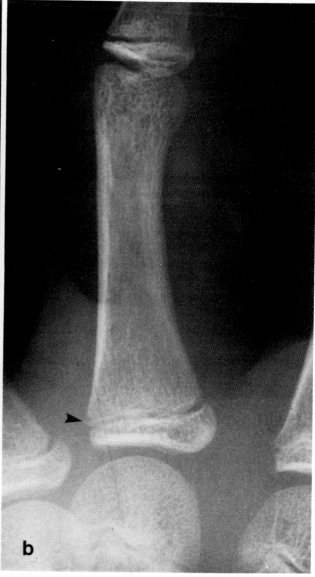

Fig. 6.16. Salter I injury of the epiphysis of the proximal phalanx of the long finger. In the frontal projection **(a)**, the long finger is swollen with the greatest swelling being about the metacarpophalangeal joint. The epiphyseal line (plate) of the proximal phalanx is wider than the other plates and a tiny fracture fragment (*arrowhead*) is present in the ulnar aspect of the epiphyseal line. In the oblique projection **(b)**, the widened epiphyseal line and the avulsion fragment (*arrowhead*) are more clearly seen.

The commonest fracture of the subungual tuft of the distal phalanx is the comminuted, minimally displaced variety (Fig. 6.17). Fractures of the tuft may be markedly displaced, particularly when the injury is severe, mangling, or caused by a sharp instrument (Fig. 6.18). Linear, minimally, or non-displaced fractures of the distal phalanx may be extremely difficult to identify and may be clearly seen on only one of multiple radiographs (Fig. 6.19).

"Baseball" or "mallet" finger are names given to a flexion deformity occurring at the distal interphalangeal joint, usually the result of a fracture of the dorsum of the base of the distal phalanx. This injury is commonly caused by a direct blow to the end of the finger producing severe, abrupt flexion at the distal interphalangeal joint. The common extensor tendon may be either avulsed from its insertion on the dorsal aspect of the base of the phalanx, or a small triangular shaped fragment containing the extensor insertion may be pulled off (Fig. 6.20). As a result, the distal phalanx is angled volarly by the unopposed action of the flexor digiti profundus tendon and the patient is unable to extend the distal phalanx.

Figure 6.21 illustrates a fracture of the dorsum of the base of the distal phalanx which is proximal to the insertion of the common extensor tendon. No mallet finger deformity exists.

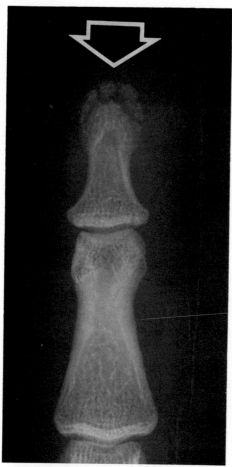

Fig. 6.17. Comminuted, minimally displaced fracture of the subungual tuft.

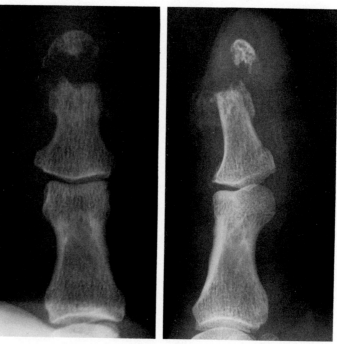

Fig. 6.18. Comminuted, displaced fracture of the subungual tuft. Note the associated soft tissue damage.

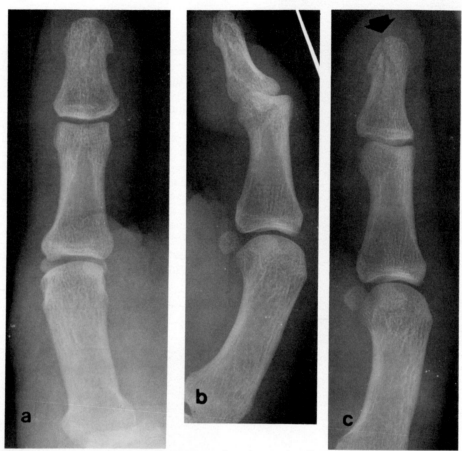

Fig. 6.19. (a, b) Multiple views are commonly necessary in order to visualize nondisplaced fractures. The comminuted fracture in the distal phalanx of the thumb is clearly seen only in the slightly oblique projection **(c)**.

Avulsion fracture of the volar aspect of the base of the middle phalanx is a common injury (Fig. 6.22). The typical fragment of this injury is very small and is frequently seen only on the lateral view. With this fracture, the associated soft tissue swelling may be the most obvious radiographic abnormality.

Even though trauma to the hand appears to be limited to a digit, radiographic examination of the entire hand in frontal projection is mandatory to ensure that an associated, but clinically unsuspected, metacarpal fracture is not overlooked (Fig. 6.23).

It has been previously stated that the routine radio-graphic examination of the hand should include not only the anteroposterior projection but an oblique view as well. The basis for this dictum is illustrated in Figure 6.24, where the complete, displaced fracture of the fourth metacarpal, which could be easily over-looked in the frontal projection, was obvious in the oblique radiograph.

Trauma to the hand may cause injury to phalanges and metacarpals simultaneously (Fig. 6.25). For this reason, also, the entire hand must be examined in frontal projection even though the clinical findings indicate only metacarpal injury.

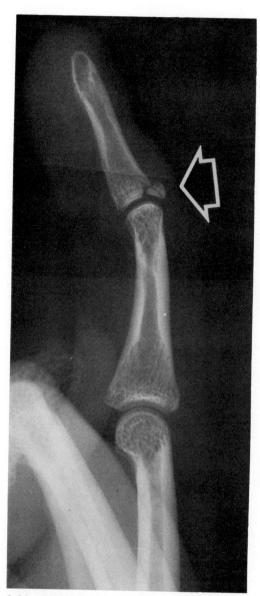

Fig. 6.20. ''Baseball'' or ''mallet'' finger. The small triangular fragment is proximally retracted by the action of the common extensor tendon. The flexion deformity results from the unopposed action of the flexor digiti profundus tendon.

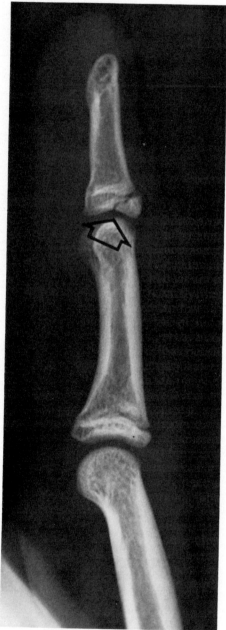

Fig. 6.21. Nondisplaced fracture of the dorsal aspect of the base of the distal phalanx. In this instance, the common extensor tendon inserted distal to the fracture fragment and a mallet deformity did not result.

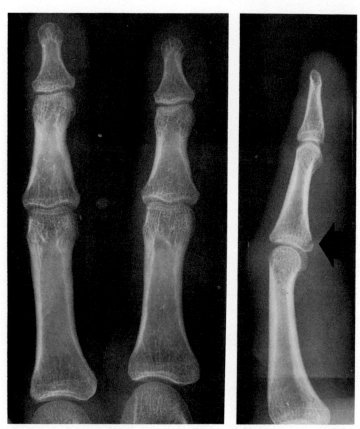

Fig. 6.22. Minimally displaced avulsion fracture of the base of the middle phalanx. This is a common fracture which is occasionally missed because of the size of the separate fragment and because the fracture, generally, can only be recognized in a true lateral projection. Note the disparity between the amount of soft tissue swelling of the digit and the size of the fragment.

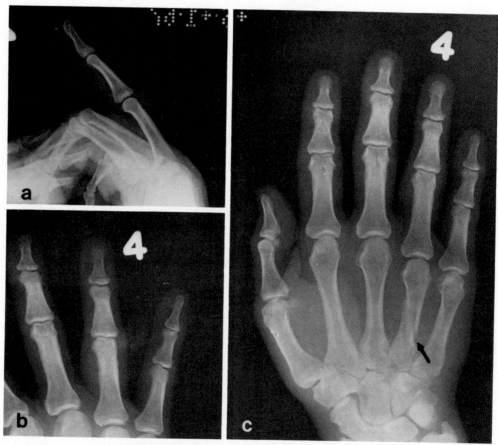

Fig. 6.23. This patient complained of pain and tenderness of the ring finger following trauma to the hand. Although the ring finger is swollen, the phalanges are all intact **(a, b)**. The fracture of the fourth metacarpal **(c,** *arrow*), which was clinically unsuspected, would have been overlooked if roentgen examination had been confined to the symptomatic digit.

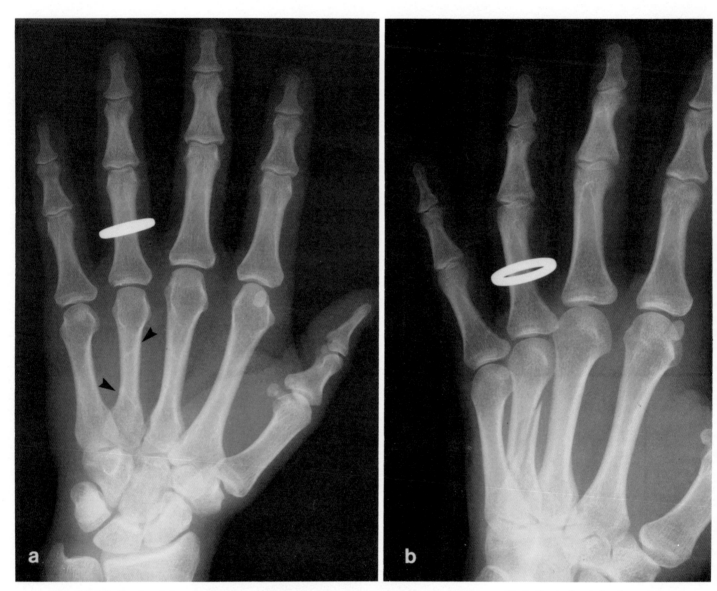

Fig. 6.24. In the frontal projection **(a)**, the fracture of the shaft of the fourth metacarpal is indicated only by the subtle, oblique linear densities (*arrowheads*). The alignment of the fragments, as seen in this projection, is anatomic. In the oblique projection **(b)**, the displaced fracture of the fourth metacarpal is obvious.

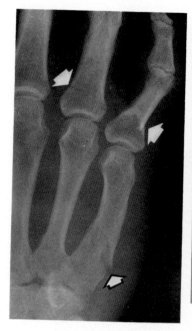
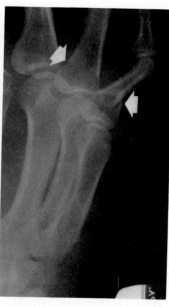

Fig. 6.25. Simultaneous fractures of the proximal phalanx of the fourth and little fingers (*top arrows*) and the base of the fifth metacarpal (*bottom arrow*).

Metacarpal fractures which occur prior to fusion of the epiphyses usually involve the metaphysis (Fig. 6.26). While the epiphyseal line may obscure the fracture, the fracture should be recognizable on the basis of roentgen characteristics of the fracture line and cortical disruption at the fracture site.

Fractures of the metacarpal shaft are more commonly spiral than transverse. Minimally displaced spiral fractures may be quite difficult to identify radiographically (Fig. 6.27).

Metacarpal shortening, usually associated with displaced fractures, is caused by the unopposed action of the intrinsic muscles of the hand.

Fractures of the base of the metacarpals are frequently obscure because of the configuration of this portion of the metacarpal, the superimposition of the adjacent bony shadows and minimal displacement of the fragments. Figure 6.12 illustrates such a fracture that might have been overlooked except for the marked soft tissue swelling in the hypothenar space.

Fractures of the base of the first metacarpal may be subtle, are associated with a hematoma of the thenar space which causes a soft tissue density between the first and second metacarpals, and are frequently imprecisely labeled as "Bennett's" fractures (Figs. 6.28 and 6.29).

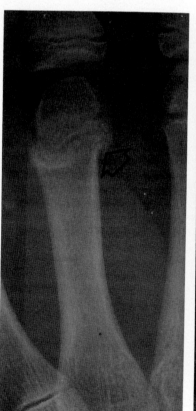
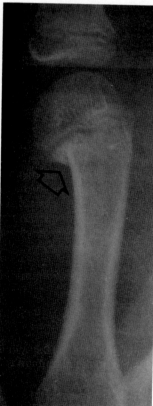

Fig. 6.26. Impacted, slightly displaced fracture in the metaphysis. The characteristics of the fracture line and the immediately adjacent epiphyseal line are readily comparable in this illustration. Note the cortical disruption and the impaction of the fragment at the fracture site indicated by the *arrows*.

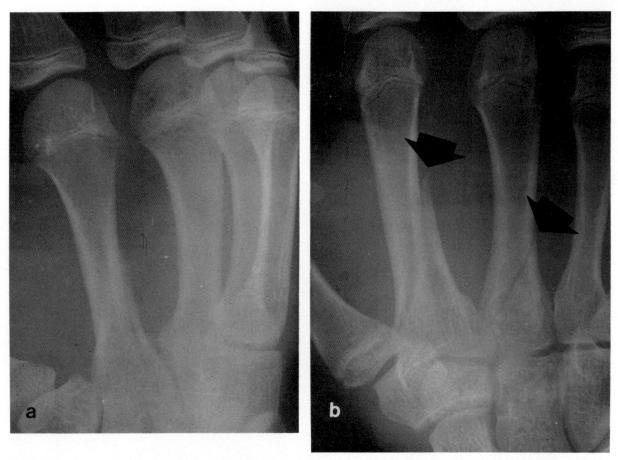

Fig. 6.27. Spiral fracture of the shaft of the second and third metacarpals. The fracture of the second metacarpal is poorly seen and that of the third metacarpal is not visible in the oblique projection **(a)**. However, each fracture (*arrows*) is clearly evident in the anteroposterior radiograph **(b)**.

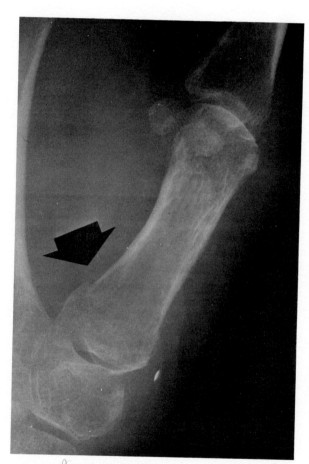 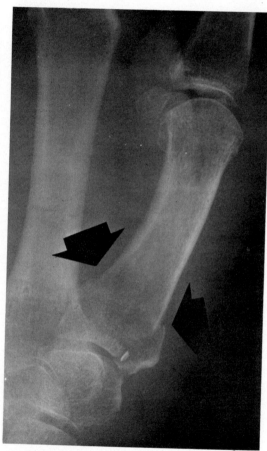

Fig. 6.28. Comminuted, nondisplaced fracture of the base of the first metacarpal.

TRANSVERSE THROUGH
BASE OF 1ST METACARPAL

COMMINUTTED #
INVOVING JOINT
SURFACE
"BENNETT'S FRACTURE"
NEED EXCELLENT
REDUCTION

PREVENT O.A.

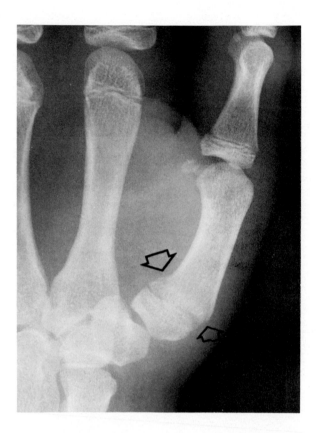

Fig. 6.29. Minimally displaced fracture in the metaphysis of the first metacarpal. Soft tissue swelling in the thenar space is indicated by the increase in density between the first and second metacarpals.

The injury first described by Bennett (2–4) is an oblique fracture through the base and proximal articulating surface of the first metacarpal *with associated proximal dislocation of the distal fragment* (Fig. 6.30). The important feature is the associated dislocation and, therefore, this injury should properly be referred to as "Bennett's fracture-dislocation." The clinical significance of this distinction rests in the management of the injury. While the dislocation can be readily reduced with traction, the pull of the abductor pollicis longus, which inserts upon the dorsal aspect of the base of the metacarpal, results in prompt proximal and radial displacement of the distal fragment as soon as traction is released.

Nontraumatic Lesions

The radiographic appearance of some normal variants (Fig. 6.31) and nontraumatic lesions may pose differential diagnostic problems. The rough edges of the site of insertion of the flexor tendon sheaths produce a cortical irregularity of the phalanges which could simulate an incomplete fracture (Fig. 6.32).

The roentgen signs of acute osteomyelitis include soft tissue swelling, irregular demineralization, and cortical disruption (Fig. 6.33). Periosteal new bone reaction usually requires approximately 3 weeks to become radiographically discernible and, therefore, is not considered an acute finding.

Fractures occurring in benign neoplastic lesions may occur spontaneously or with only minor trauma. The fracture itself is usually readily identifiable (Fig. 6.34). The commonest benign lytic lesion of the hand is the enchondroma.

Although rare, metastatic disease may involve the bones of the hand (Fig. 6.35).

WRIST

Radiographic Examination

The routine radiographic study of the wrist consists of frontal, lateral, and each oblique projections. In contrast to the lateral radiograph of the hand, the lateral examination of the wrist is extremely important, particularly in the evaluation of carpal dislocations and the position of distal radial and ulnar fracture fragments.

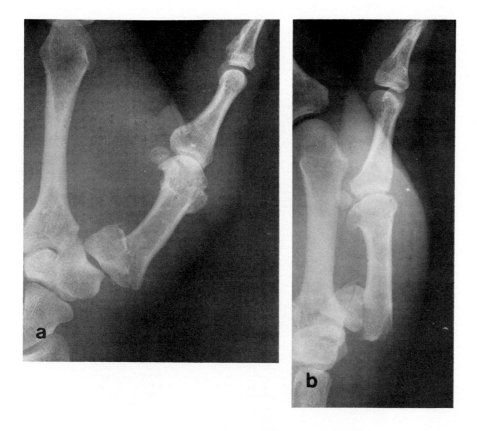

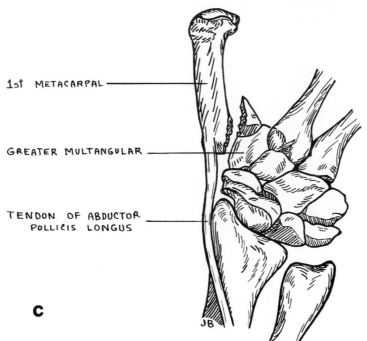

1st METACARPAL

GREATER MULTANGULAR

TENDON OF ABDUCTOR
POLLICIS LONGUS

c

Fig. 6.30. (a–c) Bennett's fracture-dislocation of the first metacarpal [(c) Modified from F. Netter: *Ciba Found Clin Symp*, 1970.]

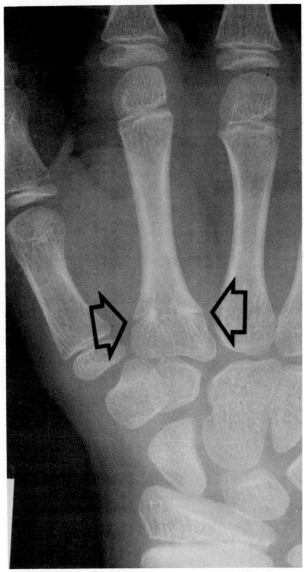

Fig. 6.31. False epiphyseal center of second metacarpal (*arrows*). This developmental variant may involve the base of the second, third, fourth, or fifth metacarpals.

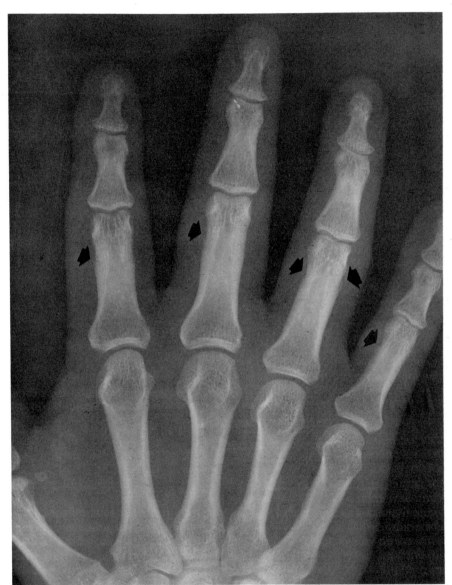

Fig. 6.32. The cortical irregularities indicated by the *arrows* represent the rough edges of the site of insertion of flexor tendon sheaths. These are normal structures and should not be misinterpreted as either nutrient artery foramina or incomplete cortical fractures.

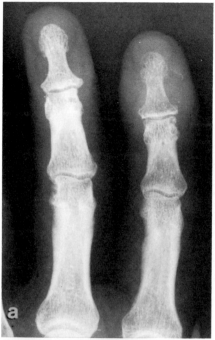

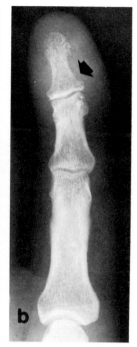

Fig. 6.33. Acute osteomyelitis of the distal phalanx of the index finger. In the frontal projection **(a)**, the digit is diffusely swollen and the distal phalanx demineralized. Cortical disruption and fragmentation (*arrow*) is present at the radial aspect of the base **(b)**. The *open arrow* indicates a soft tissue defect on the lateral roentgenogram **(c)**. Note the diffuse soft tissue swelling and moderate demineralization of the distal phalanx.

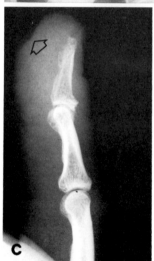

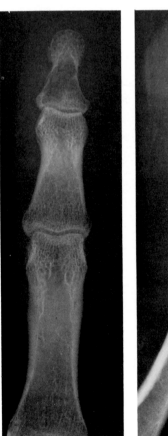

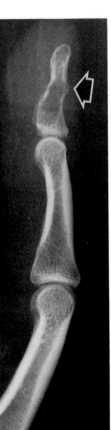

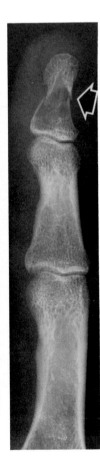

Fig. 6.34. Minimally displaced fracture of an enchondroma.

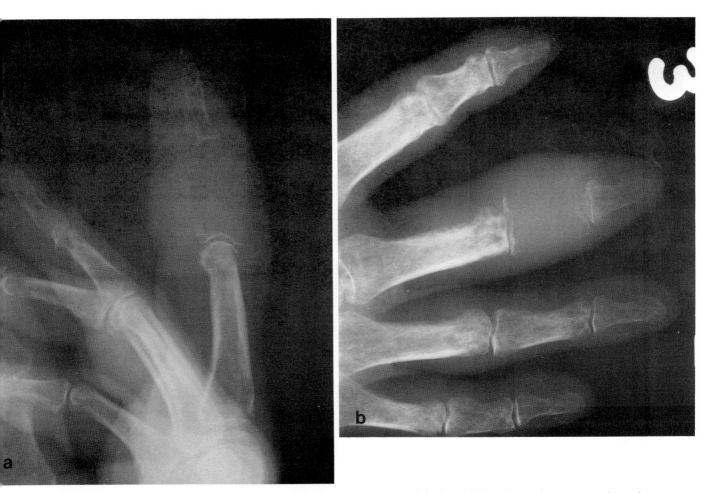

Fig. 6.35. Osteolytic metastatic disease involving multiple phalanges of the hand. The primary tumor was a bronchogenic carcinoma. The clinical impression of the hand lesion was acute osteomyelitis.

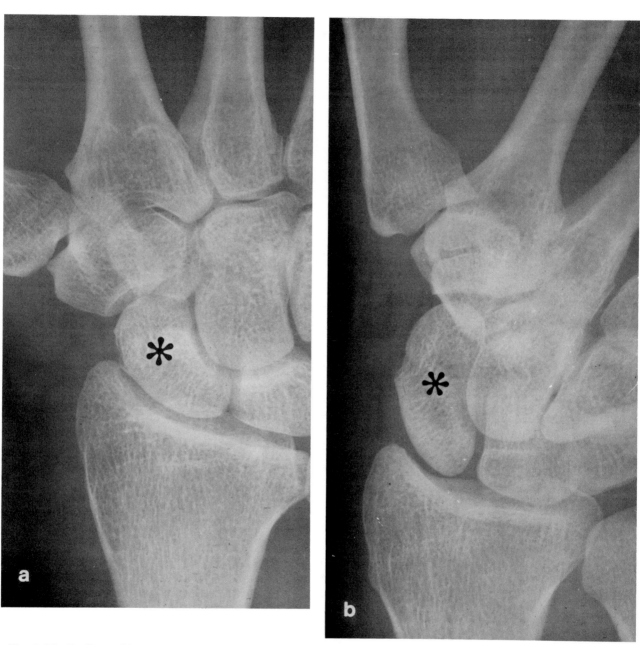

Fig. 6.36. Radiographic appearance of the navicular (scaphoid) (*) in straight frontal **(a)** and navicular **(b)** projections. In the straight frontal projection **(a)**, the scaphoid is foreshortened along its longitudinal axis and the waist is not well seen. In the navicular projection **(b)**, made with the hand and wrist in maximum ulnar deviation possible and the central beam centered upon the anatomic snuff-box and angled approximately 10° ulnarly and proximally, the longitudinal axis of the scaphoid is optimally projected.

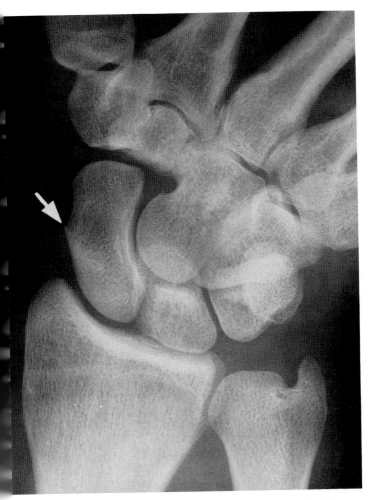

Fig. 6.37. Navicular view of the wrist. The cortical irregularity of the radial aspect of the navicular (*arrow*) is a normal structure, namely, the distal margin of the proximal articulating surface of the navicular, and should not be misinterpreted as a cortical buckling fracture.

Radiographic Anatomy

Anatomically, the wrist joint is limited to the articulation between the distal radius and proximal row of carpals. Clinically, however, the wrist is said to "include the soft parts of bones and joints over an area embracing not only the carpus, but the bony extremities of the radius and ulna and the bases of the metacarpals articulating with it. It includes the radiocarpal, midcarpal, and carpometacarpal joints" (5).

The pronator quadratus is a thin, flat, quadrilateral muscle which passes transversely from the distal radius to the distal ulna, lying on the volar aspect of the interosseous membrane and the radioulnar joint (Fig. 6.38). It has an intimate relationship with the periosteum of the distal radius and ulna. Superficially, the pronator quadratus is covered by a layer of loose connective tissue. In the lateral radiograph of the wrist, the pronator muscle produces a thin soft tissue density (*) immediately adjacent to the volar aspect of the radius (Fig. 6.39) outlined by the radiolucency of the covering connective tissue.

The frontal radiograph of the wrist should include the distal radius and ulna, the carpal bones, and the bases of the metacarpals (Fig. 6.40).

The normal radiocarpal angle and the relationship of the radial and ulnar styloid processes appears in Figures 6.40 and 6.41. Alterations of this normal relationship may be the most obvious finding in cases of impacted fracture of the distal radius (Fig. 6.42).

The roentgen appearance of the completely, or nearly completely, fused distal radial epiphyseal line

The carpal navicular view is specifically designed to permit visualization of the scaphoid bone in profile along its curved, longitudinal axis (Fig. 6.36). This projection should be routinely included in the roentgen evaluation of the acutely injured wrist. The radial surface of the navicular (scaphoid) is seen in greater detail and in a different perspective than in the anteroposterior projection. As a result, the distal margin of the radial (proximal) articulating surface of the navicular appears as a localized irregularity of the radial aspect of the navicular. This entirely normal anatomic feature (Fig. 6.37) should, therefore, be accepted as a normal structure and not confused as a cortical buckling or incomplete fracture.

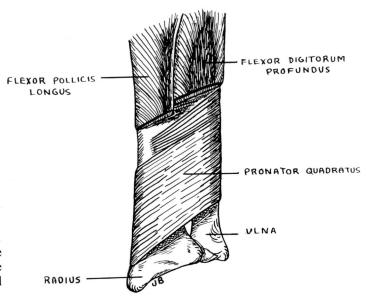

Fig. 6.38. Relationship of the pronator quadratus muscle to the volar aspect of the distal radius and ulna.

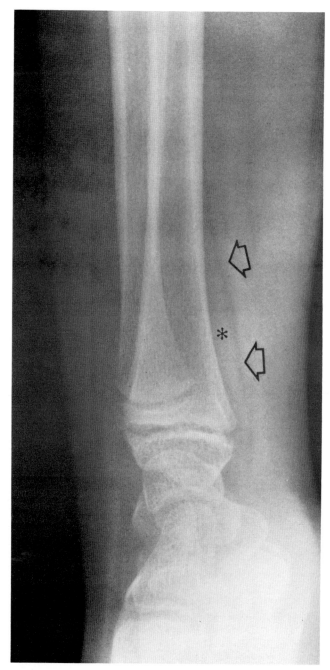

Fig. 6.39. The pronator muscle produces the thin, slightly convex soft tissue density (*) immediately adjacent to the volar aspect of the radius. The volar surface of the pronator quadratus is delineated by the lucency of the covering adipose tissue (*arrows*) within the fascial plane.

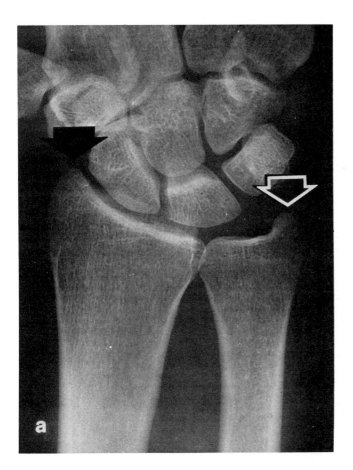

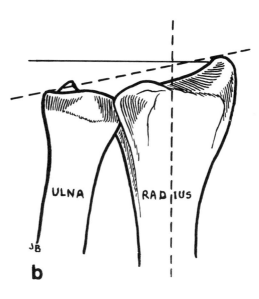

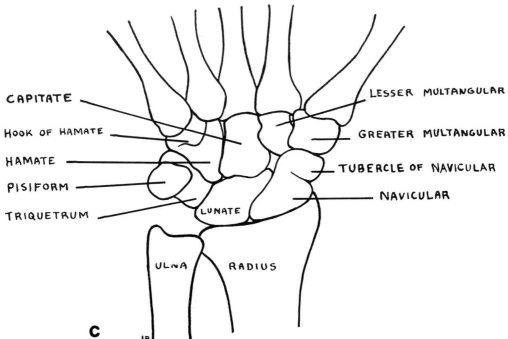

Fig. 6.40. (a) Frontal roentgenogram of an adult wrist. The radial and ulnar styloid processes are indicated by the *arrows*. **(b)** The drawing of the distal radius and ulna is intended to emphasize the relationship between the radial and ulnar styloid processes. (Modified from L. L. Ralston: *Handbook of Fractures*. C. V. Mosby, St. Louis, Mo., 1967) **(c)**. Schematic representation of the carpal bones. (Modified from F. Netter, *Ciba Found Clin Symp* 1970).

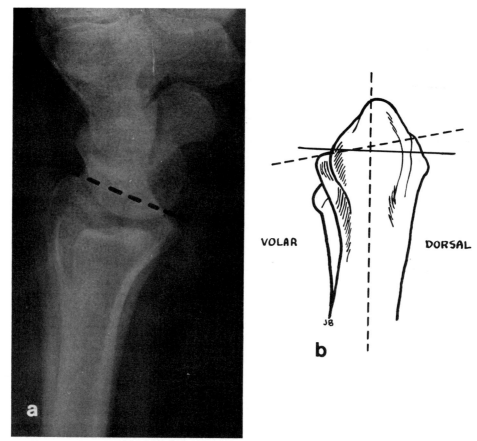

VOLAR

DORSAL

b

Fig. 6.41. (a) Lateral roentgenogram of the wrist. The volar angulation of the distal radial articulating surface is indicated by the *dotted line* on the roentgenogram and is emphasized in the drawing **(b)**. (Modified from L.L. Ralston: *Handbook of Fractures.* C. V. Mosby, St. Louis, Mo., 1967).

may simulate an impacted or incomplete distal radial fracture. Figures 6.43–6.45 are examples of the appearance of the completely fused distal radial epiphyseal line in adults. This thin, vague, sclerotic, linear transverse density, which represents the fused epiphyseal line, should not be mistaken for an impacted fracture. The absence of soft tissue swelling militates against an acute, impacted, nondisplaced fracture. Figures 6.46 and 6.47 are examples of the roentgen appearance of incomplete fusion of the radial cortical margin of the distal radial epiphysis. The smooth, sclerotic, parallel margins of the short segment of incomplete fusion, its direct extension from the thin, sclerotic, oblique density representing the fused epi-

physeal line, and its location should permit recognition of this normal structure, even in the presence of a history of an injury to the wrist and radiographic evidence of soft tissue swelling.

Radiographic Manifestations of Trauma

As has been mentioned in other chapters, it is mandatory to obtain right angle radiographs of the extremities following trauma in order to accurately assess the magnitude of injury and the true relation of the fragments. The basis of this dictum is seen in Figure 6.48, where the true extent of the injury is only

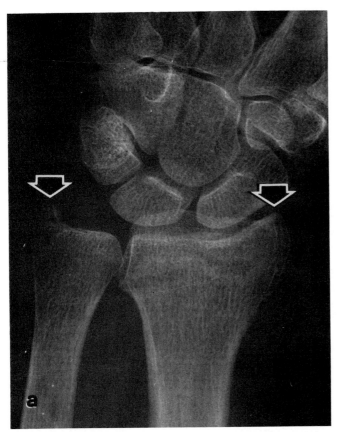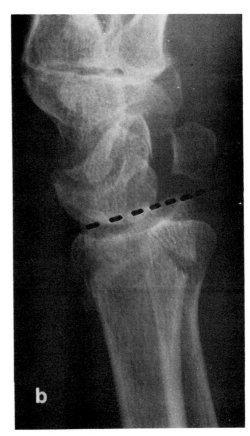

Fig. 6.42. Impacted fracture of the distal radius associated with a minimally displaced fracture of the ulnar styloid process. Note that the ulnar and radial styloid processes are on the same plane in the frontal projection **(a)**. In the lateral projection **(b)**, the normal volar inclination of the distal radial articulating surface has been reversed. These changes in the normal radiocarpal anatomy are frequently the cynosure of subtle fractures involving the distal radius.

appreciated in the lateral projection.

Localized, diffuse, nonspecific soft tissue swelling about the wrist, as elsewhere, may be the most obvious radiographic finding in instances of subtle bony injury (Fig. 6.49).

Hemorrhage beneath the pronator quadratus muscle causes the muscle to bulge volarly. This change in the normal soft tissue anatomy is clearly discernible radiographically (Fig. 6.50) and is an extremely valuable sign (6) often heralding the presence of subtle injuries of the distal third of the radius or ulna (Figs. 6.51 and 6.52).

In addition to volar bulging of the pronator quadratus muscle, the pronator quadratus sign (6) has also been described as a loss or absence of definition (Fig. 6.53) of the lucent fat stripe overlying the pronator muscle.

Dislocation of the distal radioulnar joint (Figs. 6.54 and 6.55) is frequently associated with fracture of the distal third of the radius or ulnar and is commonly either not appreciated or ignored. Isolated dislocation of the distal radioulnar joint occurs uncommonly. Volar dislocation (or subluxation) (Fig. 6.56) is more common than dorsal displacement of the ulna.

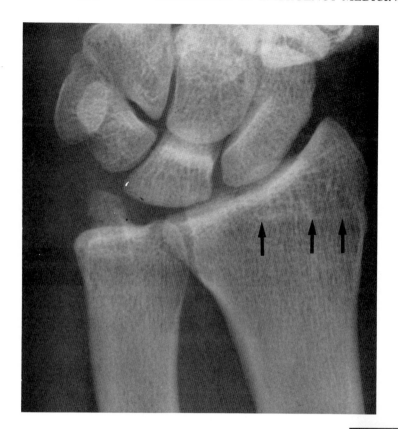

Fig. 6.43. The thin sclerotic density (*arrows*) that occasionally forms at the site of fusion for the epiphysis with the metaphysis may be mistaken for an incomplete impacted fracture. The absence of soft tissue swelling should help distinguish this normal finding from a fracture line.

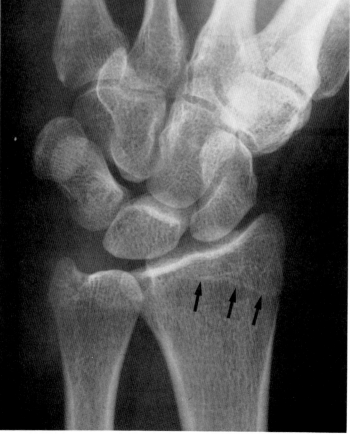

Fig. 6.44. Normal fused distal radial epiphyseal line (*arrows*) in an adult.

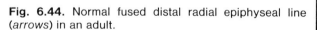

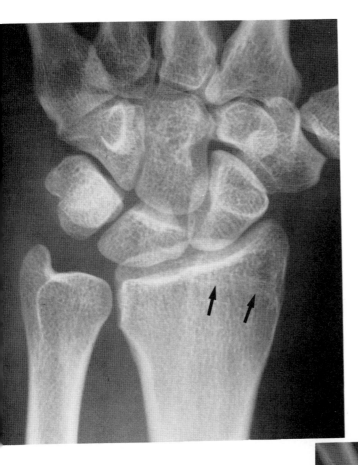

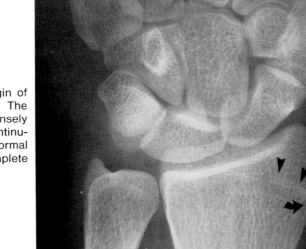

Fig. 6.45. Normal fused distal radial epiphyseal line (*arrows*) in an adult.

Fig. 6.46. Incompletely fused radial cortical margin of the distal radial epiphyseal line (*curved arrows*). The margins of the short unfused arc are smooth, densely sclerotic, and parallel. The unfused segment is continuous with the fused physis (*arrowheads*). This normal variant should not be mistaken for an acute, incomplete fracture.

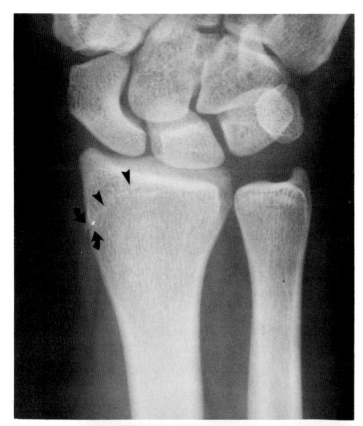

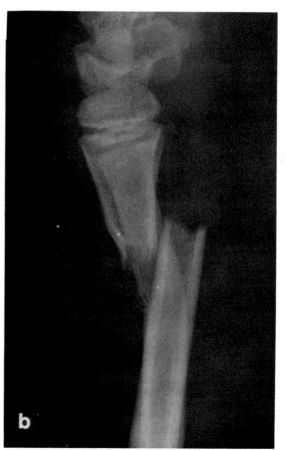

Fig. 6.47. Incompletely fused distal radial epiphyseal line (*curved arrows*). Note that the contiguous margins are smoothly sclerotic, parallel and sharply defined and that the short ununited arc is directly continuous with the already fused epiphysis (*arrowheads*).

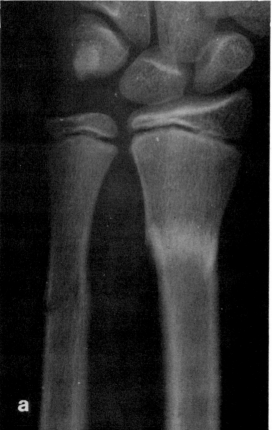

Fig. 6.48. Complete, displaced fracture of the distal radius associated with a green stick fracture of the ulna. Note the deceptive appearance of the fragments in the frontal projection (a), the difficulty in distinguishing the distal radial and ulnar fragments in the lateral projection (b), and the fact that the distal radioulnar joint is normally maintained.

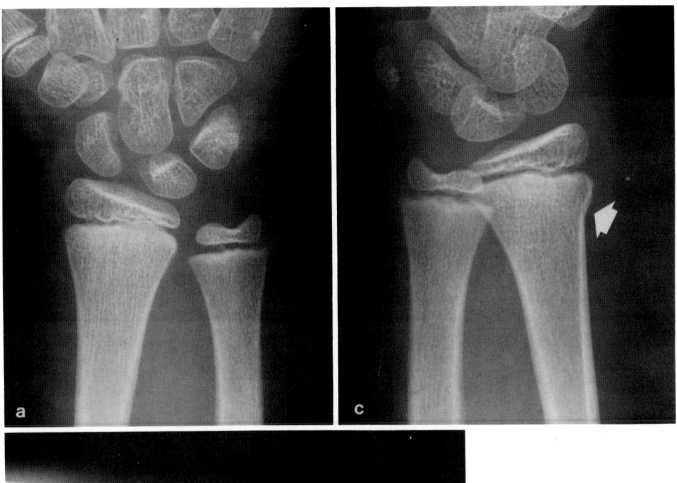

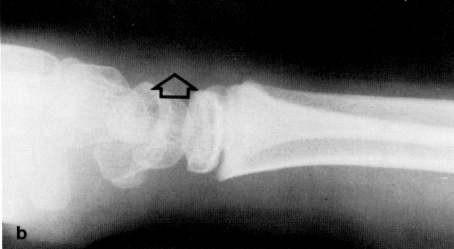

Fig. 6.49. In the frontal projection of the wrist (a), the bones appear negative. In the lateral projection (b), the most obvious abnormality is soft tissue swelling of the dorsum of the wrist. A cortical buckling fracture in the distal radial metaphysis is indicated by the *arrow* in (c).

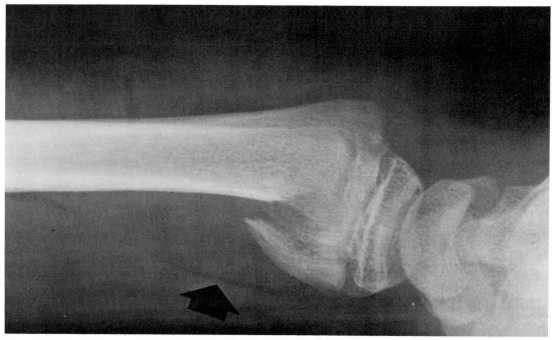

Fig. 6.50. This patient has an obvious, displaced fracture in the distal radial metaphysis. Note the marked increase in the size of the pronator quadratus muscle shadow (*arrow*) and compare with Figure 6.39. The volar bulging of the pronator quadratus reflects the presence of a periosteal hemorrhage.

Fig. 6.51. Salter-Harris II epiphyseal-metaphyseal injury of the distal radius. In the frontal projection **(a)**, the distal radial physis is widened radially and narrowed ulnarly. In the oblique projection **(b)**, an oblique fracture line is evident in the ulnar aspect of the radial metaphysis (*open arrows*). In the lateral radiograph **(c)**, the metaphyseal fracture is evident dorsally (*open arrow*). The most prominent roentgen sign of injury, however, is the abnormal pronator quadratus sign (*solid arrow*).

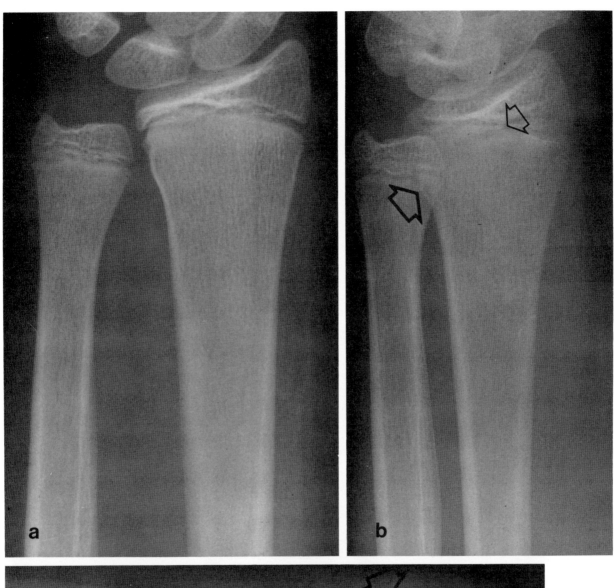

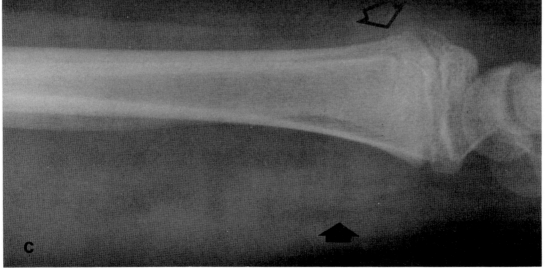

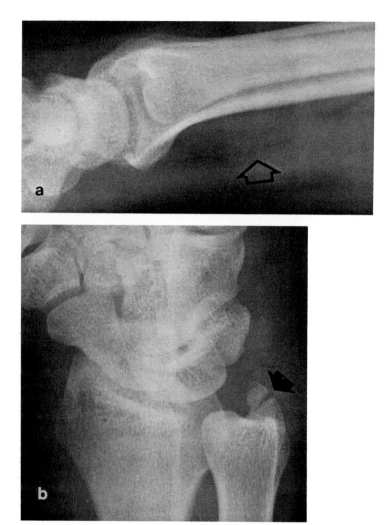

Fig. 6.52. The distended pronator quadratus shadow (**a**, *open arrow*) is associated with an oblique fracture through the base of the ulnar styloid process (**b**, *solid arrow*).

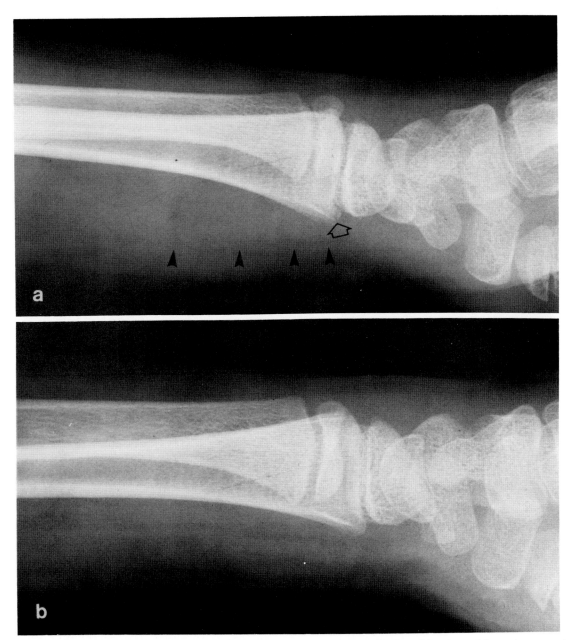

Fig. 6.53. (a) Positive pronator quadratus sign associated with a minimally displaced fracture of the volar aspect of the distal radial metaphysis (*open arrow*). Not only is the pronator muscle shadow wider than normal, but also the overlying fascial plane is obscured (*arrowheads*). **(b)** Lateral radiograph of uninjured opposite wrist. Note the normal thickness of the pronator muscle mass and the normal lucency of the overlying fascial plane.

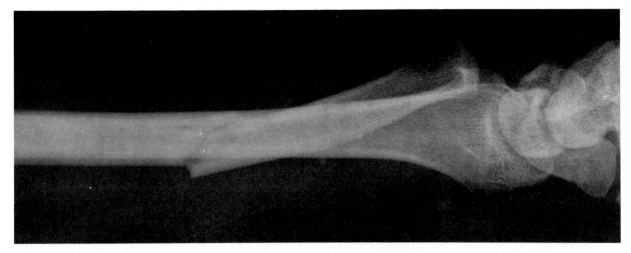

Fig. 6.54. Distal radioulnar dislocation caused by dorsal angulation of the distal *ulnar* fragment.

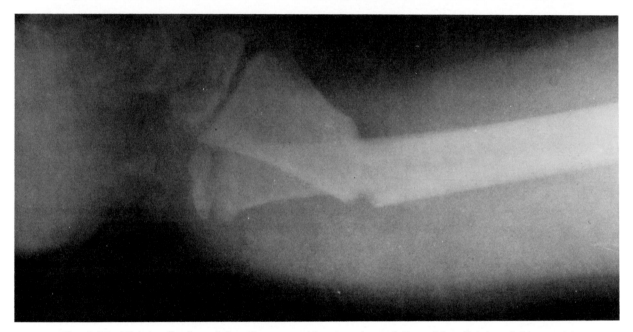

Fig. 6.55. Distal radioulnar dislocation caused by dorsal angulation of the distal *radial* fragment.

Dislocations of the radiocarpal joint are rare (Fig. 6.57). Generally, the ulnar styloid processes remain intact.

Epiphyseal injuries, particularly the Salter I (Fig. 6.58) and Salter II types (Figs. 6.50 and 6.59), commonly involve the distal radius.

It is possible for a separated epiphysis to return to its normal position so completely that the presence of a separation cannot be definitely established (Salter I epiphyseal injury). If the pronator quadratus muscle is prominent, or if a small fracture fragment from the metaphysis can be identified (Fig. 6.53), a separation may be reasonably inferred. Calcification within the hematoma may not be radiographically visible for 2–3 weeks following the injury.

A fall on the outstretched hand, with the hand in pronation and the hand and wrist in dorsiflexion, results in a variety of injuries, depending upon the patient's age (7). In the very young child, this force produces a greenstick fracture of the distal radius which may or may not be associated with a fracture of the distal ulna. In the older child or adolescent, the distal radial epiphysis is usually displaced dorsally, along with a fragment of the dorsal aspect of the adjacent metaphysis, i.e., a Salter II injury (Fig. 6.59). In adults, the distal radial fracture usually occurs within 1 inch of the distal radial articulating surface with the distal radial fragment being dorsally and proximally displaced. Displacement of the distal radial fragment usually results in volar angulation and

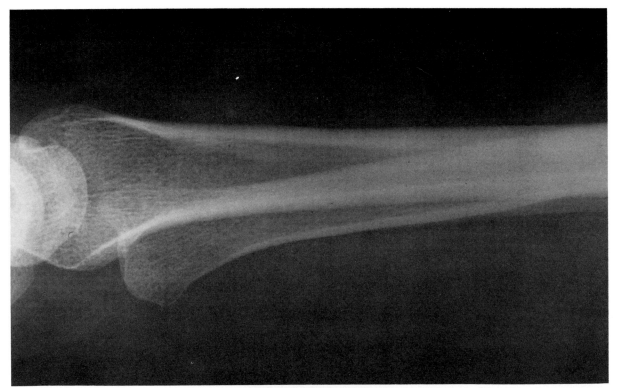

Fig. 6.56. Isolated distal radioulnar subluxation with volar displacement of the ulna.

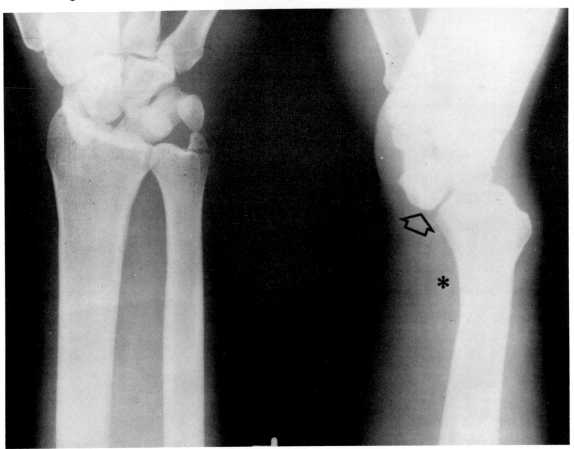

Fig. 6.57. Volar radiocarpal dislocation associated with a fracture of the base of the ulnar styloid process. The *open arrow* indicates the volarly displaced proximal row of carpal bones. The *asterisk* (*) signals the positive pronator quadratus sign, probably produced by hemorrhage associated with the ulnar styloid fracture.

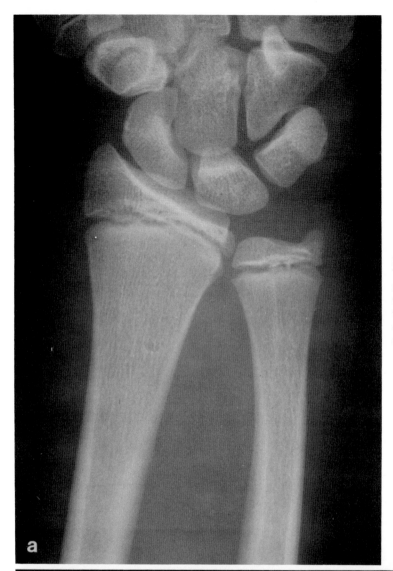

a

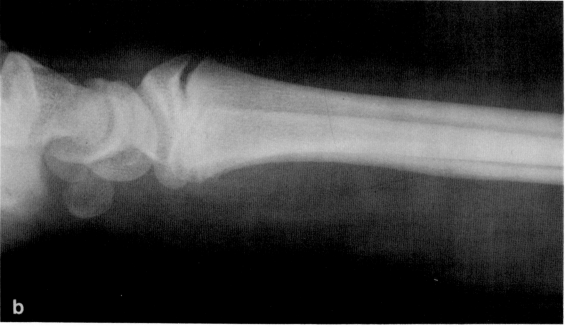

b

Fig. 6.58. Salter I injury of the distal radius. The incomplete distal radial epiphyseal separation is not recognizable in the frontal projection **(a)**. In the lateral radiograph **(b)**, however, the distal radial epiphyseal line is widened dorsally and the pronator quadratus sign, indicating subperiosteal hemorrhage, is positive.

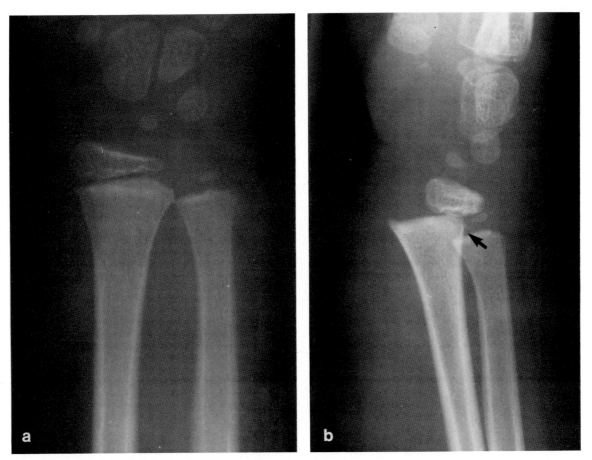

Fig. 6.59. Salter II distal radial injury. In the frontal projection **(a)**, the position of the distal radial epiphysis appears normal. In the lateral radiograph **(b)**, however, the dorsal displacement of the epiphysis is obvious. The *arrow* indicates the small distal metaphyseal fragment which establishes this injury as a Salter II type.

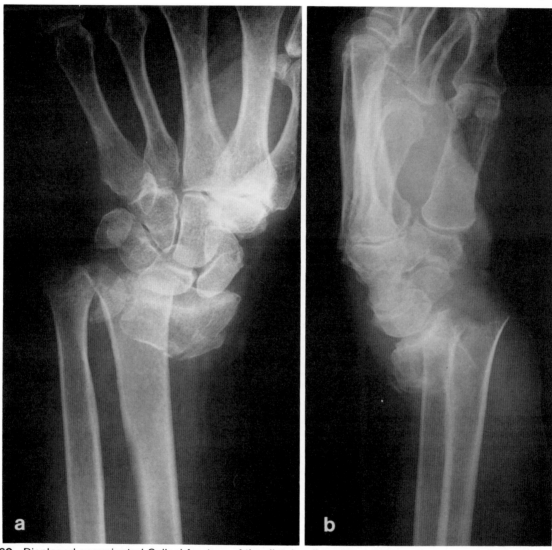

Fig. 6.60. Displaced comminuted Colles' fracture of the distal radius with a displaced fracture of the distal ulna. The distal radial *and* ulnar fragments are dorsally, proximally, and radially displaced. The normal relationship between the distal radial and ulnar fragments indicates that the articular disk (triangular fibrocartilage) is intact and that the distal radioulnar articulation is normally maintained.

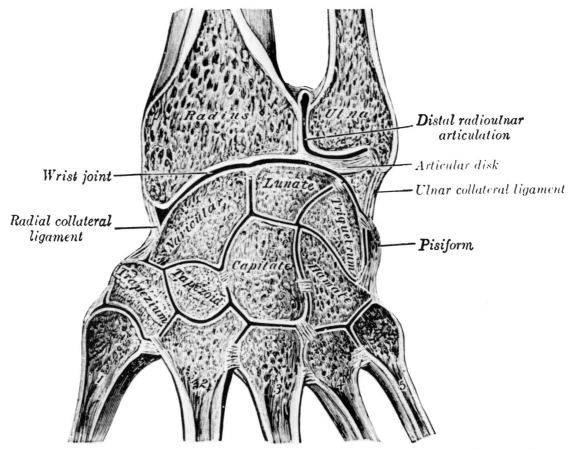

Fig. 6.61. Schematic representation of the joints of the wrist indicating the articular disk (the triangular fibrocartilage). [Reprinted with permission from C.M. Goss (Ed.): *Gray's Anatomy of the Human Body*, ed. 29 (Amer.). Lea & Febiger, Philadelphia, 1975.]

dorsal impaction of the fragments. Characteristically, the bones of the wrist and hand accompany the distal radial fragment in radial displacement as well. There may or may not be an associated distal ulnar fracture. This injury, which is the most common fracture of the wrist, is referred to as the Colles' fracture (Fig. 6.60), even though Colles' original description in 1814 referred only to a distal radial fracture (8). The condition of the distal end of the ulna is reflective of the status of the articular disk (triangular fibrocartilage) (Fig. 6.61), which extends from the radial surface of the ulnar styloid process to the ulnar aspect of the distal end of the radius and binds the distal ulna and radius firmly together. A transverse fracture through the base of the ulnar styloid process indicates that the triangular fibrocartilage is intact and has simply avulsed the ulnar styloid process. However, if the ulnar styloid process is intact, it indicates that the triangular fibrocartilage has been either avulsed from one of its attachments or disrupted. This observation is particularly valid when the distal radial fragment is displaced and the distal ulna is both intact and not displaced.

With the exception of the fracture of the distal ulna, the commonest fracture associated with a Colles' fracture involves the carpal scaphoid.

The Smith fracture, also referred to as a "reversed Colles" fracture, consists of a fracture of the distal radius in which the distal fragment is volarly and proximally displaced (Fig. 6.62). There may or may not be an associated distal ulnar fracture. The mechanism of injury is described as a fall on the back of the hand with the wrist in dorsiflexion. However, DePalma (7) states that this mechanism is rare and that the Smith fracture most commonly results from a backward fall onto the outstretched hand in supination.

Oblique fractures of the base of the radial or ulnar styloid process are the result of medial or lateral compressive force. The earlier discussion of the roentgen appearance of the fused or incompletely fused distal radial epiphyseal line emphasized the similarity of the radiographic appearance of this normal structure to that of an impacted or minimally displaced, oblique fracture of the distal radius. Figure 6.63 is an example of such a fracture. The presence of soft tissue

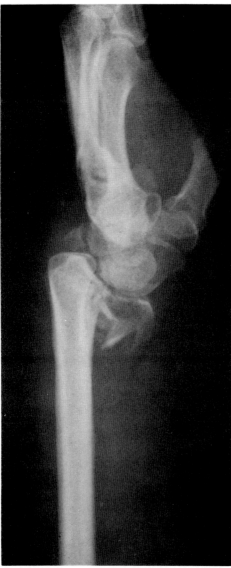

Fig. 6.62. Smith (reversed Colles') fracture.

swelling lateral to the distal end of the radius and the positive pronator quadratus sign should help in distinguishing this acute fracture from the normal epiphyseal line (Figs. 6.43–6.47).

An isolated, acute fracture of the base of the ulnar styloid process is seen in Figure 6.64. In this example, the acute, minimally displaced fracture is proximal to an old, ununited fracture of the styloid process.

The major dislocations of the carpal bones center upon the lunate-capitate relationship and are the result of either flexion or extension injuries of the wrist. The type of dislocation or fracture-dislocation is dependent upon the magnitude and direction of the force of injury and the disruption or preservation of the lunate-capitate articulation.

Displacement of the lunate, only, is referred to as volar or dorsal lunar dislocation. When the lunate retains its normal relationship to the distal radial articulating surface and the remainder of the carpal bones are displaced, the injury is called perilunar dislocation and may be either volar (anterior) or dorsal (posterior) (7, 9–12).

Carpal dislocations caused by extension (fall on the outstretched hand) are volar dislocations of the lunate or dorsal perilunar dislocations. If the hand and wrist are severely hyperextended and the force of the injury is received on the fingers and metatarsal heads, the capitate rolls dorsally on the lunate and the force transmitted through the radius drives the lunate volarly. In the process, the dorsal radiolunate ligaments are disrupted.

Radiographically, volar dislocation of the lunate (Fig. 6.65) is characterized, in frontal projection, by the triangular appearance of the dislocated lunate and by superimposition of the contiguous surfaces of the base of the capitate and the lunate. The diagnosis is established, however, in the lateral projection, where the lunate is seen to be displaced and rotated volarly out of its normal position relative to the distal radial articulating surface. The volar rotation, typically, ap-

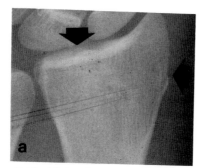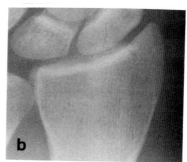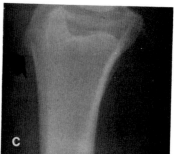

Fig. 6.63. Minimally displaced oblique fracture of the base of the radial styloid process **(a, b)**. The fracture line is indicated by the *solid black arrows*. In the lateral projection **(c)**, the positive pronator quadratus sign is indicated by the *open arrow*. The uninjured opposite wrist is shown in frontal projection **(b)**. The radiograph has been reversed for ease of comparison with part **(a)**.

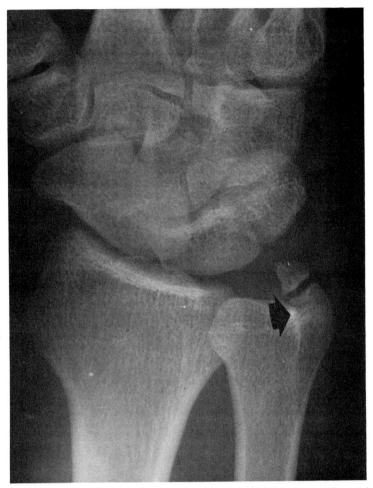

Fig. 6.64. Acute, minimally displaced fracture of the base of the ulnar styloid process (*arrow*). The triangular shaped, separate fragment with dense sclerotic cortical margins represents a previous, old, ununited fracture of the styloid process itself.

proximates 90° so that the concave, distal surface of the lunate faces volarly and its convex proximal surface is dorsally directed. The relation of all of the other carpal bones, to one another and to the radius, ulna, and metacarpals, remains normal in pure, or uncomplicated, volar dislocation of the lunate.

In some instances of pure volar dislocation of the lunate, the proximal surface of the lunate may remain in contact with the distal end of the radius. Even so, the lunate-capitate relationship is completely disrupted and the lunate is clearly dislocated anterior to the capitate and the other carpal bones (Fig. 6.66).

Dorsal perilunar dislocation occurs as the result of a fall on the outstretched hand when the hand is only moderately hyperextended and when the force of impact is on the palm of the hand such as occurs when the arms and hands are extended from the body. In this instance, the oblique force transmitted through the radius and the lunate disrupts the lunate-capitate

articulation and the capitate and all the other carpal bones are driven posteriorly. The radiolunate articulation is normally maintained. While dorsal perilunate dislocation may occur as a pure injury, it is most frequently associated with a transscaphoid fracture and, less frequently, with a scaphoid fracture and a fracture of the ulnar styloid process.

The roentgen signs of dorsal perilunate dislocation are illustrated in Figure 6.67, in which the perilunate dislocation is associated with a trans-scaphoid and ulnar styloid fracture, and in Figure 6.68, in which the perilunate dislocation is associated with a fracture-dislocation of the scaphoid (navicular).

In the frontal projection (Figs. 6.67*a* and 6.68*a*) the distal row of carpal bones is superimposed, to varying degrees, upon the lunate but the lunate retains its normal configuration and relationship to the distal radial articulating surface, in contradistinction to its triangular configuration in the volar lunate disloca-

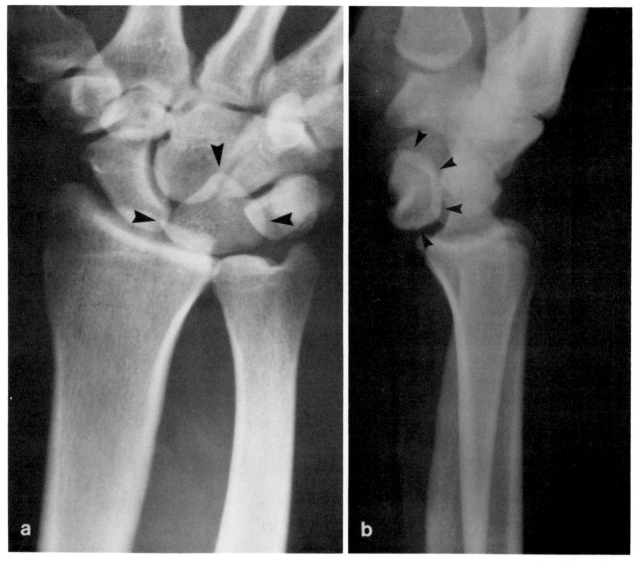

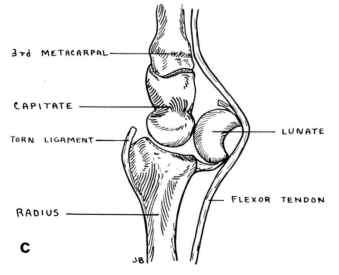

Fig. 6.65. Volar dislocation of the lunate. In the frontal projection **(a)**, the triangular configuration of the lunate (*arrowheads*) is readily apparent, as is superimposition of the contiguous surfaces of the lunate with the capitate, the hamate, and the triquetrum. In the lateral radiograph **(b)**, the volarly dislocated lunate (*arrowheads*) is clearly evident lying anterior to the other carpal bones and at 90° rotation to the long axis of the radius. **(c)** is a schematic drawing of a pure volar dislocation of the lunate.

3rd METACARPAL

CAPITATE

TORN LIGAMENT

RADIUS

LUNATE

FLEXOR TENDON

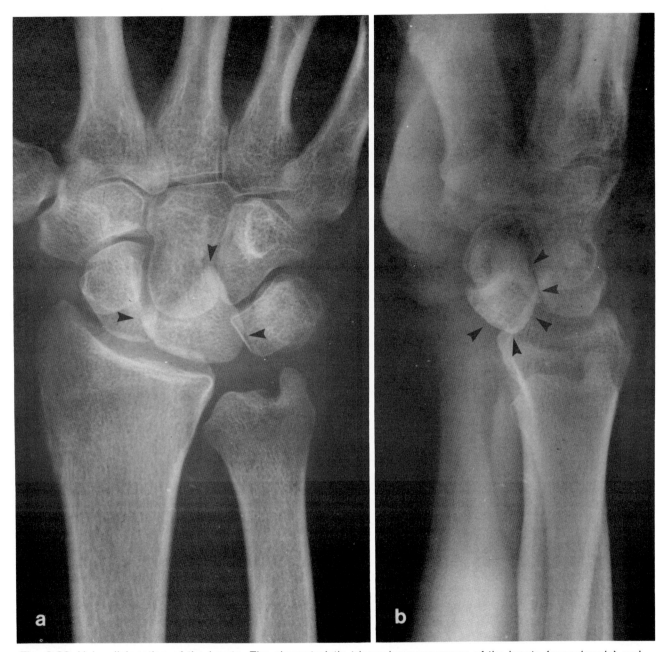

Fig. 6.66. Volar dislocation of the lunate. The characteristic triangular appearance of the lunate (*arrowheads*) and superimposition of the lunate upon adjacent portions of the triquetrum, capitate, and scaphoid are seen in the frontal radiograph **(a)**. In the lateral projection **(b)**, the proximal, convex surface of the lunate remains in partial contact with the distal end of the radius anteriorly, but the complete volar dislocation of the lunate (*arrowheads*) with respect to the other carpal bones is clearly evident.

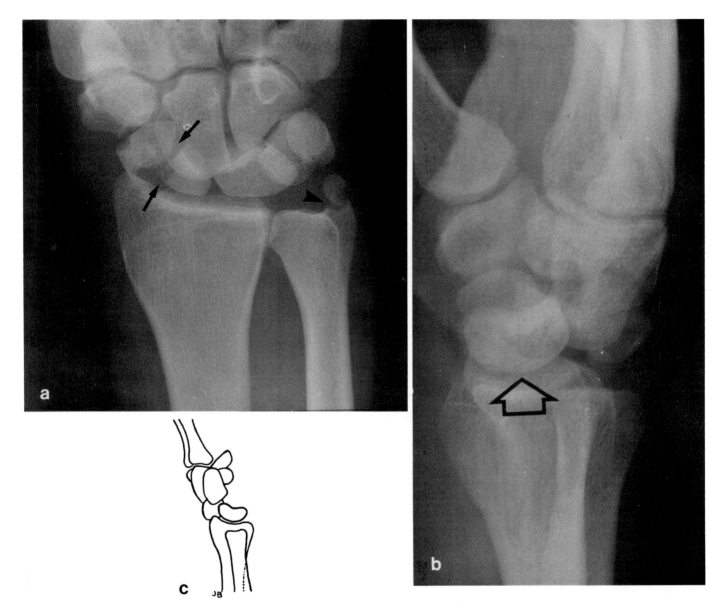

Fig. 6.67. Trans-scaphoid dorsal perilunate dislocation associated with a fracture of the base of the ulnar styloid process. In the frontal projection **(a)**, the *stemmed arrows* indicate the fracture through the waist of the scaphoid (navicular). The distal row of carpal bones is superimposed upon the proximal row, the configuration and relationship of the lunate to the radius is essentially normal, and neither fragment of the scaphoid is dislocated. The scaphoid fragments, therefore, have maintained their normal relationship to the radius and the lunate. The *arrowhead* indicates the ulnar styloid process fracture. In the lateral radiograph **(b)** the *open arrow* indicates the normal relationship between the proximal convex surface of the lunate and the distal radial articulating surface. The capitate and other carpals, except the scaphoid, are situated dorsal to the lunate. Part **(c)** is the schematic representation of a dorsal perilunate dislocation.

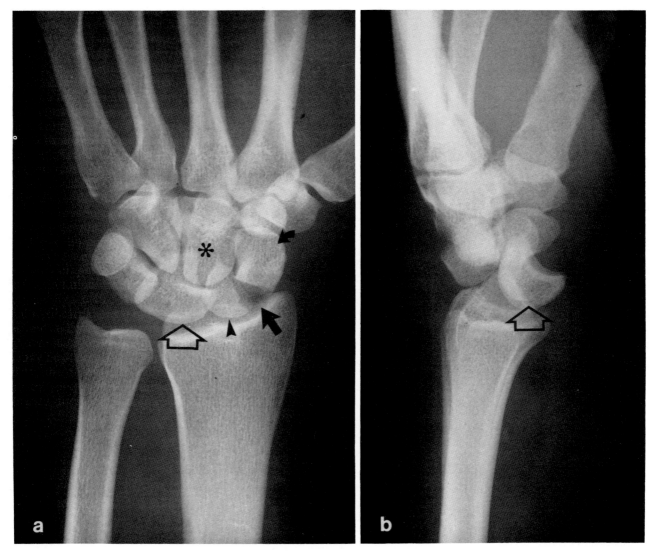

Fig. 6.68. Displaced trans-scaphoid dorsal perilunate dislocation. In the frontal projection (**a**), the scaphoid fragments are distracted (*stemmed arrow*). The lunate (*open arrow*) and proximal navicular fragment (*arrowhead*) maintain an essentially normal relationship to the distal radius, while the distal navicular fragment (*curved arrow*) relates to the capitate (*) which is superimposed upon the lunate and the proximal navicular fragment. In the lateral projection (**b**), the lunate (*open arrow*) is rotated slightly volarly but retains an essentially normal relationship to the radius. All other carpals, including the distal navicular fragment, are dislocated posteriorly to the lunate. Marked distraction of the navicular fragments carries a high probability of ischemic necrosis of the proximal fragment.

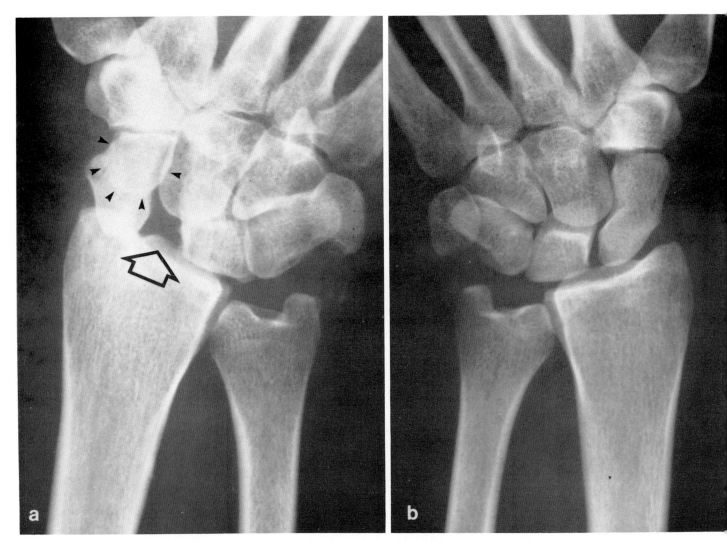

Fig. 6.69. Isolated rotary subluxation of the scaphoid **(a).** The space between the scaphoid and lunate is abnormally widened and has a truncated configuration (*open arrow*). The cortex of the distal pole of the rotated scaphoid, seen on end, results in the "ring" sign (*arrowheads*). The posteroanterior projection of the opposite, uninjured wrist **(b)** is shown for comparison. (Courtesy of Georges El-Khoury, M.D., Department of Radiology, University of Iowa.)

tion. In the lateral radiograph (Figs. 6.67*b* and 6.68*b*), the normal radiolunate relationship is maintained, i.e., the convex proximal surface of the lunate closely parallels the concave distal radial articulating surface, the transverse axis of the lunate is approximately perpendicular to the longitudinal axis of the radius, and the distal concave surface of the lunate is essentially distally directed. The remainder of the carpal bones together with the bones of the hand are dorsally dislocated relative to the lunate.

The fragments of the scaphoid fracture may, together, accompany other carpal bones in the dorsal dislocation relative to the lunate. More commonly, however, and as is illustrated in Figure 6.68, the scaphoid fragments separate with the proximal frag-

ment retaining its normal relationship to the lunate and radius (13), while the distal fragment accompanies the other carpal bones in dorsal dislocation. In this instance, the incidence of aseptic (ischemic) necrosis of the proximal fragment is nearly 100% (7).

Carpal dislocations caused by flexion are very rare and are caused by a fall on the back of the hand when the hand and wrist are severely hyperflexed. These injuries include dorsal dislocation of the lunate and, when the degree of hyperflexion is not so severe, volar perilunate dislocation.

Rotary subluxation of the scaphoid is an uncommon lesion described initially by Thompson et al. (14) and more recently by Hudson et al. (15). It is characterized by volar rotation of the scaphoid along its

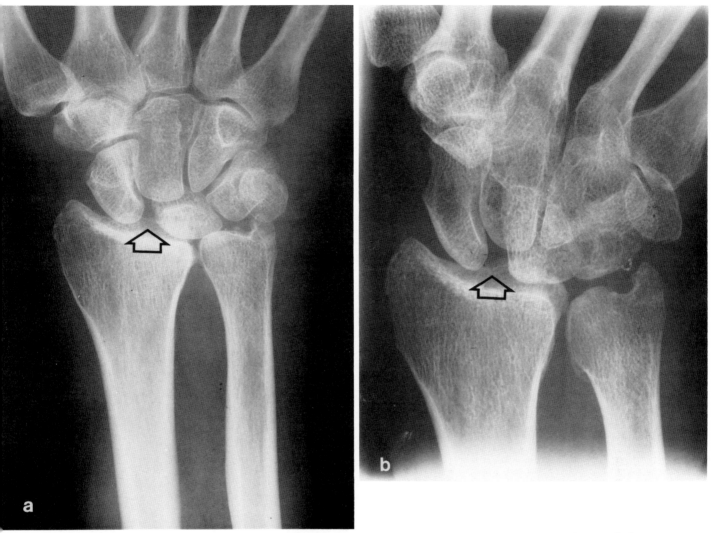

Fig. 6.70. Isolated rotary subluxation of the scaphoid. In this instance, the abnormal widening of the scapholunate space (*open arrow*) is not as striking as in Figure 6.69. However, it is abnormal and has the typical truncated configuration in the frontal radiograph **(b)**. The navicular view **(b)** confirms the abnormal scapholunate space (*open arrow*) and establishes that the navicular is intact.

long axis. In the absence of an obvious fracture, radiographically, and with only minimal to modest clinical findings, rotary subluxation of the scaphoid is commonly not recognized and is usually diagnosed as a "sprain." The clinical significance of the injury is the post-traumatic arthritis which develops if the subluxation is not reduced.

Radiographically, rotary subluxation of the scaphoid is characterized by abnormal widening of the space between the scaphoid and lunate and by the ring-like appearance of the cortex of the distal pole of the scaphoid. The latter results from the volar rotation of the scaphoid which causes the distal pole to be seen, radiographically, end-on (Figs. 6.69 and 6.70).

Fractures of the scaphoid (carpal navicular) are common, usually occurring in young males. They produce pain and tenderness in the region of the anatomic snuff box. However, these clinical signs are not specific for a scaphoid fracture and may be produced by injury to any of the structures along the radial aspect of the wrist. Additionally, scaphoid fractures may be extremely subtle and not discernible on the frontal or oblique projections of the wrist. For these reasons, therefore, it seems prudent to obtain a navicular view in any patient who has sustained an acute, significant injury to the radial aspect of the wrist. Even under optimum circumstances, a scaphoid fracture may not be initially visible radiographically. If symptoms persist and there is strong clinical suspicion of a navicular fracture, the radiographic study

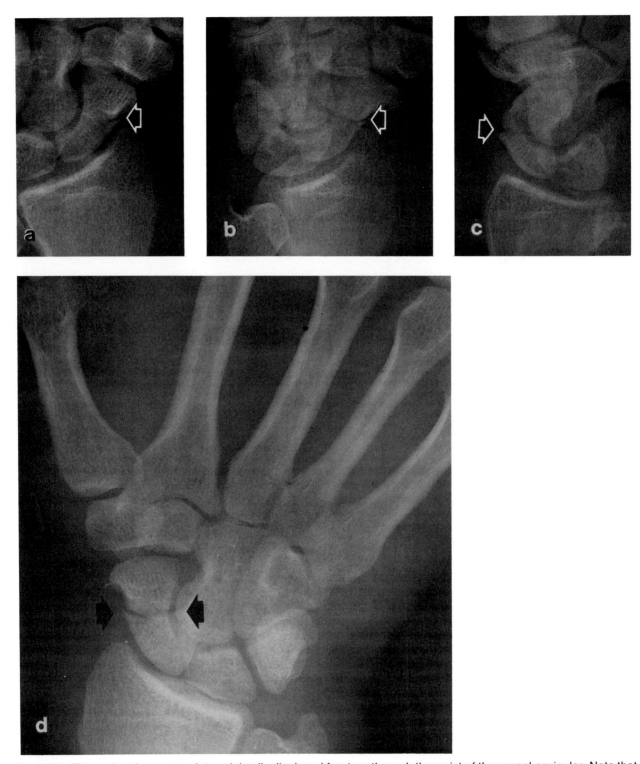

Fig. 6.71. This patient has a complete, minimally displaced fracture through the waist of the carpal navicular. Note that in the anteroposterior (**a**) and the oblique views (**b, c**) only a short arc of the fracture line is radiographically discernible and there is no indication that the fracture is complete. Only the navicular view (**d**) demonstrates the true extent of this fracture.

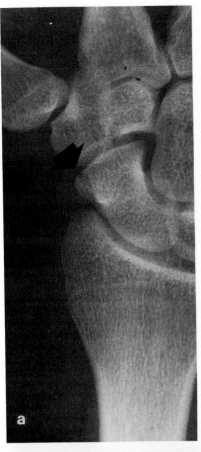

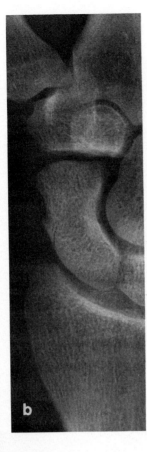

Fig. 6.72. This patient has a minimally displaced fracture of the tubercle of the navicular which could have been overlooked in the anteroposterior radiograph (a), was not visible in the navicular view (b), but was clearly evident in an oblique view of the wrist (c). Figures 6.71 and 6.72 emphasize the fact that no single radiograph will demonstrate every fracture of any given bone and that multiple views of every peripheral joint must be obtained.

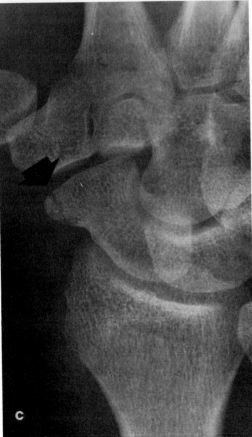

should be repeated in 7–10 days when the fracture line will be visible because of bony resorption associated with healing. Obliteration or displacement of a lucent area representing adipose tissue normally interposed between the radial convex surface of the scaphoid and the tendon of the extensor pollicis brevis has been described as being due to hemorrhage associated with a navicular fracture (16).

DePalma (7) states that the incidence of avascular necrosis of the proximal fragment of a nondisplaced navicular fracture approximates 50% and of a displaced fracture, almost 100%. Because the blood supply to the proximal portion of the scaphoid enters the waist of its convex surface, the more proximal the fracture line, the greater the incidence of avascular necrosis (11).

Eighty percent of scaphoid fractures involve its waist (Fig. 6.71) (7). Fractures of the tubercle of the scaphoid (Fig. 6.72) represent less than 5% of navicular fractures and are usually minimally displaced and, consequently, radiographically subtle. Fractures of the proximal pole (Fig. 6.73), as indicated previously, have a very high incidence of nonunion and avascular necrosis.

Scaphoid fractures occur more frequently as isolated injuries or, less frequently, in association with perilunate dislocations. Rarely, scaphoid fractures may occur in association with fractures of other bones of the wrist (Fig. 6.74).

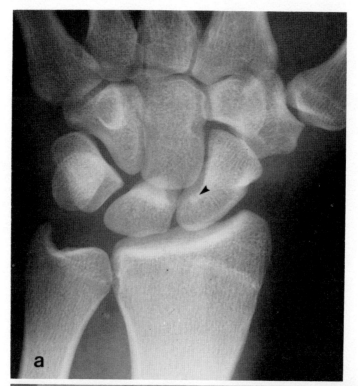

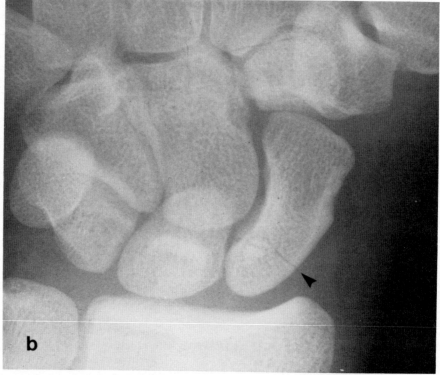

Fig. 6.73. Minimally displaced complete fracture of the proximal pole of the scaphoid. In the routine frontal projection (**a**), the fracture is almost imperceptible (*arrowhead*). The fracture line is considerably more evident in the navicular view (**b**, *arrowhead*), however. The lucent area normally present adjacent to the convex radial surface of the scaphoid has been replaced by a soft tissue density (*) which represents hemorrhage into the adipose tissue. This finding is the positive navicular fat stripe (NFS) sign (16).

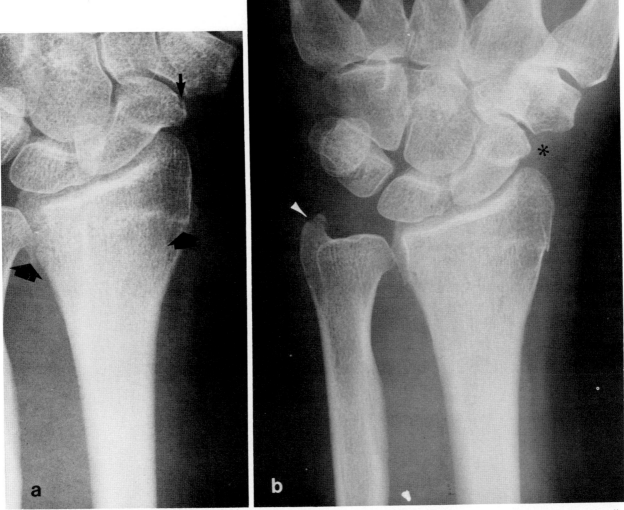

Fig. 6.74. Minimally displaced fracture of the tubercle of the scaphoid (*stemmed arrow*) associated with a minimally displaced, complete fracture of the radius (*arrows*) and a fracture of the ulnar styloid process (*arrowhead*). In the frontal projection (**b**), the NFS sign is positive (*), indicating blood into the adipose tissue normally present lateral to the scaphoid.

Fractures of other individual carpal bones (Figs. 6.75–6.79) are rare. Of these, the most common is the isolated fracture of the triquetrum (Fig. 6.80). This fracture is generally seen only in the lateral radiograph of the wrist. The separate fragment is typically a thin piece of cortical bone arising from the dorsum of the triquetrum. Soft tissue swelling of the dorsum of the wrist is invariably present.

Metacarpocarpal dislocations are unusual. In this injury, the bases of the metacarpals are displaced dorsally and override the distal row of carpal bones (Fig. 6.81).

Figure 6.82 illustrates a fundamental observation regarding the forearm, which in this instance involves the wrist. The basic axiom is that the shortening of only one of the bones of the forearm caused by either angulation or overriding of fracture fragments can only be accommodated by an associated proximal or distal radioulnar dislocation. In the patient in question, the radius is shortened as a result of impaction and displacement of the radial fracture fragments. The consequent and usually overlooked concomitant injury in this patient is the distal radioulnar dislocation. The ulnar styloid fracture is an incidental injury. Had the distal radioulnar articulation been normal, roentgen examination of the proximal portion of the forearm, including the elbow, would be mandatory to demonstrate the proximal dislocation. In the patient

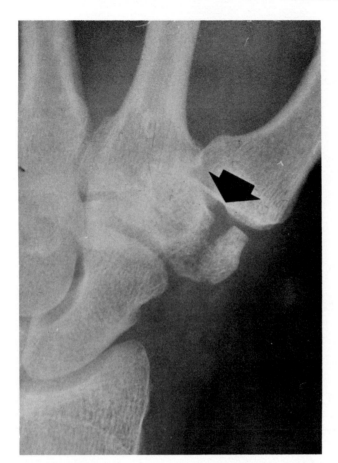

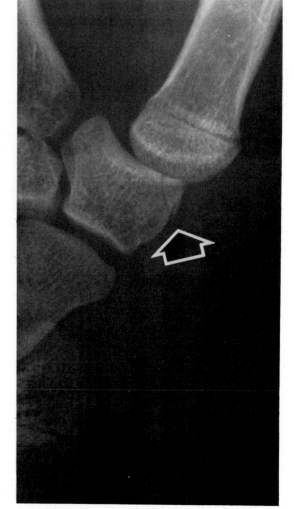

Fig. 6.75. Comminuted, distracted frature of the greater multangular.

Fig. 6.76. Minimally displaced, complete fracture of the greater multangular (*arrow*). This fracture was not visible on either the frontal or lateral radiograph of the wrist. It is, however, clearly evident on this navicular view.

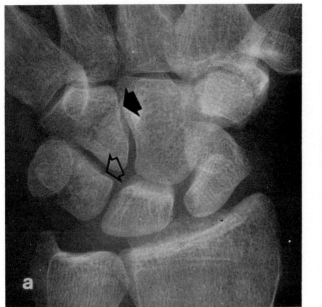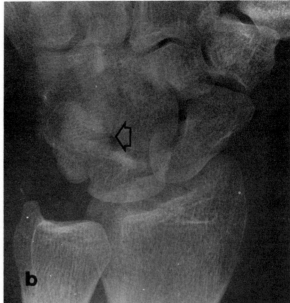

Fig. 6.77. (a,b) Complete, nondisplaced fracture of the triquetrum (*solid arrow*) and of the hamate (*open arrows*).

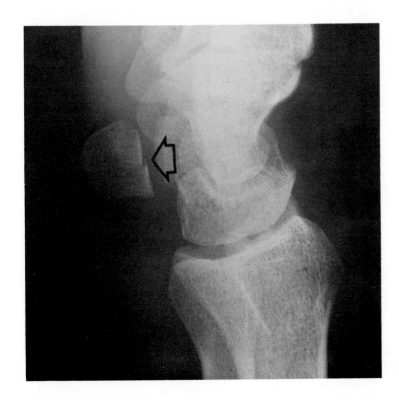

Fig. 6.78. Isolated fracture of the pisiform.

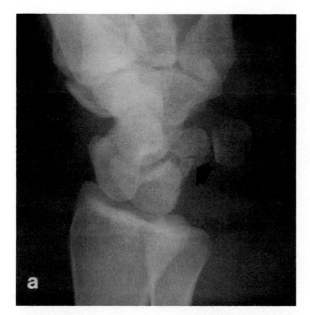
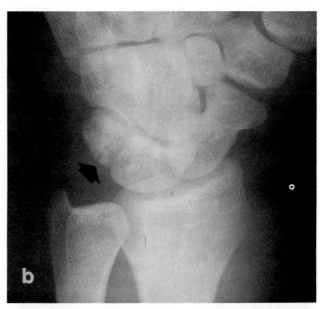

Fig. 6.79. (a,b) Isolated fracture of the hamate.

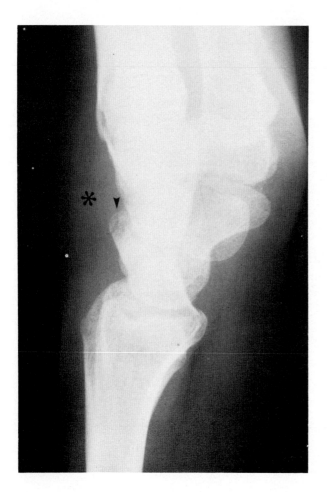

Fig. 6.80. Isolated "chip" fracture of the dorsal aspect of the triquetrum (*arrowhead*). Soft tissue swelling (*) is present in the dorsum of the wrist.

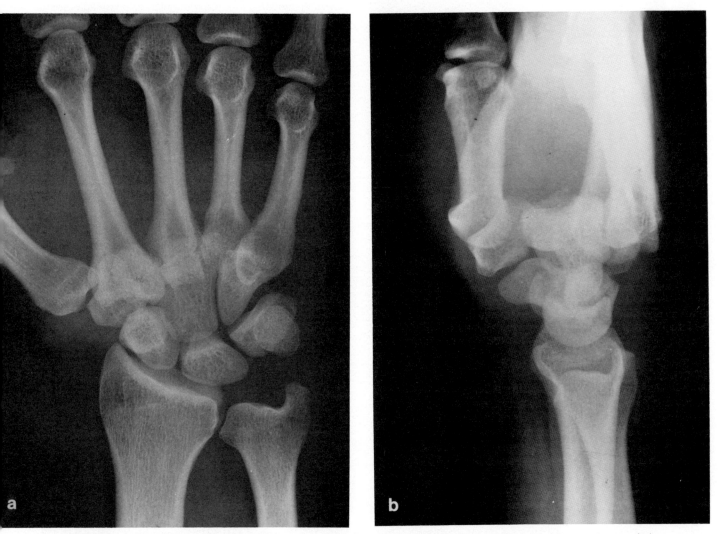

Fig. 6.81. Dorsal metacarpocarpal dislocation. In the frontal projection **(a)**, the base of the lateral four metacarpals is superimposed upon the distal row of carpal bones. In the lateral projection **(b)**, the dorsal and proximal dislocation of the metacarpals is obvious.

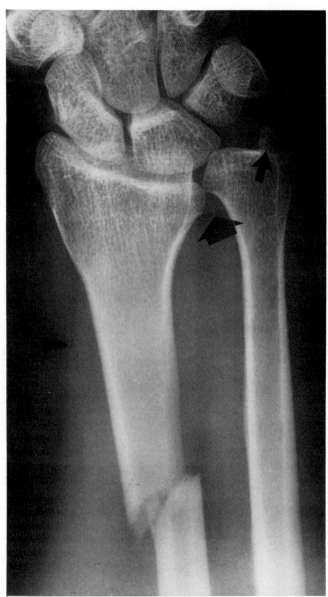

Fig. 6.82. The radius is shortened as a result of the impaction and displacement of the fragments of the fracture at the junction of its mid and distal thirds. The radial shortening has, in this patient, caused a distal radioulnar dislocation (*arrow*). Radial displacement of the distal fragment of the ulnar styloid process fracture (*stemmed arrow*) indicates that the triangular fibrocartilage (articular disk) is intact.

illustrated in Figure 6.82, the fracture in the distal third of the radius coupled with the distal radioulnar dislocation constitutes a Galeazzi fracture.

References

1. SALTER RB: *Textbook of Disorders and Injuries of the Musculoskeletal System.* Williams & Wilkins, Baltimore, 1970.
2. BENNETT EH: Fractures of the metacarpal bones. *Dublin J Med Sci* 73:72, 1882.
3. BENNETT EH: On fractures of the metacarpal bone of the thumb. *Br Med J* 2:12, 1886.
4. BENNETT EH: Fracture of the metacarpal bone of the thumb. *Trans R Acad Med, Ireland* 15:309, 1897.
5. CALLANDER CL: *Surgical Anatomy,* ed. 2. W.B. Saunders, Philadelphia, 1950.
6. MacEWAN DW: Changes due to trauma in the fat plane overlying the pronator quadratus muscle: A radiologic sign. *Radiology* 82:879, 1964.
7. DePALMA AF: *The Management of Fractures and Dislocations,* ed. 2. W.B. Saunders, Philadelphia, 1970.
8. SHULTZ RJ: *The Language of Fractures.* Williams & Wilkins, Baltimore, 1972.
9. NELSON SW: Some important diagnostic and technical fundamentals in the radiology of trauma with particular emphasis on skeletal trauma. *Radiol Clin North Am* 4:241, 1966.
10. RUSSELL TB: Inter-carpal dislocations and fracture-dislocations: A review of 59 cases. *J Bone Joint Surg (Brit.)* 31:524, 1949.
11. KAYE J: Fractures and dislocations of the hand and wrist. *Semin Roentgenol* 13:109, 1978.
12. MARASCO JA Jr: Essential facets of radiological diagnosis of extremity trauma. *CRC Crit Rev Diagn Imaging* 9:105, 1977.
13. WORLAND RL, DICK HM: Transnavicular perilunate dislocation. *J Trauma* 15:407, 1975.
14. THOMPSON TC, CAMPBELL RD Jr, ARNOLD WD: Primary and secondary dislocation of the scaphoid bone. *J Bone Joint Surg* 46-B:73, 1964.
15. HUDSON TM, CARAGOL WJ, KAYE JJ: Isolated rotary subluxation of the carpal navicular. *AJR* 126:601, 1976.
16. TERRY DW, RAMIN JE: The navicular fat stripe. *AJR* 124:25, 1975.

chapter seven

Chest

General Considerations

For purposes of this discussion, the chest shall be defined as the thoracic cage, including the soft tissues of the anterior chest wall, portions of the shoulder girdles, and the intrathoracic contents. The diaphragm has been discussed in conjunction with the abdomen and the thoracic spine in Chapter 3.

Whenever possible, roentgen examinations of the chest should be made with the patient in the erect position because physiologic alterations of intrathoracic structures inherent in the recumbent position may simulate organic disease on the supine radiograph of the chest.

The technical factors employed in the production of a chest roentgenogram are probably more critical than in the radiographic examination of any other part of the body. Pulmonary interstitial disease may be simulated by the prominent vascular and parenchymal markings on an underexposed radiograph. Conversely, gross pulmonary or cardiovascular pathology may be obscured or obliterated by radiographic overexposure, poor screenfilm or patient-film contact, or patient motion.

The roentgen study of the chest may provide valuable information regarding the etiology or extent of acute intra-abdominal disease or trauma. Furthermore, intrathoracic abnormalities may produce symptoms referable to the upper abdomen. For these reasons, radiographic examination of the chest should always be considered in the evaluation of acute symptoms which appear to originate in the abdomen.

Radiographic Examination

The routine radiographic study of the adult chest consists of erect posteroanterior and lateral projec-tions made in deep inspiration. Clinical situations occur in which it is impossible to obtain an erect (standing) posteroanterior (PA) roentgenogram of the chest. In those instances, and when possible, an erect (sitting) *anteroposterior* projection is preferable to a supine examination.

Radiographs made in expiration may be misinterpreted as showing cardiomegaly and parenchymal densities at each base, suggesting atelectasis or developing pneumonitis (Fig. 7.1). As a general rule, if the posterior portion of the right ninth rib is visible above the diaphragmatic surface in the PA radiograph, an adequate degree of inspiration may be assumed.

Deep inspiration is particularly important in chest roentgenograms of infants and children (Fig. 7.2) because the poorly aerated lung produces a radiographic appearance that closely resembles pneumonia.

The lateral radiograph is essential for the accurate localization of pulmonary lesions (Fig. 7.3), mediastinal masses, evaluation of cardiac size and configuration, and detection of posteriorly situated pleural effusions. Up to 500 cc of fluid may accumulate in the posterior costophrenic sulcus and not be visible in the frontal projection because of the configuration of the diaphragm. Unless dictated by the patient's condition, a single frontal roentgenogram constitutes an inadequate examination of the chest for the practice of emergency medicine.

In infants and young children, the routine examination of the chest should include each oblique projection in addition to the frontal and lateral views. In patients of this age group, lower lobe pneumonias are commonly obscured by the cardiac shadow in the frontal projection and by the spine in the lateral radiograph. Oblique examinations will generally project the area of involvement into clear view (Figs. 7.4 – 7.6).

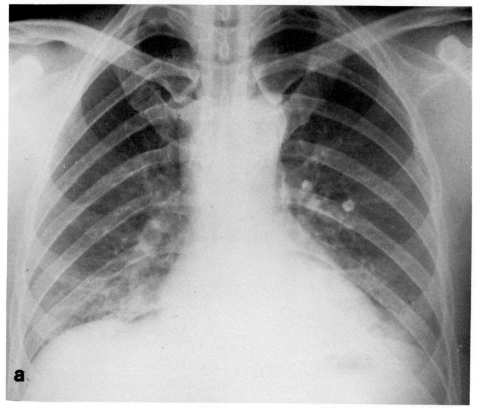

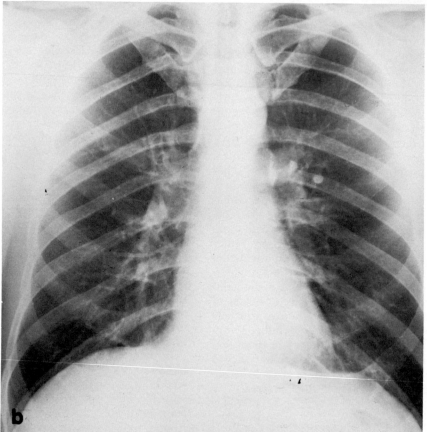

Fig. 7.1. PA radiograph of the chest of a healthy young male made in forced expiration **(a)** and deep inspiration **(b)**. In the expiratory examination **(a)**, the heart appears enlarged and the superior mediastinum widened. Bilateral basilar areas of hypoventilatory subsegmental atelectasis are clearly evident. All of these changes are physiologic during forced expiration. The effect of deep inspiration upon the radiographic appearance of the chest is dramatically recorded in **(b)**.

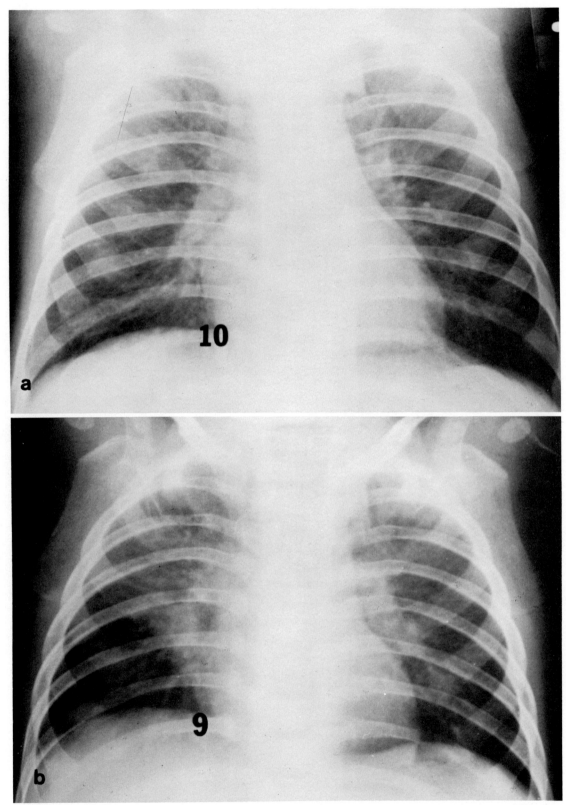

Fig. 7.2. The effect of deep inspiration (a) and forced expiration (b) upon the radiographic appearance of the chest of a young child. In the inspiratory roentgenogram (a), the right hemidiaphragm is at the level of the 10th rib. In the expiratory examination (b), the right hemidiaphragm is well above the level of the ninth rib posteriorly. Note the change in the appearance of the pulmonary parenchyma in the expiratory radiograph (b) and its resemblance to a bilateral upper lobe pneumonitis.

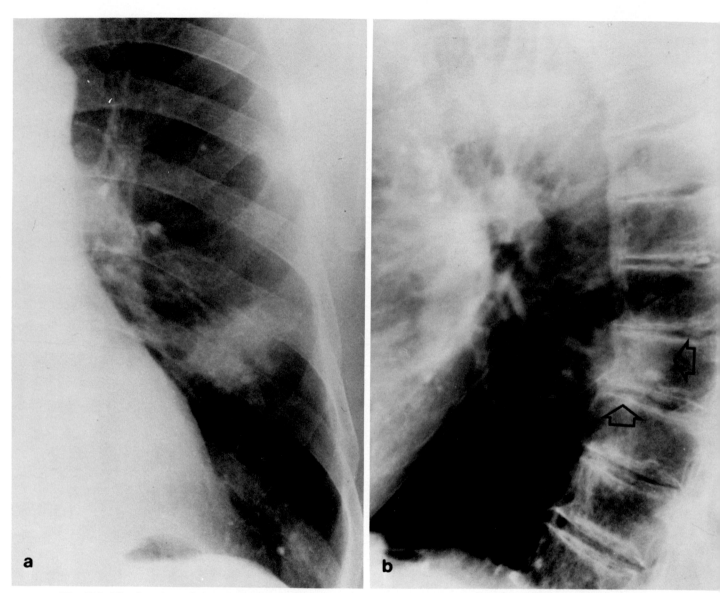

Fig. 7.3. The location of the carcinoma in the left midlung field cannot be determined on the basis of the frontal projection **(a)** alone. In the lateral radiograph **(b)**, the lesion (*arrows*) is clearly seen in the superior segment of the left lower lobe, superimposed upon the thoracic spine.

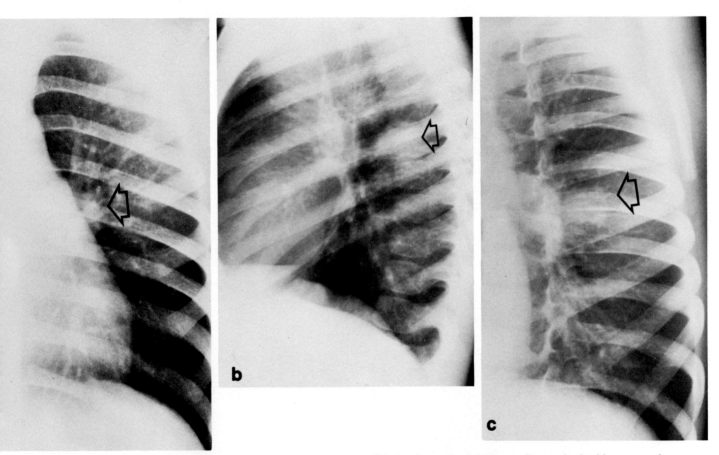

Fig. 7.4. In the frontal radiograph **(a)**, the subsegmental consolidation (*arrow*) could be easily overlooked because of the superimposed hilar structures. In the lateral projection **(b)**, the area of consolidation is largely obscured by the superimposed density of the thoracic spine and ribs. In the oblique projection **(c)**, however, the pneumonic process (*arrows*) is clearly seen in the apical segment of the left lower lobe, separate from the hilum.

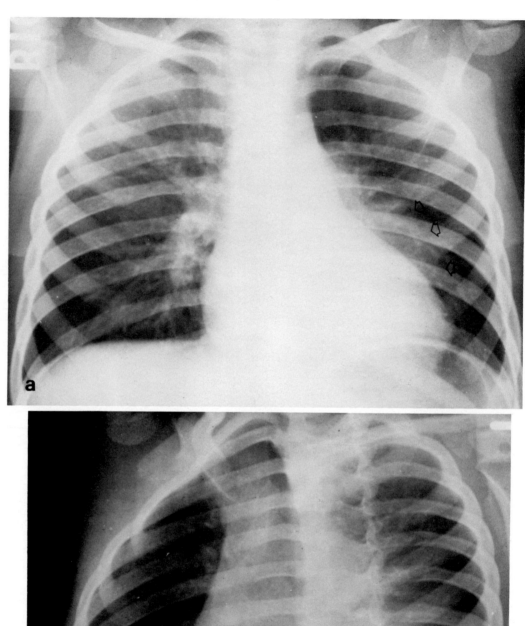

Fig. 7.5. (a) The left lower lobe pneumonia (*arrows*) is largely obscured by the density of the cardiac shadow in the frontal projection. The oblique projection **(b)** provides a more accurate assessment of the magnitude of left lower lobe consolidation.

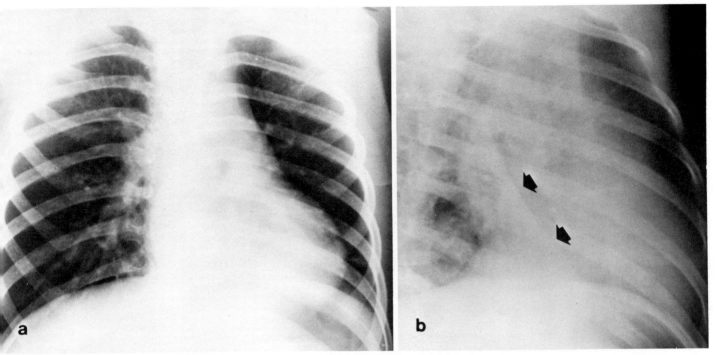

Fig. 7.6. The frontal projection of the chest **(a)** gives little indication of the left lower lobe atelectasis (*arrows*) seen the oblique projection **(b)**.

In the presence of major trauma, radiographic examination of the chest may be possible only in the supine position. Physiologically, in the supine posture, the mediastinum widens and the cardiac shadow increases in transverse diameter. Although the superior mediastinum is wider, its margins remain distinct, and normal anatomic landmarks remain identifiable (Fig. 7.7). Therefore, mediastinal widening alone, in the supine examination of the chest, does not constitute a radiographic sign of mediastinal hemorrhage.

The supine chest roentgenogram has serious diagnostic limitations that must be considered when the examination is requested and interpreted. Small or moderate pleural effusions that spread out in the posterior gutter in the recumbent posture may not be discernible in the supine projection. Pneumothorax may be impossible to detect in the supine radiograph because of migration of the air into the anterior (uppermost) pleural space.

Frontal examination of the chest made in forced expiration is valuable in the detection of a tiny pneumothorax and in evaluation of tension pneumothorax.

Lateral decubitus roentgenograms of the chest are invaluable in the detection of small pleural effusions. With the affected side down, the fluid will be visible along the lateral chest wall. In the opposite decubitus position, the fluid migrates into the mediastinal pleural space (Fig. 7.8).

The apical lordotic view (Fig. 7.9) provides maximum visualization of the apices of the lungs. This examination is, as its name implies, made with the patient in the lordotic position and is designed to project the anterior ends of the upper ribs and the clavicle away from the underlying apical pulmonary parenchyma.

Oblique views of the chest provide a different perspective to the cardiac silhouette, the mediastinal structures, and the lungs.

Fluoroscopic examination of the chest permits a qualitative evaluation of pulmonary aeration, appraisal of rate and amplitude of cardiac pulsation, and assessment of diaphragmatic excursion.

Aortography and pulmonary arteriography are the definitive (radiographic) studies for the detection of degenerative or traumatic lesions of the aorta and pulmonary embolization.

Laminography rarely has application in the radiographic evaluation of chest lesions in the emergency patient.

Radiographic Anatomy

The erect PA and lateral radiograph of the normal chest is seen in Figure 7.10. The intrathoracic portion of the trachea and the carina are obscured by the density of the mediastinal structures and the spine in the PA projection.

The aortic arch and the descending thoracic aorta (Fig. 7.10, *solid arrow*) lie to the left of the midline. The descending aorta passes obliquely from above

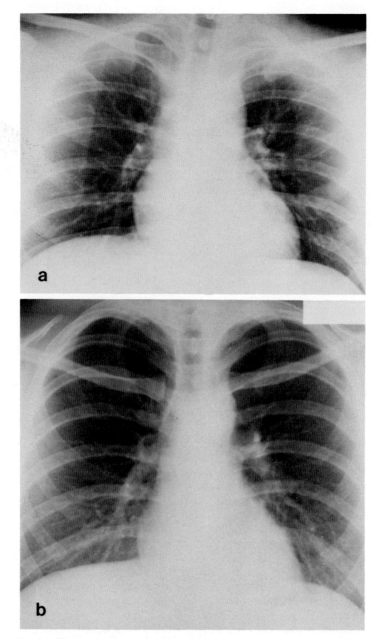

Fig. 7.7. Effect of the supine position upon the radiographic appearance of the chest. In the supine radiograph **(a)**, the superior mediastinum is wide but its margins are sharp and the lateral border of the aortic arch and the right stem bronchus are identifiable. The transverse diameter of the heart is increased and upper lobe pulmonary veins are discernible. These are characteristic physiologic changes that occur in recumbency. Part **(b)** is the erect PA radiograph of the same patient's chest made minutes following the supine examination **(a)**.

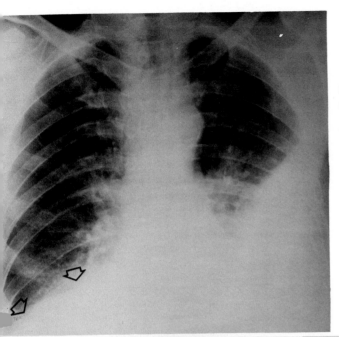

Fig. 7.8. The value of decubitus projections in the evaluation of a small pleural effusion. In the frontal projection **(a)**, it is evident that the patient has a large left pleural effusion. The *right* hemidiaphragm (*arrows*) is ill defined and the possibility of a small infrapulmonary effusion exists. The lateral radiograph **(b)** provides no assistance regarding a possible small right effusion because of the density of the larger left effusion. In the right lateral decubitus projection **(c)** a right pleural effusion is clearly evident extending along the lateral chest wall and obliterating the right costophrenic angle (*arrows*). In the opposite (left) decubitus position **(d)**, the right pleural effusion has migrated into the mediastinal space, leaving the costophrenic angle and lateral chest wall clear.

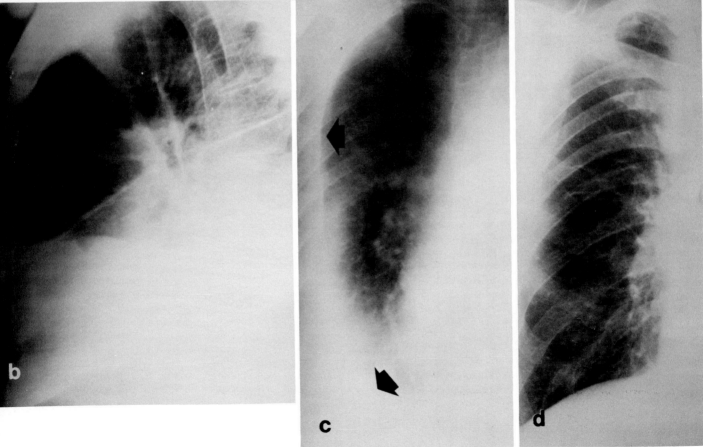

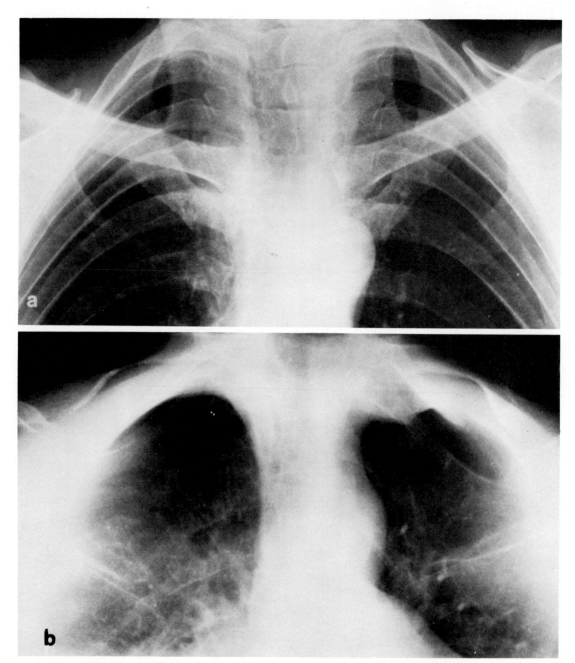

Fig. 7.9. In the routine frontal projection of the chest **(a)**, the apices of the lungs are obscured by superimposed soft tissue and bony densities. The apical lordotic view **(b)** is designed to project the lung apices free from the superimposed densities of the chest wall.

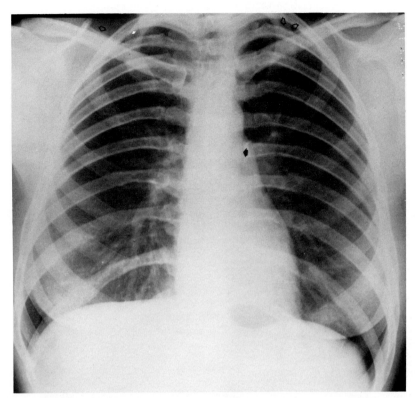

Fig. 7.10. Erect frontal radiograph of the normal chest. The lateral margin of the arch and the descending portion of the thoracic aorta are indicated by the *solid arrow*. The "companion" shadow above the clavicle (*open arrows*) is caused by the density of the skin and subcutaneous tissues which pass over the superior margin of the clavicle.

downward and slightly medially behind the heart. The shadow of the aorta must not be confused with the posterior mediastinal pleural reflection of the left lower lobe which extends *parallel* to the thoracic spine, described in Chapter 3.

The "aortic-pulmonary mediastinal stripe" (Fig. 7.11) (1) represents the mediastinal pleural reflection of the left upper lobe as it crosses the aortic arch and extends to the left hilum.

The cardiophrenic angles are normally acute. A pericardial fat pad frequently occupies the right cardiophrenic angle. This normal structure may obscure the angle, but the cardiac and diaphragmatic margins are usually visible through it. The density of the fat pad is not as great, nor its margins as sharply defined, as a pericardial cyst (Fig. 7.12).

The medial segment of the right middle lobe and the lingular segment of the left upper lobe wrap around the lateral cardiac walls. Consolidation of the middle lobe (Fig. 7.13) or the lingular segment (Fig. 7.14) will obscure the contiguous arc of the heart border on the roentgenogram. This is referred to as the "silhouette" sign by Felson and Felson (2). A corollary of the silhouette sign is that a density which is superimposed upon, but which does not obscure or obliterate, the heart border lies posterior to the heart (Figs. 7.15 and 7.16).

The hilar shadows are composed principally of the pulmonary arteries and veins, the walls of the stem bronchi and their segmental divisions, lymph nodes, and areolar tissue. Calcification of hilar nodes is a frequent finding and usually is of no clinical significance.

The sternum is not well seen in the PA radiograph of the chest because it is almost completely obscured by the superimposed density of the mediastinal structures and the spine.

The thin, sharply defined homogeneous soft tissue density located above and parallel to the superior cortex of the clavicles is called the "companion shadow" (Fig. 7.10). This density represents the skin and subcutaneous tissue that pass over the clavicle and dip into the concavity of the supraclavicular fossa. Medially, the companion shadow is continuous with the density of the lateral margin of the inferior portion of the sternocleidomastoid muscle. The companion shadow is effaced or obliterated when the supraclavicular fossa is filled with enlarged lymph nodes, such as in lymphomas or metastatic disease.

An important radiographic anatomic observation is the fact that apices of the upper lobe extend well above the level of the clavicles (Fig. 7.10).

The lateral radiograph of the chest (Fig. 7.17) dramatically illustrates the depth of the posterior costo-

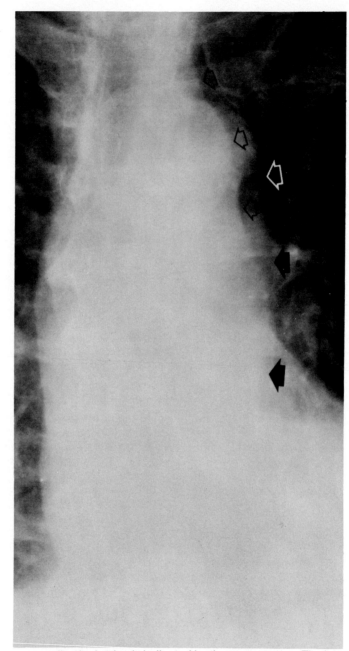

Fig. 7.11. The aortic-pulmonary mediastinal stripe is indicated by the *open arrows*. The lateral margin of the descending thoracic aorta is indicated by the *solid arrows*.

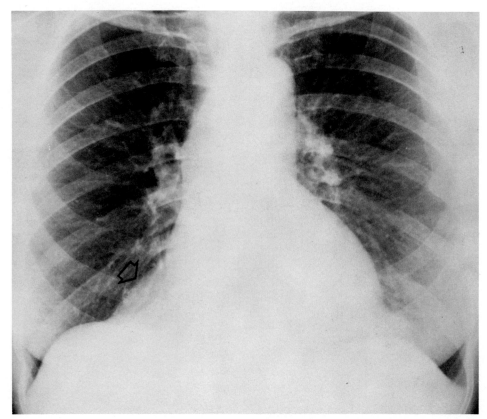

Fig. 7.12. The right cardiophrenic angle is obscured by a homogeneous, sharply defined density (*arrow*) which, at thoracotomy, was proven to be a pericardial cyst.

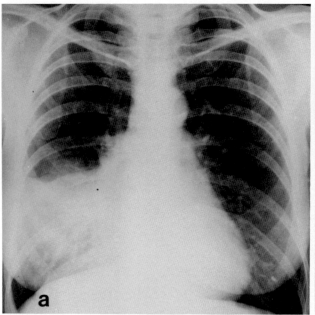

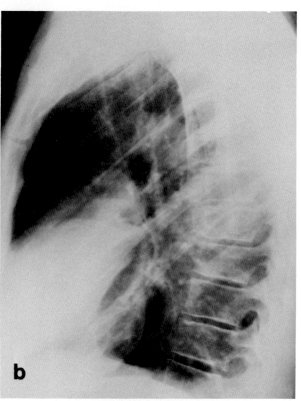

Fig. 7.13. The "silhouette" sign of right middle lobe consolidation. In the frontal projection **(a)**, the right heart border is obscured by the consolidation at the right base. Note also that the lung tissue in the right costophrenic angle (lateral basilar segment of the lower lobe) is spared. The configuration of the consolidation coincides with the anatomic distribution of the right middle lobe. In the lateral projection **(b)**, the density of the middle lobe consolidation is superimposed upon the cardiac shadow and is obscured by it.

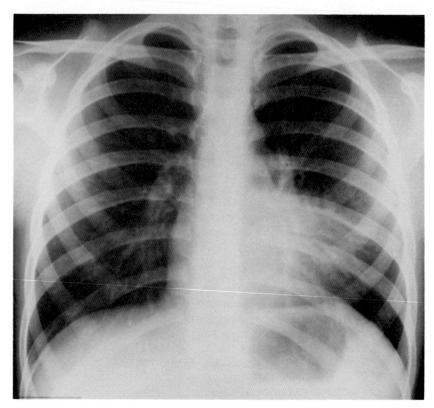

Fig. 7.14. Silhouette sign of the left heart border caused by pneumonia of the lingular segment of the left upper lobe.

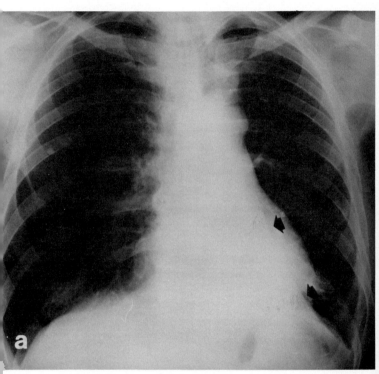
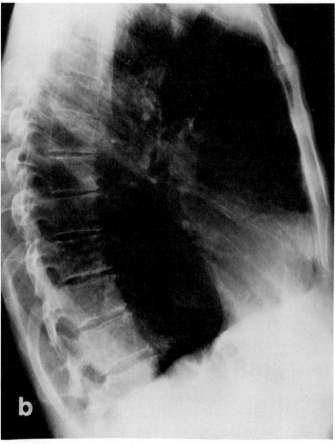

Fig. 7.15. Atelectasis of the left lower lobe. In the frontal projection **(a)**, the sharp margin of the atelectatic left lower lobe (*arrows*) is seen behind the density of the left heart border. In the lateral projection **(b)**, the density of the left lower lobe atelectasis is superimposed upon the lower thoracic vertebral bodies.

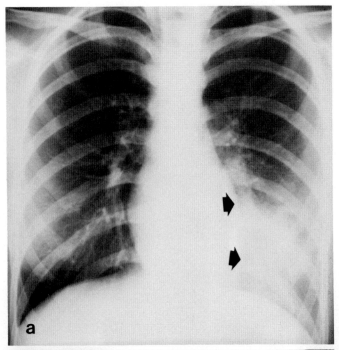

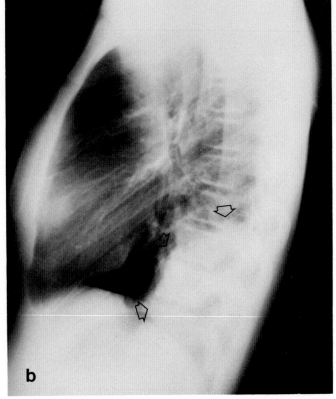

Fig. 7.16. Pneumonic consolidation of the left lobe. In the frontal radiograph **(a)**, the left heart border (*arrows*) is clearly evident through the large area of parenchymal density of the left base. This observation indicates that the density, which is superimposed upon but does not obliterate the left heart border, involves the lower lobe rather than the lingular segment of the left upper lobe (compare with Fig. 7.14). The presence of the consolidation in the posterior basilar segment of the left lower lobe is confirmed by its location (*arrows*) in the lateral radiograph **(b)**.

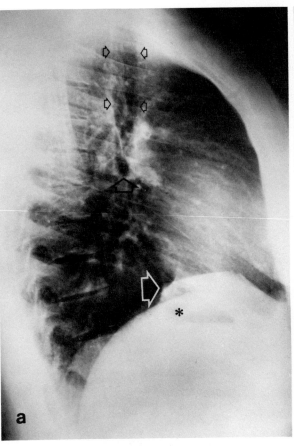

a

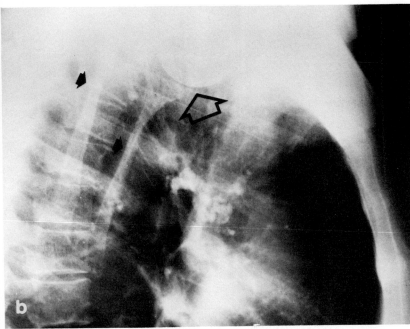

b

Fig. 7.17. (a) Lateral radiograph of the chest of a normal patient. The walls of the trachea and the carina are indicated by the *open arrows*. The *solid arrow* denotes the inferior vena cava. Gas in the fundus of the stomach (*) identifies by normal anatomic relationship the left hemidiaphragm. **(b)** In this lateral roentgenogram of the chest, the lateral borders of the scapulae are indicated by the *solid arrows* and the glenoid fossa and humeral head by the *open arrow*.

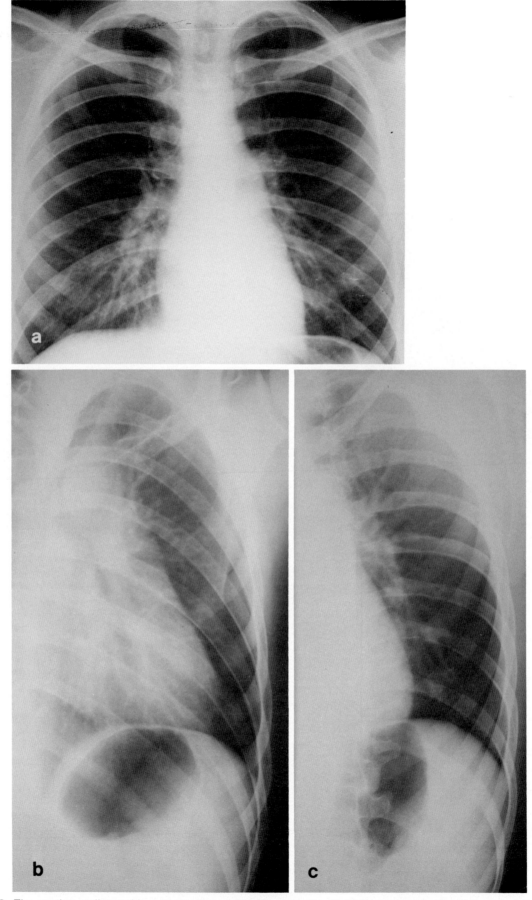

Fig. 7.18. The routine radiographic examination of the ribs includes the PA erect projection **(a)** and each oblique projection **(b, c)** of the affected side. The purpose for the oblique projections is to visualize all segments of the ribs, particularly those segments which are obscured by superimposition in the frontal projection.

phrenic sulcus and the volume of the lower lobe that lies posterior to the dome of the diaphragm.

The posterior margin of the cardiac shadow is composed of the left atrium above and the left ventricle inferiorly.

The trachea is usually visible to the level of the carina (Fig. 7.17a, *open arrows*). The inferior vena cava (*solid arrow*) is frequently seen as a sharply defined, curved soft tissue density superimposed upon the diaphragm and extending to the right atrium at the inferior arc of the posterior surface of the heart.

The diaphragmatic surfaces can usually be identified in the lateral chest roentgenograms by the fact that air in the gastric fundus [Fig. 7.17(*)] is normally closely related to the left hemidiaphragm.

When the arms are elevated for the lateral examination of the chest, the scapulae rotate anterolaterally and their lateral margins become superimposed upon the posterior third of the chest. Frequently, the glenoid fossa and the humeral head are projected upon the superior mediastinum. These normal structures should not be considered as representing abnormal radiographic densities.

Ribs

The routine examination of the ribs, when the patient's condition will permit, must include an erect PA radiograph of the chest and each oblique projection of the affected side (Fig. 7.18).

The indications for the erect frontal examination of the chest include the detection of possible pneumothorax, pulmonary contusion, or pleural effusion primarily and secondarily recognition of pre- or co-existing disease, i.e., left heart failure (Fig. 7.19).

The purpose for examination of the affected hemithorax in each oblique position is to visualize all segments of the ribs. Incomplete or minimally displaced rib fractures may be difficult, or impossible, to identify on the posteroanterior radiograph alone and frequently may be recognizable only in one of the oblique views (Fig. 7.20).

Portions of the lower ribs are obscured by the density of the upper abdominal contents in the routine rib views described above. When the clinical findings suggest an abnormality of the ribs below the diaphragm, an anteroposterior radiograph of the lower

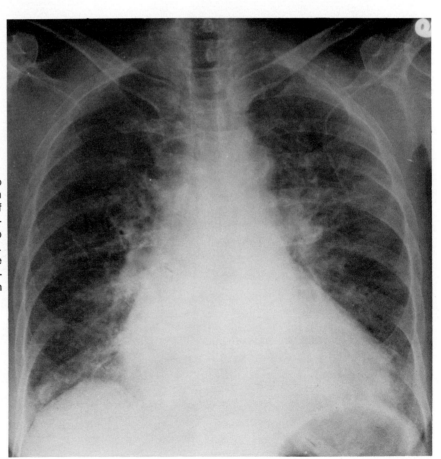

Fig. 7.19. This elderly female, who sustained trauma to the chest in an automobile accident, complained of chest pain, orthopnea, and dyspnea. The clinical impression was rib fracture and pulmonary contusion. Radiographic examination of the chest and ribs revealed only pre-existent cardiac decompensation with early frank pulmonary edema.

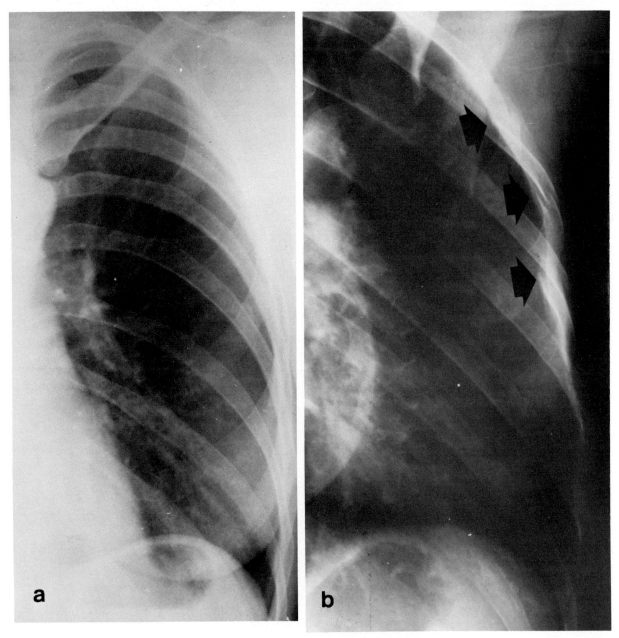

Fig. 7.20. The frontal **(a)** radiograph of the left hemithorax is negative. In the oblique projection **(b)**, complete, displaced fractures (*arrows*) are seen in the anterior axillary line of three of the left upper ribs.

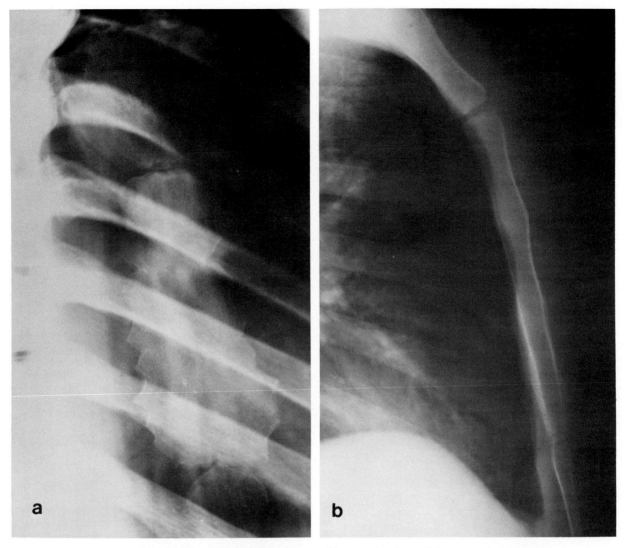

Fig. 7.21. Frontal (**a**) and lateral (**b**) radiographic examinations of the normal sternum.

portion of the chest and the upper portion of the abdomen using either abdominal or lumbar spine radiographic technique is required to evaluate the lower ribs as well as the lower thoracic and upper lumbar vertebrae.

Sternum

The routine roentgen study of the sternum consists of frontal views, made with the patient prone and rotated slightly off the midline in each direction, and a lateral projection (Fig. 7.21). Laminograms of the sternum, made in lateral projection, may be needed if the routine studies are not definitive.

Radiographic Manifestations of Trauma

Radiography is not usually needed to establish the presence of soft tissue abnormality of the chest wall. Occasionally, however, small amounts of subcutaneous emphysema can only be detected on the chest roentgenogram (Fig. 7.22).

Skeletal Injuries

The manubrium and corpus of the sternum are united by cartilage at the sternal synchondrosis (the sternal angle). Blunt trauma to the anterior chest wall can result in dislocation at this site (Fig. 7.23).

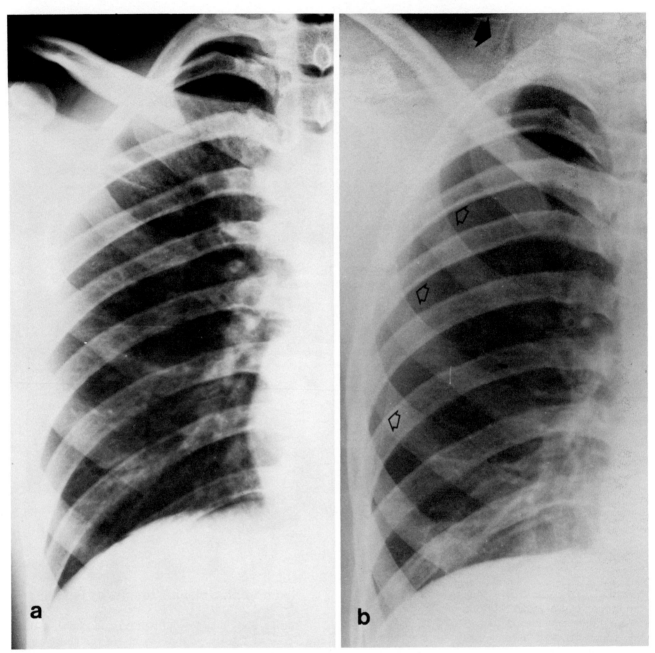

Fig. 7.22. This patient was stabbed in the posterior portion of the right hemithorax inferiorly. The supine examination of the chest **(a)** was negative. The pneumothorax (*open arrows*) and the clinically unrecognized subcutaneous emphysema in the neck (*solid arrow*) were visible on the erect frontal radiograph **(b)**.

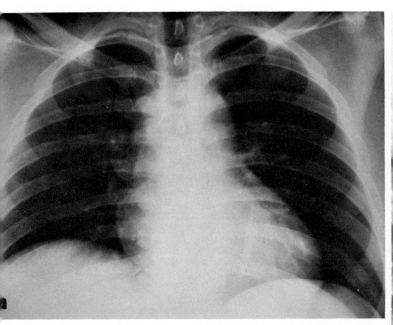

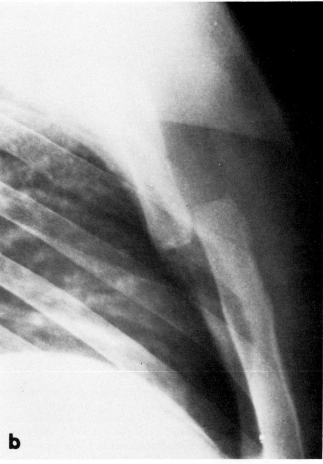

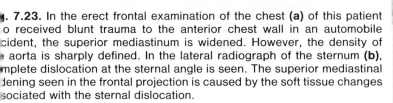

7.23. In the erect frontal examination of the chest **(a)** of this patient o received blunt trauma to the anterior chest wall in an automobile cident, the superior mediastinum is widened. However, the density of aorta is sharply defined. In the lateral radiograph of the sternum **(b)**, mplete dislocation at the sternal angle is seen. The superior mediastinal ening seen in the frontal projection is caused by the soft tissue changes sociated with the sternal dislocation.

Fracture of the sternum usually occurs in the body. Clinically, the significance of sternal fractures lies in the 25–45% mortality rate (6), which results not from the fracture per se but from associated injuries within the chest, such as rupture of the aorta, trachea, diaphragm, myocardial or pulmonary contusion, or rupture of the pulmonary vessels. Gibson et al. (7) report a 75% incidence of head trauma associated with sternal fractures caused by automobile accidents. Therefore, the clinician must maintain a high index of suspicion regarding sternal fractures so that this injury is not overlooked in patients with head trauma and so that a sternal fracture, when present, may serve to alert the clinician to possible associated serious intrathoracic injury. The essential radiograph required to establish the diagnosis of significant sternal injury is the lateral projection, which may be obtained with the horizontal beam when the patient must be examined in the supine position.

Radiographically, the significance of sternal fracture lies in the *similarity* of the roentgen changes produced by this injury to those produced by traumatic rupture of the aorta or other major vessel in the mediastinum. Figure 7.24*a* demonstrates what appears to be ill defined mediastinal widening in the PA radiograph. The patient was not in shock and none of the clinical findings of ruptured thoracic aorta were present. The lateral radiograph (*b*) clearly demonstrates the displaced fracture of the corpus of the sternum and the peristernal soft tissue changes that resulted in the apparent ill defined superior mediastinal widening seen in the frontal projection.

Anomalies of the ribs are easily recognized as such and should not constitute a diagnostic problem radiographically.

Rib fractures are usually the result of either compression of the chest or a direct blow to the chest wall. The former type of injury, resulting in a decrease in the arc of the ribs, causes an outward break at the site of greatest compression. This "spring fracture" is rarely associated with puncture of the lung. Direct, localized trauma to the chest wall, when of sufficient force, results in fracture at the site of impact. In this circumstance, the fracture ends are more likely to penetrate the chest wall, producing a hemo- or pneumothorax.

Blunt trauma to the chest may produce incomplete, nondisplaced rib fractures that are not discernible on the initial radiographic study. If rib fracture is suspected clinically, or if pain persists, roentgenograms

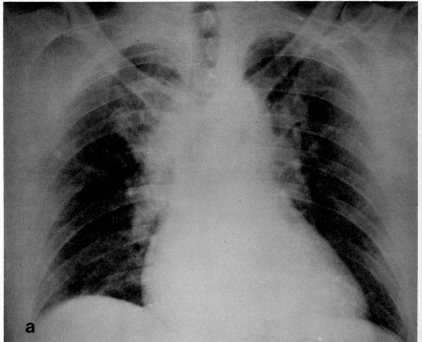
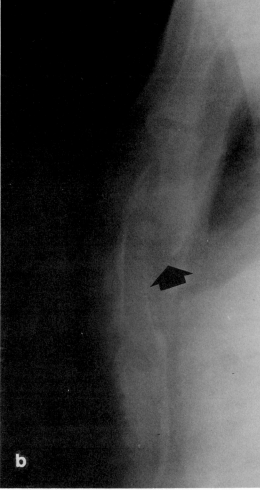

Fig. 7.24. The erect frontal radiograph of the chest **(a)** of this patient who received significant blunt trauma to the anterior chest wall discloses apparent gross, ill defined widening of the superior mediastinum. In the lateral radiograph of the sternum **(b)**, a complete, comminuted, displaced fracture of the sternum is seen (*arrow*). The **apparent** superior mediastinal widening seen in the frontal projection represents instead the soft tissue abnormalities associated with the sternal fracture.

of the ribs in 10–14 days will usually demonstrate callous formation at the fracture site, thereby establishing the diagnosis. Costal cartilage injury and incomplete costochondral separation are not detectable radiographically.

Rib fractures are uncommon in children because of the resiliency of the thoracic cage. However, with a history of appropriate trauma, the possibility of a rib fracture in a child should not be ignored (Fig. 7.25).

A localized pleural effusion (hematoma) seen along the lateral chest wall in the frontal projection frequently identifies the site of a minimally displaced fracture which may not be visible in the PA radiograph but which may be visible only in an oblique projection (Fig. 7.26).

Fractures of the upper ribs are uncommon because they are relatively protected by the clavicle, scapula, and the large muscle masses of the anterior and posterior chest walls. When present, either alone or in conjunction with fracture of the bones of the shoulder girdle, these fractures connote an injury of considerable magnitude and are frequently associated with pneumo- or hemothorax, subcutaneous or mediastinal emphysema (Fig. 7.27), pneumopericardium (Fig. 7.28), or pulmonary contusion (Fig. 7.33). The lower ribs, being less securely attached anteriorly, are more mobile and less susceptible to fracture by blunt trauma. These ribs may be fractured by a forceful direct blow and, when such a fracture occurs posteriorly on the left, evidence of associated splenic or renal trauma should be sought.

"Flail" chest injury occurs when multiple ribs are fractured on each side of the point of injury, resulting in a segment of chest wall that is no longer firmly attached (Fig. 7.29) and which moves freely and paradoxically with respect to the thorax during res-

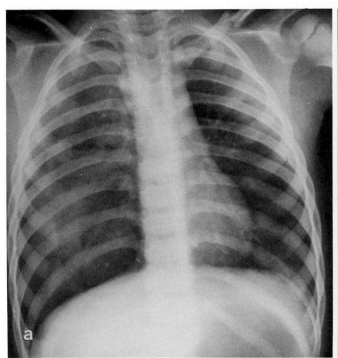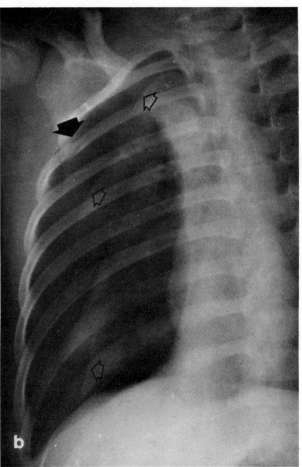

Fig. 7.25. This 4-year-old child sustained blunt trauma to the chest. In addition to the displaced fracture in the mid-third of the left clavicle, the erect PA radiograph of the chest **(a)** revealed right pulmonary contusion and a right pneumothorax. The pneumothorax (*open arrows*) is seen to best advantage in the oblique **(b)** radiograph of the chest. The only skeletal abnormality was a complete, minimally displaced fracture in the midaxillary line of the right third rib (*solid arrow*).

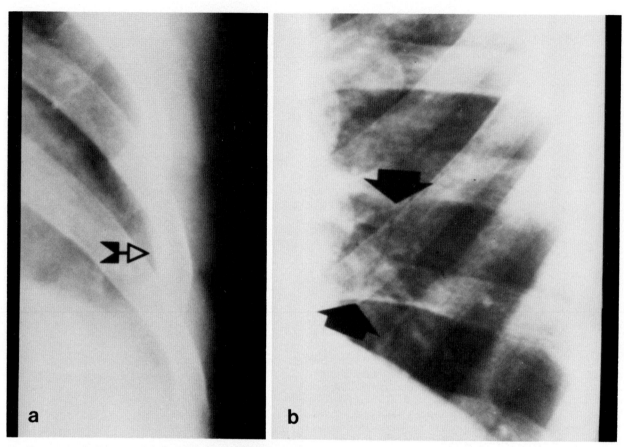

Fig. 7.26. In the frontal projection **(a)**, the localized pleural hematoma (*arrow*) marks the site of a rib fracture which is only radiographically visible in an oblique **(b)** projection (*arrows*).

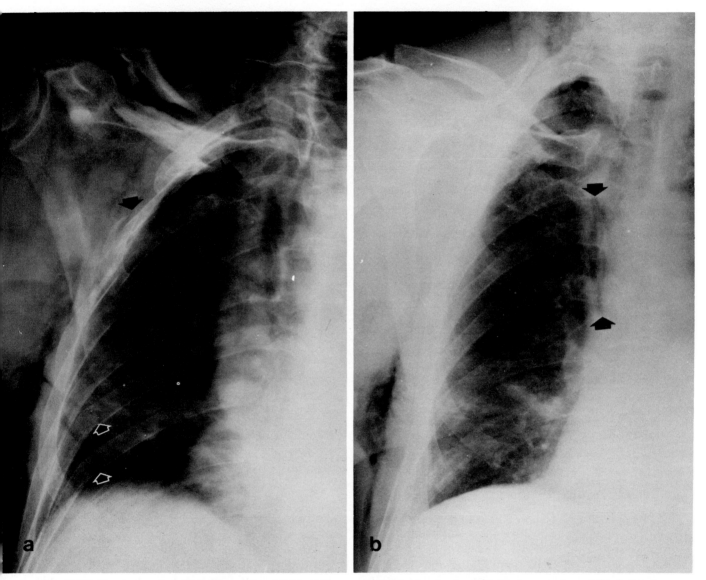

Fig. 7.27. Fractures of multiple ribs of the right hemithorax, including fractures of the first, second, and third ribs. In addition, the patient sustained a comminuted fracture of the right clavicle and extensive subcutaneous emphysema **(a)**. Mediastinal emphysema (*arrows*) is seen in the frontal projection of the chest **(b)**.

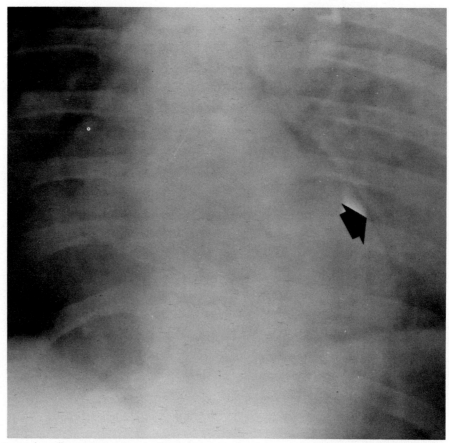

Fig. 7.28. Pneumopericardium (*arrow*) in a patient who sustained massive anterior chest wall trauma and a fracture of the left first rib.

piration. Flail chest is the result of a major trauma, is usually associated with multiple injuries, and has a relatively high mortality rate (8).

Pulmonary Contusion

Pulmonary contusion results from blunt trauma to the chest, most commonly caused by an automobile accident or a fall. The parenchymal changes, which consist of intra-alveolar, perivascular and peribronchial hemorrhage and transudate (3–5), are caused by transmission of the force of the parenchyma through the chest wall and by compression and recoil of the lung.

Although pulmonary contusion is usually associated with some degree of chest wall injury, it must be recognized as a separate injury distinct from that of the chest wall (9–11). Pulmonary contusion occurs in 30–75% of patients with blunt chest trauma (10), is usually mild, usually clears without producing significant respiratory disturbance, and may be clinically masked by more serious conditions such as flail chest or pneumo- or hydrothorax. Even when more severe,

the extent and significance of the lesion, which is commonly not initially appreciated either clinically or radiographically, is recognized only by arterial pO_2 levels reflecting hypoxia (<70 mm Hg breathing room air).

Pathophysiologically, the blast effect of blunt chest trauma, which compresses the lung tissue, results in parenchymal hemorrhage and edema. When the initiating force is released, the lung rebounds, producing an abrupt negative pressure on the already damaged tissue. The hemorrhage occurs at the alveolar capillary level, resulting in both intra-alveolar and interstitial extravasation of blood and edema. The ensuing cellular response to tissue damage combine with the hemorrhage and edema to produce a progressive O_2 diffusion barrier and, initially at least, hypoxemia, which may be paradoxical with respect to the clinical and radiographic appearance of the patient or which may be progressively severe. Mortality rates due to pulmonary contusion of approximately 31% have been reported by Keller et al. (12) and by Perry and Galway (13). Pulmonary contusion plays a major role in 25% of automobile accident fatalities (10).

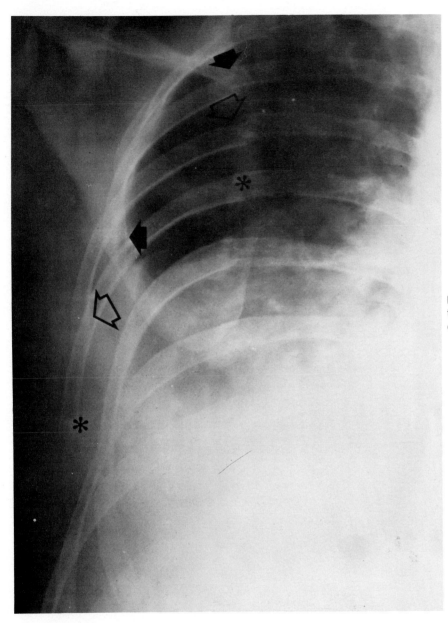

Fig. 7.29. Multiple fractures of multiple ribs constitute the radiographic evidence of a ''flail'' chest.

Radiographic signs of pulmonary contusion may not be present immediately but are usually (70%) visible within 1–2 hours following injury (10). In the remaining 30%, roentgen evidence of pulmonary contusion may not appear until 6 (10) to 24 (11) hours postinjury. For this reason, serial roentgenograms of the chest are indicated in those patients whose initial chest radiographs do not demonstrate changes of pulmonary contusion following significant blunt chest trauma.

The parenchymal lesions usually progress during the first 24 hours and, except in instances of massive contusion or complication, begin to clear by 48–72 hours (Figs. 7.30 and 7.31). Rib fractures are commonly (Figs. 7.32 and 7.33), but not necessarily (Fig. 7.34), associated with pulmonary contusion. Massive pulmonary contusion may occur without associated thoracic wall fracture (Fig. 7.35).

The radiographic appearance of pulmonary contusion consists of patchy, ill defined areas of parenchymal density which may be either solitary (Fig. 7.36) and localized, multiple, or diffuse (Fig. 7.33). Multiple foci of contusion in adjacent portions of the lung may coalesce. The area of contusion does not respect anatomic divisions of the lung and, therefore, the changes seen on chest roentgenograms do not coincide with any of the anatomic divisions of the lung. Further, as stated earlier, except in the instance of massive con-

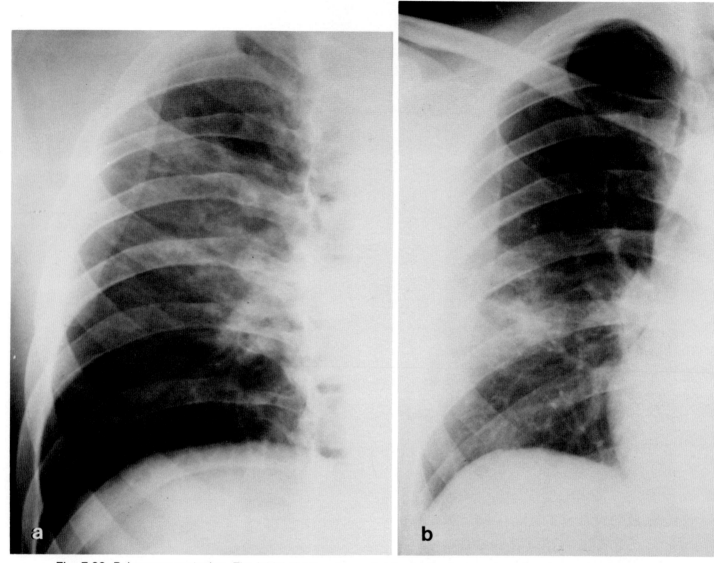

Fig. 7.30. Pulmonary contusion. The initial chest radiograph **(a)**, obtained approximately 1 hour postinjury, demonstrates an extensive, ill defined area of patchy interstitial density which represents contusion of the right upper lobe. Chest roentgenogram of the same patient **(b)**, 48 hours later, demonstrates marked resolution of the contusion.

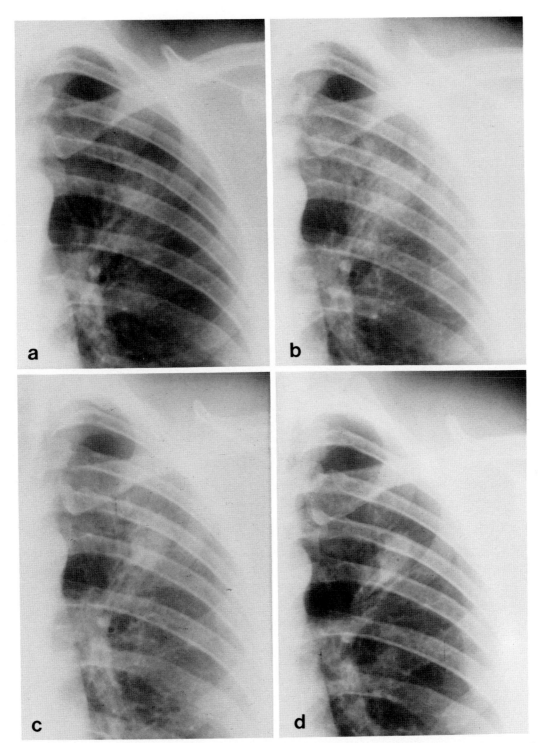

Fig. 7.31. Pulmonary contusion complicated by pulmonary laceration and hemorrhage. The ill defined patchy density in the left upper lobe on the initial chest roentgenogram **(a)**, obtained shortly following blunt left upper chest trauma, represents a pulmonary contusion. Twelve hours later **(b)**, the area of contusion had increased in size radiographically. By 36 hours **(c)**, the contusion had partially resolved, but within the area of contusion, a smaller, more dense discrete lesion began to emerge. This represented the frank pulmonary laceration and hemorrhage which persisted after the roentgen signs of contusion had completely cleared **(d)**, 5 days postinjury.

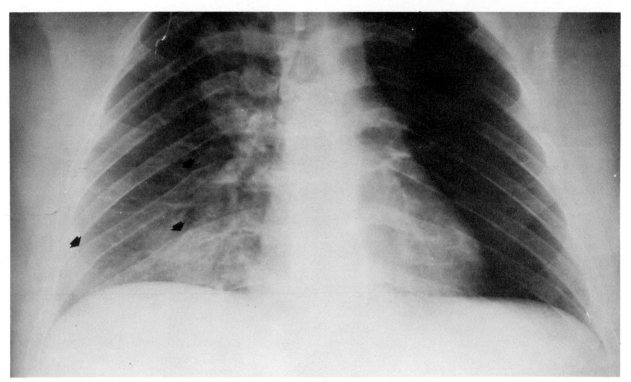

Fig. 7.32. Right lower lobe pulmonary contusion associated with minimally displaced fractures (*arrows*) of the posterior aspect of multiple right lower ribs.

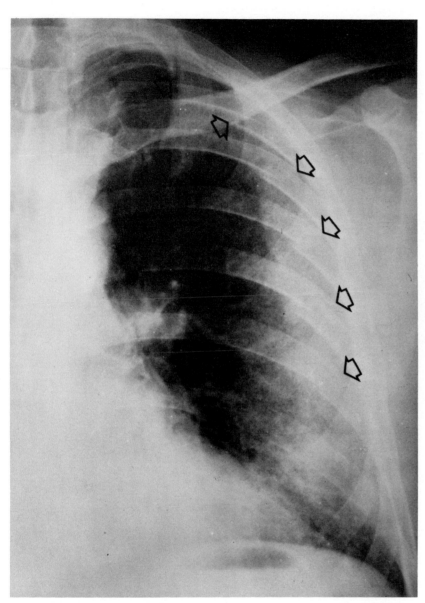

Fig. 7.33. The diffuse haziness in the peripheral portion of the left lung represents early pulmonary contusion associated with multiple rib fractures (*arrows*).

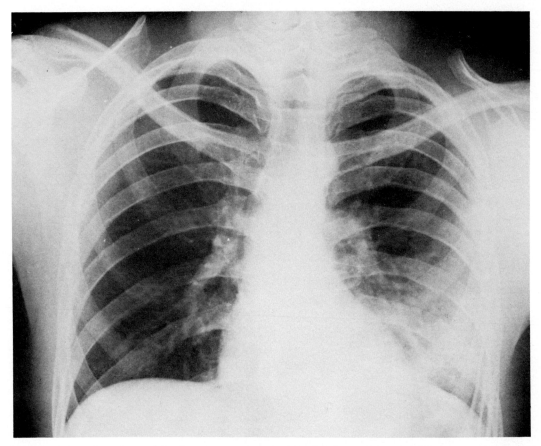

Fig. 7.34. Contusion of portions of the lingular segment and the left lower lobe without demonstrable rib fracture.

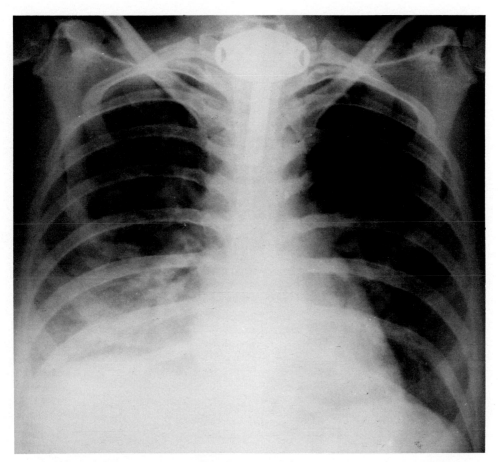

Fig. 7.35. Massive contusion of the right lower lobe without associated rib fracture.

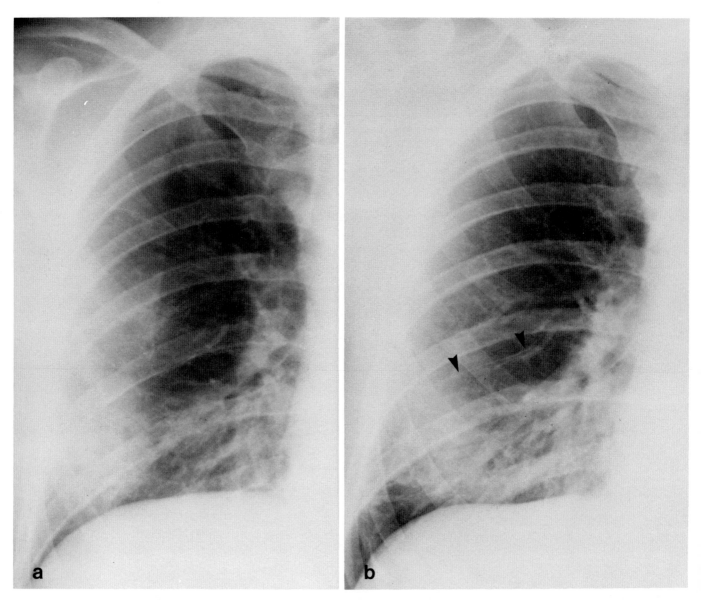

Fig. 7.36. Diffuse, solitary area of pulmonary contusion in the distribution of the lateral segment of the right middle lobe **(a)**. Three days postinjury **(b)**, the contusion had partially cleared. Depression of the minor fissure (*arrowheads*) indicates associated partial atelectasis of the right middle lobe.

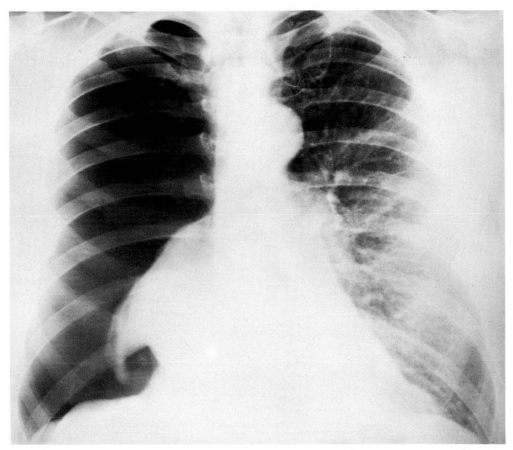

Fig. 7.37. Massive right pneumothorax.

tusion, the radiographically visible parenchymal abnormalities may not reflect the extent of the parenchymal damage nor the magnitude of the gaseous
diffusion barrier and resultant hypoxemia.

Cyst-like "pneumatoceles" developing in areas of
pulmonary consolidation following blunt injury to the
chest have been described by Greening et al. (14).
These unusual roentgen signs of chest trauma should
not be mistaken for cavities caused by tuberculosis or
other granulomatous diseases.

Pneumothorax

Pneumothorax may occur spontaneously or be
caused by blunt or penetrating trauma. A "closed"
pneumothorax occurs with an intact chest wall. An
"open" pneumothorax is also referred to as a "suck-
ing" wound of the chest. Pneumothorax may also be
classified on the basis of magnitude of collapse into
marginal (Fig. 7.22), moderate, or massive (Figs. 7.37
and 7.38).

Tension pneumothorax (Fig. 7.39) occurs when the
communication which permits air to enter the pleural
space acts as a flap valve so that air enters the pleural
space during inspiration and cannot escape during
expiration. The mediastinal structures are forced to
the contralateral side, producing compression of the
contralateral lung and impairment of venous circulation. If allowed to persist, a tension pneumothorax is
rapidly fatal because of ventilatory and circulatory
collapse.

Spontaneous pneumothorax most commonly results from rupture of a bleb immediately beneath the
visceral pleura. In over 50% of patients, the etiology
of the rupture is unknown. Many diseases have been
associated with spontaneous pneumothorax, including
such disparate conditions as spasmodic asthma, staphylococcic pneumonia (Fig. 7.40) and metastatic
disease (Fig. 7.41).

The roentgen diagnosis of pneumothorax depends
upon demonstration of the very thin density of the
visceral pleura. When the magnitude of collapse is
moderate or massive, or if an associated hydrothorax

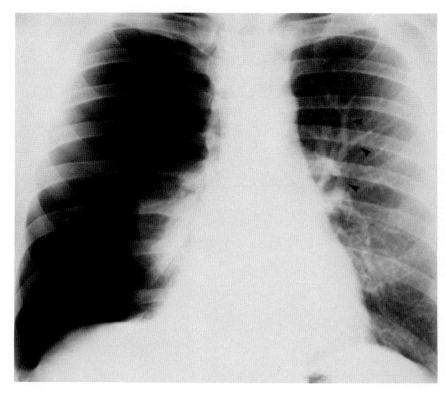

Fig. 7.38. Massive pneumothorax with complete collapse of the right lung. Shunting of the right pulmonary blood volume into the left lung has caused left pulmonary hypervolemia and abnormal distention of the left upper lobe veins (*arrowheads*).

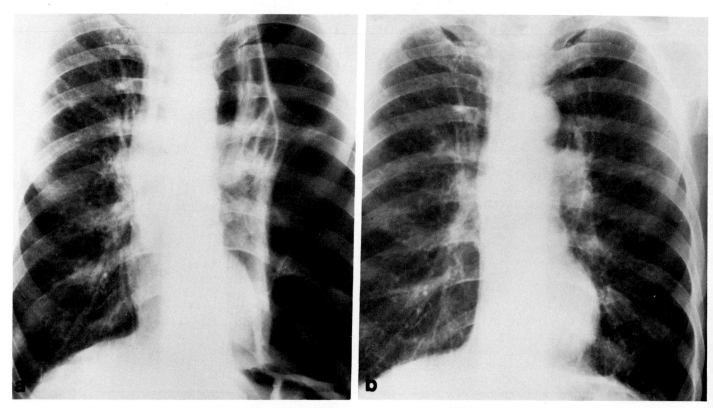

Fig. 7.39. Left tension pneumothorax with displacement of the mediastinal structures to the right **(a)**. Following re-expansion of the left lung **(b)**, the mediastinal structures have returned to the midline.

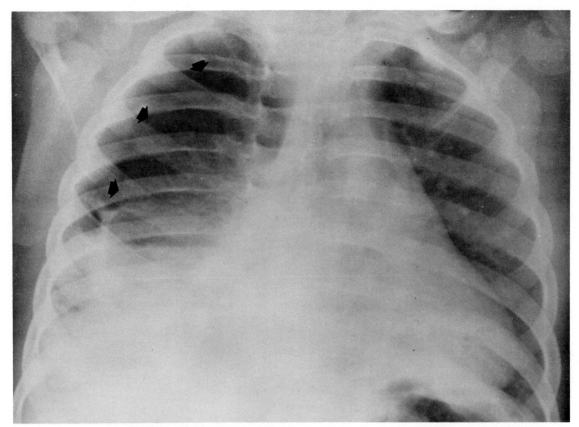

Fig. 7.40. Right pneumothorax associated with staphylococcic pneumonia.

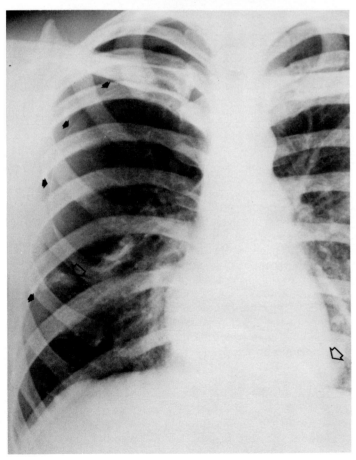

Fig. 7.41. Spontaneous pneumothorax (*solid arrows*) associated with pulmonary metastasis (*open arrows*).

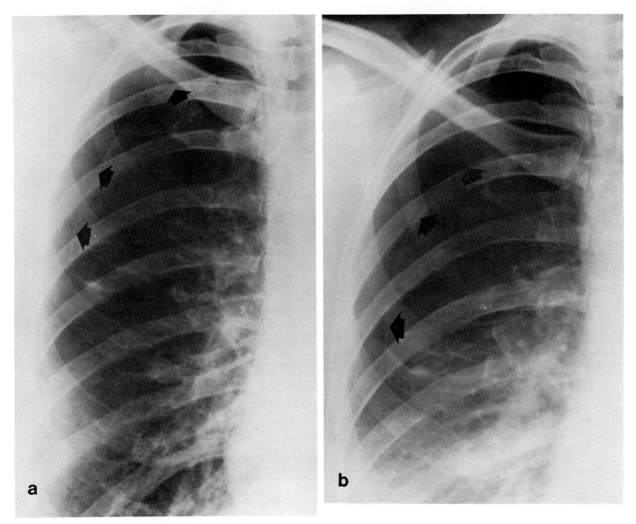

Fig. 7.42. The effect of inspiration **(a)** and expiration **(b)** on the volume of pneumothorax.

produces an air-fluid level within the pleural space, the diagnosis is readily apparent.

The diagnosis of marginal pneumothorax may be exceedingly difficult because of superimposed skeletal shadows or problems in perceiving the faint density of the pleural surface. The pneumothorax may be enhanced in a PA radiograph exposed in forced expiration (Fig. 7.42). The basis of this phenomenon is that the collapsed lung decreases in volume during expiration while the air in the pleural space stays constant. The lung draws away from the chest wall, rendering the pneumothorax more obvious. If patients who cannot assume the erect posture are placed in the decubitus position with the affected side up, air will gravitate to the uppermost portion of the pleural space and will be perceptible in the lateral decubitus roentgenogram.

As previously noted, a marginal pneumothorax is likely to be unrecognized in supine examination of the chest because the air migrates to the anterior pleural space while the pleural surfaces, laterally, remain in apposition. Thus, a negative supine radiograph of the chest does not exclude the presence of a pneumothorax (Fig. 7.22).

It is important to remember that wounds in the neck or the lower portion of the chest cage or upper abdomen may penetrate the pleural space, producing a pneumothorax.

Pneumomediastinum

Air in the mediastinum is relatively common in infants and rare in adults. Pneumomediastinum oc-

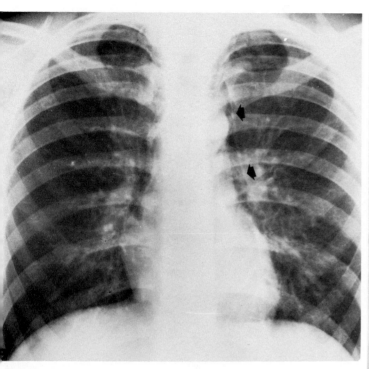

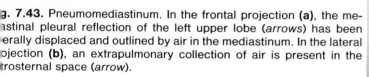

Fig. **7.43.** Pneumomediastinum. In the frontal projection **(a)**, the mediastinal pleural reflection of the left upper lobe (*arrows*) has been laterally displaced and outlined by air in the mediastinum. In the lateral projection **(b)**, an extrapulmonary collection of air is present in the retrosternal space (*arrow*).

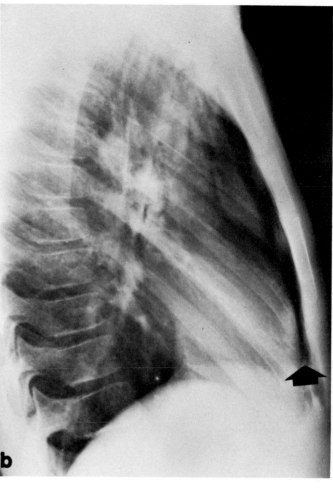

curs most frequently spontaneously. Other etiologies include trauma, rupture of the esophagus, and gas entering the mediastinum from below the diaphragm following diagnostic or therapeutic installation of air.

Spontaneous pneumomediastinum results from rupture of an alveolus distal to a check valve bronchiolar obstruction such as caused by inflammatory edema or asthmatic spasm. The gas migrates along peribronchial planes to the hila and enters the mediastinum.

The radiographic identification of pneumomediastinum is usually not difficult. The mediastinal pleura is displaced laterally and appears as a sharp, oblique, linear density that parallels the heart border. This shadow is usually more apparent on the left. In the lateral projection, an extrapulmonary collection of gas is characteristically seen in the retrosternal space (Fig. 7.43). Dissection of mediastinal air into the neck and the chest wall is more common in adults (Fig. 7.44) than in children.

Cardiovascular Injury

Cardiac injury is common in patients who sustain significant blunt trauma to the chest. Rapid deceleration injuries, such as steering wheel accidents or falls from a height, constitute the most common cause of this type of injury. Pathologically, cardiac contusion is the most frequently encountered lesion. Myocardial rupture is the most rapidly fatal cardiac injury. Damage to the valve leaflets and to the chordae tendineae are not common, usually occur simultaneously, and rarely produce radiographic signs.

Radiology plays a minor role in the diagnosis of penetrating injuries of the heart. Patients who survive penetrating cardiac injuries may show increase in the size of cardiac silhouette and blunting of the right cardiophrenic angle due to hemopericardium.

Traumatic rupture of the aorta, due to blunt chest trauma, is one of the most common injuries in high speed automobile accidents. The most frequent site of

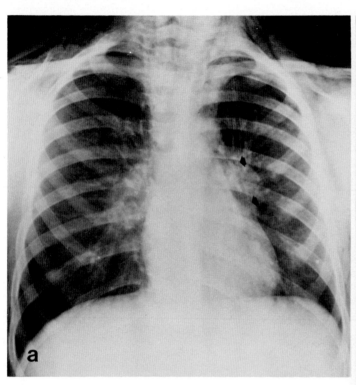

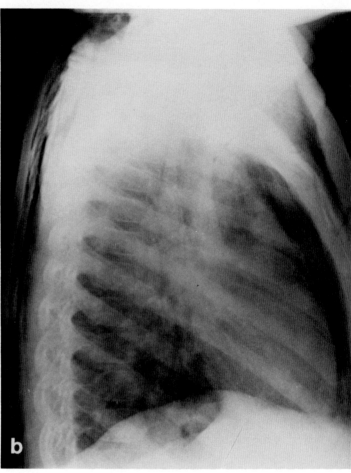

Fig. 7.44. Extensive subcutaneous emphysema of the chest wall and neck of a patient with pneumomediastinum. In the frontal projection **(a)**, the mediastinal pleural surface of the left lung is indicated by the *arrows*. In the lateral projection **(b)**, a large accumulation of air is seen in the retrosternal space.

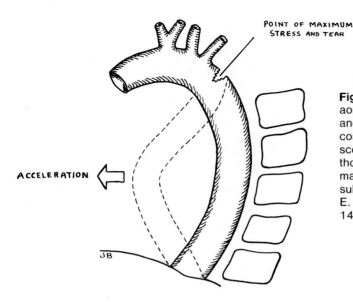

POINT OF MAXIMUM
STRESS AND TEAR

ACCELERATION

JB

Fig. 7.45. Most frequent site of traumatic rupture of the aorta. The aorta is fixed proximally by the great vessels and the ligamentum arteriosum and distally by the intercostal arteries and the diaphragm. The intervening descending portion of the aorta, being relatively mobile, is thought to swing forward during rapid deceleration with maximum stress and tear occurring just distal to the left subclavian artery. (Modified from G. J. Schonholtz and E. J. Jahnke: *Journal of Bone and Joint Surgery* 46: 1421, 1964.)

rupture is the descending aorta distal to the origin of the left subclavian artery and proximal to the level of the ligamentum arteriosum (Fig. 7.45). Although this lesion is usually rapidly fatal, Parmley et al. (15) report that approximately 11% of all patients with this injury live as long as 6 hours following arrival at the hospital. As many as 20% of all patients with isthmus rupture survive to reach the hospital (15). The second most common site of aortic rupture, which is more frequently associated with falls, is at the root of the ascending arch. Survival following this injury is usually brief (16), with only approximately 7% of patients reaching the hospital alive (15).

The significant number of patients with traumatic rupture of the aorta who survive the initial injury do so because the resultant hematoma is temporarily contained by the aortic adventitia and the mediastinal pleura. This type of rupture has been called "lethal delay rupture" by Naclerio (17). The tamponade usually ruptures during the first 24–48 hours following trauma. It is in this "grace period" that a high index of suspicion can lead to prompt diagnosis and lifesaving thoracotomy and repair of the defect.

The diagnosis of traumatic rupture of the aorta depends upon a high index of suspicion regarding the presence of the lesion. As many as one-third of patients with traumatic rupture have only minimal clinical evidence of blunt chest trauma (18). Conversely, many of these patients have more clinically impressive concomitant injuries which detract from the potentially lethal vascular injury. For these reasons Blair et al. (19) state that "the consistently most dramatic and lethal missed diagnosis in blunt chest trauma is transection of the aorta." As a screening device, Wilson et

al. (18) believe that traumatic rupture of the aorta *must* be suspected in all patients who have been involved in automobile accidents in which speeds exceeded 30 miles per hour. Every road traffic accident victim seen at the Maryland Institute for Emergency Medicine is suspected of having a traumatically ruptured aorta (20). Therefore, traumatic rupture of the aorta must be considered in the differential diagnosis of any patient sustaining major blunt chest trauma and, particularly, in a patient in whom the cause of circulatory collapse is not readily apparent. However, Ayella et al. (20) have observed that 60% of traumatic aortic ruptures involve only the intima and muscularis, with the adventitia remaining intact and the superior mediastinal hematoma secondary *not* to bleeding from the aorta but to rupture of the smaller vessels. Therefore, in the majority of patients with traumatic aortic rupture, clinical signs of shock may not be present or, if present, are likely due to other injuries. This important aspect of patients who sustain, and survive, blunt traumatic aortic injury, i.e., that the lesion is usually clinically "silent" (15), is further emphasized by three patients reported by Blair et al. (19) with traumatic rupture of the aorta in whom the diagnosis was initially unsuspected because the clinical condition of each was described as "good" when first seen in the Emergency Department and by the patient illustrated in Figure 7.46 who sustained a comminuted fracture-dislocation of the left hip and a clinically unsuspected rupture of the aorta in an automobile accident.

Radiographically, the diagnosis of traumatic rupture of the aorta should be suspected in any patient who, following major trauma, demonstrates on supine

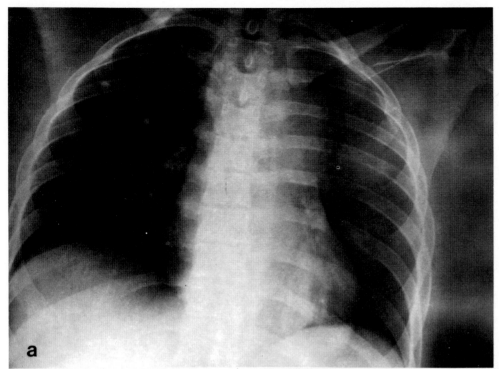

Fig. 7.46. This patient sustained a comminuted fracture-dislocation of the left hip in a high speed automobile accident. She was not in shock and had no significant chest complaints. The supine radiograph of the chest **(a)** taken prior to undergoing general anesthesia for reduction of the hip injury demonstrated *ill defined* superior mediastinal widening, obscuration of normal superior mediastinal anatomy, an extrapleural left apical cap, and a left pleural effusion—all signs of a superior mediastinal hematoma. An aortogram **(b, c)** demonstrated the aortic rupture (*).

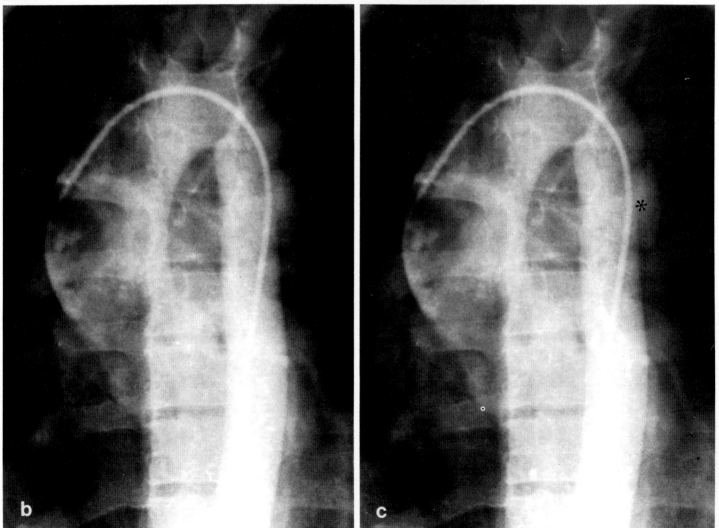

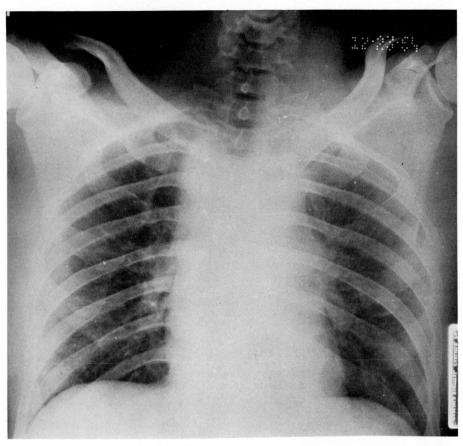

Fig. 7.47. Supine examination of the chest of a patient with acute traumatic rupture of the aorta. The mediastinum is abnormally widened by an ill defined soft tissue density which obscures all of the normal mediastinal landmarks. These changes, which must be interpreted in light of the clinical information relative to the patient, are caused by the mediastinal hematoma.

or erect chest radiograph *ill defined* widening of the superior mediastinum, which obscures the definition of the normal superior mediastinal structures and which must be confirmed by aortography. Many references appear in the literature describing the principal roentgen sign of traumatic rupture as simply "mediastinal widening" (15, 18, 21, 22). To equate mediastinal widening with the presence of a mediastinal hematoma is not only erroneous of itself but may lead to unnecessary aortography. The majority of patients who have sustained trauma sufficient to rupture the aorta are examined radiographically in the supine posture. Physiologically, the superior mediastinum widens in recumbency, and this fact is recorded in the supine chest roentgenogram (Fig. 7.7). In addition, even though the superior mediastinal density is wider in the supine posture secondary to altered hemodynamics in the superior mediastinal vasculature, the normal soft tissue anatomy of the superior mediastinum, i.e., the aortic knob, trachea, and right stem bronchus, remains visible on a properly exposed radiograph. In contradistinction, the margins of a superior mediastinal hematoma are ill defined and

indistinct and the density of the hemorrhage obscures the definition of the soft tissue structures which are normally radiographically visible (Fig. 7.47). Occasionally, it may be impossible to exclude the presence of a superior hematoma on the supine chest radiograph following major blunt trauma. Ayella et al. (20) advocate obtaining a true erect frontal radiograph of the chest in patients suspected of traumatic aortic rupture who do not have clinical evidence of spinal injury. In the experience of the Maryland Institute of Emergency Medicine (20), traumatic aortic rupture has not been present if the superior mediastinum is radiographically normal in the erect position (Fig. 7.48).

Conversely, the persistence of roentgen signs of a superior mediastinal hematoma, even in the erect projection, can not be considered as conclusive evidence of aortic rupture since in 60% of patients the aortic tear is not complete and the superior mediastinal hematoma is due to rupture of smaller vessels associated with skeletal and soft tissue injury (Fig. 7.49). Therefore, as stated previously, radiographic signs of a superior mediastinal hematoma are not

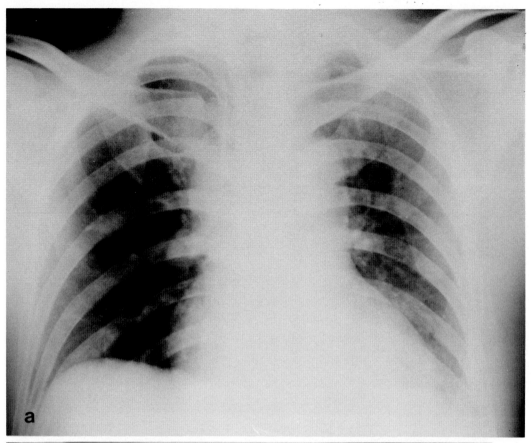

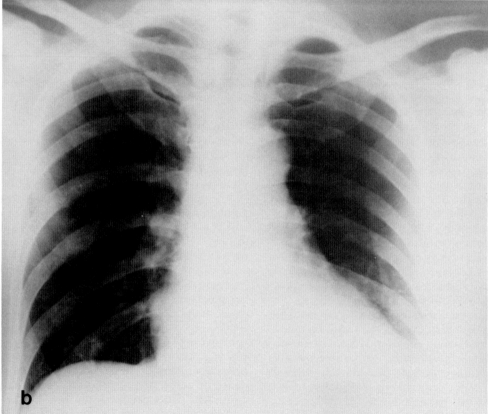

Fig. 7.48. Supine **(a)** and erect **(b)** frontal roentgenograms of the chest of a patient who sustained left lower rib fractures following blunt chest trauma. In the supine radiograph **(a)**, the superior mediastinal density is widened, and it is impossible to exclude a superior mediastinal hematoma. In the erect projection **(b)**, made minutes following the supine examination, the roentgen appearance of the superior mediastinum is normal. Splinting of the left hemithorax and the small left pleural effusion are secondary to the lower left rib fractures.

Fig. 7.49. Superior mediastinal hematoma without traumatic rupture of the aorta. This patient sustained major blunt trauma to the chest in a high speed automobile accident. In the supine examination of the chest **(a)**, the *solid arrows* indicate bilateral rib and right scapular fractures. The *open arrows* indicate the ill defined density in the superior mediastinum, which has obliterated the normal superior mediastinal soft tissue anatomy and which represents a superior mediastinal hematoma. An aortogram **(b)** demonstrated the intact thoracic aorta. Frontal and lateral radiographs of the thoracic spine **(c,d)** demonstrate displaced fractures of multiple upper ribs and **transverse processes** and fractures of multiple upper thoracic vertebral bodies. The superior mediastinal hematoma, therefore, was secondary to the skeletal and soft tissue injury and not related to traumatic aortic rupture. However, traumatic rupture of the aorta must be suspected on the basis of the history, physical findings, and supine chest roentgenogram. These all require an aortogram to establish the status of the aorta.

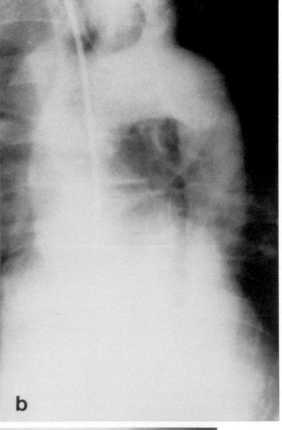

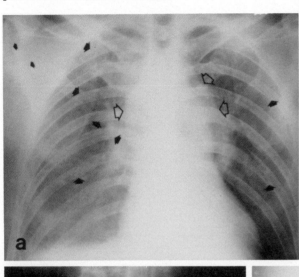

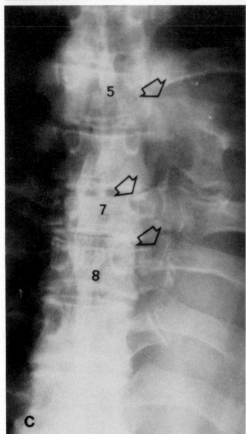

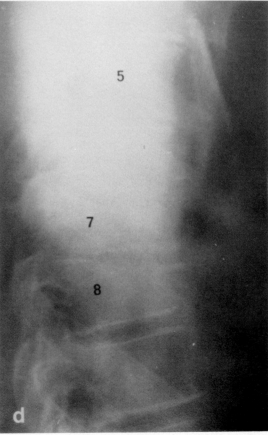

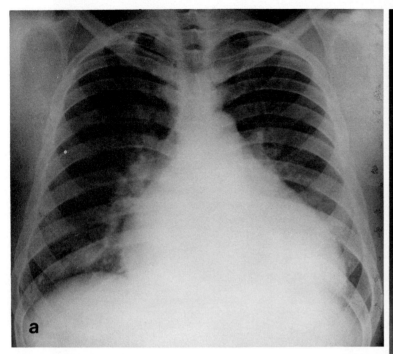

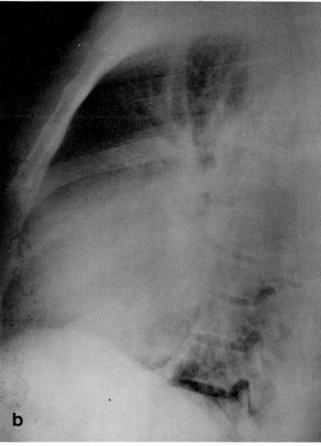

Fig. 7.50. Pericardial effusion. The cardiac silhouette is diffusely enlarged in a globular configuration. The cardiophrenic angles are obtuse in the frontal projection **(a)**. In the lateral projection **(b)**, the cardiac silhouette is grossly and diffusely enlarged, with the posterior border of the pericardium extending to the anterior borders of the thoracic vertebrae.

pathognomonic for aortic rupture and, for this reason, aortography is required to establish, or exclude, traumatic rupture of the aorta.

Other roentgen signs of superior mediastinal hematoma include extrapleural left apical cap, displacement of the trachea to the right, elevation of the left stem bronchus, and a left pleural effusion (Fig. 7.46).

Superior mediastinal hematoma (and traumatic rupture of the aorta) may be radiographically simulated by dislocation (Fig. 7.23) or fracture (Fig. 7.24) of the sternum. An erect or horizontal beam supine lateral radiograph of the chest demonstrating the sternal injury is helpful in establishing the correct diagnosis.

Injury to the pericardium may occur with blunt or penetrating trauma. Traumatic pericardial effusion is usually bloody. Acute hemopericardium, if over 250 cc, usually produces fatal cardiac tamponade. Lesser amounts of blood in the pericardial sac or nontraumatic pericardial effusions (Fig. 7.50) are difficult to diagnose radiographically. The "typical" roentgen changes of pericardial effusion include increase in the size of the cardiac silhouette, globular configuration, obtuse cardiophrenic angles, and decreased amplitude of cardiac pulsation during fluoroscopy. Unfortunately, however, all of these signs are relative and are frequently equivocal on routine radiographic examinations. The diagnosis of pericardial effusion can be definitely established by means of angiocardiography using CO_2 or iodinated contrast medium, echocardiography, or radioactive isotope heart-liver scan.

The hemopericardium following blunt trauma may take as long as a week to develop and an initial negative chest roentgenogram should not be considered as indicating the absence of either cardiac or pericardial injury.

Pneumopericardium (Fig. 7.28) may be difficult to distinguish radiographically from pneumomediastinum or a small pneumothorax. Air in the pericardial sac will be confined to the anatomic distribution of the parietal pericardium, which terminates at the point of its reflection about the great vessels. Thus, air that extends more cephalad than this level lies outside the pericardium. Air in the mediastinum does not accu-

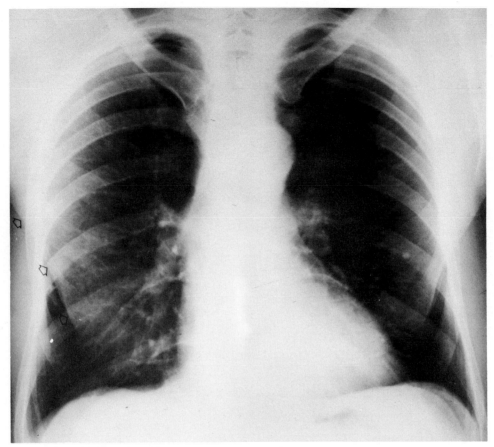

Fig. 7.51. Soft tissue density of the pectoral muscles (*arrows*).

rately parallel the heart border. The presence of a small pneumothorax simulating a pneumopericardium can usually be established by means of expiratory posteroanterior and the appropriate lateral decubitus chest roentgenograms.

Intrathoracic Evidence of Intra-abdominal Disease

The intrathoracic roentgen signs of trauma affecting abdominal contents has been discussed elsewhere. However, it seems appropriate to emphasize some of these findings by repetition.

The "classic" roentgen signs of rupture of the spleen include a small left pleural effusion, plate-like atelectasis at the left base, and elevation and loss of definition of the left diaphragmatic surface. The gastric air bubble may be medially displaced in the erect PA chest roentgenogram. When any, or all, of these signs are present in a patient with a history of left upper abdominal trauma, the radiologic diagnosis of ruptured spleen may be reasonably entertained. However, it is extremely important to be aware that the chest radiograph will be negative in a high percentage of patients with splenic rupture, particularly when subcapsular. (23).

Nontraumatic Lesions

Chest Wall

The radiographic importance of chest wall soft tissues is that these structures occasionally produce radiographic densities that may be misconstrued as abnormal findings.

The shadow of well developed pectoral muscle mass produces a hazy density (Fig. 7.51) that resembles pneumonia. Folds in the skin, when strategically situated, may suggest a pneumothorax (Fig. 7.52). Male (Fig. 7.53) and female (Fig. 7.54) nipple shadows may produce rounded densities on the PA radiograph that suggest metastatic nodules. Repeating the frontal study with a small amount of barium paste applied to the nipple will confirm when the shadow is caused by the nipple.

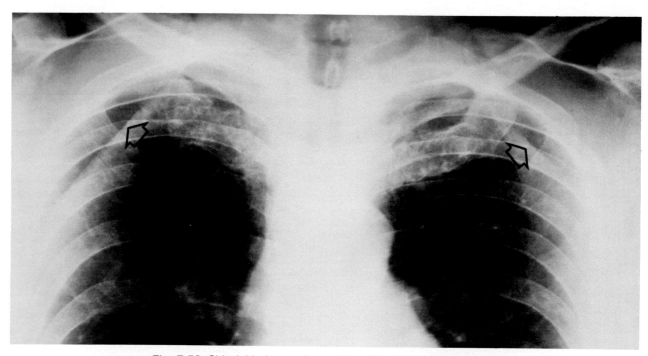

Fig. 7.52. Skin folds (*arrows*) simulating bilateral pneumothorax.

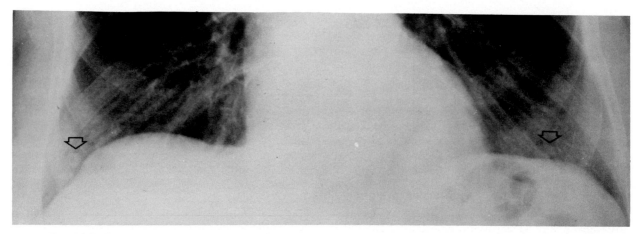

Fig. 7.53. The faint round densities (*arrows*) are caused by the enlarged nipple of the breast of a male.

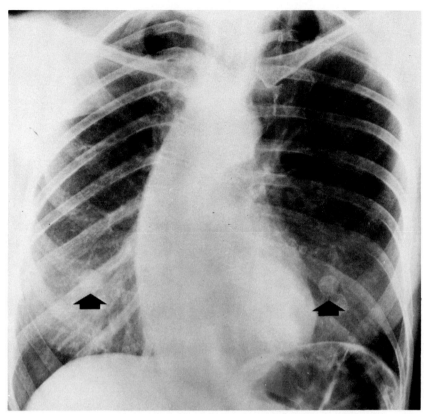

Fig. 7.54. Female nipple shadows.

The breast shadow itself may produce an ill defined haziness at either base, suggesting an inflammatory process (Fig. 7.55). The difference in density of the inferior portion of the lung fields following a radical mastectomy (Fig. 7.56) may be misleading if the observer is not aware of the absence of the breast shadow on the operated side.

The medial border of the scapula may be superimposed upon the peripheral third of the chest in such a fashion as to simulate a minimal pneumothorax (Fig. 7.57).

Rib Cage

The several ossification centers of the body of the sternum fuse at a variable rate from ages 6 to 25 years. Ununited epiphyseal lines occurring in the corpus are distinguishable from fracture lines by their location, the characteristics of their margins (Fig. 7.58), and the patient's age.

Primary tumors of the sternum are rare. Metastatic involvement of the sternum, however, is relatively common, particularly from primary breast carcinoma in females and primary lung carcinoma in males (Fig. 7.59).

The radiographic detection of primary rib tumors may be difficult. Clinically, these lesions are the source of chest wall pain and, frequently, a palpable mass. When the tumor involves the anterior end of a rib, the radiographic changes secondary to lysis of the bone are frequently subtle and may be easily overlooked. The associated soft tissue mass may be the most obvious roentgen sign of the tumor (Fig. 7.60). Multiple myeloma commonly involves the rib cage, producing irregular areas of varying degrees of demineralization, cortical disruption, pathologic fracture, and soft tissue mass (Fig. 7.61). Osteolytic and osteoblastic rib metastasis is a common cause of chest wall pain with or without a pathologic fracture.

Pleura

The "azygos lobe" is a normal variant caused by an anomalous position of the azygos vein as it passes

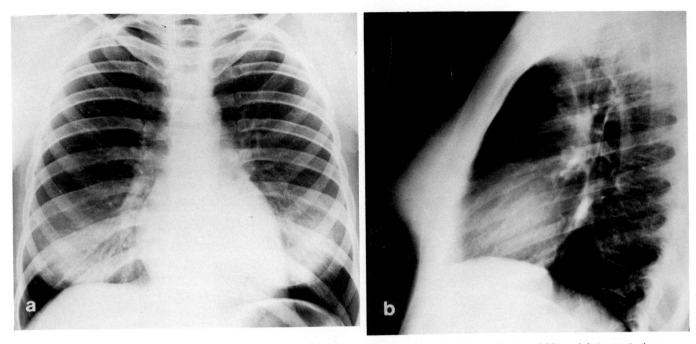

Fig. 7.55. Normal female breast shadow producing ill defined density at the right base that could be misinterpreted as an inflammatory process.

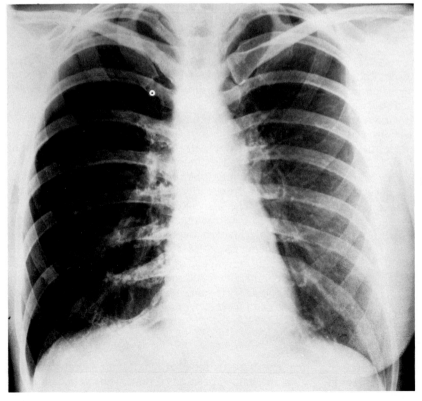

Fig. 7.56. Note the difference in density of the lung fields following right radical mastectomy.

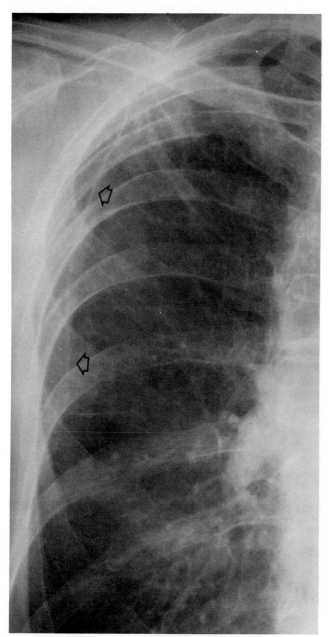

Fig. 7.57. Medial border of the scapula (*arrows*) simulating a minimal right pneumothorax.

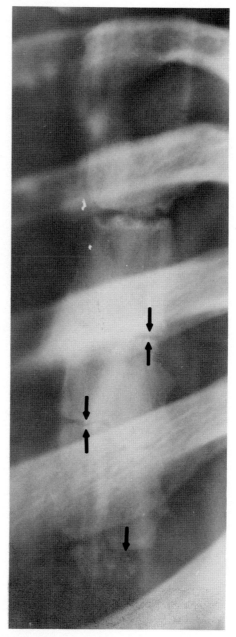

Fig. 7.58. Normal epiphyseal lines of the sternum (*arrows*).

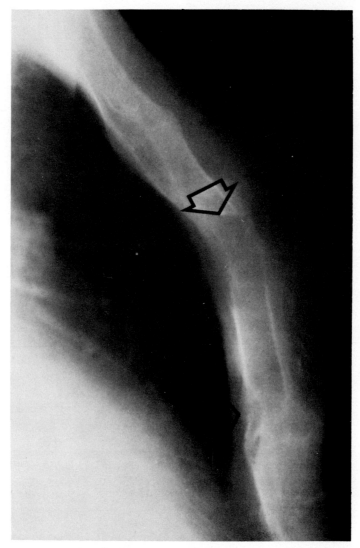

Fig. 7.59. Osteolytic metastatic desease of the sternum (*arrows*).

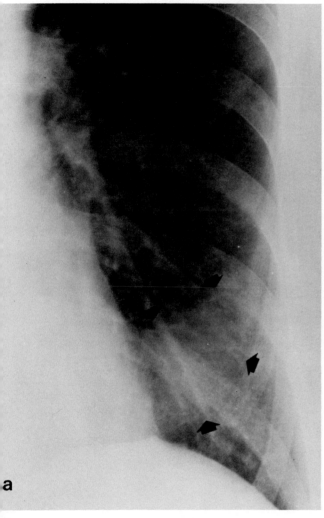

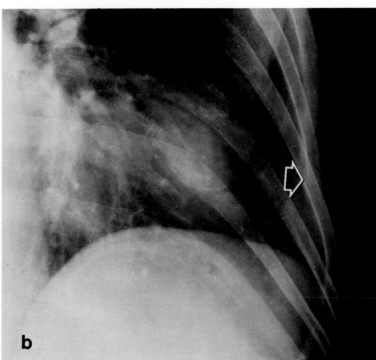

Fig. 7.60. Multiple myeloma of the anterior end of the left seventh rib. In the frontal projection **(a)**, an ill defined, homogenous, soft tissue density (*arrows*) has replaced the rib. In the oblique projection **(b)**, the anterior end of the rib has been amputated by the lytic process (*arrow*).

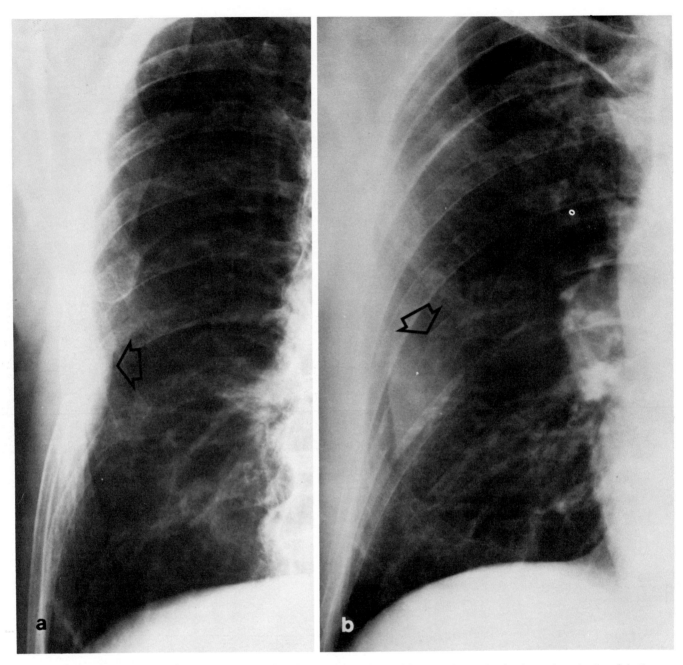

Fig. 7.61. The irregular demineralization of the ribs is caused by multiple myeloma. In the frontal projection **(a)**, the *open arrow* indicates a soft tissue mass of the right lateral chest wall. In the oblique projection **(b)**, the extensive lytic destruction of the rib and the tumor mass are clearly demonstrated.

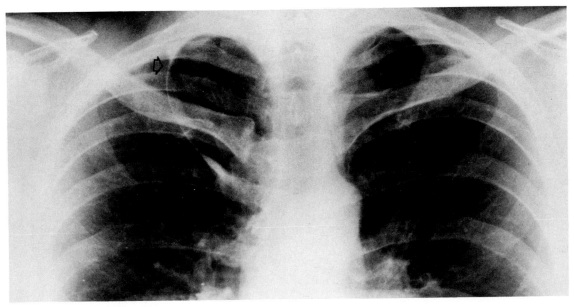

Fig. 7.62. Azygos lobe (*arrow*).

anteriorly to enter the superior vena cava. The azygos fissure (Fig. 7.62) is formed by invagination of the visceral and parietal pleura of the right upper lobe by the course of the vein. The site of the fissure is quite variable. It has no clinical significance.

The pleura is usually not radiographically visible because it is very thin and because a long enough segment of pleura is rarely "seen" end-on by the central x-ray beam to produce a radiographic shadow. Occasionally, however, an arc of lung surface, postinflammatorily thickened pleura, small interlobar effusions, or subpleural edema will be visible radiographically and will outline portions of the pulmonary lobes (Fig. 7.63). Pleural thickening is occasionally seen at the right base, extending in an oblique course for a variable distance above the diaphragmatic surface (Fig. 7.64). This linear density represents either the inferior extent of the major interlobar fissure or an anomalous fissure.

Pleural thickening may blunt the costophrenic angle and may be indistinguishable from a small effusion. The distinction is based on fluoroscopic observation of the chest and radiographs made in decubitus positions. Thickened pleura will not change in configuration regardless of position. A loculated pleural effusion is practically indistinguishable from thickened pleura. A free pleural effusion, on the other hand, will change location in decubitus films and, fluoroscopically, configuration during respiration.

An encapsulated interlobar effusion may simulate a pulmonary mass on the frontal radiograph (Fig. 7.65). In the lateral view, the true nature of the "mass"

is obvious. Because encapsulated effusions characteristically accumulate and disappear, they are referred to as "phantom" or "vanishing" tumors.

Infrapulmonary effusion may be extremely difficult to diagnose radiographically (24). Because the effusion collects between the convexity of the diaphragm and the concavity of the diaphragmatic surface of the lung, its superior surface is frequently sharply defined and parallels the arc of the diaphragmatic surface (Fig. 7.66). Because of this appearance, the infrapulmonary effusion is frequently mistaken for elevation of the diaphragm. The diagnosis is made on the basis of a high index of suspicion and decubitus chest roentgenograms.

Lungs

Inflammation

The radiographic signs of inflammatory disease involving intrathoracic structures are protean, and there is no attempt to describe them here with any degree of thoroughness. Rather, some examples of useful roentgen signs indicative of inflammatory disease, examples of the roentgen appearance of some infrequently encountered, serious disease entities, and some examples of less familiar radiographic changes of common disease entities will be presented. For a more exhaustive discussion of the radiographic findings produced by inflammatory disease within the chest, the reader is referred to any of the well known texts on the subject.

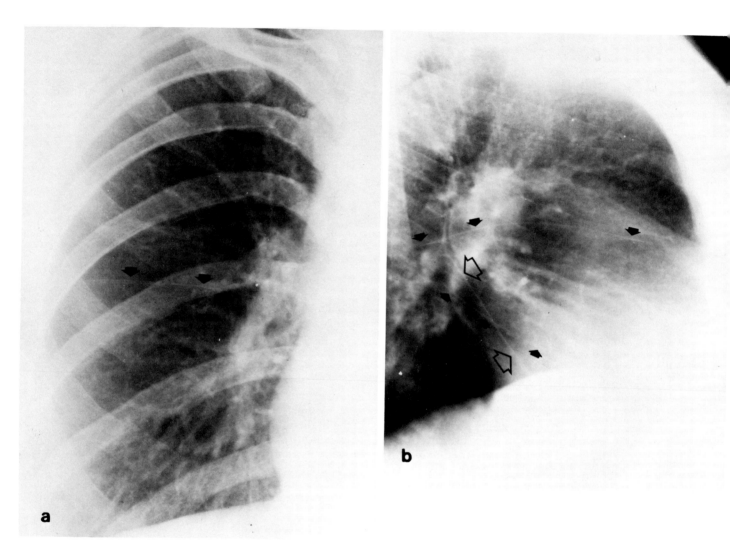

Fig. 7.63. In the frontal projection **(a)**, the *arrows* indicate pleura in the minor fissure. In the lateral projection **(b)**, the pleura of the minor (horizontal) fissure and the inferior portion of the major interlobar fissure, which together define the volume of the right middle lobe is indicated by the *small solid arrows*. The inferior portion of the interlobar fissure of the left lung is indicated by the *open arrows*.

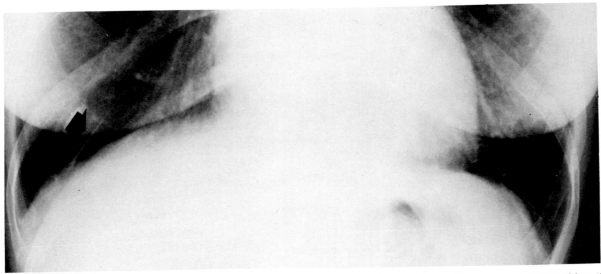

Fig. 7.64. The *arrow* indicates a short segment of thickened pleura at the right base. This may represent either the inferior extent of the major interlobar fissure or an anomalous fissure.

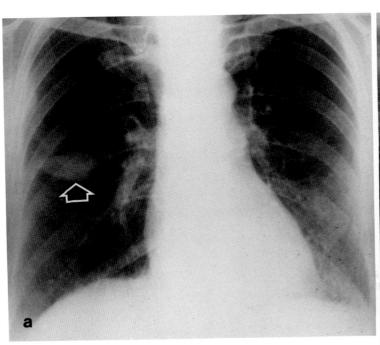

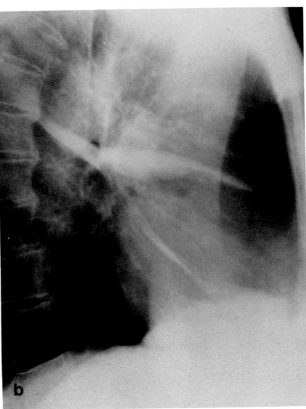

Fig. 7.65. Interlobar effusion **(a,b)** simulating a tumor of the right lung in the frontal projection **(a)**.

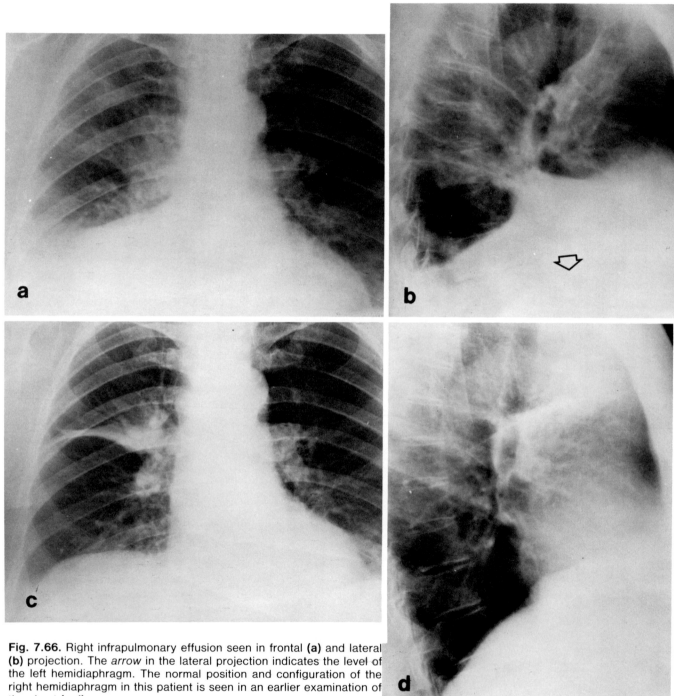

Fig. 7.66. Right infrapulmonary effusion seen in frontal **(a)** and lateral **(b)** projection. The *arrow* in the lateral projection indicates the level of the left hemidiaphragm. The normal position and configuration of the right hemidiaphragm in this patient is seen in an earlier examination of the chest **(c,d)**.

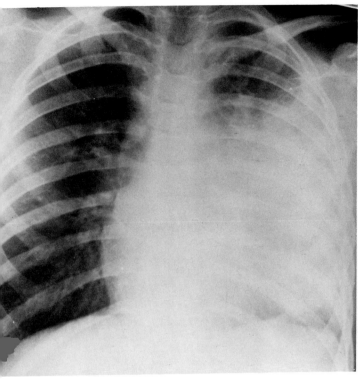

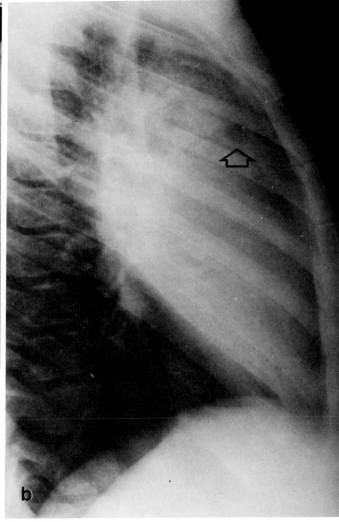

7.67. (a) Staphylococcal pneumonia of the left upper lobe. The *w* in the lateral projection **(b)** indicates a small abscess within the solidation.

In the pediatric age group, staphylococcal pneumonia produces a major threat to the patient because of the frequently overwhelming nature of the disease itself and the high incidence of complications such as septicemia, pleural effusion (55%), pneumothorax (21%), and lung abscess (13%) (25).

The early recognition of staphylococcal pneumonia bears a direct relationship to the success of therapy. The typical roentgen appearance of staphylococcal pneumonia is a dense, homogeneous consolidation of a segment, lobe, or entire lung. Characteristically, a pleural effusion is present. Early, the effusion is small and may only be visible on oblique projections as a thin linear density resembling pleural thickening along that portion of the chest wall corresponding to the area of parenchymal involvement. The presence of an abscess within the consolidation (Fig. 7.67) together with the pleural effusion and/or pneumotho-

rax constitutes the sine qua non of a staphylococcal pneumonia (Fig. 7.40).

Other bacterial pneumonia also usually produce consolidation of the involved lung tissue. Radiographically, this appears as an area of parenchymal density which closely mirrors the extent of involvement and the stage of the infection.

Viral pneumonia, such as influenza, however, produces frank consolidation in less than 10% of patients (26). In most patients with viral pneumonitis, therefore, the chest roentgenogram will be inconsistent with the clinical findings relative to the chest. Frequently, the only radiographic abnormality will be a tiny pleural effusion and engorgement of the interlobular septal lymphatic channels (Kerley "B" lines) (Fig. 7.68). Conte et al. (27) have described six different roentgen patterns attributable to viral pneumonia. These are neither precisely defined nor static, but may

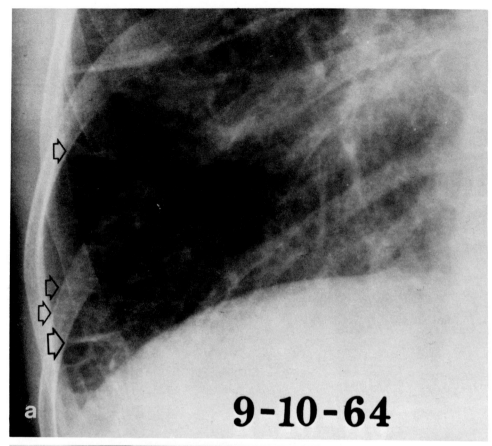

9-10-64

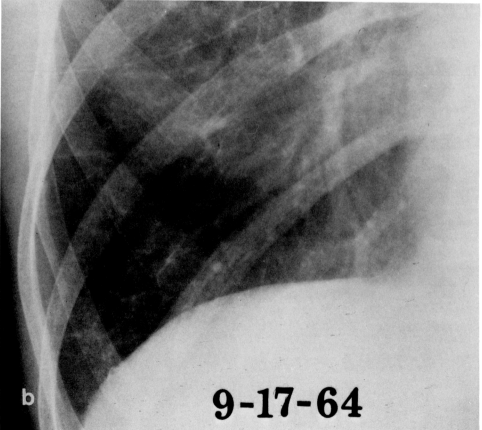

9-17-64

Fig. 7.68. (a) Viral pneumonia represented by the ill defined haziness at the right base. The presence of edema in the interlobular septal lymphatic channels (Kerley ''B'' lines) is indicated by the *arrows*. **(b)** Same patient 1 week later, asymptomatic following treatment. The inflammatorily induced interlobular septal edema is no longer present.

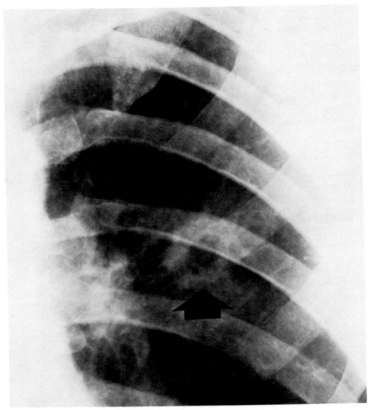

Fig. 7.69. Acute pulmonary abscess (*arrow*). Communication with the bronchus can be seen at the 7 o'clock position.

change from one to the other depending upon the stage of the disease. Of the six, however, the most frequent is peribronchial infiltrate that extends out from the hilum. The margins of the process are vague, the hila are usually prominent because of lymph node enlargement, and segmental bronchi are visible for a greater distance than normally because of the peribronchial infiltrate.

Acute lung abscess is no longer a common entity due to the use of antibiotics in the treatment of pneumonia. The cause of tissue necrosis is usually due to virulence of the causative organism. If the intrapulmonary abscess does not communicate with the bronchial tree, it appears as a homogeneous density, radiographically. When communication with a bronchus permits expulsion of necrotic material, the lesion should more correctly be referred to as a "cavity." If some necrotic material remains in the cavity, the presence of an air-fluid level will establish the nature of the lesion. If the opening into the bronchus is situated so that all necrotic contents are expelled, the cavity will be recognizable as an air-filled space surrounded by a thick, irregular wall (Fig. 7.69). The

radiographic appearance of a cavitating pulmonary lesion is not sufficiently characteristic to distinguish between a cavity caused by a common bacterial pathogen, tuberculosis, or a cavitating bronchogenic carcinoma. While in many instances the clinical findings, the location of the lesion, and the appearance of its wall may suggest the etiologic agent, the correct etiologic agent can only be established by the appropriate laboratory tests.

Bronchopleural fistula (Fig. 7.70), when loculated, may resemble a lung cavity because of the air space containing an air-fluid level. The extreme peripheral location and demarcation of extension to the pleural space in oblique and decubitus roentgenograms should establish the correct diagnosis.

Pulmonary reactions to chemical poisons are most commonly caused by the actual aspiration of kerosene or gasoline during ingestion or vomiting. The tissue response to hydrocarbons inhaled directly into the lungs consists of edema, hemorrhage, and cellular infiltration. The magnitude and severity of the tissue response, as well as the prognosis, varies directly with the amount of poison aspirated. The roentgen ap-

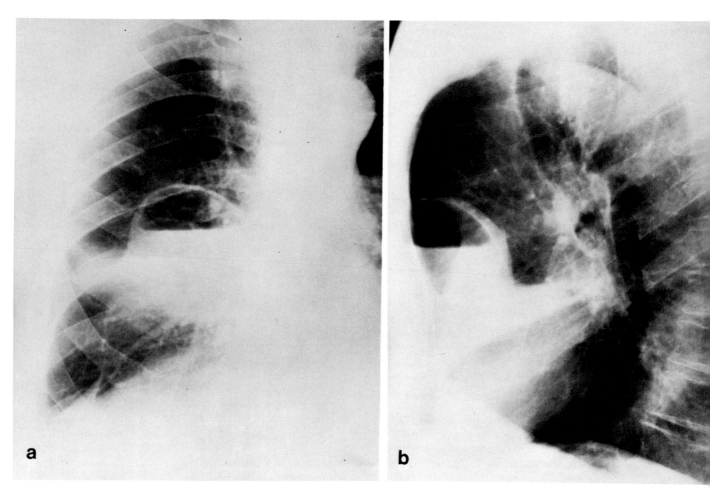

Fig. 7.70. Bronchopleural fistula which, in the frontal projection **(a)**, suggests a thin walled pulmonary abscess. In the lateral projection **(b)**, the pleural location of the air-fluid level is clearly demonstrated.

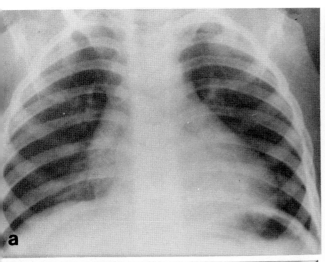

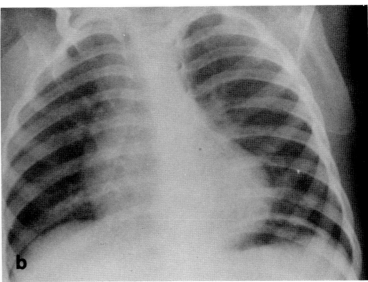

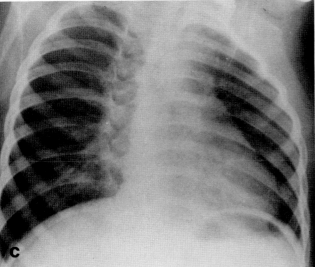

Fig. 7.71. (a-c) Chemical pneumonitis of the left lower lobe secondary to kerosene aspiration.

pearance of the lung reflects the distribution, amount, and severity of the tissue response.

Radiographic abnormalities develop rapidly and may be present within 30 minutes after the inhalation. The roentgen changes are not specific for hydrocarbon inhalation but are characteristic enough to suggest the etiology. Bilateral, perihilar or basilar patchy, mottled, ill defined areas of increased density are typically seen in mild cases (Fig. 7.71). In more severe cases, segments or entire lobes of both lungs may be obscured by the densities. It is of practical importance that the radiologic findings are commonly present when the physical examination of the chest is negative, that the roentgen picture develops rapidly, and that it is a reasonably accurate indication of the magnitude and severity of the aspiration.

Bronchial Obstruction

Diffuse

Diffuse bilateral pulmonary hyperlucency caused by air trapping (Fig. 7.72) is the radiographic abnormality of acute asthma. It is also frequently the only roentgen sign of tracheobronchitis or asthmatic bronchitis in infants and children. Spasm of the alveolar ducts and small bronchioles, which acts as a ball valve obstruction to the egress of air during expiration, is the pathologic basis of this radiographic finding. The ribs become horizontally situated, the intercostal spaces bulge, and the diaphragms become depressed.

In adults, moderate or severe diffuse obstructive type pulmonary emphysema is not difficult to diag-

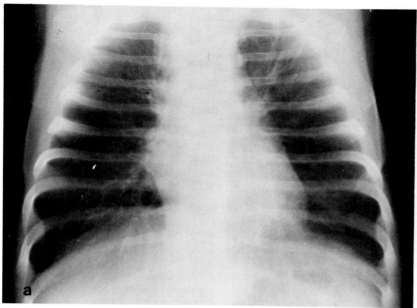
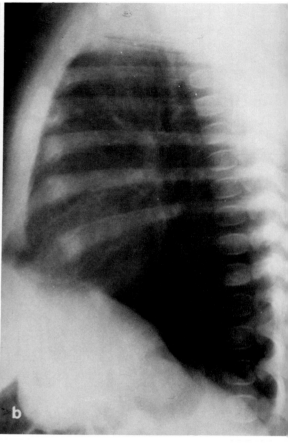

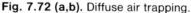

Fig. 7.72 (a,b). Diffuse air trapping.

nose radiographically because of the obvious hyper-lucency of the lungs, flattened and depressed diaphragmatic surfaces, elongated cardiac silhouette and paucity of vascular shadows in the periphery of the lungs, and increase in width of the retrocardiac and retrosternal spaces (Fig. 7.73). Emphysematous bullae may be discernible (Fig. 7.74).

Early in the disease, however, before the structural changes described above become established, the roentgen appearance of the chest of a patient with early or mild obstructive emphysema may resemble that of a patient with asthenic habitus. The distinction between these possibilities can only be made by fluoroscopic observation demonstrating limited or restricted diaphragmatic excursion and decreased aeration of the lungs in the emphysematous patient.

Diffuse bronchial (or bronchiolar) obstruction in infants and children is most commonly secondary to bronchial asthma or asthmatic bronchitis and is caused by bronchiolar spasm initially. During the acute episode of bronchiolar spasm, air enters the alveoli during inspiration but is denied egress by the bronchiolar spasm. This is referred to as air trapping. Radiographically, during an acute episode of air trap-ping, the lungs will be diffusely distended and hyper-lucent, frequently in all four projections. The intercostal spaces usually bulge and the ribs, particularly in infants, tend to be horizontally situated. Diaphragmatic depression is usually best appreciated in the lateral radiograph (Fig. 7.72). When the acute episode has subsided, the radiographic signs of air trapping are reversed and the chest is radiographically normal.

Should the initiating cause of bronchiolar spasm persist or be recurrent, muscular hypertrophy develops in the bronchial walls leading to persistent air trapping, disruption of alveoli, and persistent roentgen signs of chronic obstructive pulmonary disease (COPD).

Localized

Congenital lobar emphysema is a life-threatening emergency occurring during the 1st year of life (28, 29). It is more common in boys than girls and usually involves the right upper or lower lobe. The etiology of congenital lobar emphysema is unknown, but the altered pulmonary dynamics of the involved lobe(s) result in retention of air following expiration due to

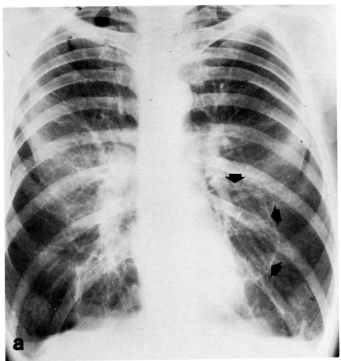

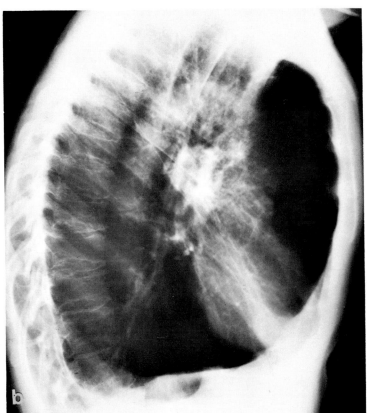

Fig. 7.73. Chronic obstructive pulmonary disease with bleb formation (*arrows*) in the lingular segment of the left upper lobe. In both frontal (a) and lateral (b) projections, the diaphragmatic surfaces are depressed and flattened. The lungs are hyperlucent and the pulmonary vascular shadows are crowded into the inner third of the lung fields. There is a paucity of vascular shadows peripherally. The heart is elongated and vertically situated. The retrosternal and retrocardiac spaces are markedly increased in anteroposterior diameter.

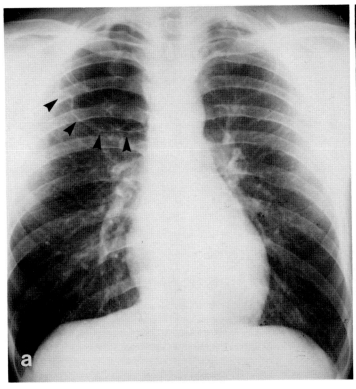

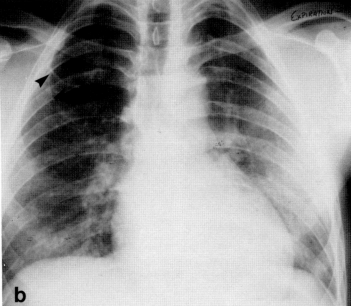

Fig. 7.74. Large emphysematous bleb in the apical segment of the right upper lobe (*arrowheads*). Note the sharp, thin, lobulated margins of the bleb(s) and the absence of parenchymal or vascular markings within the air filled sac (a). In expiration (b), the area of bleb formation remains hyperlucent because of the inability of the damaged portion of the lung to collapse or expel the air within its walls.

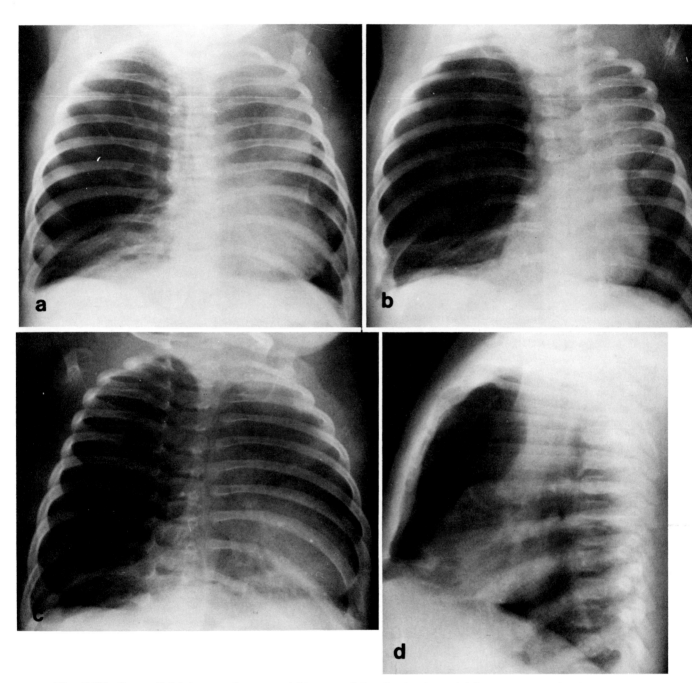

Fig. 7.75. Congenital lobar emphysema, right upper lobe. In the frontal **(a)** and oblique **(b,c)** projections, the geographic distribution of the right upper lobe is hyperlucent and there is compression atelectasis of the right middle and lower lobes. The distended right upper lobe has caused shift of the heart and mediastinal structures to the left. In the lateral radiograph **(d)**, the overdistended, hyperlucent right upper lobe is seen herniating into the retrosternal anterior mediastinum.

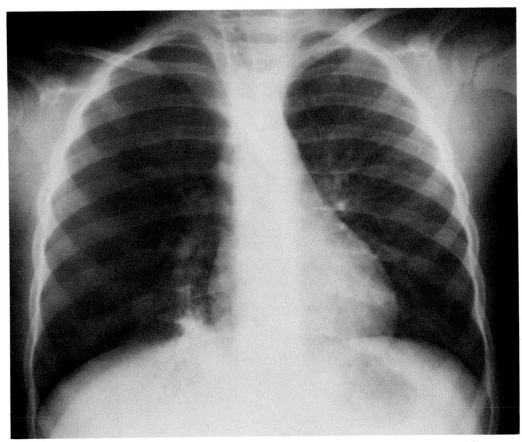

Fig. 7.76. Frontal inspiratory radiograph of the chest of an infant who aspirated a peanut into the right lower lobe stem bronchus. The right lung is hyperlucent relative to the left and the mediastinal structures are only slightly, if at all, shifted to the left. Subsegmental atelectasis and chemical pneumonitis are present in the anterior base of the segment of the right lower lobe just lateral to and separate from the right heart border.

an inability of the lobe to deflate. The symptoms are nonspecific and include respiratory distress, tachypnea, cough, and cyanosis. The treatment is surgical excision of the involved lobe.

Radiographically, congenital lobar emphysema produces marked overdistention of the abnormal lobe, compression of the adjacent lobes, depression of the ipsilateral diaphragm, displacement of the mediastinal structures to the side opposite the involved lobe and, in the lateral radiograph, herniation of the overdistended lobe into the retrosternal space (Fig. 7.75).

Air trapped behind (distal to) a nonopaque endobronchial obstruction such as an aspirated nonopaque foreign body (peanut) or a mucous plug may be difficult to appreciate in the frontal radiograph of the chest made in inspiration. The classic roentgen signs in inspiration include hyperlucency of the obstructed lung and normally situated mediastinal structures. Following expiration, however, the mediastinal structures shift toward the opposite side, i.e., the side *away*

from the obstructed bronchus. The rationale for this is that during inspiration the normal ingress of air into the nonobstructed lung results in a similar volume of air in each lung. Consequently, the lungs are of similar lucency and the mediastinal structures remain in the midline. Therefore, in the inspiratory frontal radiograph, the only sign of endobronchial obstruction may be only a relative hyperlucency of the afflicted lung (Fig. 7.76). Following expiration, however, the free escape of air from the nonobstructed lung decreases the tension in that lung compared to the tension of the obstructed lung and the mediastinal structures shift toward the nonobstructed side. Additionally, the obstructed lung remains hyperlucent, while the nonobstructed lung demonstrates hypoventilatory subsegmental atelectasis.

If frontal inspiratory and expiratory chest radiographs are inconclusive, decubitus examinations of the chest are useful in confirming, or establishing, the presence of a ball valve endobronchial obstruction.

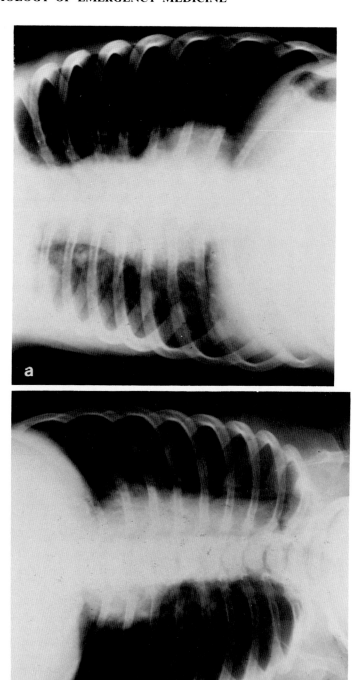

Fig. 7.77 Endobronchial ball valve obstruction, left stem bronchus. In the right lateral decubitus projection **(a)**, the dependent right lung is physiologically partially atelectatic secondary to compression and hypoventilation. In the left lateral decubitus projection **(b)**, the left lung, instead of being hypoventilated, remains hyperventilated and hyperlucent because of the air trapped by the left stem bronchial obstruction. At bronchoscopy, a mucous plug was removed from the left stem bronchus.

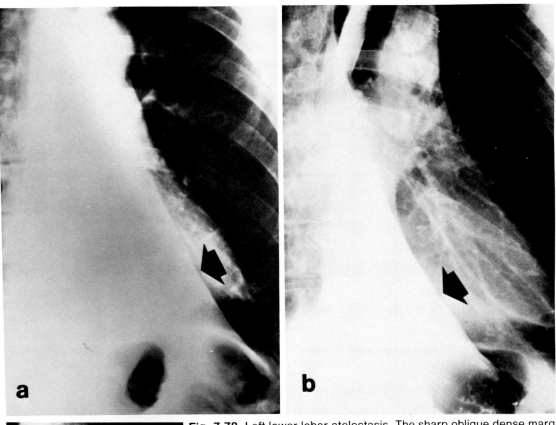

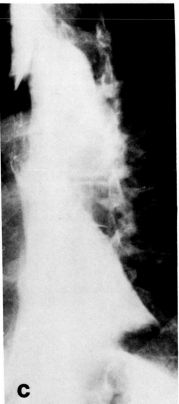

Fig. 7.78. Left lower lobar atelectasis. The sharp oblique dense margin projecting through the density of the left heart border in the frontal projection **(a)** represents the interlobar surface of the completely atelectatic left lower lobe. The margins of the atelectatic lobe (*arrows*) seen in the oblique projections **(b,c)** are a characteristic roentgen sign of atelectasis.

Normally, the dependent lung in the horizontal beam decubitus radiograph of the chest is atelectatic. In the presence of a ball valve endobronchial obstruction with peripheral air trapping, the obstructed lung remains hyperlucent even when it is the dependent lung in the decubitus radiograph (Fig. 7.77).

Basilar atelectasis, even when an entire lobe is involved, may be a very difficult radiographic diagnosis. On the left, the completely atelectatic lower lobe may be obscured by the density of the heart shadow in the frontal projection. In the lateral projection, the thickness of the atelectatic tissue lying against the heart and mediastinal structures may be insufficient to produce a radiographic shadow (Fig. 7.15). If complete collapse is suspected on the routine roentgenograms, the diagnosis can be confirmed by the typical, triangularly-shaped, sharply defined, homogeneous density seen in the overpenetrated PA and oblique radiographs (Fig. 7.78).

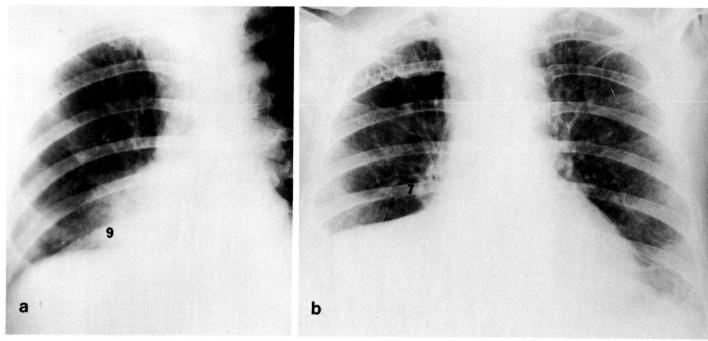

Fig. 7.79. Pneumonia of the right lower lobe. Note that the right diaphragmatic surface is normally situated relative to the ninth rib posteriorly. Same patient who subsequently developed complete atelectasis of the entire right lower lobe secondary to a mucous plug. Note that the striking similarity between the margin of the atelectatic right lower lobe **(b)** and the normal appearance of the diaphragmatic surface **(a)** makes the radiographic distinction extremely difficult.

The radiologic liability of atelectasis of the right lower lobe (Fig. 7.79) resides in its frequently striking similarity to the contour of the right hemidiaphragm or an infrapulmonary effusion. In the former instance, the distinction might be suggested by the configuration and location of the major fissure in comparison with the normal location and configuration of the right hemidiaphragm. The pleural surface of the atelectatic lobe is usually sharply defined, whereas the superior margin of an infrapulmonary effusion may be irregular and indistinct. However, the roentgen distinction is extremely difficult, particularly if the condition of the patient will not permit lateral or decubitus examination to be made.

Intrathoracic Manifestations of Intra-abdominal Disease

The role of the erect PA and lateral radiograph in the evaluation of patients with intra-abdominal disease has been described in Chapter 8. However, it merits re-emphasis by brief repetition here.

Not only may basilar pneumonia with diaphragmatic pleurisy produce clinical signs and symptoms of an acute abdomen, i.e., acute cholecystitis, but some intra-abdominal lesions frequently produce intrathoracic abnormalities on the chest roentgenogram. (A note of caution is also necessary, however, to emphasize that the radiographic examination of the chest may be entirely negative in the presence of rupture of the spleen.)

Subdiaphragmatic abscess (Fig. 7.80) may occur with equal frequency beneath either diaphragm, may occupy the anterior or posterior subphrenic spaces equally, may only develop after the passage of considerable time following the causative episode, and may produce elevation of the ipsilateral hemidiaphragm, restriction of fixation of diaphragmatic motion, pleural effusion, and basilar atelectasis or pneumonia in over 70% of patients (30).

Ultrasound, computed tomography, and nuclear medicine studies are all extremely valuable in the detection of subdiaphragmatic collections.

Pneumoperitoneum is almost always visible in the erect frontal chest roentgenogram. Rarely, however, air trapped in the anterior subphrenic space may not be discernible in the frontal projection and may be visible only in the erect lateral examination (Fig. 7.81). Therefore, both PA and lateral examinations of the chest in erect position are indicated when radiographic evidence of pneumoperitoneum is sought.

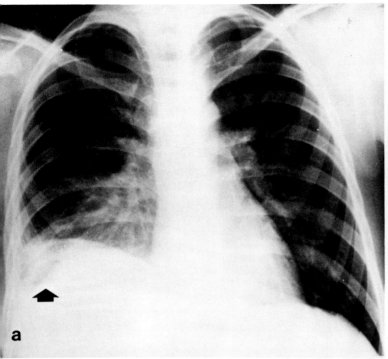

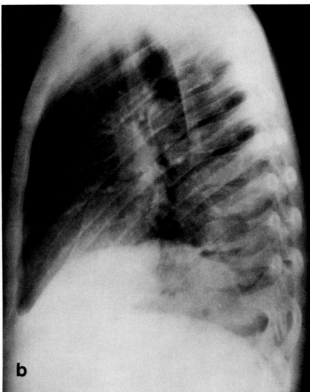

Fig. 7.80. Right subdiaphragmatic abscess. The right diaphragm is elevated and indistinct and the costophrenic angle obscured by a small pleural effusion. In both the frontal **(a)** and lateral **(b)** projections, gas can be seen within the abscess (*arrow*).

Rupture of the Esophagus

Spontaneous rupture of the esophagus [Boerhaave's syndrome (31)] is a medical emergency. The typical clinical picture is characterized by severe chest and abdominal pain, following vomiting, frequently associated with shock. The mortality of nonsurgically treated patients with spontaneous rupture of the esophagus approaches 100% with approximately 90% dying within the first 48 hours (32). The clinical diagnosis of spontaneous rupture of the esophagus is commonly missed (33). Delayed diagnosis is probably the result of a low index of suspicion on the part of the attending physician, atypical presenting signs and symptoms, and the similarity of the symptoms of esophageal rupture to those of other intrathoracic and intra-abdominal major insults such as myocardial infarction, pulmonary embolism, pneumothorax, perforated intra-abdominal hollow viscus, or acute pancreatitis. However, the relationship of severe chest and abdominal pain, dyspnea, and shock following vomiting in a previously well individual should create a high degree of probability for the diagnosis of spontaneous rupture of the esophagus.

The site of rupture is typically located in the left posterolateral aspect of the distal portion of the esophagus just proximal to the diaphragm.

Radiographically, the earliest sign of spontaneous rupture of the esophagus is widening of the mediastinum by the presence of an irregular, coarsely mottled, streaky or floccular density caused by the presence of air and gastric contents in the paraesophageal tissues. Left pleural effusion is common, as is atelectasis of the left lower lobe (Fig. 7.82). Pneumomediastinum and subcutaneous emphysema of the neck are common and may be the only discernible radiographic signs in the immediate postrupture period (34).

Pulmonary Embolus

Pulmonary thromboembolism is a common cause of death, with the mortality of unrecognized (untreated) pulmonary embolic disease being approximately 30% (35). Pulmonary embolization with hemorrhage or infarction is usually associated with intravenous thrombosis of the pelvis or lower extremities, which may be caused by any condition of the patient

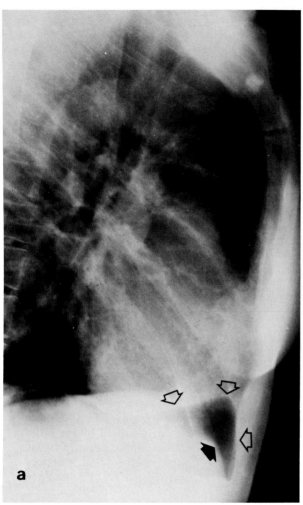

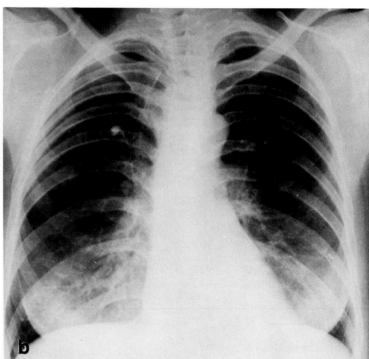

Fig. 7.81. Pneumoperitoneum. In the lateral projection **(a)**, the air is seen in the anterior subdiaphragmatic space (*open arrows*). The *solid arrow* indicates the anterior surface of the dome of the liver. The pneumoperitoneum was not radiographically discernible in the frontal projection of the chest **(b)**.

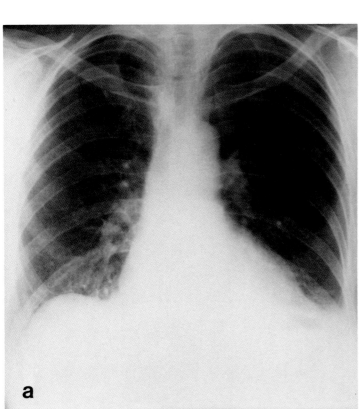

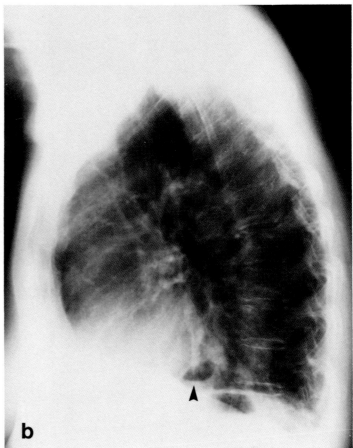

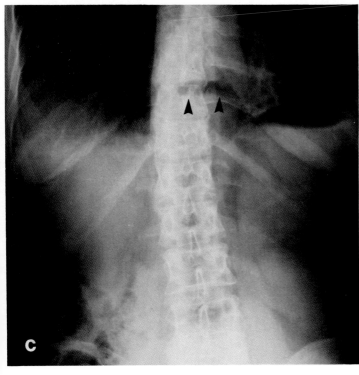

Fig. 7.82. Spontaneous rupture of the esophagus. In the frontal projection of the chest **(a)**, the only abnormality visible is a small left pleural effusion. However, in the lateral radiograph of the chest **(b)** and the erect radiograph of the abdomen **(c)**, an air-fluid interface (*arrowheads*) is present in the left lower mediastinum and signs of atelectasis of the medial basilar segment of the left lower lobe are evident.

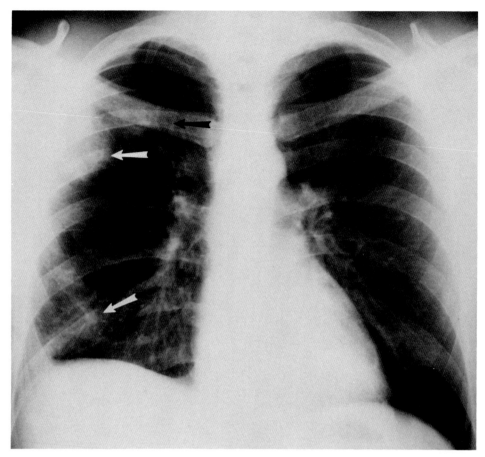

Fig. 7.83. Multiple emboli of the right lung. Several parenchymal densities, some of which are peripheral, wedge-shaped, and pleural based (*arrows*), are present in the right lung. These are associated with a pleural effusion which has obliterated the costophrenic angle and elevation of the right diaphragm.

which results in slowing of the circulation, the presence of trauma, or infection in the vicinity of the pelvic veins. It is important to be aware that there appears to be an increased incidence of pulmonary embolization in young healthy females using oral contraceptives in comparison to those in the same age group who do not employ this form of contraception (36, 37).

It has been established that the clinical, laboratory, and plain chest radiographic signs of pulmonary embolism are variable, unreliable and, even when present, nonspecific (38–40). The diagnosis of pulmonary embolism, therefore, depends largely upon a high index of suspicion and the appropriate use of radiographic procedures.

At the outset, it is necessary to be aware that the traditionally "classic" or "characteristic" plain film signs of pulmonary embolism occur infrequently and are nonspecific. Particularly, the classic roentgen description of a peripheral wedge-shaped, pleural based parenchymal density (Figs. 7.83 and 7.84) (41) is

infrequently seen and, if assumed to be the "typical" or sole plain chest radiographic appearance of a pulmonary embolism, will, because of its low incidence, result in failure to suggest the diagnosis in the majority of patients with this disease. Similarly, Westermark's sign (42), which is an absence of pulmonary arterial shadows distal to a central pulmonary embolism (Fig. 7.85), is seen infrequently and is nonspecific. A similar change in the pulmonary arterial pattern may be seen in pulmonary arterial hypertension or bulbous emphysema.

Another subjective and infrequent sign of pulmonary embolism seen on the plain frontal chest roentgenogram is increased width of a major hilar pulmonary artery (Fig. 7.86), which is due to dilatation of the artery proximal to an impacted embolus (43).

Usually, the initial plain chest roentgenogram obtained in a patient suspected of having a pulmonary embolus will be essentially negative (44). Figley et al. (45) have aptly described the plain chest film contribution to the diagnosis of pulmonary thromboembolic

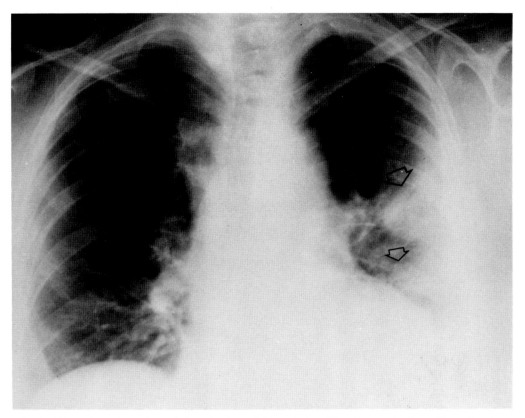

Fig. 7.84. "Typical" wedge-shaped, peripheral, pleural based densities (*arrows*) of confirmed pulmonary emboli involving the majority of the left lower lobe.

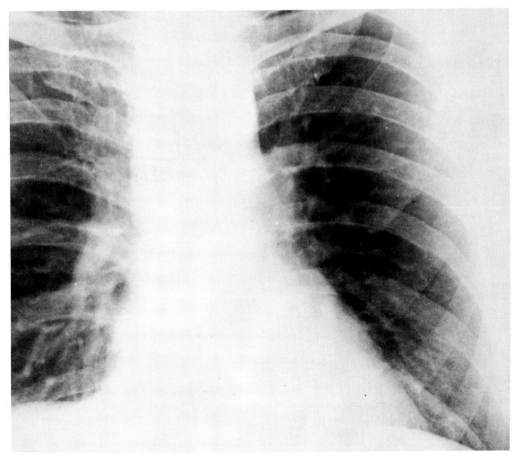

Fig. 7.85. Blood clot impacted in a major left lower lobe artery. Note the absence of pulmonary arterial shadows extending from the inferior portion of the left hilum in comparison with those arising from the right hilum.

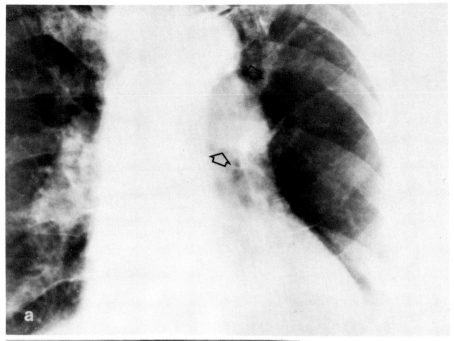

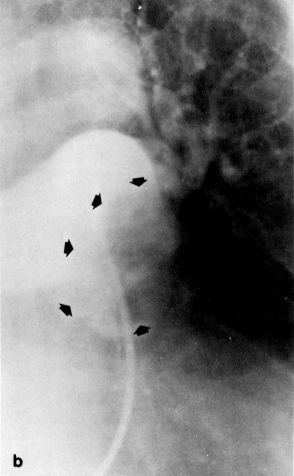

Fig. 7.86. Large embolus in the left lower lobe artery. In the frontal roentgenogram of the chest **(a)**, the left main pulmonary artery is greatly increased in diameter (*arrow*). Pulmonary arteriogram **(b)** indicates the size and location of the embolus (*solid arrows*) in the left lower lobar artery.

disease: "The principal evidence of embolus on the chest roentgenogram is often the paucity of abnormalities for a patient in such dire straits."

In those patients in whom the clinical findings are strongly suggestive of pulmonary thromboembolic disease, frontal and lateral radiographs of the chest should be obtained in hopes of demonstrating some of the plain film signs of pulmonary embolism and to rule out other conditions which may be suggested by the presenting signs and symptoms, i.e., spontaneous pneumothorax, pleural effusion, and acute pneumonia.

In the majority of patients suspected of having thromboembolic pulmonary disease, the diagnosis can be established, or excluded by a *combined* xenon-133 ventilation and technetium-99m labeled albumen microsphere perfusion scan (39, 46). Because of the physical characteristics of the isotopes, the xenon-133 ventilation scan must be performed first. While pulmonary blood flow is most simply and effectively demonstrated by the perfusion scan, and while a normal perfusion scan virtually excludes a pulmonary embolus (39), it has been demonstrated that an *abnormal* perfusion scan, while being highly sensitive, is not specific for pulmonary embolism. Abnormal perfusion scans may result from emphysema, asthma, airway obstruction, diseases which produce fluid in the alveoli such as pneumonia, edema or hemorrhage, or atelectasis.

Because ventilation abnormalities also frequently cause perfusion defects, the specificity of the perfusion scan is enhanced by combining the two studies. Therefore, a matched ventilation-perfusion defect militates against a pulmonary embolus while, conversely, a ventilation-perfusion *mismatch* (normal ventilation scan in conjunction with an abnormal perfusion scan) (Fig. 7.87) is highly suggestive of a pulmonary embolus, particularly when the chest roentgenogram is negative. Bogren et al. (46) have concluded that "approximately half of the cases with possible pulmonary embolism can be accurately diagnosed as having or not having pulmonary embolism with ventilation-perfusion scintigraphy. The remaining 50% with possible pulmonary embolism will have equal ventilation-perfusion defects. Approximately 25% of patients belonging to this latter group will have pulmonary embolism while 75% will not. Importantly, the likelihood of pulmonary embolism in the equal ventilation-perfusion group is decreased to 10% in the presence of concomitant normal chest films."

Pulmonary angiography is the definitive diagnostic procedure in the evaluation of pulmonary emboli but should be reserved for those patients in whom the ventilation-perfusion scan chest radiograph is equivocal prior to the institution of anticoagulant therapy or surgical intervention or in patients with chronic obstructive pulmonary disease.

The Heart and Pulmonary Circulation

The roentgen examination of the chest is a useful indicator of the status of cardiac function. The value of chest radiography in the patient with frank, clinically obvious left heart failure and pulmonary edema is well known. Less emphasis has been placed upon the role of the chest roentgenogram in the evaluation of patients with minimal or vague cardiopulmonary symptoms.

As the left heart decompensates, the resultant increase in pulmonary venous pressure causes a redistribution of the pulmonary blood pool from the lung bases to the apices. This cephalization of blood causes the upper lobe veins, which are normally not radiographically visible, to become discernible on the erect chest roentgenograms (Figs. 7.88 and 7.89). Distention of the upper lobe veins and pulmonary hypervascularity occur at pulmonary capillary pressures of less than 25 mm Hg. These earliest objective signs of elevated pulmonary venous pressure (cardiac decompensation) usually precede any symptoms other than easy fatigability. Physical examination of the chest is typically negative.

Pulmonary pressures in the 25–30 mm Hg range are associated with exudation of fluid into the pulmonary interstitum characterized radiographically by subpleural edema, which renders the interlobar fissures opaque, by a diffuse faint haziness in the central portions of the lungs (Fig. 7.90a), and Kerley "B" lines. The latter are short, transverse, parallel, thin linear densities which are best seen in the costophrenic angles extending into the lung from the pleura (Figs. 7.90b and 7.91). Kerley "B" lines represent interlobar septa made opaque by the exudation of fluid from the interlobular septal lymphatic channels into the perilymphatic space. These findings together with cardiomegaly are indicative of incipient or early frank pulmonary edema (Fig. 7.92).

Pulmonary capillary pressure in the 30–40 mm Hg range is accompanied by exudation of fluid into the alveolar spaces and frank pulmonary edema. Radiographically, confluent, ill defined densities are diffusely present throughout each lung and there may be either a unilateral or bilateral pleural effusion (Fig. 7.93).

Atypical distributions of pulmonary edema that may defy detection by physical examination are recognizable radiographically. "Central" pulmonary edema, which is difficult to detect clinically because of its perihilar distribution, produces a rather characteristic roentgen pattern of ill defined density about the hila (Fig. 7.94). Left heart decompensation infrequently produces pleural effusions without pulmonary edema (Fig. 7.95). Pulmonary edema associated with azotemia typically is of the perihilar variety (Fig. 7.96).

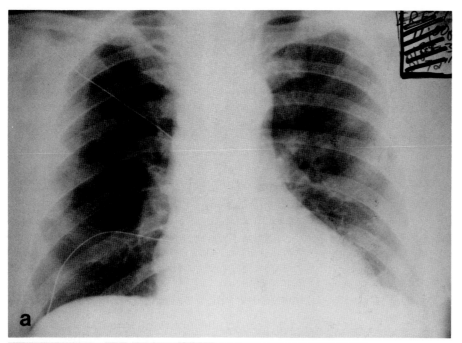

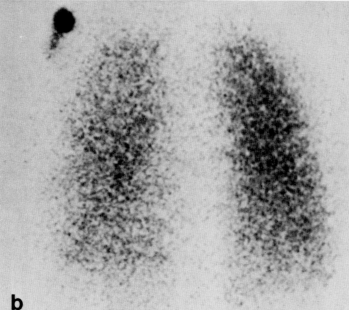

Fig. 7.87. Multiple bilateral pulmonary emboli. The frontal chest roentgenogram **(a)** reveals hyperlucency and hypovolemia of the upper and mid-thirds of the right lung and possible fullness of the right pulmonary artery. No parenchymal abnormalities are visible in either lung, and the left lung, particularly, is radiographically normal. The heart is enlarged and the aorta slightly dilated. Although not symmetrical, there is uniform distribution of the radionuclide throughout each lung in the 2 minute ventilation scan **(b)**, and there was no retention in the "wash-out" phase. Multiple bilateral perfusion defects are present in the technetium scan **(c)**. The ventilation-perfusion mismatch constitutes highly probable evidence of pulmonary emboli.

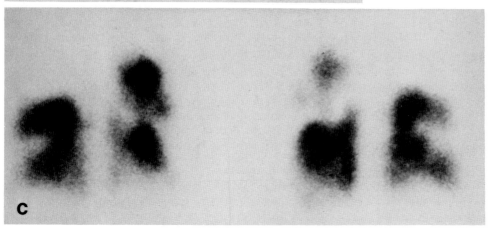

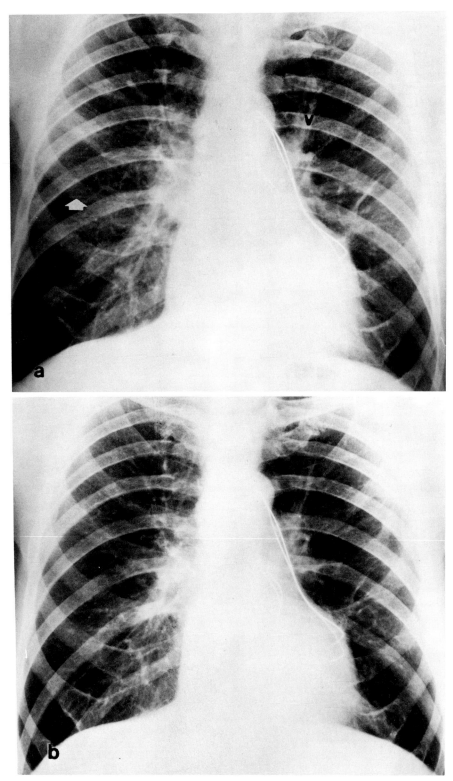

Fig. 7.88. Relative left heart decompensation with elevated pulmonary venous pressure **(a)**. Upper lobe pulmonary venous distention is evident and is most conspicuous in the left upper lobe (*V*). Subpleural edema has rendered the minor fissure of the right lung opaque (*arrow*). **(b)** Same patient following therapy. The heart has decreased in size, the subpleural fluid resorbed, and pulmonary venous pressure returned to normal levels as evidenced by the absence of upper lobe venous distention.

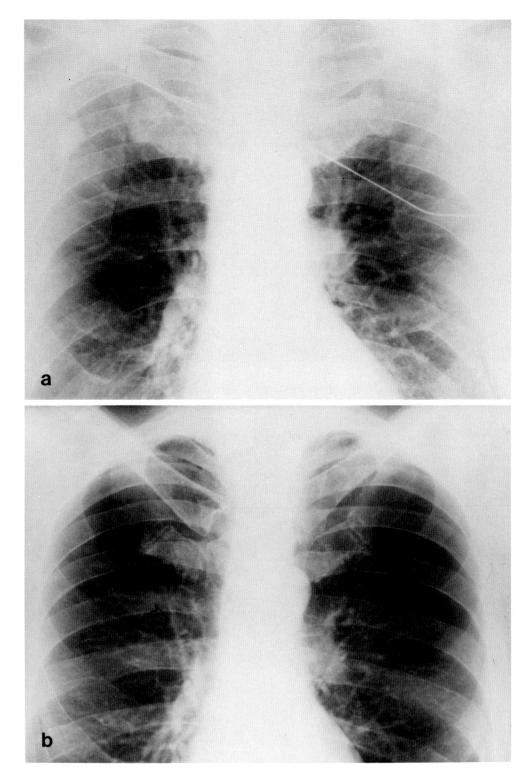

Fig. 7.89. Elevated pulmonary venous pressure without pulmonary edema. Abnormally prominent distended upper lobe veins (*arrows*) and pulmonary hypervascularity **(a)** are signs of pulmonary venous hypertension to levels less than 25 mm Hg. Following appropriate medical management, the hypervascularity has disappeared and the upper lobe veins are normal **(b)**, reflecting restoration of normal pulmonary venous pressure.

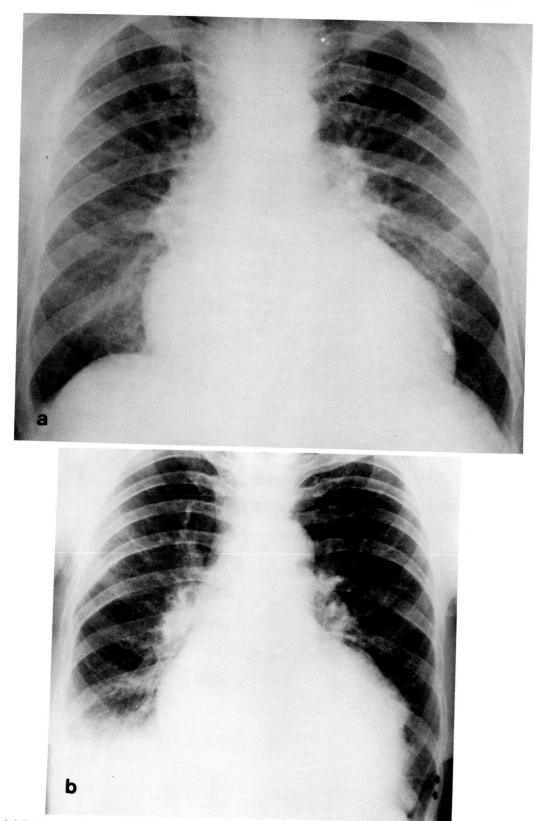

Fig. 7.90. (a) Diffuse cardiomegaly, bilateral hilar fullness, and diffuse pulmonary vascular engorgement are all signs of incipient pulmonary edema. **(b)** The *arrows* in the left costophrenic angle indicate Kerley "B" lines in a patient with left heart failure.

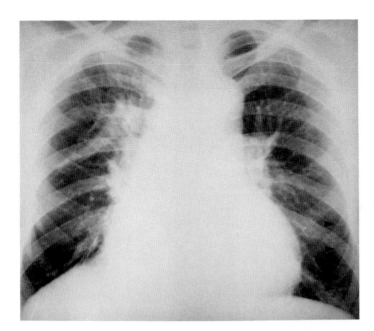

Fig. 7.91. Elevated venous pressure. The thin, short, horizontal linear densities which are best seen in the left costophrenic angle projecting from the pleural surface into the lung (*arrowheads*) are Kerley "B" lines.

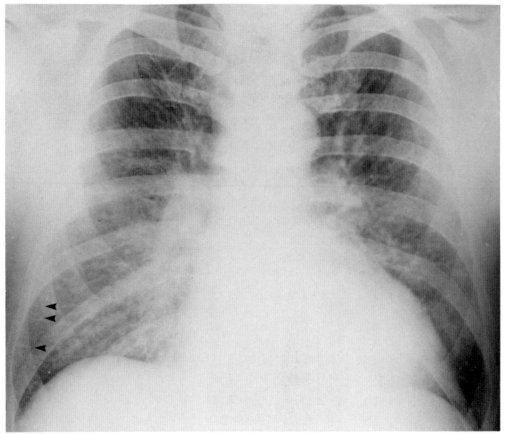

Fig. 7.92. Frank pulmonary edema with Kerley "B" lines in each costophrenic angle. This patient demonstrates all the radiographic signs of left heart failure and pulmonary edema. The heart is diffusely enlarged with left ventricular preponderance. The cardiac margins are indistinct. The aorta is dilated and tortuous. There is obvious diffuse pulmonary hypervolemia characterized by hypervascularity and distended upper lobe veins. The ill defined haziness distributed throughout each lung represents frank pulmonary edema. Kerley "B" lines are present in each costophrenic angle, more prominently on the right (*arrowheads*).

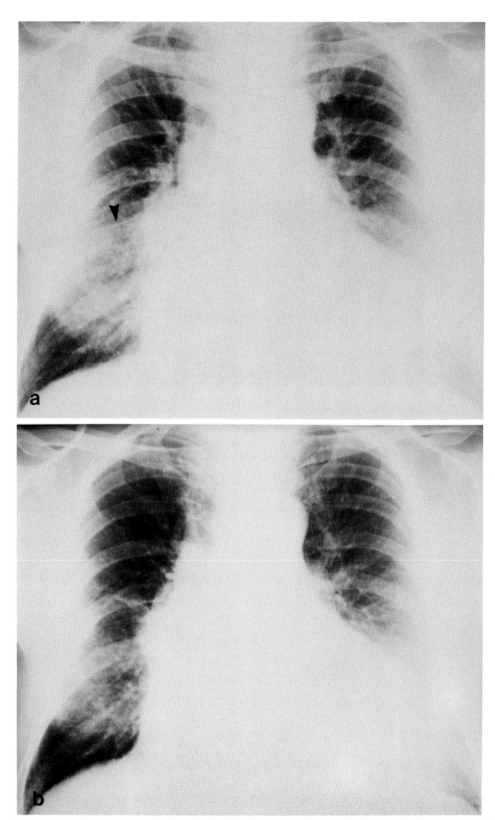

Fig. 7.93. Left heart failure with frank pulmonary edema and left pleural effusion. At the time of acute left heart failure **(a)**, the heart is enlarged and the aorta dilated and tortuous. The margins of each are indistinct. Upper lobe veins are abnormally distended and hypervascularity is evident. Conglomerate densities and diffuse haziness in each midlung field represent frank pulmonary edema. The minor fissure is visible on the right *(arrowhead)* and there is a moderate left pleural effusion. Following appropriate medical treatment, the signs of left heart failure disappeared, although the heart remains enlarged **(b)**.

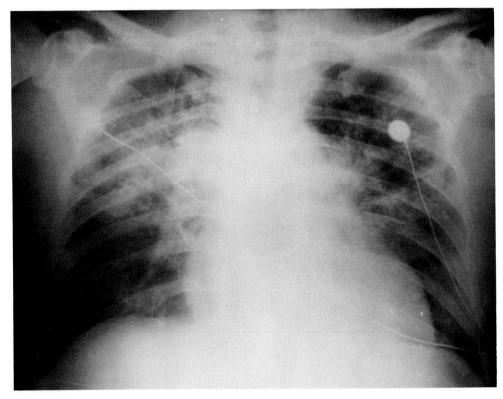

Fig. 7.94. Left heart failure with central (perihilar) pulmonary edema. The ill defined hazy density in the perihilar areas represents this atypical distribution of pulmonary edema. Note that the apices, bases, and periphery of the lungs are relatively free of fluid exudation.

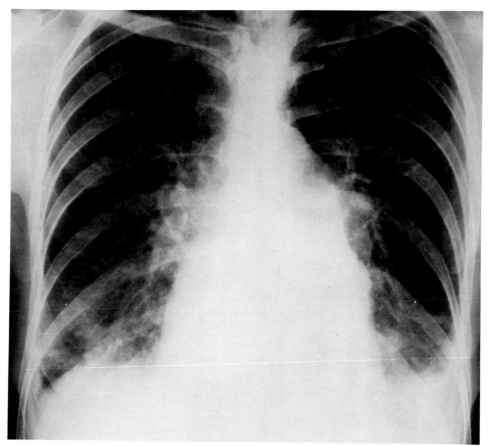

Fig. 7.95. Left heart failure with bilateral pleural effusions but without pulmonary edema.

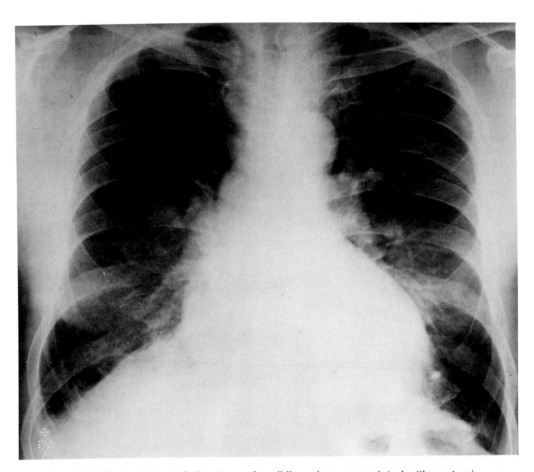

Fig. 7.96. Typical ''butterfly'' pattern of perihilar edema associated with azotemia.

Pulmonary arterial hypertension is characterized by distention of the major pulmonary arteries, a rather abrupt tapering decrease in their caliber as they leave the hila, and a paucity of vascular markings in the peripheral third of the lung fields (Fig. 7.97).

For a comprehensive review of the radiographic manifestations of altered pulmonary hemodynamics, the reader is referred to the publications of Harris (47), Shanks and Kerley (48), and Simon (49–51).

Cardiac aneurysms most commonly involve the left ventricle. Early in the development of the aneurysm, its radiographic detection is difficult (Fig. 7.98a) and may only be confirmed by fluoroscopic observation of paradoxical pulsation of the involved segment of the left ventricular wall. When fully established, the appearance of a ventricular aneurysm is characteristic (Fig. 7.98b).

Aortic aneurysms usually involve the posterior portion of the arch or the descending thoracic aorta. Aneurysms of the ascending aorta are uncommon and usually syphilitic in origin. Although usually solitary, aortic aneurysm may be multiple (Fig. 7.99).

The roentgen characteristics of an aortic aneurysm frequently so closely resemble those of a pulmonary neoplasm or abscess as to make the distinction impossible on plain chest radiographs. Fluoroscopic

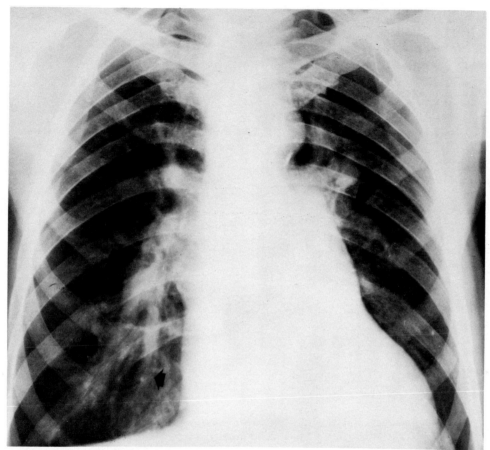

Fig. 7.97. Pulmonary arterial hypertension. The typical radiographic signs include distention of the central pulmonary arteries, abrupt decrease in their caliber just beyond the hilum, and a marked paucity of vascular markings in the peripheral portions of the lung.

evaluation of the lesion is usually equivocal because pulsations may not be observed in an aneurysm containing a mural thrombus, and a tumor or abscess situated close to the aorta may demonstrate a pulsation. Aortography usually provides data upon which the differentiation between aneurysm and a nonvascular lesion can be established (Fig. 7.100).

Pulmonary Neoplasia

Primary or metastatic pulmonary neoplasia may be the etiology of pain, hemoptysis, or dyspnea. Gener-

ally, primary bronchogenic neoplasms produce readily discernible roentgen shadows. The Pancoast tumor, which involves the mediastinal aspect of the upper lobe (Fig. 7.101), is notoriously difficult to identify on the chest roentgenogram because of the superimposed densities of the normal mediastinal soft tissues and the thoracic cage. The presenting symptoms of this tumor may be interscapular pain, dyspnea, dysphagia, or, when on the left, hoarseness due to entrapment of the left recurrent laryngeal nerve. Involvement of the phrenic nerve results in paresis of the ipsilateral hemidiaphragm, which will be elevated

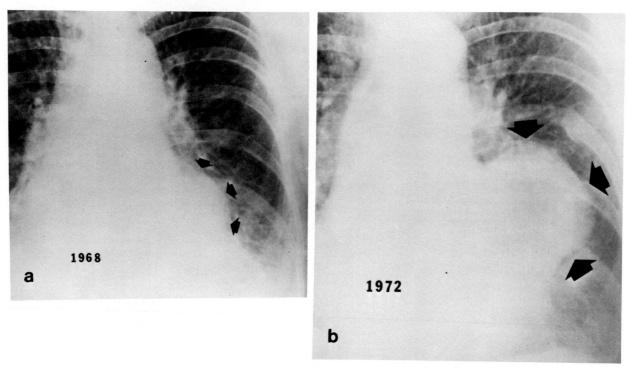

Fig. 7.98. Left ventricular aneurysm. **(a)** In 1968, the aneurysm (*arrows*) was very small and barely perceptible radiographically. **(b)** By 1972, the aneurysm had increased greatly in size.

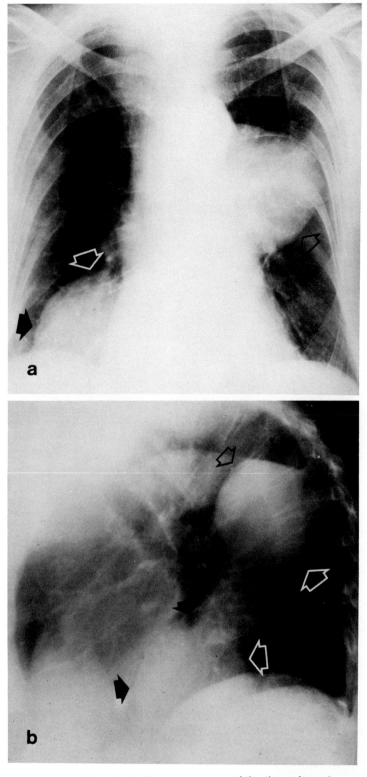

Fig. 7.99 (a,b). Multiple aneurysms of the thoracic aorta.

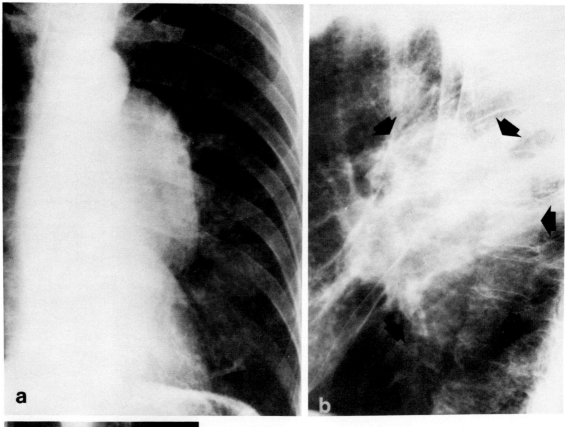

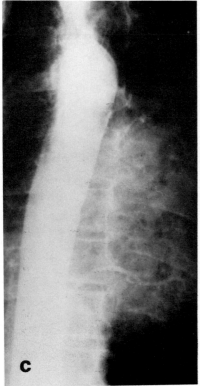

Fig. 7.100. Left hilar mass of indeterminate etiology in the frontal (a) and lateral (b) projections. The thoracic aortogram (c) demonstrates the nonvascular origin of the lesion, which was ultimately proven to be a large necrotic bronchogenic carcinoma.

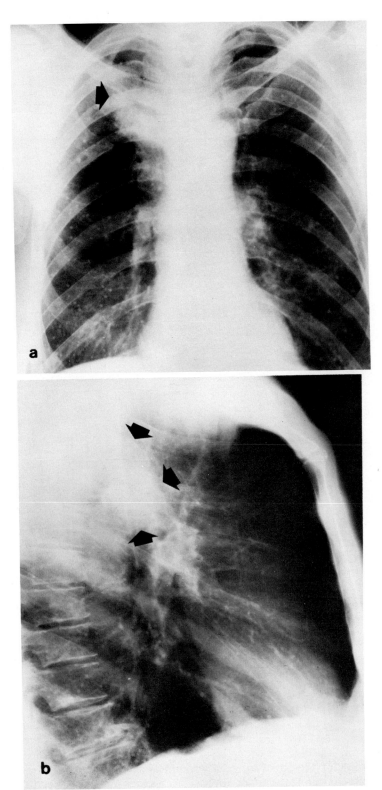

Fig. 7.101. Pancoast tumor of the mediastinal aspect of the right upper lobe. In the frontal projection **(a)**, the tumor is obscured by the superimposed density of the ribs and anterior end of the clavicle. In the lateral projection **(b)**, the mass is obscured by the density of the mediastinal structures and the upper thoracic vertebrae.

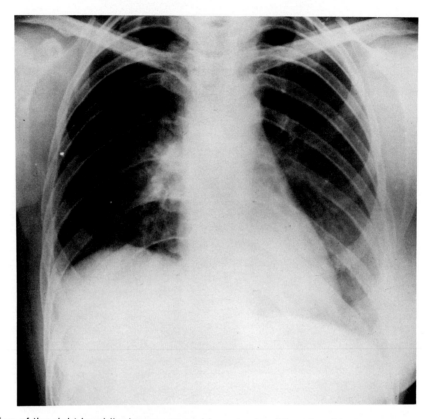

Fig. 7.102. Elevation of the right hemidiaphragm caused by paresis of the phrenic nerve secondary to the right hilar tumor.

on the chest roentgenogram (Fig. 7.102) and which moves paradoxically when the "sniff" test is observed fluoroscopically. Compression of the superior vena cava results in the typical clinical features of the superior mediastinal obstruction syndrome.

Primary carcinoma of the lung is uncommon in females who do not smoke. However, primary aden-ocarcinoma of the lung is the most common broncho-genic neoplasm of females, occurring in approxi-mately 5% (Fig. 7.103).

Dyspnea may be caused by extensive hematogenous (Fig. 7.104) or lymphangitic (Fig. 7.105) pulmonary metastasis.

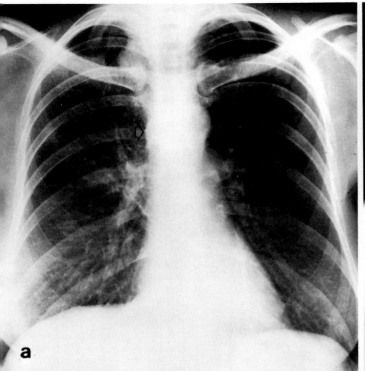

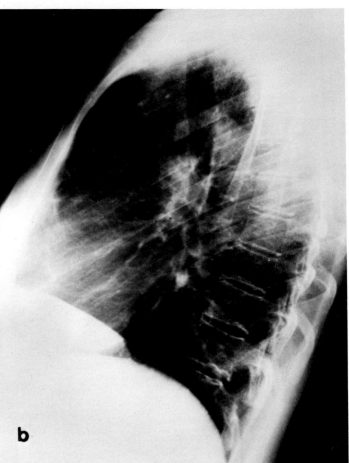

Fig. 7.103. Primary adenocarcinoma in the mediastinal aspect of the right upper lobe (*solid arrow*) with enlarged right sided paratracheal lymph nodes (*open arrow*).

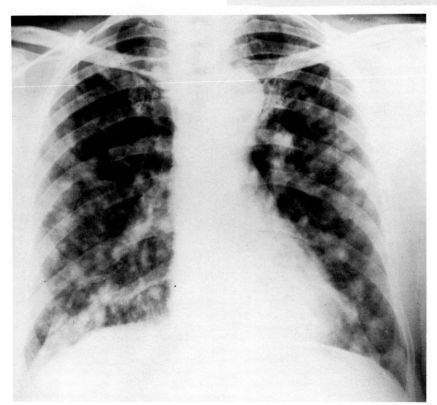

Fig. 7.104. Hematogenous pulmonary metastatic disease.

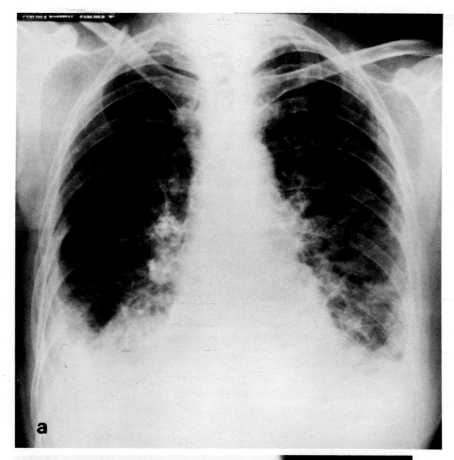

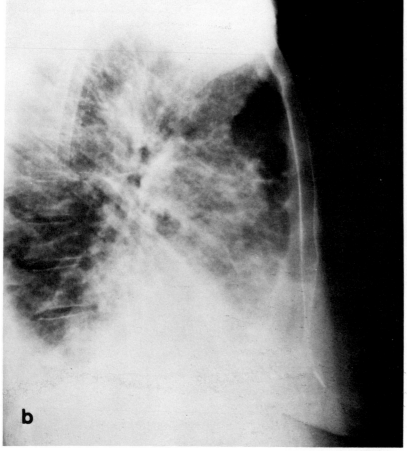

Fig. 7.105 (a,b). Lymphangitic pulmonary metastasis with bilateral pleural effusions.

References

1. KEATS TK: The aortic-pulmonary mediastinal stripe. *AJR* 116:107, 1972.
2. FELSON B, FELSON H: Localization of intrathoracic lesions by means of the postero-anterior roentgenogram. The Silhouette Sign. *Radiology* 55:363, 1950.
3. TING YM: Pulmonary parenchymal findings in blunt trauma to the chest. *AJR* 98:343, 1966.
4. STEVENS E, TEMPLETON AW: Traumatic non-penetrating lung contusion. *Radiology* 85:247, 1965.
5. WILLIAMS JR, STEMBRIDGE VA: Pulmonary contusion secondary to non-penetrating chest trauma. *AJR* 91:284, 1964.
6. BALLINGER WF, RUTHERFORD RB, ZUIDEMA GD: *The Management of Trauma.* W. B. Saunders, Philadelphia, 1968.
7. GIBSON LD, CARTER R, HINSHAW DB: Surgical significance of sternal fractures. *Surg Gynecol Obstet* 114:443, 1962.
8. RELIHAN M, LITWIN MS: Morbidity and mortality associated with flail chest injury: A review of 85 cases. *J Trauma* 13:663, 1973.
9. FULTON RL, PETER ET, WILSON JN: The pathophysiology and treatment of pulmonary contusions. *Trauma* 10:719, 1970.
10. KIRSH MM, SLOAN H: *Blunt Chest Trauma.* Little, Brown & Co., Boston, 1977.
11. ALFANO GS, HALE HW Jr.: Pulmonary contusion. *Trauma* 5:647, 1965.
12. KELLER JW, MECKSTROTH CV, SANZENBACHER L, et al.: Thoracic injuries due to blunt trauma. *J Trauma* 7:541, 1967.
13. PERRY JF Jr., GALWAY CF: Chest injury due to blunt trauma. *J Thorac Cardiovasc Surg* 49:604, 1965.
14. GREENING R, HYNETTE A, HODES PJ: Unusual pulmonary changes secondary to chest trauma. *AJR* 77:1059, 1957.
15. PARMLEY LF, MATTINGLY TW, MANION WC, JAHNKE EJ: Non-penetrating traumatic injury of the aorta. *Circulation* 17:1086, 1958.
16. SCHONHOLTZ GJ, JAHNKE EJ: Occult injury of the thoracic aorta associated with orthopedic trauma. *J Bone Joint Surg* 46:1421, 1964.
17. NACLERIO EA: *Chest Injuries.* Grune & Stratton, New York, 1971.
18. WILSON RF, ARBULU A, BASSETT JS, WALT AJ: Acute mediastinal widening following blunt chest trauma. *Arch Surg* 104:551, 1972.
19. BLAIR E, TOPUZLU C, DAVIS JH: Delayed or missed diagnosis in blunt chest trauma. *Trauma* 11:129, 1971.
20. AYELLA RJ, HANKINS JR, TURNEY SZ, COWLEY RA: Ruptured thoracic aorta due to blunt trauma. *Trauma* 17:199, 1977.
21. SUTORIUS, DJ, SCHREIBER, JT, HELMSWORTH, JA: Traumatic disruption of the thoracic aorta. *J Trauma* 13:583, 1973.
22. GAZZANIGA AB, KHURI EI, MIR-SEPASI HM, BARTLETT RH: Rupture of the thoracic aorta following blunt trauma. *Arch Surg* 110:1119, 1975.
23. McGEE RB, D'LUZANSKY JJ: Acute blunt traumatic rupture of the spleen. *Arch Surg* 99:121, 1969.
24. PETERSON JA: Recognition of infrapulmonary pleural effusion. *Radiology* 74:34, 1960.
25. REBHAN AW, EDWARDS HE: Staphylococcic pneumonia: A review of 329 cases. *Can Med Assoc J* 82:513, 1960.
26. SCANLON GT, UNGER JD: The radiology of bacteria and viral pneumonia. *Radiol Clin North Am* 11:317, 1973.
27. CONTE P, HEITZMAN ER, MARKARIAN B: Viral pneumonia. *Radiology* 95:267, 1970.
28. KEATS TE: An approach to the radiologic diagnosis of respiratory distress in the newborn. *Weekly Radiology Science Update.* Biomedia, Inc., Narberth, Pa., 1976.
29. REID, JM, BARCLAY RS, STEVENSON JG, WELSH TM: Congenital obstructive lobar emphysema. *Dis Chest* 49:359, 1966.
30. MILLER WT, TALMAN EA: Sub-phrenic abscess. *AJR* 101:961, 1967.
31. BOERHAAVE H: Atrocus, Nec Descriptiprius, Morbi Historia Secundum, Medicae Artis Leges Conscripta. Lugduni, Batavorum, Boutesteniana, 1974.
32. SYMBAS PN, HATCHER CR, HARLAFTIS N: Spontaneous rupture of the esophagus. *Ann Surg* 187:634, 1978.
33. IZAGUIRRE SFS, HAGGERTY JT, ECKERT G: Spontaneous rupture of the esophagus. *Surgery* 67:607, 1970.
34. REYNOLDS J, DAVIS JT: Injuries of the chest wall, pleura, pericardium, lungs, bronchi and esophagus. *Radiol Clin North Am* 4:383, 1966.
35. DALEN JE, ALPERT JS: Natural history of pulmonary embolism. *Prog Cardiovac Dis* 17:259, 1975.
36. VESSEY MP, DOLL R: Investigation of relation between use of oral contraceptives and thromboembolic disease. *Br Med J* 2:199, 1968.
37. INMAN WHW, VESSEY MP: Investigation of deaths of pulmonary, coronary, and cerebral thrombosis and embolism in women of child-bearing age. *Br Med J* 2:193, 1968.
38. DALEN JE: Diagnosis of acute pulmonary embolism. In *Pulmonary Embolism,* edited by JE Dalen. Medcom, New York, 1972.
39. RAVIN CE, GREENSPAN RH: Evaluation of patients with suspected pulmonary embolism. *Weekly Radiology Science Update.* Biomedia, Inc., Narberth, Pa., 1977.
40. RABIN ED: Overdiagnosis and treatment of pulmonary embolism. *Ann Intern Med* 87:775, 1977.
41. HAMPTON AO, CASTLEMAN B: Correlation of post-mortem chest teleroentgenograms with autopsy findings: With special reference to pulmonary embolism and infarction. *AJR* 43:305, 1940.
42. WESTERMARK N: On the roentgen diagnosis of lung embolism. *Acta Radiol* 19:357, 1938.
43. FRAZER RG, PARE JAP: *Diagnosis of Disease of the Chest.* W. B. Saunders, Philadelphia, 1970.
44. ISRAEL HL, GOLDSTEIN F: The varied clinical manifestations of pulmonary embolism. *Ann Intern Med* 47:202, 1967.
45. FIGLEY MM, GERDES AJ, RICKETTS HJ: Radiologic aspects of pulmonary embolism. *Semin Roentgenol* 2:389, 1967.
46. BOGREN HG, BERMAN DS, VISMARA LA, MASON DT: Lung ventilation perfusion scintigraphy in pulmonary embolism. *Acta Radiol* 19:933, 1978.
47. HARRIS JH, Jr.: The pulmonary arteries and veins: Their radiographic identification. *Med Radiogr Photogr* 29:52, 1963.
48. SHANKS CS, KERLEY P: *A Textbook of X-ray Diagnosis,* ed. 2. H. K. Lewis, London, 1951.
49. SIMON M: The pulmonary veins in mitral stenosis. *J Fac Radiol* 9:25, 1958.
50. SIMON M: The pulmonary vessels in incipient left ventricular decompensation. *Circulation* 24:158, 1961.
51. SIMON M: The pulmonary vessels: Their hemodynamic evaluation using routine radiographs. *Radiol Clin North Am* 1:363, 1963.

chapter eight

Abdomen

General Considerations

For the purpose of this discussion, the "abdomen" will include those organs and organ systems located between the diaphragm and the pelvic peritoneal reflection. The radiology of the urinary tract and of the pelvis concerned with emergency medicine each constitute separate chapters. Consequently, neither the urinary tract nor the pelvis and its contents will be discussed here.

Many of the disease processes that acutely affect the abdomen produce radiographic signs that are helpful in establishing the correct diagnosis. However, the radiographic changes may not be specific for a particular disease process or injury. For this reason, clinical data concerning the patient is extremely important in interpreting the radiographs.

It is very important to realize that the radiographic appearance of the abdomen may not be consonant with the clinical findings. This may be particularly true if the roentgenograms are obtained within a relatively short time following the onset of symptoms. The explanation lies in the fact that the radiographic changes may not be caused by the primary process itself, but represent, instead, alterations of anatomy or physiology that occur secondary to the primary entity and that require variable intervals of time to produce radiographically discernible changes.

The length of time required for these changes to develop ranges from immediate, as in the instance of free perforation of a peptic ulcer producing massive pneumoperitoneum, to delayed rupture of the splenic capsule in which the latent period from injury to the development of radiographic findings may be as long as 1 month (1). Thus, a negative radiographic examination of an "acute" abdomen should not lull the observer into a sense of complacency regarding the patient. Such a study must be evaluated as any other

laboratory data and must be judged in light of the clinical information relative to the patient. Finally, it should be remembered that, as the changes in physiology and anatomy caused by the pathologic process develop, the radiographic appearance of the abdomen will reflect these changes.

Intrathoracic pathology may produce clinical signs and symptoms suggesting an upper abdominal process. Therefore, when the clinical findings suggest upper abdominal pathology, erect posteroanterior and lateral examinations of the chest, when possible, should be obtained in addition to the appropriate abdominal films.

The effects of blunt trauma upon the abdomen are frequently masked by more obvious associated injuries that are relatively insignificant clinically. Symptoms referable to blunt intra-abdominal trauma may be so trivial as to be ignored during the early post-trauma hours. This is probably the explanation for the significantly higher mortality rate associated with nonpenetrating abdominal trauma than with penetrating wounds. Therefore, everyone involved in the diagnosis and management of patients who have sustained blunt abdominal trauma must have a high index of suspicion for the presence of significant intra-abdominal injuries, particularly in the absence of obvious clinical signs or symptoms.

Radiographic Examination

The single frontal projection of the abdomen, also referred to as AP or supine abdomen, scout or survey film, KUB (*K*idney-*U*reter-*B*ladder), constitutes the routine radiographic examination of the abdomen. This study provides only cursory information regarding the abdomen and its contents and cannot be relied upon to demonstrate a small or moderate pneumoperitoneum, nor to permit differentiation between reflex (adynamic) ileus and mechanical obstruction. Therefore, when the clinical picture suggests either a pneumoperitoneum or an intestinal obstruction or ileus, each decubitus projection and, if the patient's condition will permit, an anteroposterior roentgenogram made with the patient in full erect position must be obtained.

If only a limited examination of the abdomen is possible, for whatever reason, and pneumoperitoneum is a diagnostic possibility, the supine and right-side-up decubitus examinations constitute an adequate radiographic study. In the presence of a pneumoperitoneum, the free air will accumulate along the right lobe of the liver in this decubitus position and will be evident on the roentgenogram. Each of these studies can be made with the patient on a litter in the Emergency Department if necessary. The absence of a radiographically demonstrable pneumoperitoneum does not exclude rupture of a hollow viscus. A small perforation can occur and either seal itself or be covered by omentum or mesentery. In these circumstances, the amount of free air may be so small as to be undetectable radiographically, or it may be absorbed by the time the radiographic examination is obtained.

The patient should be placed in the erect or decubitus position for 3 or 4 minutes prior to making the radiographic exposure. This slight delay will permit air in the peritoneal space to migrate beneath the diaphragm or along the liver margin. In the event of mechanical obstruction or reflex ileus, it will permit time for the air-fluid levels in the gut to become more clearly established.

It is absolutely essential that erect radiographic studies of the abdomen be made with the patient in the completely erect position in order that the presence of the air-fluid levels, when they exist, may be established and their characteristics accurately recorded. The physical basis for obtaining a useful erect roentgenogram of the abdomen is that a horizontal x-ray beam must pass parallel to the air-fluid interface in order to demonstrate, radiographically, that an air-fluid level exists. If the patient is not completely erect, the x-ray beam will strike the air-fluid interface tangentially and the interface will not be recorded on the film, thereby decreasing the likelihood of a correct diagnosis.

The erect examination of the abdomen must include the diaphragmatic surfaces in order to be certain that small amounts of air situated immediately beneath the diaphragmatic surfaces or intrathoracic manifestations of intra-abdominal disease are not overlooked.

It is frequently difficult to determine whether a stab wound of the abdominal wall has penetrated into the peritoneal cavity. This diagnostic enigma is associated with a high incidence of negative exploratory laparotomy. A technique of injecting stab wounds of the abdominal wall, through a catheter secured within the wound of entry by a purse-string suture, has been described (2–5). If the wound penetrates the peritoneum, anteroposterior and horizontal beam lateral roentgenograms of the abdomen made with the patient supine will reveal contrast medium in the peritoneal space surrounding loops of intestine. If the peritoneum has not been violated, the opacity will remain within the soft tissues of the abdominal wall external to the peritoneum.

Ultrasound, nuclear medicine, and computed tomography all have a place in the evaluation of the patient with an acutely ill or injured abdomen. Ultrasonography has the advantages of being noninvasive and of not requiring ionizing radiation. In the "real-time" mode, ultrasound has the capability of scanning any portion of the abdomen quickly and of recording motion such as vascular pulsation. Ultrasound is particularly useful in detecting intraperitoneal fluid accumulations, of quickly evaluating the diameter of the aorta, the presence of thrombi, and the character of aortic pulsations. The detection of subcapsular hepatic and splenic hematoma is possible with sonography. Ultrasound probably makes its greatest contribution to the evaluation of the acute abdomen in patients suspected of acute cholecystitis and obstetric-gynecologic problems. Sonographic localization of the gallbladder provides precise correlation with pain and tenderness, records the increased thickness of the edematous gallbladder wall and the presence of calculi. Sonography provides rapid and accurate evaluation of those obstetrical abnormalities that produce acute pelvic symptoms during the first trimester of pregnancy and provides useful data relative to inflammatory and neoplastic processes of the female pelvis. The application of ultrasound is limited by acute injuries of the abdominal wall, the presence of surgical dressings and tubes, the inability of the patient with acute abdominal trauma to assume the necessary positions for optimum sonographic examination, and distention of the gut due to aerophagia or reflex or mechanical obstruction.

Nuclear radiology is useful in the evaluation of splenic and hepatic trauma, renal vascular injuries, particularly traumatic renal artery thrombosis, and by recording isotope flow, provides a qualitative measure of blood flow.

Computed tomography (CT) provides unique cross-sectional and, depending on the type of equipment, sagittal and coronal display of normal anatomy of the abdomen (as well as all body areas) and alterations of anatomy caused by trauma and disease. The other unique feature of CT is that by converting the radiation absorption characteristics of various tissues into a two-dimensional visual display, many organs and structures not otherwise radiographically identifiable become readily visible. Computed tomography, utilizing contemporary equipment, is not limited by surgical dressings or intestinal distention, and does not require changes of patient position. Skeletal as well as soft tissue structures are clearly delineated and areas usually inaccessible to other imaging modalities, such as the spinal canal, the retroperitoneal spaces, and the pelvis, are well displayed by computed tomography. The selection and application of these newer imaging techniques depend upon the clinical circumstances and the plain film radiographic findings of the individual patient and should be utilized following direct personal consultation with the radiologist.

Radiographic Anatomy

The normal supine radiograph of the abdomen is seen in Figure 8.1. Superiorly, the abdomen is bounded by the diaphragm, laterally by the soft tissue densities of the flank, and inferiorly by the pelvis.

The right diaphragm is usually higher than the left. Diaphragmatic surfaces on the same level, or the left higher than the right, are not necessarily pathologic. These normal variants occur in approximately 10% of individuals. The left hemidiaphragm is normally higher than the right in patients with situs inversus.

Superiorly, the diaphragmatic surfaces are sharply defined. Inferiorly, the right hemidiaphragm cannot be separated from the liver density. Anomalously, large or small bowel may be interposed between the dome of the liver and the diaphragm (Fig. 8.2). Air in the stomach produces a radiolucent shadow to the left of the midline. This is usually easily recognizable by its location and the characteristic appearance of the gastric rugae.

Congenital anomalies of the diaphragmatic musculature may produce a scalloped appearance of the dome of the diaphragm. Eventration of the diaphragm may be partial or complete (Fig. 8.3). The mediastinal structures may be displaced by the abdominal organs which reside in the thorax because of the absent hemidiaphragm (Fig. 8.4). Fetal lobulation of the liver and ectopic location of the left kidney may cause a short arc of the appropriate hemidiaphragm to project above the main sweep of the remainder of the diaphragmatic surface.

Much has been written regarding the radiographic anatomy of the flank (6,7) which is depicted in Figure 8.5. The structure of primary radiologic interest in the flank is the longitudinal radiolucent shadow which lies medial to the flank muscles (Fig. 8.6). This has

Fig. 8.1. Radiographic appearance of a normal abdomen. The rugal pattern of the body of the stomach is outlined by air in the left upper quadrant. The *large solid arrows* indicate the lateral margins of the psoas muscles. The *small solid arrows* identify the lower pole of the left kidney. The properitoneal fat lines (flank stripe) are indicated by the *open arrows*. The ascending and descending segments of the large intestine are identified by fecal debris and gas.

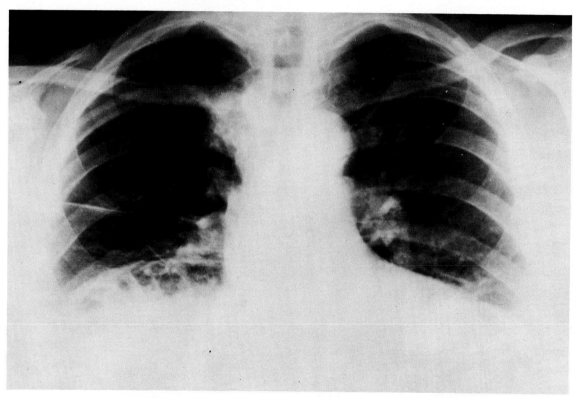

Fig. 8.2. Interposition of loops of bowel between the dome of the liver and the right hemidiaphragm.

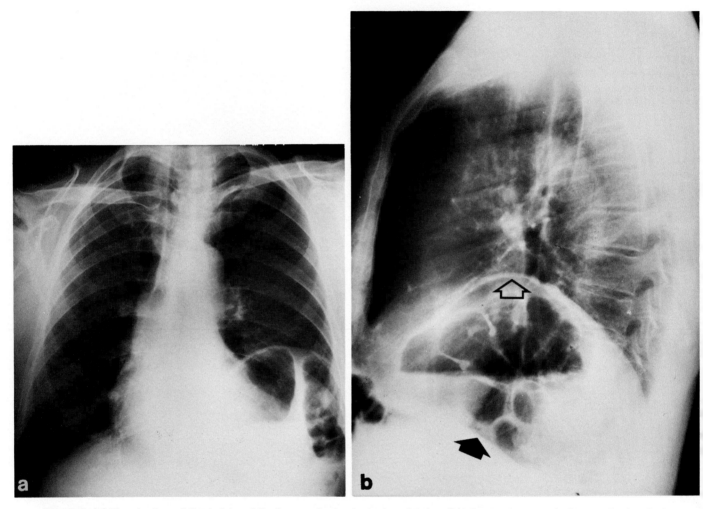

Fig. 8.3. (a) Eventration of the left hemidiaphragm. In the lateral projection **(b)**, the *open arrow* indicates the level of the anomalous left hemidiaphragm and the *solid arrow* indicates the level of the right hemidiaphragm.

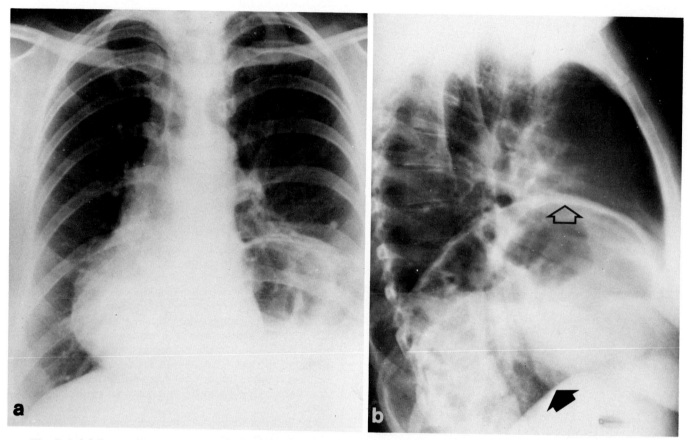

Fig. 8.4. (a) Eventration of the left hemidiaphragm with resultant displacement of the heart and mediastinal structures to the right. In the lateral projection **(b)**, the *open arrow* indicates the location of the hypoplastic left hemidiaphragm and the *solid arrow* indicates the location of the right hemidiaphragm.

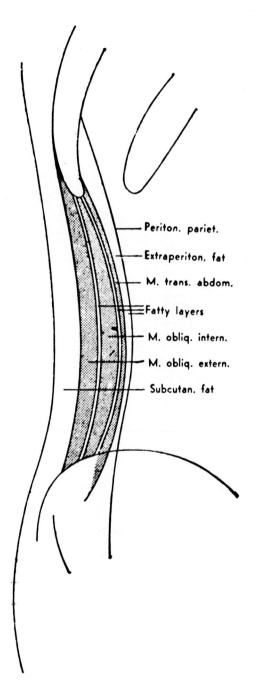

Periton. pariet.

Extraperiton. fat

M. trans. abdom.

Fatty layers

M. obliq. intern.

M. obliq. extern.

Subcutan. fat

Fig. 8.5. Schematic drawing of the soft tissues of the flank. The extraperitoneal (pre-, pro-, retroperitoneal) fat produces the lucent shadow of the "flank stripe." (Reprinted with permission from J. Frimann-Dahl: *Roentgen Examinations in Acute Abdominal Disease.* Charles C Thomas, Springfield, Ill., 1960.)

been designated the "flank stripe" by Frimann-Dahl, and represents the extraperitoneal (pro-, pre-, retroperitoneal) fat situated between the parietal peritoneum and the fascia of the transverse abdominal muscle. A flank stripe is usually not seen in infants because the properitoneal fat is obscured by intestinal content, nor in dehydrated or older patients because of scant adipose tissue.

It is important to have the clear concept that the adipose tissue forming the flank stripe lies outside the peritoneal space (Fig. 8.5), that it is continuous with the posterior pararenal fat and, inferiorly, with the adipose tissue in the pelvic extraperitoneal space, in order to understand its diagnostic radiographic significance. Also, the flank stripe may extend cephalad lateral to the lateral margin of the liver (Fig. 8.6). As such, it should not be mistaken for pneumoperitoneum in the right-side-up decubitus radiograph of the abdomen.

The medial border of the flank stripe consists, anatomically, of the parietal peritoneum (Fig. 8.5). The parietal peritoneum, per se, is not radiographically visible, but its location is precisely defined by the medial extent of the extraperitoneal fat. Normally, the serosal surface of both the ascending (Fig. 8.7) and the descending (Fig. 8.8) colon abut against the parietal peritoneum. The thickness of the lateral wall of the colon can be estimated by the gas and fecal debris outlining its mucosal surface. Therefore, the soft tissue density, which has a smooth sharp lateral margin and an irregular medial margin, represents, from lateral to medial, the parietal peritoneum, the potential (paracolic "gutter") space and the lateral bowel wall. Fluid in the paracolic "gutter" displaces the colon medially, causing an increase in the width of the soft tissue density between the extraperitoneal fat ("flank stripe") and the intraluminal colonic contents.

The inferior recess of the peritoneal cavity, the pouch of Douglas, is bounded by the pelvic peritoneal reflection, which can be conceptualized as the bottom of a paper sack containing the pelvic ileal loops, the cecum and appendix, and the ovaries. While the pelvic peritoneum, per se, is not radiographically visible, its location is frequently identifiable by virtue of the presence of a thin layer of loose areolar or adipose tissue normally present between the dome of the bladder and the pelvic peritoneum (Fig. 8.9). Radiographically, the adipose tissue interposed between the bladder and the pelvic parietal peritoneum produces a thin lucent band between the density of the bladder and that of the small bowel loops normally present in the pouch of Douglas (Fig. 8.10).

The shadows of the liver and spleen, and the retroperitoneal renal and psoas shadows are usually recorded on the supine radiograph of the abdomen (Fig. 8.1).

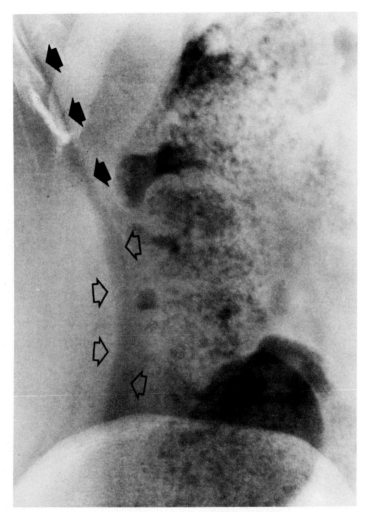

Fig. 8.6. Radiographic appearance of the soft tissues of the right flank. The extraperitoneal fat ("flank stripe") produces the sharply defined, gently curved lucent band (*open arrows*) extending from below the iliac crest to above the lateral margin of the liver (*solid arrows*). Gas and feces identify the ascending colon and, in the hepatic flexure, outline the inferior margin of the liver.

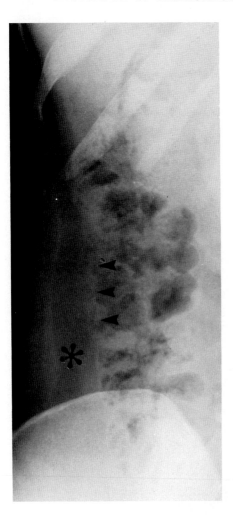

Fig. 8.7. Soft tissues of the right flank. The "flank stripe" is indicated by the (*). The lateral margin of the lucent flank stripe represents the transversalis fascia and its medial margin, the parietal peritoneum. The mucosal surface of the lateral wall of the colon is identified by colonic content. The soft tissue density between the medial margin of the flank stripe and the mucosal surface of the ascending colon (*arrowheads*) represents the parietal peritoneum, the potential paracolic "gutter," and the lateral wall of the colon. The fat of the flank stripe is visible inferior to the iliac crest as it extends into the pelvic perivesical space and, superiorly, lateral to the lateral margin of the liver.

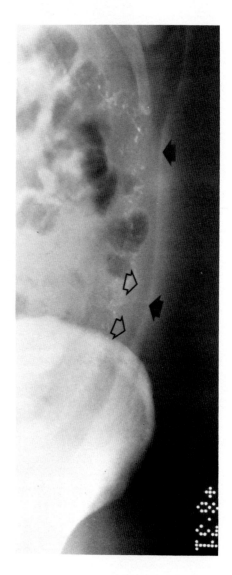

Fig. 8.8. Normal radiographic anatomy of the left flank. The *solid arrows* indicate the deep surface of the transversalis muscle (and its covering fascia), which constitutes the lateral border of the flank stripe (retroperitoneal fat). The *open arrows* indicate the lateral wall of the descending colon, which is identified by barium coating its mucosa. The lateral wall of the colon (and visceral peritoneum) constitute the medial border of the flank stripe.

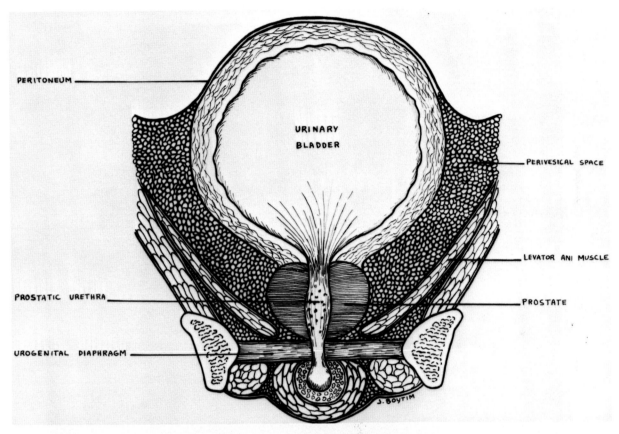

Fig. 8.9. Schematic representation of the relationship between the pelvic peritoneal reflection and the urinary bladder. Note that a thin layer of perivesical, extraperitoneal adipose or areolar tissue is located between the dome of the bladder and the peritoneum.

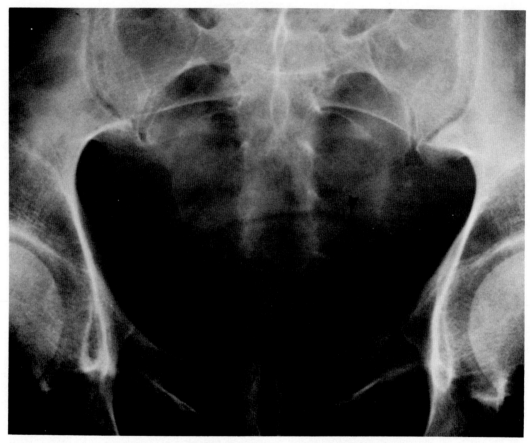

Fig. 8.10. Radiographic appearance of the adipose tissue (*arrowheads*) between the bladder and the peritoneum.

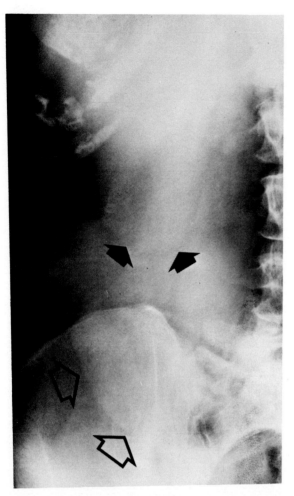

Fig. 8.11. The *solid arrows* indicate the inferior pole of the right kidney. The *open arrows* indicate the tail of the liver, which extends, in this patient, normally below the level of the iliac crest.

The size and shape of the liver shadow is extremely variable. The posterior edge of the liver may extend normally to, or below, the iliac crest in the supine examination (Fig. 8.11). The radiographic diagnosis of hepatomegaly should only be made when the liver *mass* appears to be enlarged. This usually results in displacement of the hepatic flexure, transverse colon, or stomach or in elevation of the right diaphragm (Fig. 8.12).

Normally, the pancreas cannot be seen on plain abdominal films. It is, however, visible sonographically and clearly delineated by CT.

Gas in the intestinal tract constitutes a normally present contrast medium which may serve to delineate not only the gut but, indirectly, identify the location of intra-abdominal organs.

Some air is normally present in the stomach. In the supine radiograph of the abdomen, air delineates the body of the stomach (Fig. 8.13a). In the erect position (Fig. 8.13b), the air migrates into the gastric fundus.

Figure 8.14 dramatically illustrates a basic anatomic fact related to the position of the stomach that has considerable clinical significance. With the patient supine, barium collects in the gastric fundus, which, as seen in the horizontal beam lateral radiograph, is clearly dependent with respect to the spine and the pancreas. This illustration provides the anatomic explanation for the frequent failure of intestinal decompression tubes to leave the gastric fundus unless the patient is placed in the full right lateral decubitus or the prone right anterior oblique position.

Gas is commonly seen in the duodenal bulb, but its radiographic appearance is not sufficiently characteristic to permit specific identification of the bulb.

Contrary to a commonly held belief that the small bowel should be airless, the presence of some gas irregularly distributed throughout the small intestine is a normal finding. Thus, gas will make short segments of *nondistended* small bowel visible on the plain abdominal roentgenogram. Paul and Juhl (11) believe that if a single small intestinal loop can be recognized because of the presence of gas it should be considered abnormal only if the loop is more than 8–10 cm in length and if the loop is distended.

Gas and scybala are usually seen in variable amounts throughout the colon and either is generally present in the rectum.

The radiographic examination of the abdomen includes, perforce, the lower thoracic vertebrae and some of the lower ribs. These portions of the skeleton may be injured in any instance of abdominal trauma. Such skeletal injury may be overlooked clinically, if the major effects of trauma involve abdominal soft tissue structures. Conversely, fractures of the lower ribs or lumbar transverse processes may be the most obvious radiographic sign leading to the diagnosis of trauma to the liver, spleen or kidneys. Fracture of a lower rib is the injury most frequently associated with hepatic or splenic rupture.

It is commonly helpful to be able to relate soft tissue anatomic structures to fixed bony landmarks. The renal arteries arise from the aorta at about the level of the second lumbar vertebra. The umbilicus is generally at the level of L_3 and the aortic bifurcation generally occurs at the level of L_4.

Radiographic Manifestation of Trauma

The radiographic procedure for determining whether a stab wound of the abdomen has entered the peritoneal cavity has been previously referenced but is little used because of the technical difficulties and

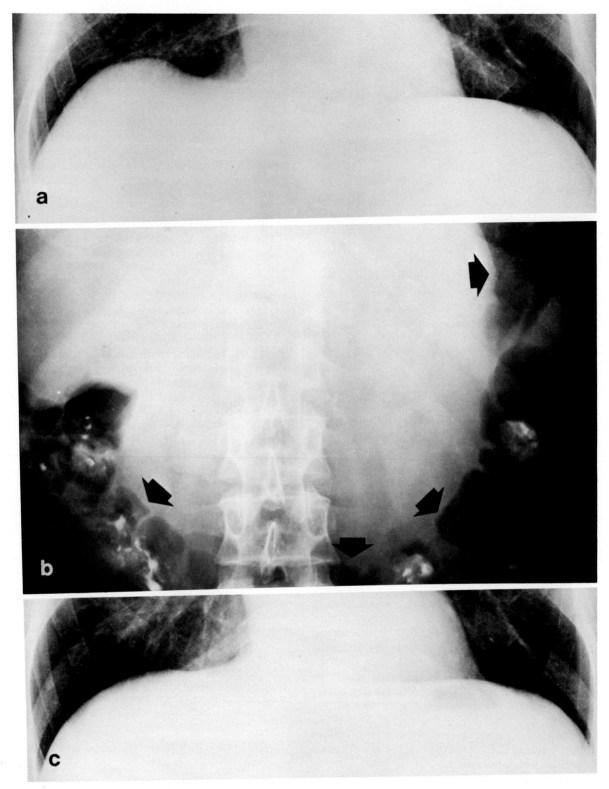

Fig. 8.12. Segmental elevation of the right diaphragm **(a)**. The size of the liver is indicated by the *arrows* **(b)**. The gastric fundus is displaced laterally, the transverse colon inferiorly, and the flexures laterally by the enlarged liver. The configuration of the right diaphragm prior to development of hepatomegaly is seen in **(c)**.

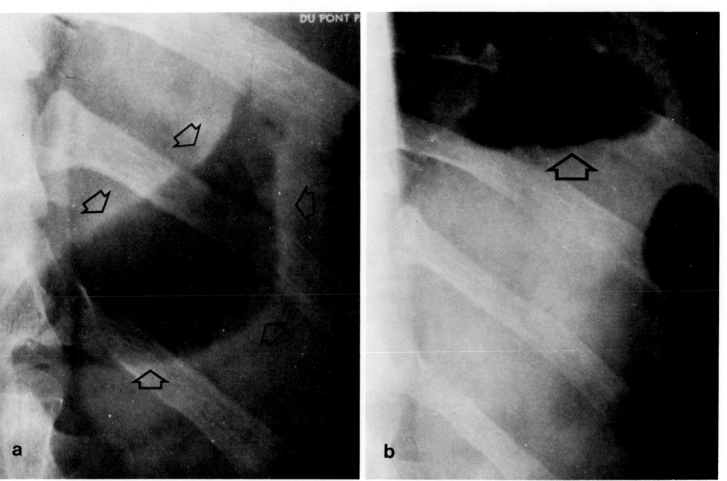

Fig. 8.13. (a) The *arrows* indicate the location and configuration of air in the body of the stomach in the supine position. **(b)** In the erect posture, the air migrates to the gastric fundus, producing an air-fluid level (*open arrow*).

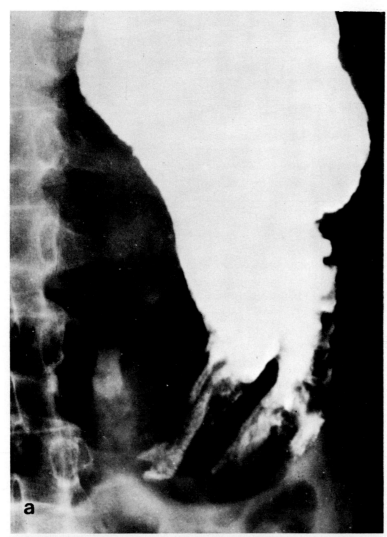

Fig. 8.14. (a) In the supine examination of the abdomen, barium fills the gastric fundus and air is seen in the antrum. In the horizontal beam lateral projection, with the patient in the supine position (b), the barium suspension occupies a very dependent position with respect to the spine and the pancreas, and air in the gastric antrum is anterior to the barium suspension in the fundus.

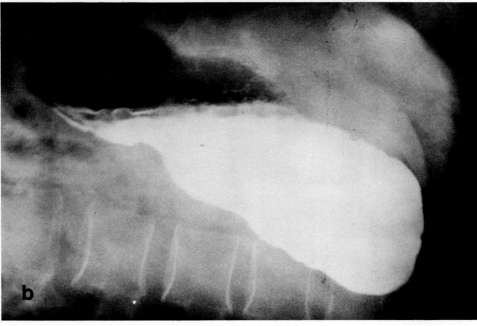

patient discomfort attendant with the procedure. If the wound is limited to the soft tissues of the abdominal wall, the contrast medium will have a characteristic appearance (Fig. 8.15) and none will be seen in the peritoneal cavity. Conversely, if the wound penetrates the peritoneum, contrast will be seen free in the peritoneal space.

Penetrating trauma to the abdomen caused by high-velocity missiles results in injuries of such magnitude that the patient's condition will generally not tolerate the time required for radiographic study. If the patient's condition does permit, however, abdominal films may be useful for localization of foreign bodies, identification of associated skeletal injury, or intra- or retroperitoneal soft tissue damage.

Upper abdominal gunshot wounds constitute a special problem in preoperative evaluation. After the necessary steps have been instituted to maintain the patient, the renal status must be evaluated in order to preclude the possibility of unknowingly removing the patient's only functioning kidney, should nephrectomy be required. This can be done by means of infusion pyelography administered in the emergency department or while the patient is on the way to the operating room. A single roentgenogram of the abdomen is sufficient to evaluate renal function on the injured side and to establish the function of the contralateral kidney (Fig. 8.16).

Blunt trauma to the abdomen can result in some of the most difficult diagnostic problems facing the emergency physician. On the one extreme, seemingly insignificant abdominal trauma can result in intraperitoneal injury of life-threatening proportion. On the other, significant damage may exist and either defy detection or specific localization, clinically, or be masked by associated lesions involving other body parts. Tovee (12) has noted that 10% of multiple injury traffic patients have an abdominal injury and that approximately 70% of traffic victims with abdominal injury have an associated injury of the head, chest, or extremity.

The various radiologic imaging procedures play a fundamental role in the evaluation of patients with blunt abdominal trauma. The physical examination of these patients is notoriously imperfect. The accuracy of peritoneal lavage, which is dependent upon hemoperitoneum (from whatever cause), ranges from 84–98% (13–15). However, a significant false negative rate has also been attributed to peritoneal lavage (13,14). In an effort to improve the diagnostic accuracy of intraperitoneal lesions caused by blunt trauma, the diagnostic laparotomy ("mini-lap") was described by Guernsey and Ganchrow (16). As originally described, the diagnostic laparotomy was reserved for patients "with multiple areas of trauma needing surgery." However, the authors clearly state that patients

"with isolated abdominal trauma are appropriately handled selectively and that such patients will likely benefit from various sophisticated procedures." In spite of the intended application of the diagnostic laparotomy, the "mini-lap" became increasingly utilized in patients with isolated blunt abdominal trauma.

The diagnostic surgical procedures just enumerated, which have supplanted the even less accurate abdominal paracentesis and four quadrant tap, are invasive, technically relatively difficult, time-consuming and have significant limitations in patients with subcapsular hepatic or splenic, retroperitoneal (17,18), or pelvic extraperitoneal (19) injury. For these reasons, plain film radiography of the abdomen (and chest), computed tomography, ultrasound, and appropriate nuclear medicine procedures should be employed in the evaluation of patients with abdominal trauma, and particularly, those patients who do not have multiple sites of injury and do not require prompt surgery.

Spleen

Rupture of the spleen is the most frequent serious injury associated with blunt upper abdominal or left lower chest trauma (4). The injury most frequently associated with splenic trauma is fracture of a lower left rib and this roentgen finding should always precipitate consideration of splenic injury. The organ most commonly injured in association with splenic trauma is the left kidney. It is usually difficult, or impossible, to establish the diagnosis of simultaneous splenic and left renal damage on plain abdominal radiographs. However, the plain radiographic findings should certainly suggest the possibility, which can then be confirmed by contrast studies, radioactive spleen scan, ultrasound, or CT.

The concepts of "delayed" (4) and "occult" (20,21) rupture of the spleen are no longer considered acceptable diagnoses (22). The appropriate clinical setting should prompt consideration of splenic injury, which can then be evaluated by very sensitive nuclear spleen scan or absolutely confirmed by splenic arteriography (23,24). Consequently, "missed" rupture of the spleen, with its tenfold greater mortality rate than that associated with the prompt recognition of splenic injury, is no longer justifiable.

The plain film signs of splenic trauma vary from "normal" appearing chest and abdominal radiographs to those of a left upper quadrant mass and frank hemoperitoneum. The roentgen signs reflect, in large measure, whether the splenic hemorrhage is subcapsular or extracapsular. It is fundamentally important to realize that, in patients with clinical evidence of

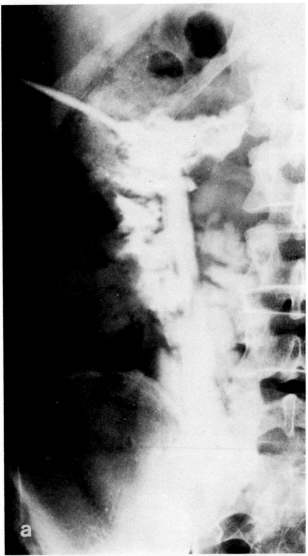

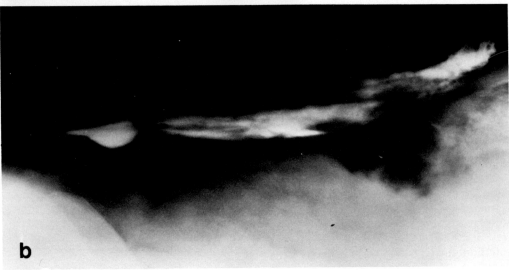

Fig. 8.15. (a, b) Contrast medium injected into a stab wound of the anterior abdominal wall. Note that the contrast medium is contained within the soft tissues of the abdominal wall and that none is seen within the peritoneal cavity.

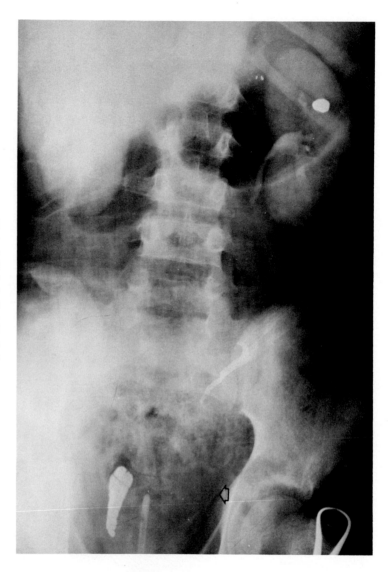

Fig. 8.16. Infusion pyelogram performed in a 13-year-old male who sustained a rifle shot of the right upper quadrant of the abdomen. The bullet traversed the abdomen and lay superimposed over the upper pole of the left kidney. This infusion was started with the patient in the emergency department and was completed by the time the patient reached the operating room at which time this roentgenogram was obtained. The patient's blood pressure was 70/0. This examination demonstrated impaired function of the right kidney and normal functioning of the left. The *open arrow* indicates the pelvic portion of the left ureter.

splenic injury, *negative plain radiographic examinations of the chest or abdomen do not exclude the possibility of splenic hemorrhage,* and that it is precisely in these circumstances that radionuclide, ultrasound, CT, or contrast studies of the spleen *must* be undertaken.

The classic triad of roentgen signs indicative of acute traumatic rupture of the spleen, i.e., elevation of the left hemidiaphragm, discoid atelectasis at the left base, and a small left pleural effusion, is uncommonly seen and should not be considered reliable. Elevation of the left hemidiaphragm occurs normally in 10% of people. However, in any patient with blunt trauma to the left upper quadrant or lower left hemithorax, elevation of the left hemidiaphragm (Figs. 8.17 and 8.18) should be considered as indicative of splenic trauma until proven otherwise. Reliable signs of a left upper quadrant mass—either subcapsular hemorrhage or extracapsular hematoma—are medial displacement of the gastric air bubble (Fig. 8.18) and inferior and medial displacement of the splenic flexure (Fig. 8.19).

Splenic size, alone, is not a reliable sign of subcapsular rupture (Fig. 8.20), because of the great normal variation in splenic size and configuration. However, if the mass of the spleen is obviously enlarged with displacement of adjacent organs (Figs. 8.19 and 8.21), intracapsular rupture is a reasonable radiographic impression which should be confirmed by radionuclide scan or ultrasonography. Schwartz (25) has described prominence of the gastric rugae and an extrinsic pressure effect of the greater curvature of the stomach as a reliable sign of a left upper quadrant mass (splenic or extrasplenic hemorrhage) in children.

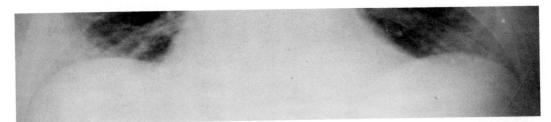

Fig. 8.17. Erect chest examination obtained in a patient with acute rupture of the spleen. The left hemidiaphragm is elevated and its margin less distinct than that of the right hemidiaphragm.

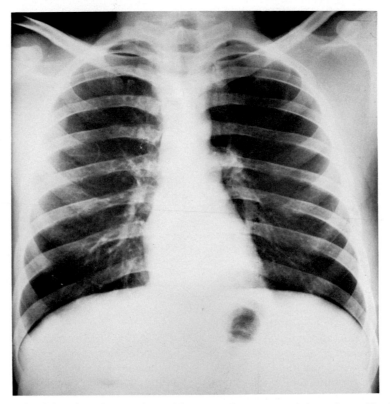

Fig. 8.18. Erect radiograph of the chest in a patient with traumatic rupture of the spleen. The left hemidiaphragm is elevated but remains sharply defined. There is neither basilar atelectasis nor a left pleural effusion. The gastric fundal air bubble is medially displaced by the left upper quadrant hematoma.

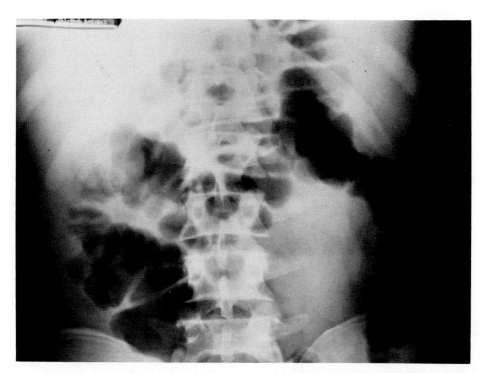

Fig. 8.19. Subcapsular hematoma of the spleen. (Same patient as Fig. 8.18.) The splenic shadow is enlarged and displaces the splenic flexure medially and inferiorly. The sharp definition of the inferomedial margin of the splenic mass and the normal relationship of the descending colon to the flank stripe indicate that the capsule is intact. A coexistent *retroperitoneal* hematoma obscures the midthird of the psoas.

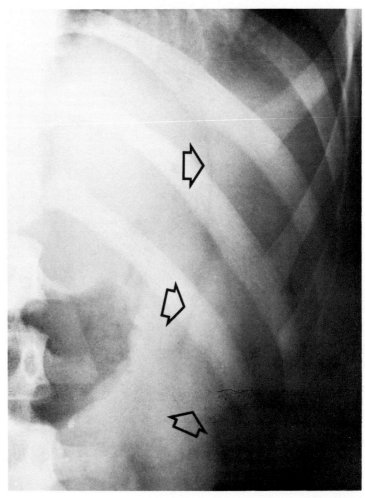

Fig. 8.20. Subcapsular rupture of a developmentally elongated spleen (*open arrows*). The weight of the surgical specimen, which included the spleen and its intact capsule, did not exceed the normal range for a teenage boy. The spleen was lacerated and approximately only 30 cc of blood was present within the capsule. The elongated configuration of the spleen was concluded, therefore, to be developmental rather than pathologic and secondary to the laceration.

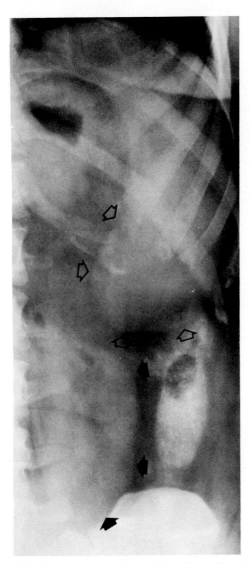

Fig. 8.21. Subcapsular rupture of the spleen. The sharply defined splenic mass is grossly enlarged (*open arrows*) and has displaced the gastric air bubble medially, the splenic flexure inferiorly. The *retro*peritoneal left kidney (*solid arrows*) has been inferiorly displaced by the *intra*-peritoneal splenic mass.

When splenic hemorrhage is contained by the splenic capsule (subcapsular rupture), the inferomedial margin of the splenic mass will be sharp and smooth (Figs. 8.19–8.21) and the relationship of the descending colon to the medial margin of the flank stripe will be normal (Fig. 8.22).

The technetium spleen scan clearly delineates the site of splenic laceration as an area of diminished radioactivity (Fig. 8.23). Sonography demonstrates the presence of an extrasplenic, intracapsular hemor-

rhage by the difference between sonographic pattern of the hemorrhage and that of the splenic paren-chyma. Splenic arteriography (Fig. 8.24) is the most definitive method of evaluating splenic injury.

The roentgen signs of extracapsular rupture of the spleen include loss of the splenic shadow and the presence of an *ill defined* left upper quadrant mass which exerts the same effect on adjacent structures as described with respect to subcapsular rupture. In addition, the free intraperitoneal blood, which accumulates in the left paracolic gutter, produces a homogeneous soft tissue density interposed between the lateral wall of the descending colon and the flank stripe, which displaces the descending colon medially (Figs. 8.25 and 8.26). Larger amounts of intraperitoneal blood will accumulate in the most dependent portion of the peritoneal space, the pouch of Douglas. The roentgen signs of *intra*peritoneal pelvic effusion (blood, ascitic fluid, or pus) consist of a midline homogeneous soft tissue density with sharply defined, convex lateral margins, which is separated from the bladder by a thin, gently curved, horizontal lucency representing extraperitoneal fat, and superimposed upon which are the pelvic ileal loops, displaced out of their normal position by the intraperitoneal blood. Additionally, the shadows of the normally present extraperitoneal soft tissue structures, i.e., the obturator internus muscles and the urinary bladder, will remain visible (Fig. 8.25).

Liver

Blunt trauma to the liver is frequently associated with injury to other intra-abdominal organs, to the skull, chest, or extremities (24). Analogous with splenic injury, trauma involving the liver should be suspected in every patient with a right lower rib fracture. Organs most commonly associated with hepatic trauma include, in order of frequency, lung, spleen, long bone, and brain (13,27). It is an interesting, and significant, observation that, of 75 patients with liver trauma reviewed by Corica and Powers (13), 18 (24%) had concomitant splenic injury and that a similar number, 14 (18%), had no signs or symptoms of abdominal trauma. The latter represent those patients with liver parenchymal damage and intact hepatic capsule.

Isolated blunt hepatic trauma, resulting in either intra- or extracapsular rupture, occurs in from 8 to 36% of injuries to a single organ (28). The mortality rate of patients with blunt hepatic trauma, only, has been reported from 25% (29) to 47% (27). In these patients, the cause of death is massive hepatic hemorrhage (13).

Traumatic lesions of the liver resulting from blunt abdominal trauma include (1) laceration (rupture) of

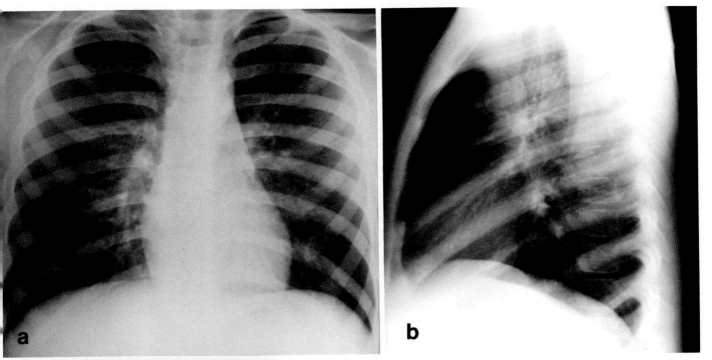

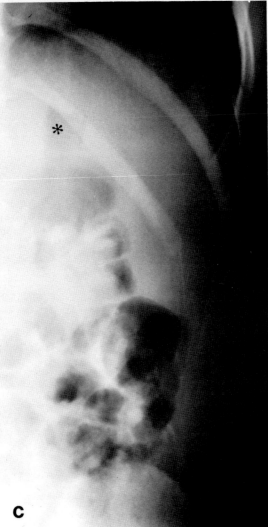

Fig. 8.22. Subcapsular rupture of the spleen. In the frontal **(a)** and lateral **(b)** radiographs of the chest, the left hemidiaphragm is elevated, but there is neither basilar atelectasis nor a left pleural effusion and the left diaphragm is sharply defined. In the supine radiograph of the abdomen **(c)**, a sharply defined, homogeneous mass, representing the subcapsular splenic hematoma, has displaced the gastric air bubble (*) medially and the splenic flexure medially and inferiorly. The relationship of the lateral wall of the descending colon to the retroperitoneal fat of the flank stripe is normal.

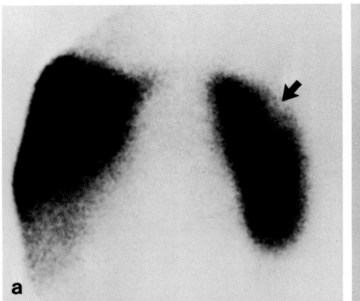

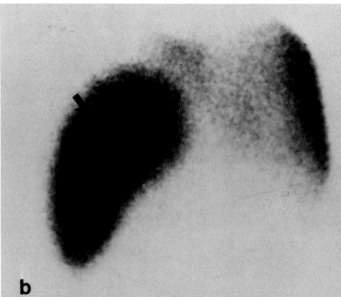

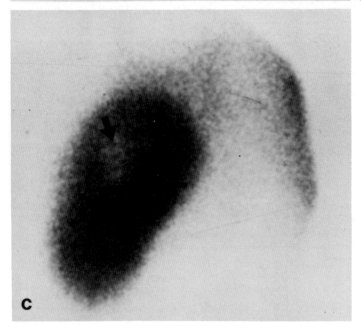

Fig. 8.23. ^{99m}Tc sulfur colloid spleen scan in frontal **(a)**, posteri
(b), and oblique **(c)** positions. The area of diminished radioactiv
(*arrow*) represents the site of a splenic laceration.

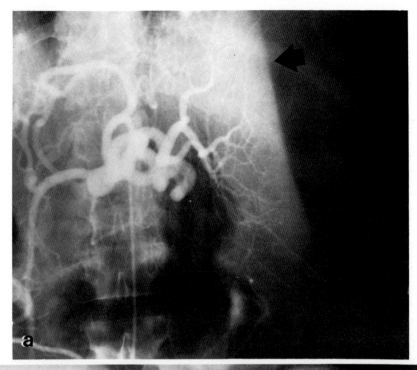

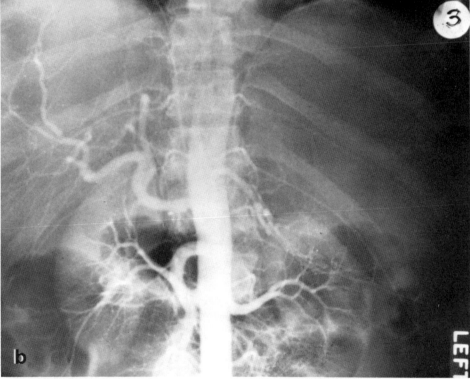

Fig. 8.24. Angiographic demonstration of splenic trauma. **(a)** is a celiac arteriogram demonstrating medial displacement and compression of the spleen by a large subcapsular hematoma (*arrows*). **(b)** is an aortogram demonstrating inferior displacement of the splenic artery by an avascular mass in the left upper quadrant which represents a large hematoma. (Reprinted with permission from *Emergency Radiology Syllabus*, American College of Radiology, Chicago, 1979.)

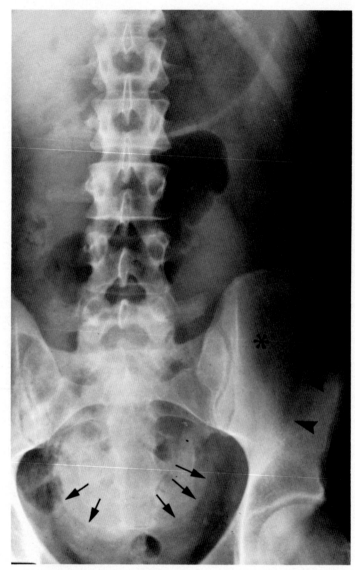

Fig. 8.25. Extracapsular rupture of the spleen. The margin of the spleen is lost. An ill defined soft tissue mass is present in the left upper quadrant. The left transverse colon is displaced superiorly and medially. Both the stomach and the left transverse colon are dilated, presumably on a reflex ileus basis. A homogeneous soft tissue density is interposed between the descending colon (*) and the flank stripe (*arrowheads*). This represents blood in the left paracolic gutter. In addition, a homogeneous soft tissue density with sharp convex lateral margins (*stemmed arrows*) is present in the center of the pelvis. This represents blood accumulated in the most dependent portion of the peritoneal space, the pouch of Douglas.

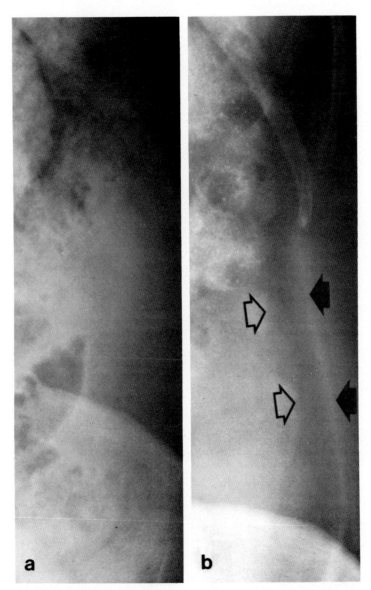

Fig. 8.26. Traumatic rupture of the spleen with massive hemoperitoneum **(a)**. The margin of the inferior pole of the spleen is obliterated by the homogeneous density of the free blood which has also filled the left paracolic gutter, displacing the descending colon medially. The flank stripe is not visible because of abdominal distention. **(b)** Radiographic appearance of the normal flank of the same patient two years earlier. The *solid arrows* indicate the lateral border of the flank stripe and the *open arrows*, its medial border, which is the lateral wall of the descending colon. (Reprinted with permission from J. H. Harris, Jr.: The significance of soft tissue injury in the roentgen diagnosis of trauma. *CRC Critical Reviews in Clinical Radiology and Nuclear Medicine* 6:295, 1975.)

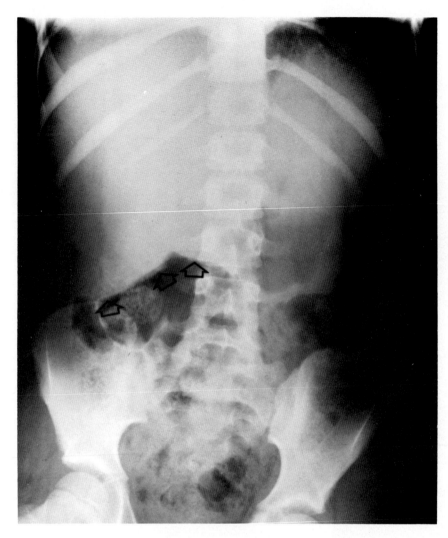

Fig. 8.27. Subcapsular rupture of the liver. The liver mass is grossly enlarged with a sharply defined inferior margin. The indentation caused by the falciform ligament is clearly evident. The hepatic flexure is displaced inferiorly and medially and the relationship between the colon and the flank stripe remains normal.

the capsule and liver parenchyma, (2) subcapsular rupture of parenchyma with intact capsule, (3) central rupture without injury to the periphery or capsule, and (4) "bursting" injury characterized by massive parenchymal and capsular disruption and, usually, profound hemorrhagic shock (25,31). The first three types of hepatic injury may be associated with minimal or no hemoperitoneum. Patients with subcapsular rupture or central laceration of the liver who do not develop hemoperitoneum are not identifiable by peritoneal lavage. It is precisely in this group of patients that the various radiographic imaging modalities are more likely to provide the correct diagnosis than physical examination or diagnostic surgical procedures.

The plain film roentgen signs of hepatic trauma with an intact capsule include enlargement of the liver mass with inferior and medial displacement of the hepatic flexure, a sharply defined inferior liver margin, and no evidence of blood in the right paracolic gutter, i.e., the relationship between the lateral margin of the ascending colon and the extraperitoneal fat (the "flank stripe") is normal (Fig. 8.27).

The angiographic appearance of a central laceration of the liver is seen in Figure 8.28.

The classic radiographic signs of extracapsular rupture of the liver and hemoperitoneum are seen in Figure 8.29. These include fracture of a lower right rib, indistinctness or loss of definition of the inferior margin of the liver, loss of definition of the inferior angle of the liver by a homogeneous soft tissue density interposed between the lateral wall of the ascending colon and the flank stripe which represents blood in the right paracolic gutter.

Larger accumulations of blood in the paracolic gutters flow into the most dependent portion of the peritoneal space, the pouch of Douglas. Blood or

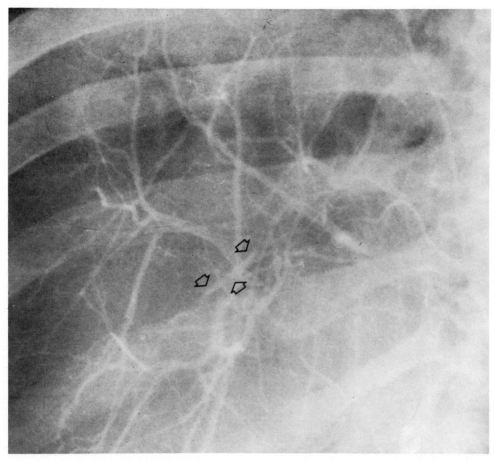

Fig. 8.28. Late arterial phase of hepatic arteriogram demonstrating contrast medium within the liver parenchyma (*arrows*) in a patient suspected of rupture of the liver.

other fluid in the pelvic peritoneal recess produces a central pelvic homogeneous density with sharply defined convex lateral margins which displaces the pelvic ileal loops up out of their normal position in the pelvis (Fig. 8.30). The laterally convex margins of the pelvic hemoperitoneum represent the bulging pelvic peritoneum. Another characteristic which establishes the intraperitoneal location of fluid within the pouch of Douglas is the fact that the extraperitoneal soft tissue structures, i.e., the obturator internus muscles (Fig. 8.30) and the bladder (Fig. 8.31), remain radiographically visible. These structures are obscured by an extraperitoneal effusion (see Ch. 10).

Small Intestine

Lesions of the small intestine resulting from blunt trauma occur both intra- and retroperitoneally, include both rupture and intramural hematoma, are difficult to diagnose preoperatively, and are often associated with other injuries, particularly rupture of the spleen. While rupture of the intestinal tract is uncommon, the small intestine is the hollow viscus most frequently ruptured by blunt trauma, with the site of rupture occurring most frequently in the third portion of the duodenum (31).

Patients with a history of upper abdominal trauma and signs of peritoneal irritation should have supine and erect or right-side-up decubitus radiographs of the abdomen. Although not a frequent finding, air in the retroperitoneal space surrounding the right kidney (Fig. 8.32), outlining the psoas shadow, or appearing under the right crus of the diaphragm is characteristic of rupture of the retroperitoneal duodenum (32).

Colon

Colon injuries are rarely caused by blunt trauma. Most are the result of penetrating injuries and, in

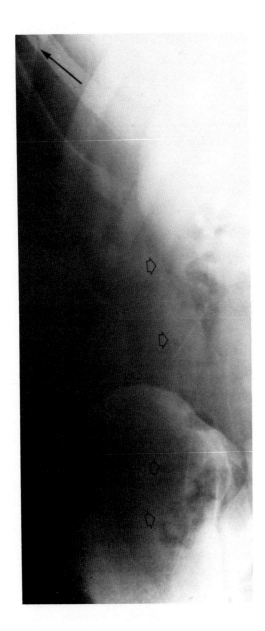

Fig. 8.29. Extracapsular rupture of the liver with hemoperitoneum. The right 10th rib is fractured posteriorly (*arrow*). The definition of the inferior margin of the liver is obscured. The outline of the inferior angle of the liver is lost by a homogenous soft tissue density which extends inferiorly between the lateral wall of the ascending colon (*open arrows*) and the flank stripe. This density (*) represents free blood in the right paracolic gutter which displaces the colon medially from the extraperitoneal fat. (Reprinted with permission from J. H. Harris, Jr.: The significance of soft tissue injury in the roentgen diagnosis of trauma. *CRC* 6:295, 1975.)

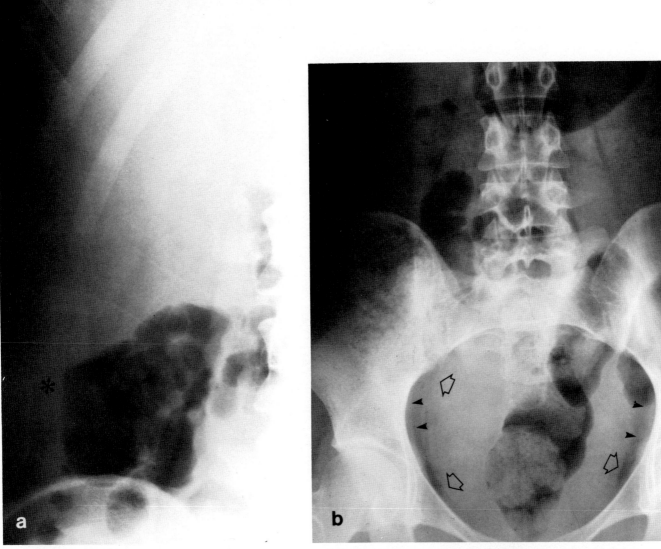

Fig. 8.30. Extracapsular rupture of the liver with massive hemoperitoneum and blood in the pelvic peritoneal recess. The supine radiograph of the upper abdomen **(a)** demonstrates enlargement of the liver mass with loss of definition of its inferior margin and depression of the hepatic flexure. The inferior angle of the liver is not visible and a soft tissue density (blood) (*) is interposed between the flank stripe and the lateral wall of the ascending colon. The supine radiograph of the lower abdomen and pelvis of the same patient **(b)** discloses a midline, homogeneous pelvic density with symmetrical, sharply defined, laterally convex margins (*open arrows*), which has displaced the pelvic small bowel loops up out of their normal position in the pelvis. This density, through which rectal gas and scybala are visible, represents the blood in the pouch of Douglas. The extraperitoneal obturator internus muscle shadows (*arrowheads*) remain radiographically visible.

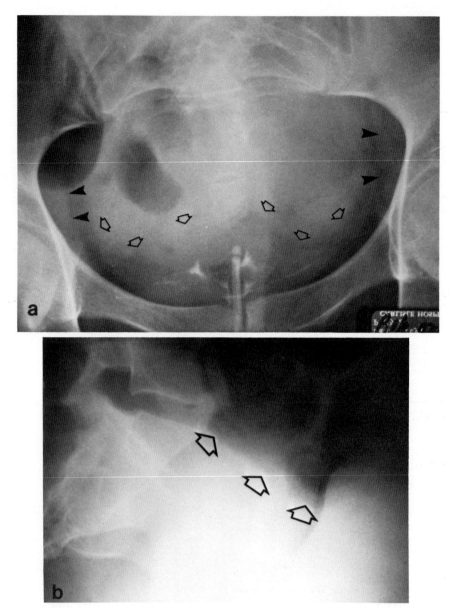

Fig. 8.31. Frontal and lateral radiographs of the pelvis of a 30-year-old woman with a septic abortion and 1000 cc of frank pus in the pouch of Douglas. In the anteroposterior view of the pelvis **(a)**, fluid in the pelvic peritoneal recess produces the homogeneous midline pelvic density with sharp, bulging lateral margins and the centrally concave inferior margin. The floor of the pouch of Douglas is separated from the bladder and uterus by a thin, radiolucent layer of adipose tissue (*open arrows*). The bladder is identified by the Foley catheter and small amounts of contrast medium. The shadows of the obturator internus muscles (*arrowheads*), also extraperitoneal structures, are clearly visible, confirming that the midpelvic fluid accumulation is intraperitoneal. The lateral radiograph of the pelvis **(b)**, shows the homogeneous density of the fluid (pus) filling the pouch of Douglas (*open arrows*) and indenting the posterior aspect of the bladder.

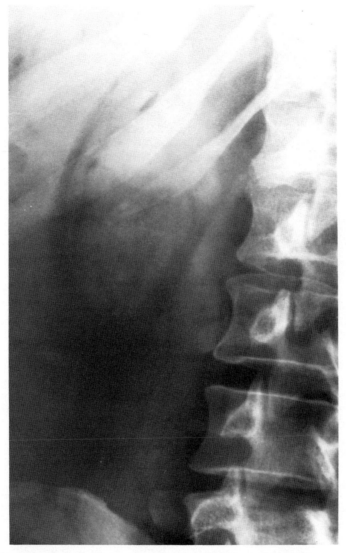

Fig. 8.32. Retroperitoneal air surrounding the right kidney and outlining the psoas muscle.

civilian practice, most of these are caused by low velocity missiles. The transverse colon is most commonly involved and over 70% of patients with colon injuries have other associated injuries as well (33).

Inferior Vena Cava

Injury to the inferior vena cava can be caused by stabbing, gunshot wounds, or blunt trauma. The latter has the highest mortality because of the increased association of trauma to the other abdominal organs. Over 50% of patients with injuries to the inferior vena cava die before they reach the hospital (34). Those patients who survive this injury do so usually on the basis of a retroperitoneal hematoma acting as a tamponade and occluding the inferior vena cava. If the

posterior peritoneum is disrupted, massive intraperitoneal hemorrhage and death usually ensue.

The commonest site of inferior vena cava lacerations occurs below the level of the renal veins, while laceration at the level of the renal veins carries the highest fatality rate. Roentgenographic examination of the abdomen is of limited value. Occasionally, a retroperitoneal mass with obliteration of the renal and psoas shadows will be seen.

Retroperitoneal Hemorrhage

This subject will also be discussed in Chapter 9.

The normal appearance of the retroperitoneal structures is seen in Figure 8.33. The psoas muscles produce a characteristic, usually well defined, soft tissue

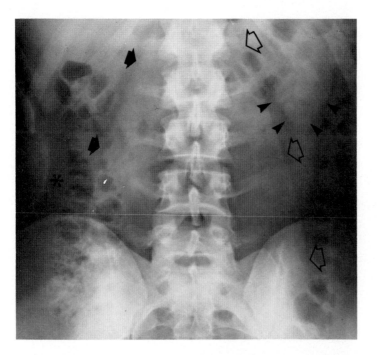

Fig. 8.33. The radiographic appearance of the retroperitoneal soft tissues in a *normal* adult. The left psoas (*open arrows*) is sharply defined and visible well below the iliac crest. Conversely, the right (*solid arrows*) is not as sharply defined and is partially obscured by intestinal content. Its course cannot be followed below the iliac crest. The inferior pole of the right kidney is obscured by gas and scybala; the left (*arrowheads*) is visible. The *asterisk* (*) indicates the right flank stripe.

mass which extends obliquely downward and laterally from the upper lumbar vertebrae, crossing the iliac wing to insert on the lesser trochanter of the femur. The distinctness of the psoas shadow may not be the same on each side, normally, and it is not unusual for a segment of either psoas shadow to be partially obscured by superimposed intestinal content. Minor variations in the appearance of the psoas shadows, therefore, should be expected and not be misinterpreted as signs of a retroperitoneal hematoma.

The lateral margin of the psoas is made radiographically visible by the retroperitoneal adipose tissue covering its fascia. In the absence of the covering fat, as in dehydrated or debilitated patients, or athletes on strenuous weight reduction programs (Fig. 8.34), the psoas shadows may not be visible.

The plain film signs of retroperitoneal hematoma include bulging of the lateral margin of the psoas due to hemorrhage within the muscle contained by the fascia (Fig. 8.35) or obliteration of the psoas shadow due to free blood in the retroperitoneal space (Fig. 8.36). The retroperitoneal hemorrhage may, as indicated above, arise from several sources, such as a lacerated or shattered kidney, as in Figure 8.36, or from laceration of the psoas muscle itself, as may occur with displaced or multiple lumbar transverse process fractures (Fig. 8.37).

Other findings commonly associated with retroperitoneal hematoma include lumbar scoliosis with the concavity on the side of the hematoma (Figs. 8.36 and 8.37), loss of definition of the renal shadow, and fracture of lumbar transverse processes (Fig. 8.37) or lower ribs (Fig. 8.36) on the affected side.

The presence and location of a retroperitoneal hematoma and its relation to retroperitoneal structures is clearly and precisely established by computed tomography (Fig. 8.38).

Intraperitoneal Hemorrhage

Intraperitoneal hemorrhage, which may result from penetrating or blunt abdominal injuries, produces radiographic findings that should permit distinction between intra- and retroperitoneal bleeding. Intraperitoneal blood does not cause obliteration of the psoas or renal shadows and is not associated with lumbar scoliosis. Hemoperitoneum produces flotation of small bowel loops, separation of the loops, unsharpness of radiographic shadows, and medial displacement of the colon from the flank stripe.

Diaphragm

Traumatic rupture of the diaphragm may be caused by blunt or penetrating injury. Direct laceration of the diaphragm is produced by the penetrating object. While the diaphragm may also be lacerated by rib fragments associated with blunt trauma, it is more commonly ruptured as the result of an abrupt increase in intra-abdominal pressure associated with blunt abdominal injury.

Rupture of the diaphragm by blunt abdominal trauma is not a common lesion and, unless it is of such magnitude as to severely affect respiration, it may be overlooked, being masked by shock or the

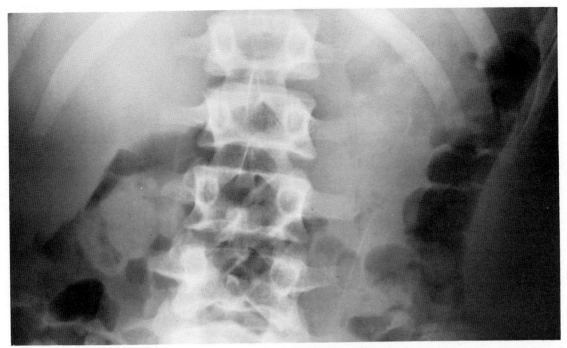

Fig. 8.34. Radiograph of the upper abdomen of an interscholastic wrestling champion who underwent a vigorous weight reduction program. There is an almost total absence of fatty tissue. Only the upper portion of the left psoas is barely visible. No fat is seen around either kidney nor in the left flank. There is no radiographically visible extraperitoneal fat. The liver is visible only by virtue of gas in the transverse colon.

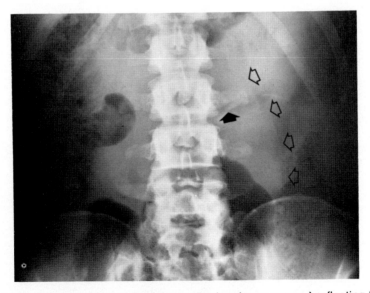

Fig. 8.35. Localized bulge in the midthird of the left psoas shadow (*open arrows*) reflecting the contained hematoma secondary to the fracture of the left third lumbar transverse process (*solid arrow*).

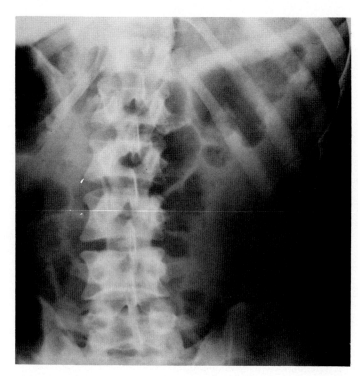

Fig. 8.36. Left retroperitoneal hematoma caused by shattered left kidney. The concavity of the lumbar scoliosis is to the left. The left psoas shadow is obscured; the right (*open arrow*) is sharply defined. The *solid arrow* indicates a fracture in the anterior axillary line of the left ninth rib.

Fig. 8.37. Right retroperitoneal hematoma caused by laceration of the psoas muscle associated with displaced lumbar transverse process fractures. The concavity of the lumbar scoliosis is to the right. The right psoas shadow is obliterated. *Solid arrows* indicate displaced fractures of the right second and third lumbar transverse processes and a minimally displaced fracture of the fourth. The inferior pole of the right kidney is visible (*open arrows*). Portions of the left psoas shadow can be identified (*arrowheads*).

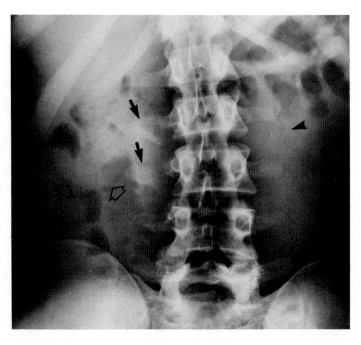

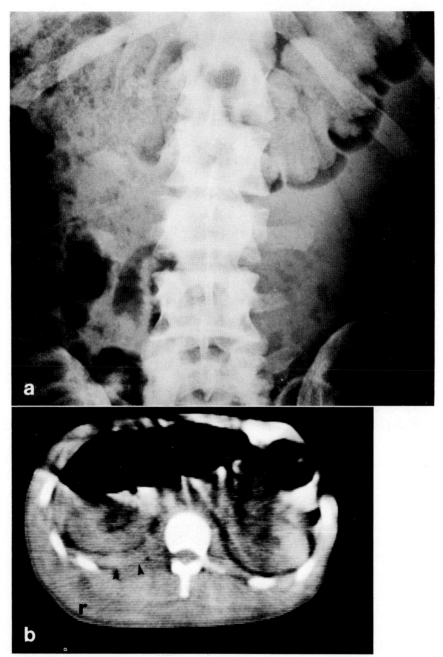

Fig. 8.38. Right retroperitoneal hematoma. The right psoas shadow is obliterated in the supine radiograph of the abdomen **(a)**. The computed tomogram **(b)** demonstrates the hematoma in the right posterior pararenal space (*arrowheads*). The hematoma obliterates the fat which delineates the psoas muscle.

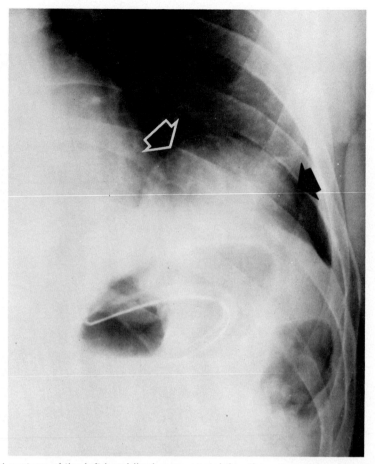

Fig. 8.39. Focal rupture of the left hemidiaphragm containing the upper pole of the spleen (*arrows*).

signs and symptoms of other frequently associated injuries such as rib fractures, splenic rupture, or other extra-abdominal injuries. The left hemidiaphragm is the site of approximately 90% of diaphragmatic ruptures (35–37), the right being protected by the mass of the liver. Similarly, the majority of traumatic diaphragmatic herniation occurs on the left. On the right, the diaphragmatic rent is usually blocked by the liver, which prevents herniation of other abdominal viscera.

If the supine, erect, and left-side-up decubitus radiographs of the abdomen are inconclusive, fluoroscopic examination of the abdomen will usually establish the presence of diaphragmatic rupture. A single swallow of barium or one of the water-soluble contrast media will disclose the status of the esophagus. If the esophagus is intact, additional contrast medium, either ingested or placed into the stomach by means of a nasogastric tube, will outline the location of the gastric fundus. The position of the splenic flexure can be established by means of a barium enema.

Rupture of the left hemidiaphragm may be small and permit herniation of only a single loop of bowel or the spleen (Fig. 8.39), left kidney, or it may be complete, eliminating the thoracoabdominal barrier. The stomach, splenic flexure, small bowel, spleen, left kidney, and omentum may herniate through the left hemidiaphragm (Fig. 8.40).

The roentgen diagnosis of rupture of the left diaphragm is based upon loss of definition of the diaphragmatic surface, elevation of the diaphragm, a pleural effusion, the presence of loops of bowel, the gastric fundus, or ill defined soft tissue densities above the normal level of the diaphragm, displacement of mediastinal structures to the right, and plate-like areas of subsegmental atelectasis in the left lower lobe.

Right pleural effusion may be the only roentgen sign of acute rupture of the right hemidiaphragm. This is particularly true when the tear is small and does not permit herniation of congenitally interposed bowel. Lacerations of the right hemidiaphragm are

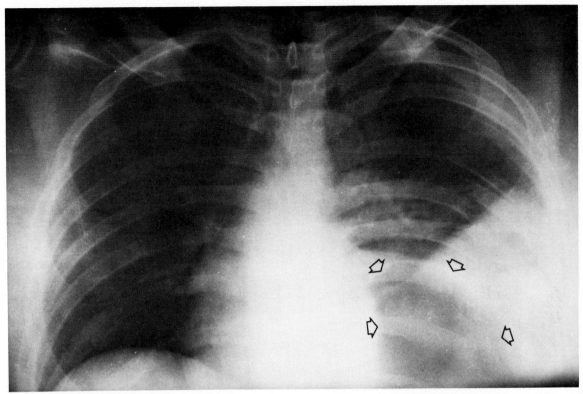

Fig. 8.40. Acute traumatic rupture of the left hemidiaphragm. In addition to atelectasis of the left lower lobe and the left pleural effusion, the *open arrows* indicate the presence of the gastric air bubble in the left pleural space.

usually not large enough to permit herniation of the liver. Occasionally, however, when the diaphragmatic rent is large, the liver may be found in the thoracic cavity together with loops of large and small intestine (Fig. 8.41).

Miscellaneous

A high incidence of association of pancreatic trauma with duodenal intramural hematoma has been reported by Cleveland and Waddell (38). There are no direct radiographic signs of pancreatic injury and, as has been stated, even the radiographic signs of duodenal trauma that might, by association, be considered secondary evidence of pancreatic injury, are rarely encountered.

Ingested foreign bodies may penetrate the wall of the stomach and initiate an inflammatory response in the adjacent portion of the abdomen. Figure 8.42 illustrates a large left upper quadrant abscess secondary to penetration of the greater curvature of the stomach by a chicken bone. The radiographic findings in this instance are characteristic of a left upper quadrant mass, namely elevation of the left hemidiaphragm, the presence of a small left pleural effusion,

and downward and medial displacement of the gastric fundus by the abscess.

The difficulty of establishing the diagnosis of pneumoperitoneum and the necessity of obtaining erect or right-side-up decubitus radiographs of the abdomen have been previously discussed. An additional roentgen sign of pneumoperitoneum may be present on the supine examination of the abdomen. This consists of air on both sides of the wall of small intestinal loops (Fig. 8.43).

Nontraumatic Lesions

Abnormal accumulations of gas and fluids in the distended intestinal tract occur in both mechanical obstruction of the small or large gut or in reflex (adynamic) ileus.

Reflex (paralytic, adynamic, inhibition) ileus, unless otherwise specified, implies a diffuse process producing uniform dilatation of the entire intestinal tract, frequently including the stomach, and is usually a manifestation of generalized peritonitis. Radiographically, distended loops of gut containing air-fluid levels on the same plane are seen in erect and decubitus films. Because peristaltic activity is decreased or

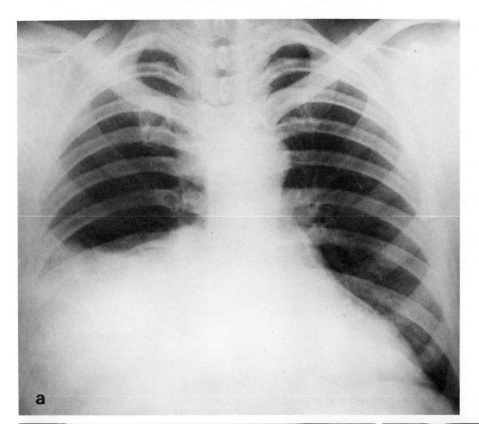

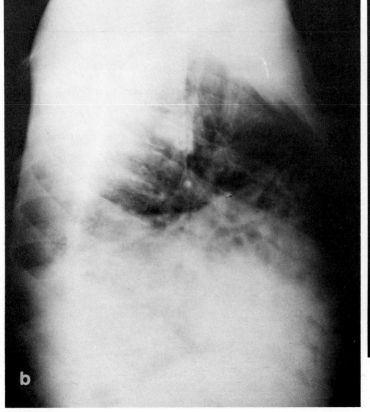

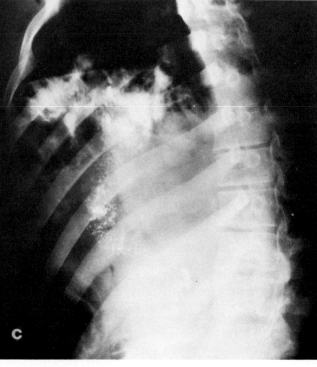

Fig. 8.41. Traumatic rupture of the right hemidiaphragm. At the time of laparotomy, the liver, small bowel, gallbladder, and large intestine were located in the right thorax. In the frontal projection of the chest **(a)**, the right hemidiaphragm cannot be identified and there is a right pleura effusion. In the lateral examination of the chest **(b)**, air-filled loops of intestine are seen above the level of the diaphragm. Following the ingestion of barium, the presence of small intestine in the right hemithorax was confirmed **(c)**.

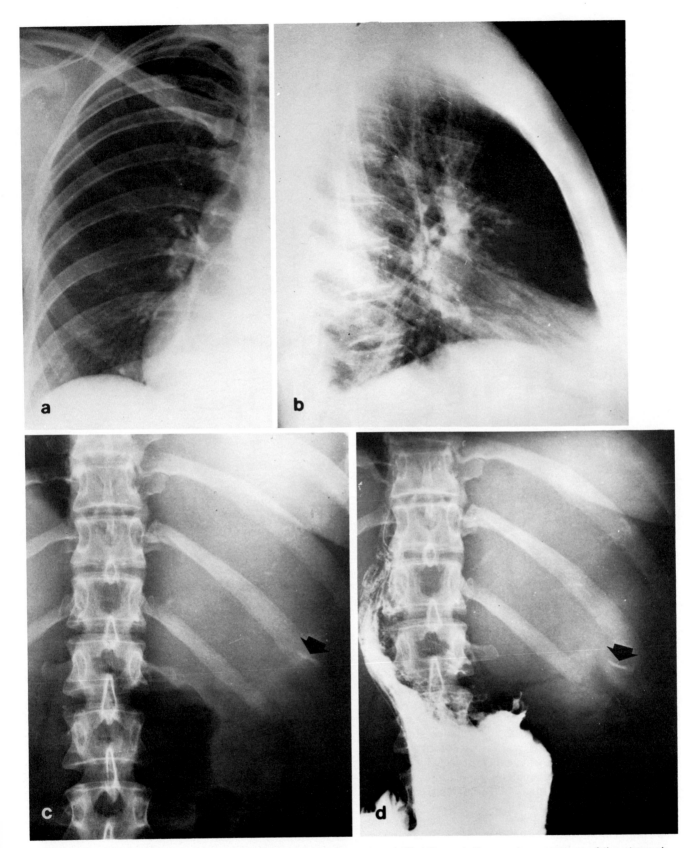

Fig. 8.42. This patient, in whom an ingested chicken bone penetrated through the greater curvature of the stomach and formed a left upper quadrant abscess, demonstrates all of the classic signs of a left upper quadrant abdominal mass, abscess, or ruptured spleen. The heart is displaced to the right. The left hemidiaphragm is elevated and its surface ill defined. There is a small left pleural effusion which is mainly posteriorly situated **(a, b)**. The stomach is displaced medially and inferiorly. The renal outline and psoas muscle shadow are obscured and the splenic flexure of the colon is displaced inferiorly. The chicken bone **(c, d)**, is indicated by the *arrow*.

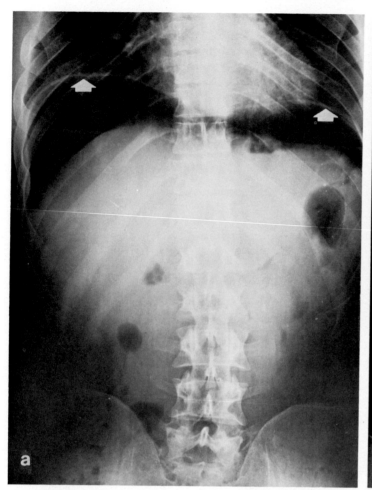
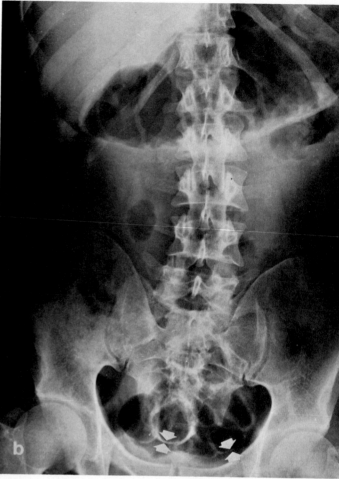

Fig. 8.43. This patient has a massive pneumoperitoneum which is obvious in the erect examination of the abdomen (a). In the supine examination (b), more subtle, but equally definitive, signs of pneumoperitoneum are seen. These consist of air on both sides of the wall of small intestinal loops in the pelvis (*arrows*) and the presence of air outlining the mucosal and serosal surfaces of the greater curvature of the stomach.

absent, the fluid settles at the same level within the limbs of a given loop in the same fashion that water seeks the same level in the limbs of a hollow "U"-shaped tube.

"Localized" ileus is associated with a localized inflammatory process, such as acute cholecystitis, pancreatitis, or appendicitis, and consists of distention of a single loop of gut—generally the small intestine. This single, distended, small intestinal loop containing air-fluid levels on similar planes is referred to as a "sentinel" loop (Fig. 8.44).

Mechanical obstruction may be the result of either a complete or partial organic occlusion of the lumen of the intestine. The site of obstruction can occur any place from the gastric outlet to the distal sigmoid colon. Therefore, obstruction may involve only the small or only the large intestine. Small intestinal loops

may be distinguished from the colon on the basis of the transverse linear densities which represent the valvulae conniventes and which extend completely across the diameter of the loop (Figs. 8.45 and 8.46).

The colon is peripherally situated in the abdomen, is larger in diameter than the small intestine, and is characterized by haustral sacculations which are identified by short, blunt thick projections that arise from the colonic wall and extend only a short distance into the gas-filled lumen (Fig. 8.45).

The etiology of mechanical obstruction is protean. Distention of the gut develops proximal to the site of obstruction as gas and fluid accumulate within the dilated loops. During the acute phases of mechanical obstruction, peristalsis becomes hyperactive as the gut attempts to work against the site of occlusion. Therefore, in erect and decubitus roentgenograms of the

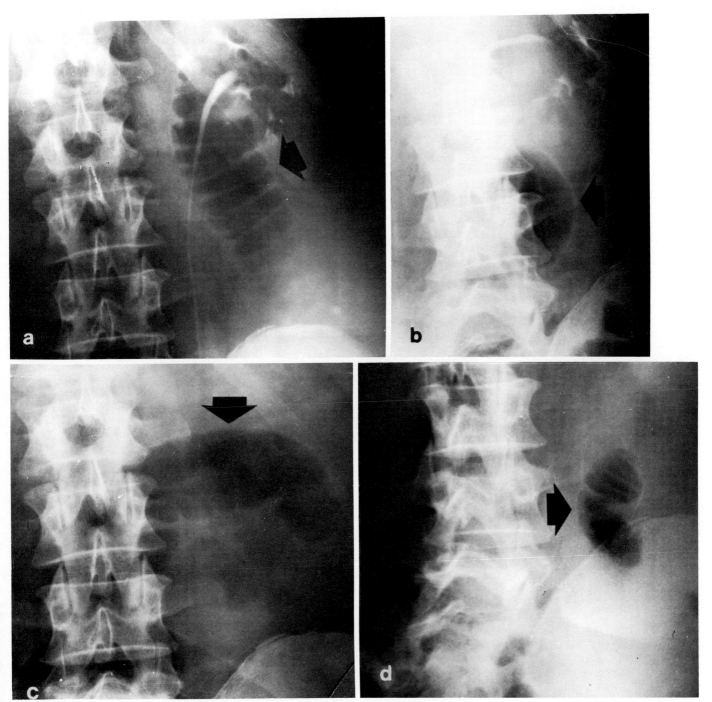

Fig. 8.44. (a–d) The localized dilatation of a single loop of small intestine (*arrows*), represents a ''sentinel'' loop. In this patient, the etiologic factor was acute cholecystitis.

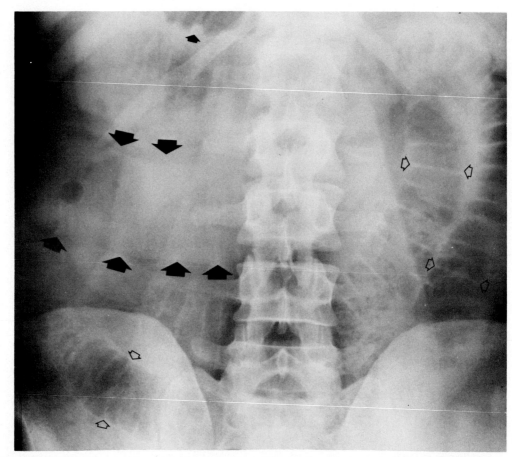

Fig. 8.45. Complete small bowel mechanical obstruction. The *open arrows* indicate distended loops of small bowel containing primarily air. Note that the valvulae conniventes extend across the diameter of the distended loops. The *large solid arrows* indicate a dilated loop of small intestine which is primarily fluid-filled. The *small solid arrow* indicates a haustral marking of the colon.

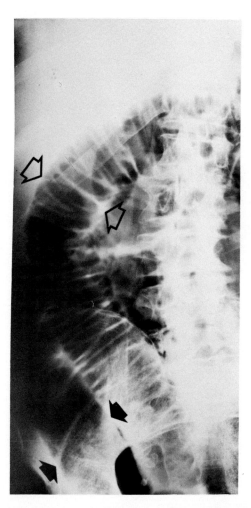

Fig. 8.46. Mechanical small bowel obstruction. The abnormally distended small intestine (*open arrows*) can be identified by the thin, transverse linear densities, representing the valvulae conniventes, which extend across the diameter of the small intestine. The *solid arrows* indicate the cecum which can be identified by means of its location and the absence of valvulae.

abdomen, air-fluid levels will be on uneven planes (Fig. 8.47) within the same loop due to the "fighting" peristalsis. Should the obstruction be complete and persistent, the gut will eventually decompensate and become atonic. Then, the radiographic appearance of the intestine will assume the characteristics of an adynamic ileus.

Abnormal accumulations of gas and fluid in the distended intestinal tract occur in both mechanical obstruction or reflex (adynamic) ileus. If the gut is largely fluid-filled, the abdomen will have a diffuse, hazy appearance, soft tissue anatomy will be obscured, and, on decubitus views, small droplets of gas may accumulate within the recesses between the valvulae

conniventes, producing a series of small, round radiolucent shadows. This distribution of gas within the small intestine has been referred to as the "string of pearls" sign (Fig. 8.48). Failure to be aware that the distended bowel may be almost completely filled with fluid, and contain very little gas, can result in failure to recognize the presence of intestinal obstruction, radiographically (Fig. 8.49).

Incomplete mechanical obstruction, as its name implies, is a partial occlusion of the lumen of the gut. Because the intestine proximal to the obstruction is distended while, simultaneously, some gas and some intestinal content pass through the obstructed point into the distal loops of bowel, it is radiographically very difficult to distinguish between an incomplete or an early complete mechanical obstruction.

The commonest cause of mechanical obstruction of the colon is carcinoma, with the obstructing sites most frequently occurring in the sigmoid, descending, and transverse colons (39). A competent ileocecal valve which prevents reflux of gas into the small intestine, in the face of an obstructing lesion of the colon, results in a "closed-loop" obstruction of the colon. The wall of the cecum, being thinner and weaker than the wall of the remainder of the colon, distends more rapidly and to a greater degree than the remainder of the colon. Therefore, rupture of the obstructed colon is most likely to occur at the cecum. It is generally agreed that should the cecum exceed 10 cm in diameter, as seen radiographically, active measures to decompress the colon are indicated.

If the ileocecal valve is incompetent and gas refluxes into the small intestine proximal to an obstructing colon lesion, rupture of the cecum is not a likely complication. Because both the large and small bowel are distended to a similar degree and each contains air-fluid levels, the radiographic appearance of the intestine resembles an adynamic ileus. Early, the distinction is based upon the appearance of the uneven air-fluid levels. Later, as the gut decompensates and becomes atonic, a complete mechanical obstruction of the distal colon cannot be radiographically distinguished from an adynamic ileus. Under these circumstances, identification of the constricting lesion by barium enema will establish the diagnosis.

Closed-loop obstruction may occur in either the small (Fig. 8.50) or large intestine. A closed-loop obstruction is one which is completely occluded, both proximally and distally, from the remainder of the gut. Volvulus is the commonest cause of closed-loop obstruction and may involve the stomach, the small intestine, or the colon. Torsion of the gut occurs most frequently where the mesentery is longest. In the small bowel, the ileum is the most frequent site, while in the colon, the sigmoid and the cecum are most commonly involved. Volvulus of the duodenum, jejunum, and transverse colon is rare.

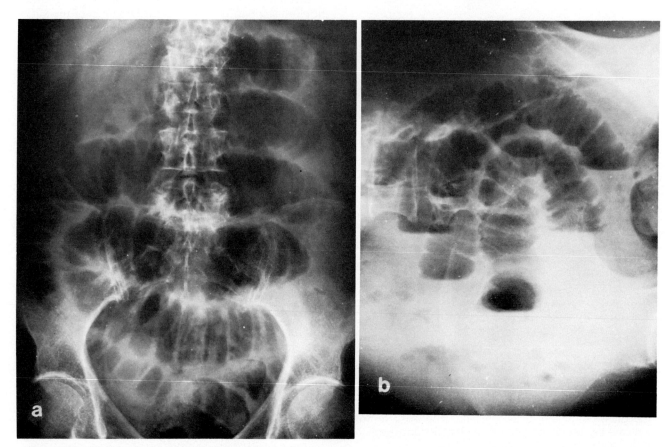

Fig. 8.47. Complete mechanical obstruction of the small bowel. In the supine examination of the abdomen **(a)**, the dilated loops of small intestine are primarily air-filled and are arranged in the typical stepladder configuration. In the decubitus examination of the abdomen **(b)**, air-fluid levels within the individual loops are on uneven planes.

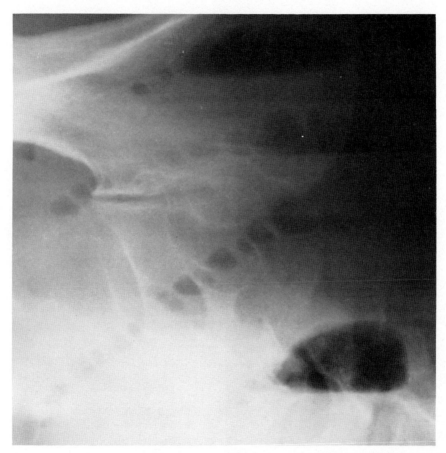

Fig. 8.48. Left lateral decubitus radiograph of the abdomen demonstrating the ''string of pearls'' sign which represents gas trapped in the recesses between the valvulae conniventes in a largely fluid-filled, mechanically obstructed small intestine.

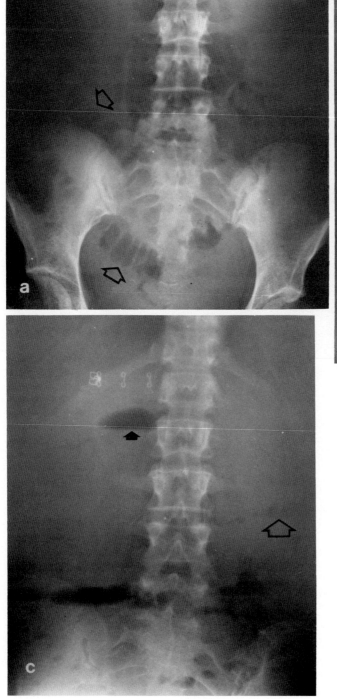

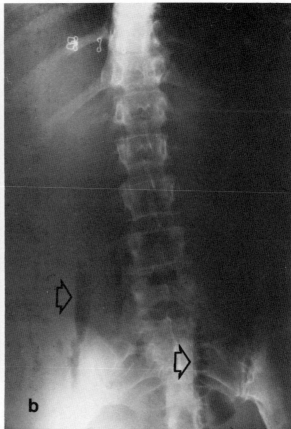

Fig. 8.49. Mechanical small bowel obstruction which the dilated loops are mainly fluid filled. In the supine radiograph **(a)**, short collections of gas in small bowel can be identified (*open arrows*). In the decubitus **(b)** and erect **(c)** radiographs, small amounts of gas accumulate in the apex of dilated loops and present short air-fluid interfaces (*open arrows*) which could be mistaken for adynamic ileus. The *solid arrow* **(c)** indicates an air-fluid interface in the gastric antrum.

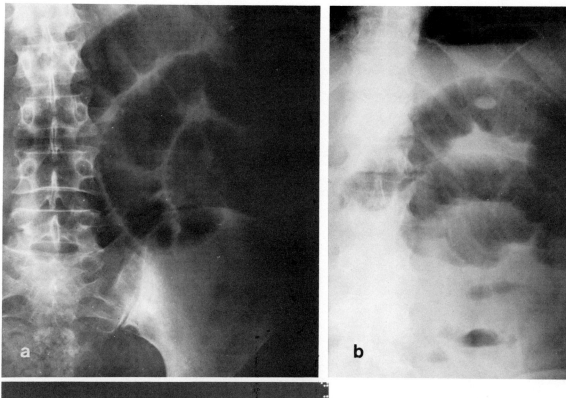

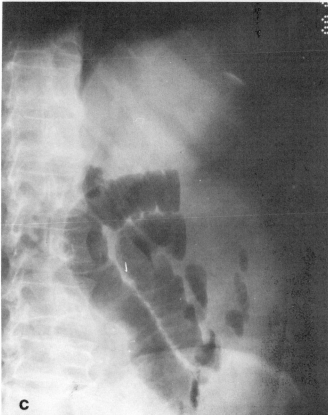

Fig. 8.50. Closed-loop, high mechanical small bowel obstruction. In the supine **(a)**, erect **(b)**, and decubitus **(c)** examinations, dilated loops of proximal small intestine are seen in the left upper quadrant of the abdomen. The air-fluid levels are on uneven planes, indicating a mechanical obstruction. The presence of valvulae conniventes, and the location of the abnormally dilated loops identify them as being in the proximal small intestine.

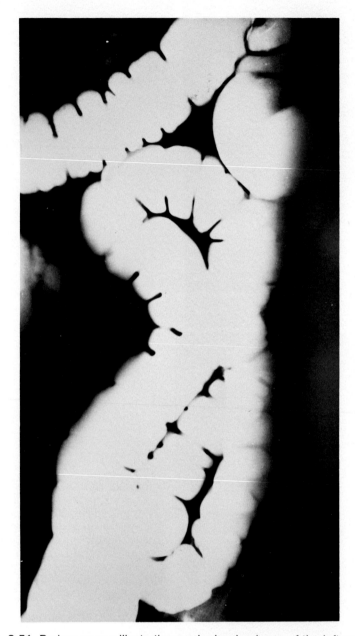

Fig. 8.51. Barium enema illustrating marked redundancy of the left colon.

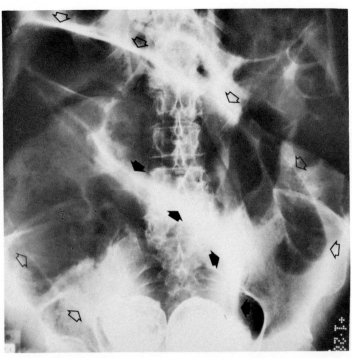

Fig. 8.52. Volvulus of the sigmoid colon. The *open arrows* indicate the antimesenteric walls of the volvulated sigmoid colon. The "central stripe" produced by the adjacent, edematous walls of the involved loop is indicated by the *solid arrows*.

Volvulus of the right colon is not limited to the cecum alone. The torsion may involve the ascending colon and even the proximal right transverse colon (40). This lesion has its greatest frequency in males between the ages of 20 and 40 years (39). The cecum is distended and is usually found in the mid- or upper abdomen toward the left. The wall of the dilated cecum is kidney-shaped in configuration, with the twisted mesentery resembling the renal hilum. This radiographic appearance is typical and usually diagnostic. If the plain film study is not definitive, a barium enema will disclose displacement of the ascending colon toward the left upper quadrant. The tapered end of the barium column points toward the torsion.

Redundancy of the sigmoid colon (Fig. 8.51) is the commonest predisposing factor to volvulus of this portion of the large intestine. The long, loose, mesentery of the redundant sigmoid predisposes to torsion of this segment upon itself. The classic radiographic picture (Fig. 8.52) consists of a greatly dilated loop of colon arising from the left side of the pelvis and projecting obliquely upward toward the right side of the abdomen. The loop may be so large as to fill the entire abdomen. The walls of the volvulated loop are readily identified as curved, linear densities separated by large amounts of gas. The "central stripe" is a characteristic finding and is produced by the edema-

tous, adjacent walls of the loop lying in close apposition.

Other etiologies of closed-loop obstruction include congenital bands or webs, congenital or acquired adhesions, anomalies or malrotation of the gut, and internal hernias. None of these causative agents produce a pathognomonic radiographic appearance.

"Gallstone ileus" is the term given to mechanical obstruction caused by a gallstone which has entered the gut by eroding through the wall of the gallbladder and an adjacent loop of small intestine. The usual site of impaction of the calculus is the pelvic or terminal ileum. The characteristic radiographic findings are those of small bowel obstruction, air in the gallbladder or biliary ductal system, and the presence of a calculus in the pelvic or terminal ileum (Fig. 8.53). The offending gallstone is frequently non-opaque or obscured by distended loops of bowel (Fig. 8.54). Even though air in the biliary ductal system is difficult to perceive (Figs. 8.55 and 8.56), it is invariably present and may be the most important clue leading to the diagnosis. The detection of this extremely significant roentgen sign requires a careful study of the right upper quadrant of the abdominal roentgenogram.

Intussusception occurs in both children and adults. As high as 75% of cases occur in children under the age of 2 years. Intussusception occurring in adults is usually led by a polyp. The clinical picture of child-

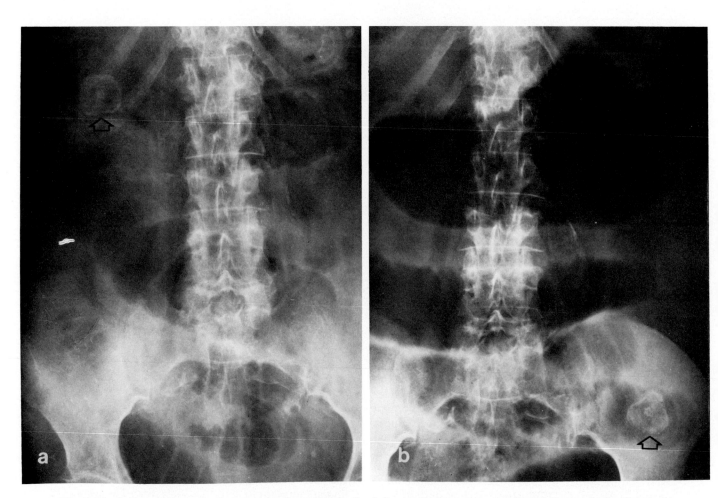

Fig. 8.53. Gallstone ileus. Supine examination of the patient demonstrating a large solitary biliary calculus **(a)**. In the supine examination of the abdomen of the same patient 1 year later **(b)**, the stomach and proximal small intestine are dilated. On this examination the biliary calculus, which was previously located in the gallbladder, is now seen in the left lower quadrant of the abdomen (*arrow*). Gas is present in the biliary ductal system.

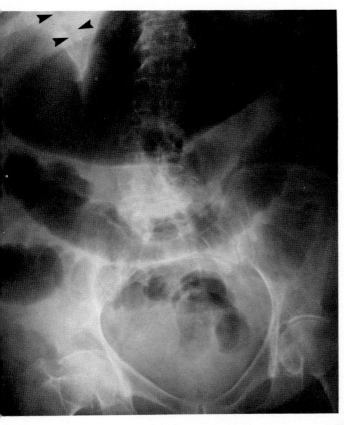

Fig. 8.54. Gallstone ileus. The gallstone causing the small bowel obstruction is nonopaque. The roentgen diagnosis can be reasonably established on the basis of the proximal small intestine obstruction and air in the common bile duct (*arrowheads*).

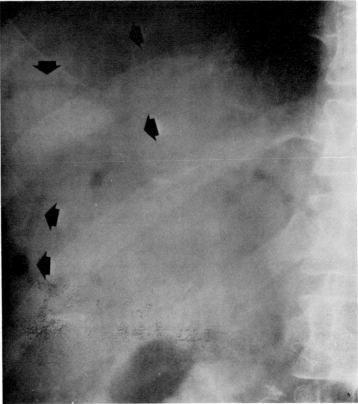

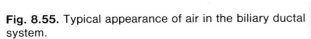
Fig. 8.55. Typical appearance of air in the biliary ductal system.

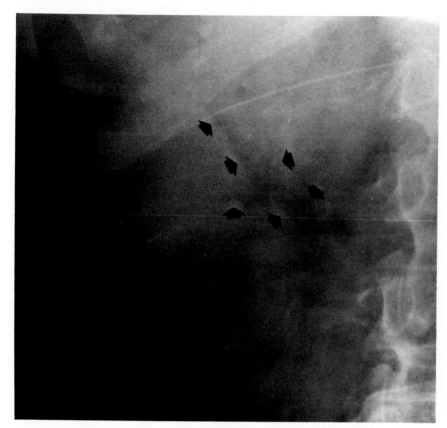

Fig. 8.56. Air in the intrahepatic bile ducts in a patient with gallstone ileus.

hood intussusception consists of brief episodes of crampy abdominal pain which cause the child to cry out sporadically. A mass is frequently palpable in the right lower quadrant of the abdomen and bright red blood is usually mixed with the stool. Radiographically, there is a paucity of intestinal gas in the right lower quadrant and an ill-defined mass may be recognized. The diagnosis is established by the characteristic appearance seen on barium enema (Figs. 8.57 and 8.58).

Intestinal infarction most commonly follows occlusion of the superior mesenteric artery or one of its branches by thrombosis or embolus. The superior mesenteric artery supplies the small intestine and the large intestine to the right midtransverse colon. The area of infarction depends upon the site of the vascular occlusion. If the superior mesenteric artery itself is blocked, many feet of small intestine, as well as portions of the right colon will be involved. If the occlusion involves only a distal branch of the superior mesenteric artery, the infarction will be limited to a short segment of bowel.

While the same pathologic processes may involve the inferior mesenteric artery, infarction of the left half of the colon is infrequent because of its rich collateral circulation.

The radiographic findings of vascular occlusion reflect the phase of the process in the intestine at the time the examination is made. If the patient is seen early, the involved loops will be distended and contain air-fluid levels on uneven planes, thereby resembling a mechanical obstruction. As the effects of vascular occlusion progress and gangrene of the bowel develops, the involved loops become more distended, hypotonic, and edematous. Radiographically, the thickened bowel wall may be apparent. The air-fluid levels assume the characteristic of an adynamic ileus (Fig. 8.59). In decubitus examinations, the affected segments of gut are dilated while the uninvolved segments are of relatively normal caliber.

Mesenteric thrombosis is commonly a difficult diagnosis to establish because of the variability of clinical and radiographic findings. In those patients in whom the etiology of the abdominal symptoms cannot

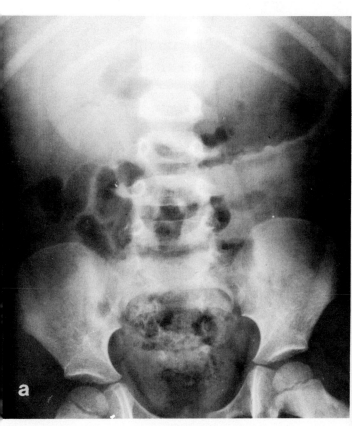

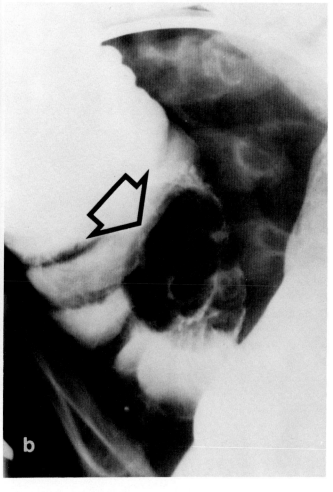

Fig. 8.57. Ileocolic intussusception. In the supine examination of the **(a)**, there is an absence of gas shadows in the right lower quadrant of the abdomen and a soft tissue mass in the region of the cecum may be identifiable. At the time of barium enema **(b)**, the intussusceptum (*arrow*) was encountered in the midascending colon.

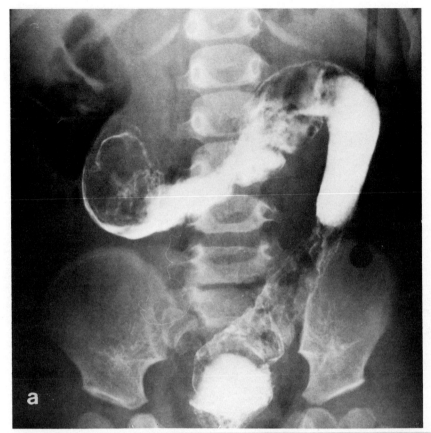

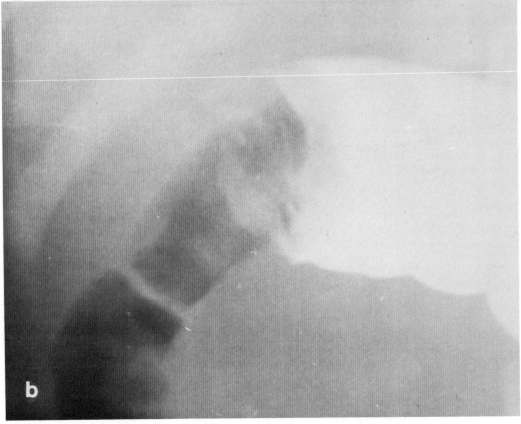

Fig. 8.58. Acute ileocolic intussusception. There is complete obstruction in the proximal transverse colon by a large filling defect which is peripherally surrounded by a thin layer of barium which is located between the head and the sleeve of the invagination. (a). In a radiograph made during the fluoroscopic examination (b), gas delineates the invaginated intussusceptum. Barium defines the lumen of the intussusciptiens, and the barium can be seen surrounding the head of the intussusception.

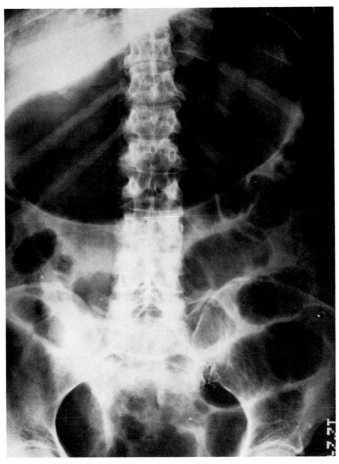

Fig. 8.59. Typical radiographic appearance of occlusion of the superior mesenteric artery. There is uniform dilatation of the small intestine. Minimal separation of the dilated small bowel loops is present. The marked distention of the stomach is not caused by thrombosis of the superior mesenteric artery.

be determined, and in whom intestinal infarction is considered, angiographic evaluation of the abdominal aorta or the superior mesenteric artery is a definitive diagnostic procedure.

Peritonitis is inflammation of the peritoneum. Histologically, peritonitis, in its earliest stages, is manifest by edema of the peritoneum, an inflammatory cellular response and an exudate. All of these changes occur prior to the development of frank pus or ascites in the peritoneal cavity. The cellular changes may be generalized or localized. Even early inflammation and edema of the peritoneum produce recognizable changes in the flank stripe on an optimally exposed abdominal radiograph because the parietal peritoneum constitutes the medial wall of the flank stripe. Swelling of the parietal peritoneum secondary to edema and the inflammatory cellular response causes the medial margin of the flank stripe to become indistinct. Exudation of edema fluid into the retroper-

itoneal space becomes admixed with the retroperitoneal fat, causing the flank stripe to become irregularly and heterogeneously dense and poorly defined. These roentgen signs of early peritonitis are illustrated in Figures 8.60 and 8.61.

Plain film radiography of the abdomen and barium enema make valuable contributions to the diagnosis of acute appendicitis (42–49). The presence of a fecalith in the right lower abdomen (Fig. 8.62) or right side of the pelvis is a reliable, but not absolute, sign of acute appendicitis. A calcified coprolith is present in over 50% of patients with a perforated appendix.

Signs of acute appendicitis include either a relatively airless intestine due to antecedent nausea, vomiting, diarrhea, and dehydration, or generalized minor small intestinal dilatation secondary to aerophagia, localized ileus in the right lower quadrant, lumbar or lumbosacral scoliosis with the concavity to the right, absence or loss of definition of portions of the psoas

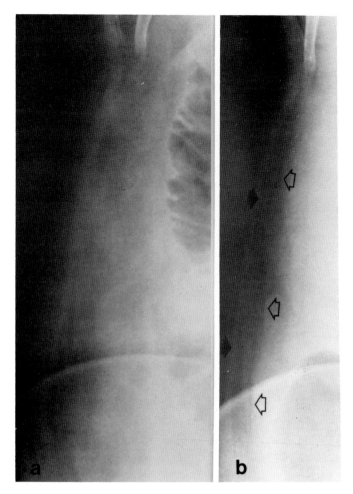

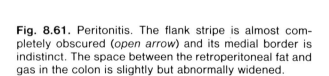

Fig. 8.60. Peritonitis. The retroperitoneal flank stripe is irregularly dense. In some portions, the lateral margin of the flank stripe (the transversalis fascia) is faintly visible. The medial margin is completely obscured **(a)**. The radiographic appearance of the same patient's right flank stripe two years earlier is seen in **(b)**.

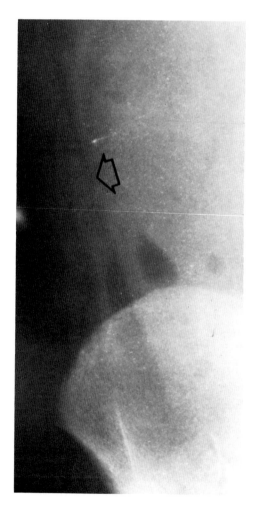

Fig. 8.61. Peritonitis. The flank stripe is almost completely obscured (*open arrow*) and its medial border is indistinct. The space between the retroperitoneal fat and gas in the colon is slightly but abnormally widened.

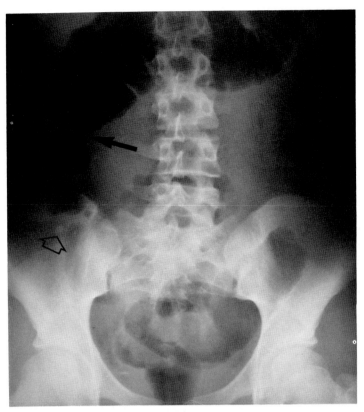

Fig. 8.62. Perforated appendix with a fecalith in the right lower quadrant (*open arrow*), "cut-off" sign in the mid-ascending colon (*stemmed arrow*), principally fluid-filled, dilated small intestine and lumbosacral scoliosis with the concavity to the right.

shadow, or a "cut-off" sign of the right colon (Figs. 8.62 and 8.63).

Plain film radiography is particularly useful in cases of acute retrocecal appendicitis where the clinical signs and symptoms are commonly atypical. The inflammatory response in the retrocecal space usually causes reflex ileus of the ascending colon, an increase in width of the distance between the flank stripe and the lumen of the colon, thickening and indistinctness of the lateral wall of the colon, loss of definition of the medial margin of the flank stripe, and some degree of obscuration of the flank stripe itself (Fig. 8.64).

The signs of an appendiceal abscess include loculated, extraluminal air (Fig. 8.65), medial displacement of the ascending colon by a soft tissue mass (Fig. 8.66), or by distortion of the cecum and displacement of the terminal ileal loop on barium enema (Fig. 8.67).

The diagnosis of right subdiaphragmatic abscess is extremely difficult to establish either clinically or radiographically. The most reliable signs of right-sided subdiaphragmatic collection include elevation of the right hemidiaphragm, indistinctness of its margins (Fig. 8.68), and decreased diaphragmatic excursion during respiration. While the roentgen signs of subdiaphragmatic collection closely mimic an infrapulmonary effusion, the distinction can usually be made on the basis of the clinical information regarding the patient and the fact that an infrapulmonary effusion will change its location and characteristics on decubitus radiographs of the chest, while signs of a subdiaphragmatic collection will not be altered by change in position. Subdiaphragmatic collections are clearly delineated by computed tomography, gallium nuclear medicine scanning, and ultrasound.

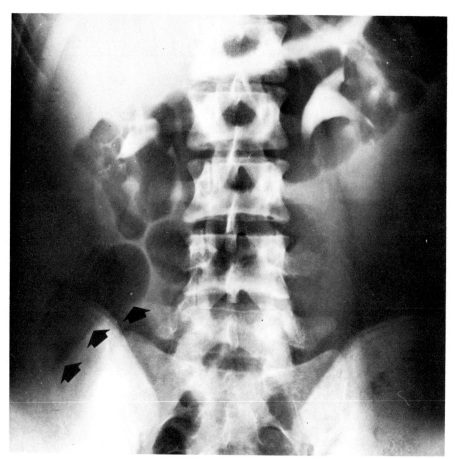

Fig. 8.63. ''Cut-off'' sign in the cecum (*solid arrows*) caused by acute appendicitis. The antegrade urogram was performed because of obscure clinical findings and microscopic hematuria. The urogram was negative. The inflamed appendix lay adjacent to the right ureter as it crossed the sacral wing.

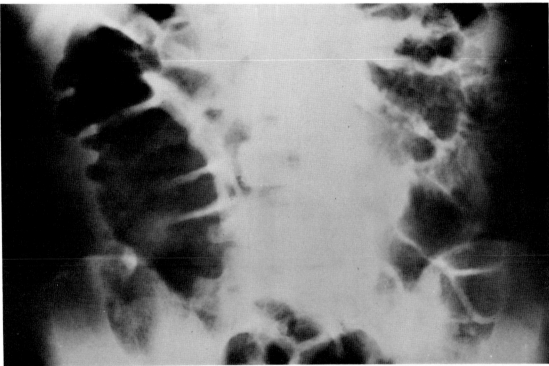

Fig. 8.64. Acute retrocecal appendicitis. The ascending colon is distended, reflexly. The distance between the flank stripe and the lumen of the colon is widened and the lateral wall of the colon is thickened and indistinct. The medial margin of the flank stripe is indistinct and the flank stripe itself is obscured. All these signs are those of an acute inflammatory process in the retrocecal ''space.''

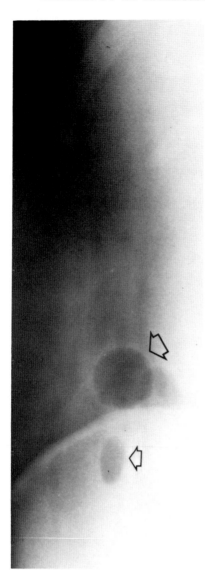

Fig. 8.65. Appendiceal abscess. The abnormal, extraluminal collections of air in the right lower quadrant (*arrows*) were located in an appendiceal abscess. Signs of peritonitis are seen in the mid- and lower portions of the flank stripe.

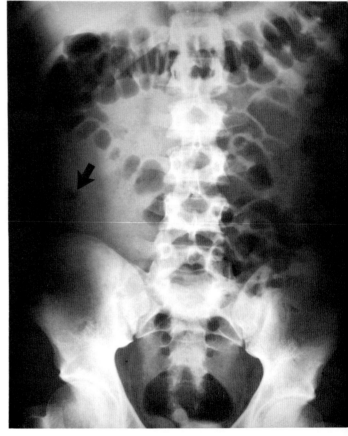

Fig. 8.66. Paracolic appendiceal abscess. The ascending colon is medially displaced by a large ill defined soft tissue density which contains an abnormal collection of gas (*arrow*). These abnormalities represented a large abscess about a perforated retrocecal appendix.

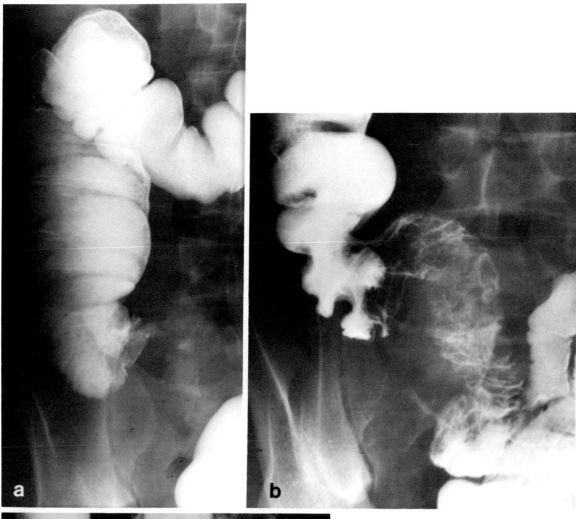

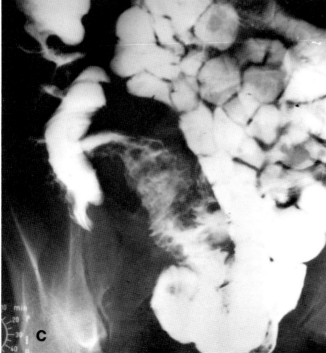

Fig. 8.67. (a–c) The appendiceal abscess has caused extrinsic distortion of the cecum. The terminal ileal loop is displaced superiorly and medially and its mucosal pattern distorted by the abscess.

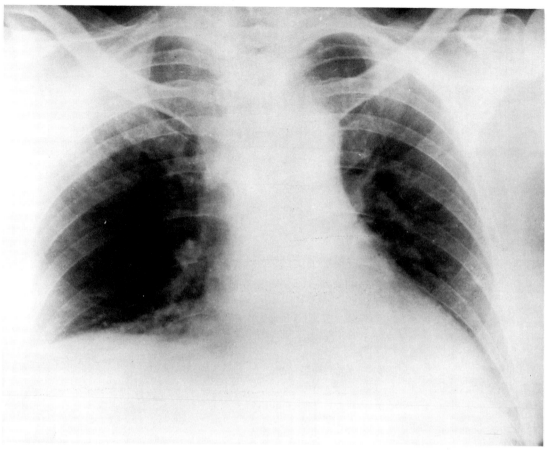

Fig. 8.68. Right subdiaphragmatic abscess. The right hemidiaphragm is elevated, its margin indistinct, and focal areas of subsegmental atelectasis are present at the right base. The right costophrenic angle is obscured by small pleural effusion.

Infrahepatic collections, being separated from the diaphragm by the liver, usually do not produce radiographic changes involving the diaphragm (Fig. 8.69).

Chronic impaction of a gallstone in the ampulla of the gallbladder causes obstruction of the cystic duct. As bile within the gallbladder becomes inspissated, the calcium carbonate becomes concentrated, thereby rendering the sludge within the gallbladder opaque. This is called "milk of calcium" bile. The typical radiographic appearance of an impacted calculus and milk of calcium bile as seen on a supine abdominal radiograph, without prior ingestion of contrast medium, is illustrated in Figure 8.70. In this form of chronic cholecystitis, the gallbladder is small and contracted.

Diffuse calcification of the wall of the gallbladder, the so-called "porcelain gallbladder," may be associated with acute cholecystitis (Fig. 8.71).

Aneurysms of the abdominal aorta usually appear to the left of the midline in the supine radiograph of the abdomen, and anterior to the spine in the lateral projection. The presence of calcification within the wall of an aneurysm is variable. When present, the calcification permits an appraisal of the length and dilatation of the aneurysm. When clinical signs suggest an abdominal aortic aneurysm, both supine and lateral radiographs of the abdomen may be necessary to establish the presence of calcification within the aneurysmal wall and to evaluate the length and diameter of the aneurysm (Figs. 8.72 and 8.73). CT or ultrasonography is required to measure the caliber of the lumen of the aneurysm or to determine the characteristics of noncalcified, pulsatile, midline abdominal masses.

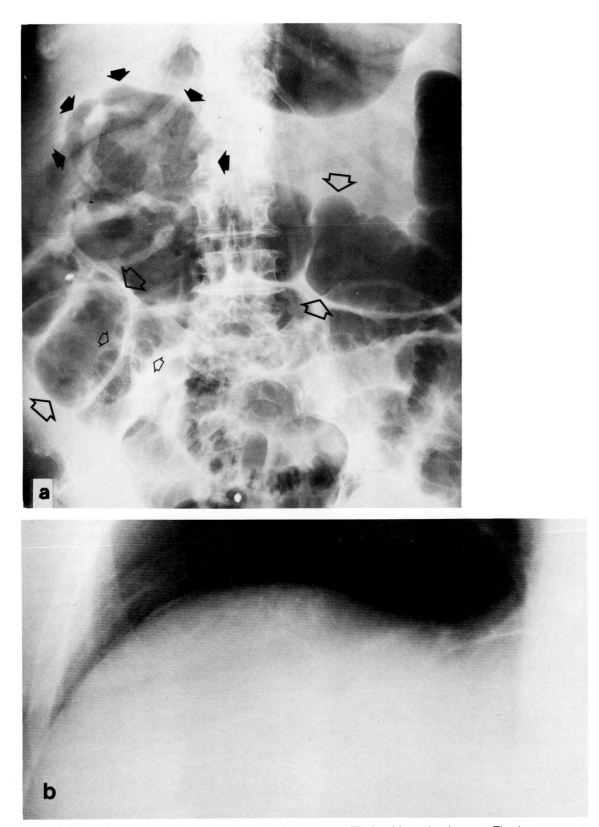

Fig. 8.69. Subhepatic abscess. The *solid arrows* indicate a gas-filled subhepatic abscess. The *large open arrows* indicate distended colon. The *small open arrows* indicate dilated small intestine. The abscess produced peritonitis and resultant adynamic ileus **(a)**. The right diaphragmatic surface, being shielded from the abscess by the mass of the liver, is normal in appearance **(b)**.

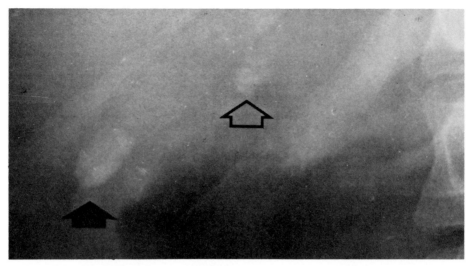

Fig. 8.70. ''Milk of calcium'' bile. The *open arrow* indicates the calculus impacted in the ampulla of the gallbladder. The *solid arrow* indicates the inspissated bile made opaque by concentration of the calcium carbonate within the small, contracted gallbladder.

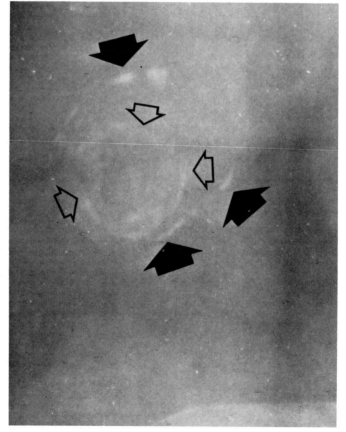

Fig. 8.71. ''Porcelain gallbladder.'' Diffuse calcification within the wall of the gallbladder is indicated by the *solid arrows*. A multilaminated solitary calculus (*open arrows*) lies within the lumen of the gallbladder.

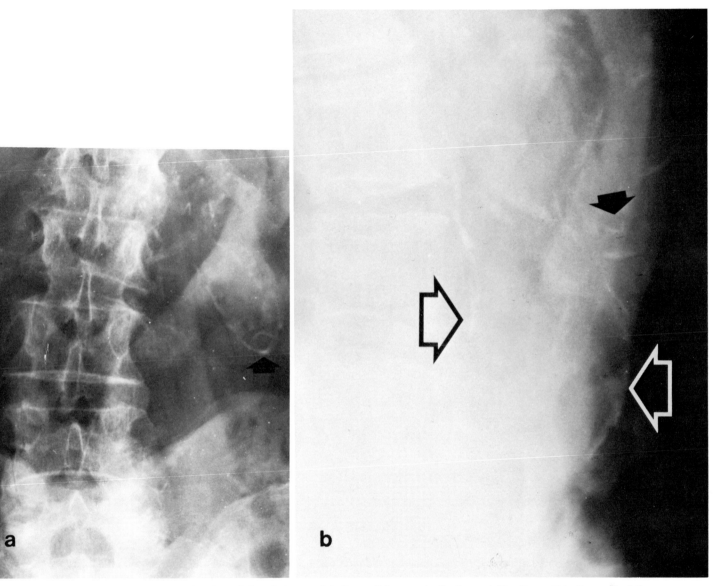

Fig. 8.72. In the supine examination of the abdomen **(a)**, the *solid arrow* indicates calcification within the wall of the tortuous, dilated splenic artery. There is no evidence of aortic aneurysm on this examination. In the lateral examination of the abdomen **(b)**, however, the calcified walls of the fusiform abdominal aortic aneurysm are clearly seen (*open arrows*). The *solid arrow* indicates the calcified splenic artery.

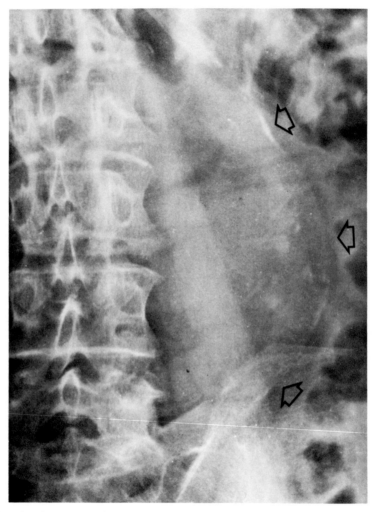

Fig. 8.73. In the frontal projection faint, diffuse calcification can be seen in the wall of the large abdominal aneurysm (*open arrows*).

References

1. DRURY ED, RUBIN BE: Computed tomography in the evaluation of abdominal trauma. *J Comput Assist Tomogr* 3:40, 1979.
2. VISCOMI GN, GONZALEZ R, TAYLOR KJW, GRADE M: Ultrasonic evaluation of hepatic and splenic trauma. *Arch Surg* 115:320, 1980.
3. FORTUNATO R, HESSEL SJ: Blunt abdominal trauma: Roentgenographic, angiographic, ultrasonic and computed tomographic evaluation.
4. SIZER JS, WAYNE ER, FREDERICK PL: Delayed rupture of the spleen. *Arch Surg* 92:362, 1966.
5. STEICHEN FM, PEARLMAN DM, DARGON EL, PROMMAS DC, WEIL PH: Wounds of the abdomen: radiographic diagnosis of intra-peritoneal penetration. *Ann Surg* 196:77, 1967.
6. CARTER JW, SAWYERS JL: Abdominal stab wound study by injection of contrast medium. *Surgery* 63:597, 1968.
7. TOBIAS S, DECLEMENT FA, CLEVELAND JC: Management of stab wounds of the abdomen. *Arch Surg* 95:27, 1967.
8. CORNELL WP, EBERT PA, ZUIDEMA GD: X-ray diagnosis of penetrating wounds of the abdomen. *J Surg Res* 5:142, 1965.
9. FRIMANN-DAHL J: *Roentgen Examinations in Acute Abdominal Diseases*, ed. 2. Charles C. Thomas Publishing Co., Springfield, Ill., 1960.
10. MCCORT JJ: *Radiographic Examination in Blunt Abdominal Trauma*. W.B. Saunders, Philadelphia, 1966.
11. PAUL L, JUHL JH: *The Essentials of Roentgen Interpretation*, ed. 2. Harper & Row, New York, 1965.
12. TOVEE EV: Blunt abdominal trauma. *J Trauma* 10:72, 1970.
13. CORICA A, POWERS SR: Blunt liver trauma: An analysis of 75 treated patients. *Trauma* 9:751, 1975.
14. BIVENS BA, JONA JZ, BELIN RP: Diagnostic peritoneal lavage in pediatric trauma. *Trauma* 16:739, 1976.
15. ENGRAV LH, BENJAMIN CI, STRATE RG, PERRY JF: Diagnostic peritoneal lavage in blunt abdominal trauma. *Trauma* 15:854, 1975.
16. GUERNSEY JM, GANCHROW MI: Diagnostic laparotomy in the patient with multiple injuries. *Trauma* 15:1053, 1975.
17. OLSEN WR, HILDRETH DH: Abdominal paracentesis and peritoneal lavage in blunt abdominal trauma. *Trauma* 11:824, 1971.
18. ROAB HD, in discussion of Engrav, et al: Diagnostic peritoneal lavage in blunt abdominal trauma. *Trauma* 15:854, 1975.
19. HUBBARD SG, BIVINS BA, SACHATELLO CR, GRIFFIN WO JR.: Diagnostic errors with peritoneal lavage in patients with pelvic fractures. *Arch Surg* 114:844, 1979.
20. LORIMER WS JR.: Occult rupture of the spleen. *Arch Surg* 89:434, 1964.
21. DRAPANAS T, YEATES AJ, BRICKMAN R, WHOLEY M: The syndrome of occult rupture of the spleen. *Arch Surg* 99:298, 1969.
22. SOLHEIM, K: Radionuclide imaging of splenic laceration in trauma. *Clin Nucl Med* 4:528, 1979.
23. THOMPSON DP, SHULTZ EH, BENFIELD JR: Celiac angiography in the management of splenic trauma. *Arch Surg* 99:494, 1969.
24. LOVE L, GREENFIELD GB, BRAUN TW, MONCADA R, FREEARK, RJ, BAKER RJ: Arteriography of splenic trauma. *Radiology* 91:96, 1968.
25. SCHWARTZ SS, BOLEY SJ, MCKINNON WMP: The roentgen findings in traumatic rupture of the spleen in children. *AJR* 82:505, 1959.
26. BAKER RJ, TAXMAN P, FREEARK RJ: An assessment of the management of non-penetrating liver injuries. *Arch Surg* 93:84, 1966.
27. OWENS MP, WOLFMAN EF, CHUNG GK: The management of liver trauma. *Arch Surg* 103:211, 1980.
28. OLINDE HDH: Nonpenetrating wounds of the abdomen. *South Med J* 53:1270, 1960.
29. BYRNE RV: The surgical repair of major liver injuries. *Surg Gynecol Obstet* 119:113, 1964.
30. MAYS ET: Bursting injuries of the liver. *Arch Surg* 93:92, 1966.
31. CERISE EJ, SCULLY JH JR.: Blunt trauma to the small intestine. *J Trauma* 10:46, 1970.
32. RESNICOFF SA, MORTON JH, BLOCH AL: Retroperitoneal rupture of the duodenum due to blunt trauma. *Surg Gynecol Obstet* 125:77, 1967.
33. HAYNES CD, GUNN CH, MARTIN JD JR.: Colon injuries. *Arch Surg* 96:944, 1969.
34. WEICHERT RF III, HEWITT RL: Injuries to the inferior vena cava: Report of 35 cases. *J Trauma* 10:649, 1970.
35. BARTHEY O, WICHBOM I: Roentgen diagnosis of rupture of the diaphragm. *Acta Radiol* 53:33, 1960.
36. DESFORGES G, STREIDER JW, LYNCH JP, MADOFF IM: Traumatic rupture of the diaphragm. *J Thorac Cardiovasc Surg* 34:779, 1957.
37. CARTER BN, GIUSEFFI J, FELSON B: Traumatic diaphragmatic hernia. *AJR* 65:56, 1951.
38. CLEVELAND HC, WADDELL WR: Retroperitoneal rupture of the duodenum due to non-penetrating trauma. *Surg Clin North Am* 43:413, 1963.
39. MARGULUS AR, BURHENNE HJ: *Alimentary Tract Roentgenology*. C. V. Mosby, St. Louis, Mo., 1967.
40. FRIMANN-DAHL J: Volvulus of the right colon. *Acta Radiol* 41:141, 1954.
41. SWISCHUK LE: *Emergency Radiology of the Acutely Ill or Injured Child*. Williams & Wilkins, Baltimore, 1979.
42. BRADY B, CARROLL D: The significance of the calcified appendiceal enterolith. *Radiology* 68:648, 1957.
43. FAEGENBURG D: Fecaliths of the appendix: Incidence—significance. *AJR* 89:752, 1963.
44. CASPAR RB: Fluid in the right flank as a roentgenographic sign of acute appendicitis. *AJR* 110:352, 1970.
45. MEYERS MA, OLIPHANT M: Ascending retrocecal appendicitis. *Radiology* 110:295, 1974.
46. CHIN R, GAMBACH R: Radiographic ureteral changes with appendicitis. *J Can Assoc Radiol* 25:154, 1974.
47. FIGIEL LS, FIGIEL SJ: Barium examination of the cecum in appendicitis. *Acta Radiol* 57:469, 1962.
48. SOTER CS: The contribution of the radiologist to the diagnosis of appendicitis. *Semin Roentgenol* 8:375, 1973.
49. VAUDAGNA JS, MCCORT JJ: Plain film diagnosis of retrocecal appendicitis. *Radiology* 117:533, 1975.

chapter nine

Kidneys and Ureters

General Considerations

Although well protected by the surrounding tissues and the skeletal and soft tissue components of the thoracoabdominal wall, the kidneys are subject to the effects of the force of injury. It is noteworthy that seemingly insignificant trauma may be the cause of severe renal damage. Thus, the detection of renal injury is dependent upon a high degree of suspicion and the prompt institution of appropriate laboratory tests and roentgen examinations.

Every renal injury should be considered to be of major significance until proven otherwise. There is no correlation between the magnitude of thoracoabdominal trauma or the degree of hematuria and the type, or extent, of renal damage. Therefore, every patient clinically suspected of having sustained renal trauma should have an infusion pyelogram as promptly as the patient's condition will permit (1). The purpose of prompt antegrade pyelography is not only to detect renal vascular injuries which are surgical emergencies but also to assess the location and status of the function of the opposite kidney.

Radiographic Examination

The fundamental roentgen study of the kidneys and ureters of the acutely ill or injured patient is the infusion pyelogram (2,3). The purpose of this examination is (1) to evaluate the nature and extent of involvement of the affected kidney and ureter and (2) to determine the location and function of the contralateral kidney. Opacification of the ureters provides useful information relative to retroperitoneal and pelvic hemorrhage, the location of ureteral calculi, and the presence of mass lesions.

Infusion pyelography is recommended over all other variations of antegrade urography, even in children (4), because of the excellent opacification of the urinary tract in face of extensive intestinal artifacts and severe hypotension (Fig. 9.1). With this technique, the urinary tract may remain opaque for as long as 1 hour, allowing sufficient time to obtain oblique, erect, prone, or body section roentgenograms when indicated.

Renal arteriography is the definitive roentgen study of the acutely injured kidney. Olsson and Lunderquist (5) described the angiographic changes of acute and subacute renal trauma in 1963. Since then, the role and value of renal angiography in the evaluation of renal trauma has become well established. Renal arteriography is indicated by persistent hematuria, decreased or absent opacification of the kidney on infusion pyelography, and roentgen signs of retroperitoneal hemorrhage (6–9).

Computed tomography provides excellent delineation of the kidneys, the opacified ureters (following enhancement), and the retroperitoneal space and its contents.

Persistent hematuria may be a sign of traumatic involvement of the renal pedicle.

Decreased or absent renal function on infusion pyelography associated with a normal appearing collecting system on retrograde pyelography in a patient who has sustained blunt abdominal trauma is the classic roentgen sign of renal artery injury. The underlying pathologic process may include circumferential intimal tear, avulsion of the renal artery, or thrombosis.

Roentgen signs of retroperitoneal hemorrhage—presence of a soft tissue mass, loss of definition of the renal or psoas shadow, and displacement of the kidney or ureter—may be caused by bleeding from other retroperitoneal structures, as well as being due to major kidney damage. Renal arteriography is not indicated in most patients with a history of blunt renal trauma, microscopic hematuria, and a normal infusion pyelogram (10).

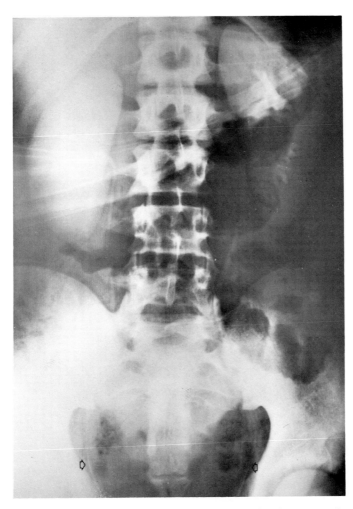

Fig. 9.1. Infusion pyelogram performed in a patient in deep shock following a gunshot wound through the upper abdomen. At the time this examination was performed, the patient's blood pressure was 60/0. The right nephrogram is the result of the shock wave concussion of the right kidney. At laparotomy, the right kidney had not been penetrated by the bullet. The infusion pyelogram demonstrates that the left kidney is present and functioning normally. The ureters are seen throughout their extent.

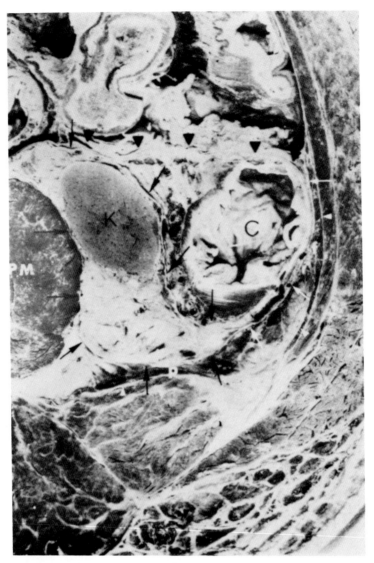

Fig. 9.2. Cross sectional anatomy of the retroperitoneal space at the level of the left kidney. The *arrowheads* indicate the posterior peritoneum. The *stemmed arrows* indicate the anterior and posterior perirenal fascia, which define the perirenal space containing the kidney (*K*) and the perinephric fat. The perirenal fasciae fuse laterally to form the lateroconal ligament (*white stemmed arrows*), which passes posterior to the colon (*C*) and is continuous with the parietal peritoneum in the flank. The space bounded by the posterior peritoneum anteriorly (*black arrowheads*) and the anterior perirenal fascia posteriorly (*black stemmed arrows*) is the anterior *para*renal space which contains fat and the colon. The posterior *para*renal space (*P*) is bounded anteriorly by the posterior perirenal fascia (*black stemmed arrows*) and the transversalis fascia posteriorly (*white arrowheads*). This space is continuous, anterolaterally, with the lateral extraperitoneal space ("flank stripe"). *PM* indicates the psoas muscle. (Reprinted with permission from M. A. Meyers, J. P. Whalen, K. Peelle, A. S. Berne: *Radiology* 104:249, 1972.)

Radiographic Anatomy

The anatomy of the retroperitoneal space, at the level of the kidneys, is clearly defined in Figure 9.2. The anterior and posterior renal fascia define the perirenal space, which contains the kidney and peri-renal fat. The anterior and posterior renal fascia fuse laterally to form the lateroconal ligament which, as it continues anteriorly lateral to the colon, is continuous with the parietal peritoneum. The anterior *para*renal space lies between the anterior renal fascia and the peritoneum and contains fat and the colon. The pos-

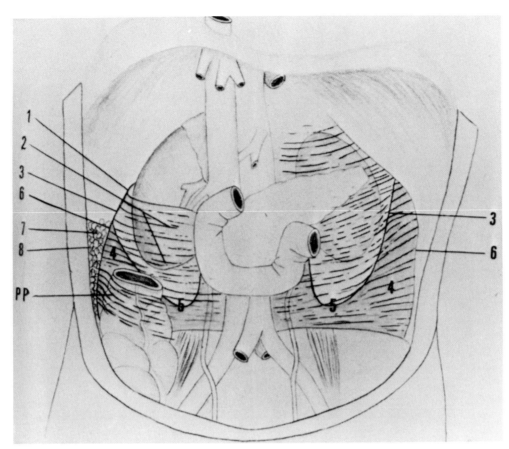

Fig. 9.3. Schematic representation of the retroperitoneal compartments. This drawing clearly illustrates the conical configuration of the inferior portion of the perirenal space (5). Other extraperitoneal structures represented include the posterior renal fascia (1), anterior renal fascia (2), line of fusion of anterior and posterior renal fascia (3), lateroconal fascia (4), line of fusion of lateroconal fascia with posterior parietal peritoneum (6), posterior *para*renal fat extending into the flank stripe (7), and transversalis fascia (8). (Reprinted with permission from M. A. Meyers, J.P. Whalen, K. Peelle, and A. S. Berne: *Radiology* 104:249, 1972.)

terior *para*renal space lies between the posterior renal fascia and the lateroconal ligament anteriorly and the transversalis fascia posteriorly. The fat of the posterior *para*renal space is continuous with that of the flank stripe (11).

The fused anterior and posterior renal fasciae form a cone-shaped space with its lateral margin extending inferomedially with the apex of the cone directed toward the lower lumbar vertebra and psoas muscles (Fig. 9.3). The inferior conical extension is an enclosed and noncommunicating space, and blood and/or urine accumulating within this space produces a characteristic coneshaped, homogeneously dense shadow which identifies its location on the abdominal radiograph (see Figs. 9.13c and 9.15).

The radiographic anatomy of the retroperitoneal space is seen in Figure 9.4. The left kidney is normally higher than the right. Anomalously, the right kidney may be at the same level as, or higher than, the left in approximately 10% of patients. Congenital absence or ectopic location (Fig. 9.5) of a kidney occurs in approximately 1 of 700 persons (12). Agenesis or hypoplasia of one kidney is usually associated with compensatory hyperplasia of the contralateral kidney (Fig. 9.6).

The adult renal shadows measure 12–14 cm in length, and normally the disparity in length between the kidneys does not exceed 1.5–2.0 cm radiographically. The upper poles are closer to the spine than the lower pole so that the long axis of each kidney is directed inferolaterally. The renal silhouette is made radiographically visible by virtue of the radiolucency of the perinephric fat enclosed within the renal fascia.

The ureters arise from the renal pelvis and promptly

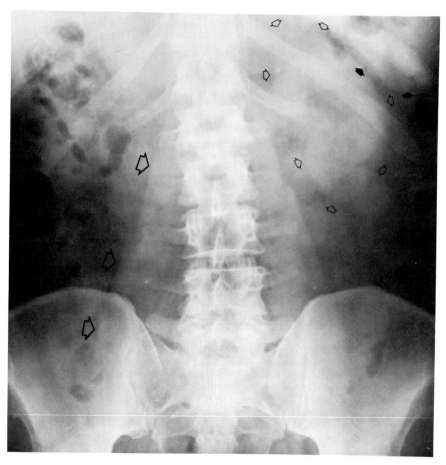

Fig. 9.4. The *large open arrows* indicate the density of the lateral margin of the right psoas muscle. Its counterpart is clearly visible on the left. The right renal shadow is largely obscured by intestinal artifacts. The left renal shadow is indicated by the *small open arrows* and the tip of the spleen by the *solid arrows*.

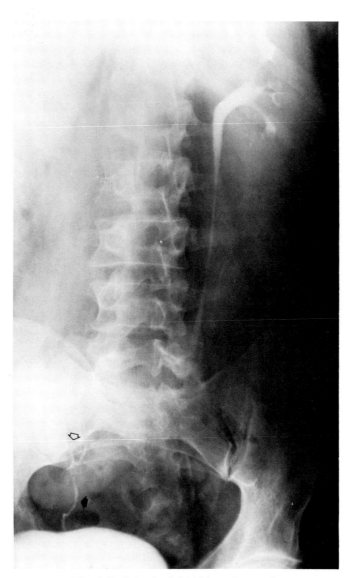

Fig. 9.5. Ectopic right kidney (*arrows*).

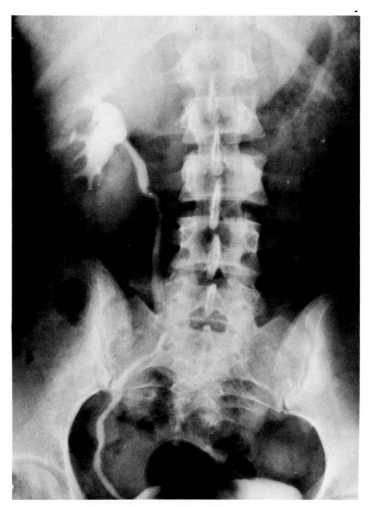

Fig. 9.6. Congenital absence of the left kidney. The right kidney is compensatorily hypertrophied.

cross the superior portion of the psoas muscle. At this point, the opacified ureter may appear to be slightly medially displaced due to the mass of the muscle. The ureter then proceeds in a slightly inferomedial course to the level of the sacral promentory. The distal portion of the ureter follows a gently convex course through the pelvis to the bladder wall.

Radiographic Manifestations of Trauma

In civilian practice, most renal injuries are caused by blunt trauma, although penetrating injuries caused by gunshot wounds and stabbings are frequent in urban settings (13).

Several classifications of renal injury have been described (9, 13–15). The classification proposed by Sargent and Marquadt (16), which consists of contusion, major fracture, and shattered kidney, seems to correlate the closest with the most common urographic patterns of renal trauma.

Contusion is the most frequent renal injury and consists of parenchymal damage without loss of integrity of the collecting system and without disruption of the renal cortex. The roentgen appearance of renal contusion may include extremely subtle changes such as an increase in size of a portion of the kidney with increase in density of the nephrogram and minor distortion of the corresponding segment of the collecting system (Fig. 9.7), severe constriction of a minor calyx (Fig. 9.8), gross distortion of a portion of the collecting system with puddling of contrast medium in the adjacent parenchyma (Fig. 9.9) or diffuse, slight renomegaly with incomplete visualization and minor distortion of the entire collecting system (Figs. 9.10 and 9.11). The contour of the renal shadow is usually unremarkable.

Fracture (laceration) of the kidney consists of parenchymal disruption which extends through the renal capsule, into the collecting system, or both. On the plain radiograph of the abdomen, extravasated blood

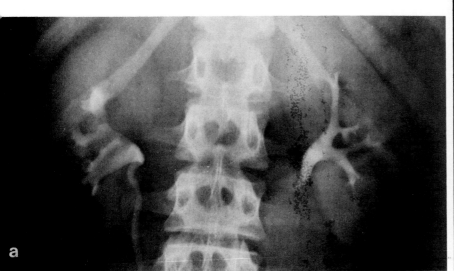
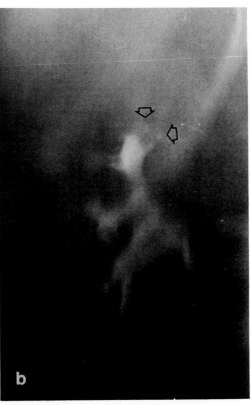

Fig. 9.7. Contusion of the upper pole of the right kidney resulting in increase in size and density of the right upper pole and subtle distortion of the right upper pole minor calyx (**a**). Nephrotomogram (**b**) demonstrates the distortion of the upper pole minor calyx as well as small accumulations of contrast medium in the renal parenchyma (*arrows*).

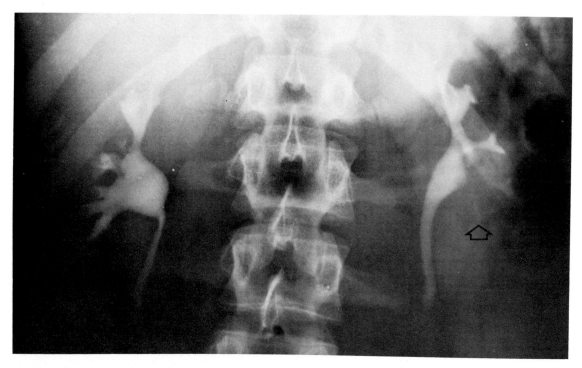

Fig. 9.8. Contusion of the left kidney. The left lower pole minor calyces and infundibulae are pinched off, only faintly opacified, and distorted.

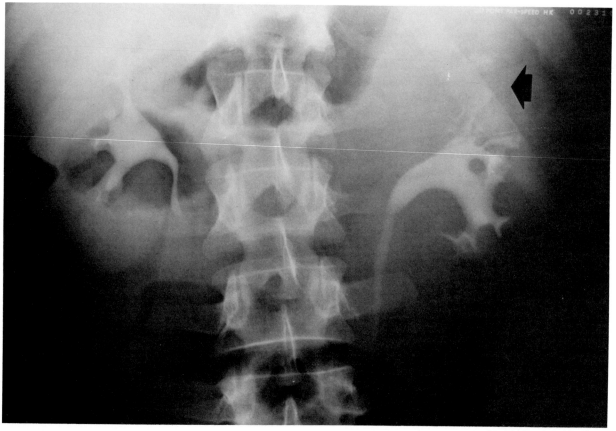

Fig. 9.9. Contusion of the upper pole of the left kidney has resulted in increase in its size, distortion of the upper pole minor calyx and infundibulum, and puddling of contrast medium within the renal parenchyma (*arrow*).

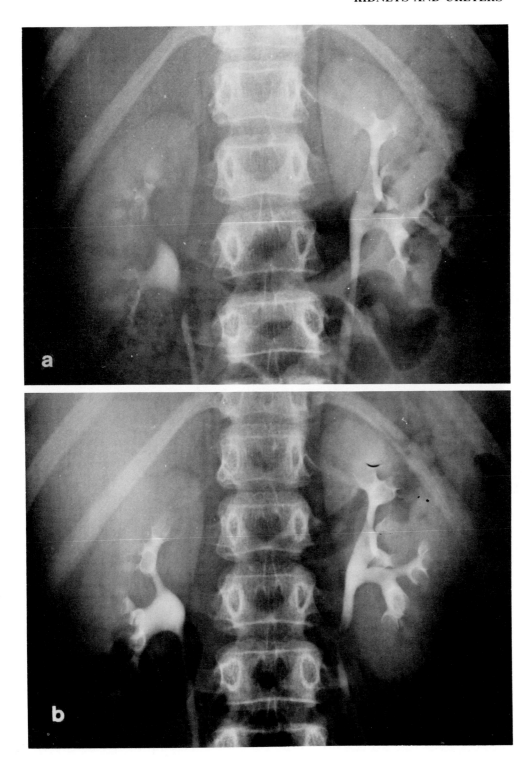

Fig. 9.10. Right renal contusion. Infusion pyelogram at the time of acute injury (**a**) reveals impaired visualization and spasm of the right collecting system as well as opacification of the renal tubules. One month later (**b**), the right collecting system was normal.

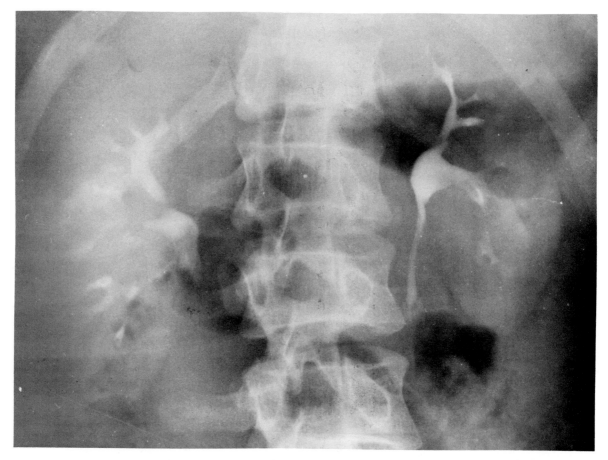

Fig. 9.11. Contusion of the right kidney. The right kidney is swollen and the nephrogram abnormally dense. The entire collecting system is diffusely distorted.

and urine may obscure the renal outline and the psoas shadow. Blood or urine which accumulates within the inferior portion of the perirenal space produces a cone shaped, sharply defined "mass" which displaces the colon laterally.

The collecting system of the lacerated kidney is recognizable on infusion pyelography, in contradistinction to the "shattered" kidney, where there is total loss of definition of the pelvocalyceal system. Early in the antegrade urogram, renal laceration may be indicated by a peripheral, nonopacified wedge shaped defect (Fig. 9.12) or by the absence of the upper (Fig. 9.13) or lower (Fig. 9.14) pole infundibulum or minor calyx. Abnormal collections of contrast may be seen in the renal parenchyma outside the collecting system (Fig. 9.13) or in the perirenal tissues (Fig. 9.14). When the laceration involves the upper pole, the extravasated blood and opacified urine in the perinephric fat medial to the upper pole of the kidney displaces the kidney and proximal ureter laterally (Fig. 9.13). When the fracture occurs in the medial or inferior pole, the blood and urine collects in the inferior perirenal space,

displacing the renal pelvis and proximal ureter medially (Fig. 9.14). Regardless of the location of the laceration, in the delayed radiograph of the urogram, blood and opacified urine will be seen in the conical inferior perirenal space as a homogeneous density which obliterates the psoas shadow and whose convex lateral margin extends from above downward inferiorly and medially as defined by the inferolateral wall of the inferior perirenal space (Figs. 9.13–9.15).

Shattered kidney is an uncommon lesion and consists of complete destruction or pulpifaction of the kidney with complete disruption of the intrarenal morphology. Because the kidney is completely disrupted, there is no renal image on the affected side. Irregular collections of contrast medium are present in the disorganized renal parenchyma and outside the renal capsule. Blood and/or urine in the inferior portion of the perirenal space displaces the ureter medially (Figs. 9.15 and 9.16).

Traumatic renal vascular lesions include renal artery thrombosis, renal vein thrombosis, and transection of the renal pedicle.

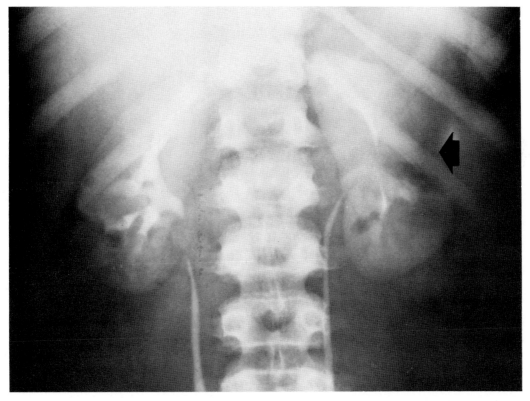

Fig. 9.12. Renal laceration. The triangular shaped defect (*arrow*) in the mid-third of the left kidney represents the area of laceration.

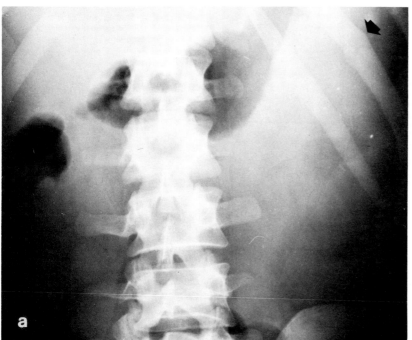

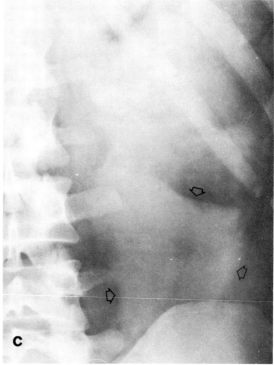

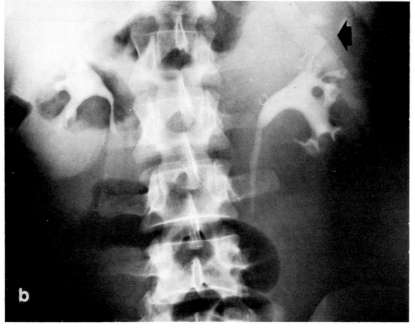

Fig. 9.13. Picture of the left kidney with large left retroperitoneal hematoma. In the supine radiograph of the abdomen (**a**), the soft tissue anatomy of the left retroperitoneal space is completely obliterated. A minimally displaced fracture is present in the left 10th rib (*arrow*). Infusion pyelography (**b**) demonstrates distortion of the left upper pole collecting system and puddling of contrast medium within the renal parenchyma (*arrow*). Opacified urine (*open arrows*) is present in the conical inferior portion of the perirenal space (**c**).

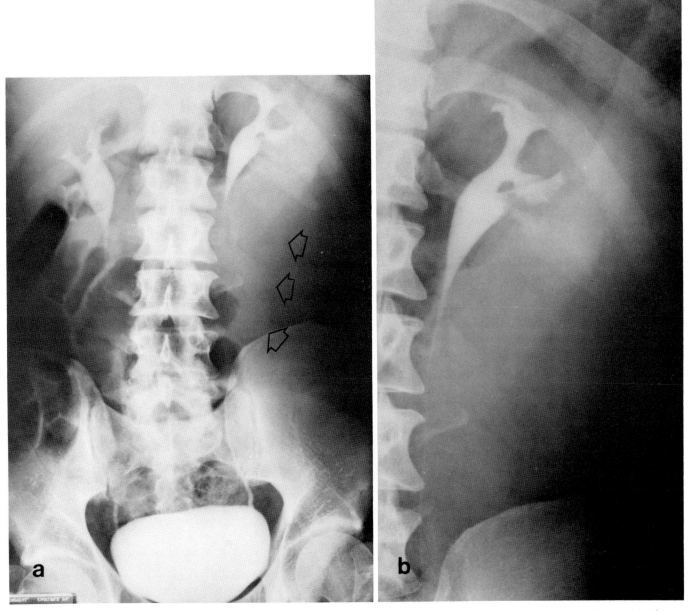

Fig. 9.14. (a, b) Fracture (laceration) of the left kidney. The middle infundibulum and minor calyx are distorted and only partially visible. The lower pole infundibulum and minor calyx are completely destroyed by the lower pole laceration. The renal pelvis and the proximal portion of the left ureter are medially displaced by a conical, homogeneous density which represents blood and urine in the inferior portion of the perirenal space (*open arrows*).

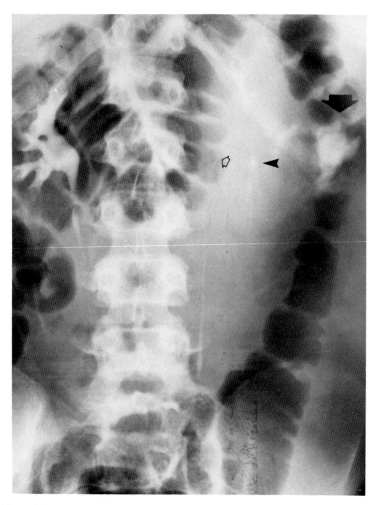

Fig. 9.15. Shattered kidney. The renal shadow is not discernible. The collecting system is completely disrupted and not visible. A small collection of contrast medium is present in the region of the lower pole (*arrowhead*) and large collections of contrast are present in the perirenal tissue lateral to the kidneys (*solid arrow*). The ureter (*open arrow*) is displaced medially and the descending colon laterally by the blood and urine in the inferior portion of the perirenal space.

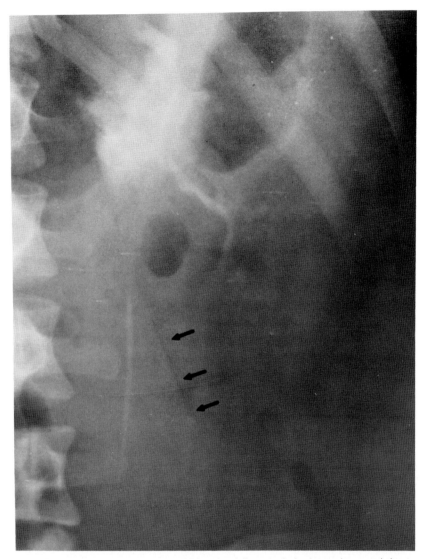

Fig. 9.16. Shattered kidney. The renal outline is completely obliterated. An irregular serpiginous collection of contrast is present in the disrupted renal substance. The collecting system is not identifiable. A large extrarenal collection of contrast medium is present adjacent to the superior portion of the psoas muscle. The ureter is circumferentially narrowed by extravasated blood and urine surrounding it within the perirenal space. Segments of the superior portion of the psoas shadow are visible through the density of the perinephric collection. This observation indicates that the extrarenal blood and urine are not free in the retroperitoneal space but are confined to the perirenal space.

Renal artery thrombosis occurs infrequently, involves the left kidney more commonly than the right, and is usually the result of abrupt deceleration injury. Pathologically, it consists of laceration of the intima just distal to the take-off of the renal artery, intimal dissection, and subintimal hemorrhage. Thrombosis of the renal artery may then occur consequent to these changes. Renal artery thrombosis is a potentially surgically curable lesion. Successful management of renal artery thrombosis depends, initially, at least, upon an awareness of the entity and its roentgen signs. He-

maturia, even microscopic, following blunt abdominal trauma, together with a fracture of a lower rib or upper lumbar transverse process should suggest that diagnosis and initiate a prompt infusion pyelogram. In renal artery thrombosis, if the renal shadow is visible, it will be of normal size and configuration and the kidney will be nonfunctioning on infusion pyelography. These circumstances demand immediate aortography or renal arteriography, which will demonstrate occlusion of the renal artery (Fig. 9.17).

Renal *vein* thrombosis, conversely, is characterized

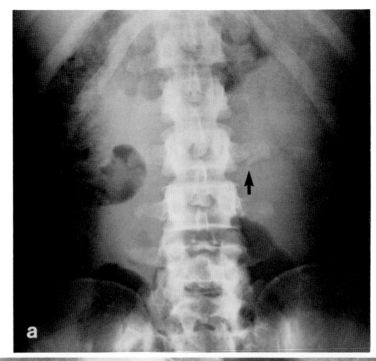

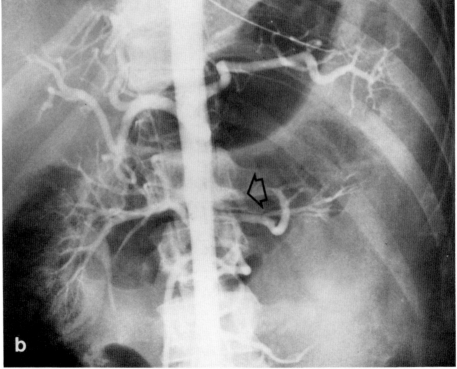

Fig. 9.17. Renal artery thrombosis. The plain radiograph of the abdomen **(a)** demonstrates a fracture of the left transverse process of L₃ (*arrow*) and focal bulging of the left psoas muscle. The left kidney was not visualized on infusion pyelography and complete occlusion of the left renal artery (*open arrow*) was established on the abdominal aortogram **(b)**.

by an enlarged renal shadow, a dense nephrogram, and delayed and impaired renal function on antegrade urography. Renal arteriography demonstrates a normal arterial phase, a dense and prolonged nephrogram, and the absence of contrast medium in the collecting system (Fig. 9.18).

Impaired or absent visualization of a kidney by antegrade urography following blunt abdominal trauma requires immediate renal angiography.

Transection of the renal pedicle is a rare injury, usually associated with massive trauma. If the renal shadow is not obscured by retroperitoneal hemorrhage, it will be laterally displaced and may be rotated along its longitudinal axis (Fig. 9.19).

Hepatic and splenic injuries are the most common nonskeletal lesions associated with renal trauma. The frequency of associated hepatic and splenic rupture with renal injury is directly proportional to the severity of the renal injury (17). The plain abdominal radiograph will demonstrate the signs of both intra- and extraperitoneal hemorrhage and the hepatic or splenic shadows will be either enlarged (subcapsular hematoma) or obscured (extracapsular hemorrhage) (Fig. 9.21).

The roentgen appearance of penetrating injuries of the kidneys depends largely upon the direction, nature, and velocity of the penetrating foreign body. The rapid dissipation of energy associated with the passage of a high velocity missile close to, but not directly injuring, the kidney may be sufficient to temporarily impair renal function to the degree that only a nephrogram may be seen on infusion pyelography (Fig. 9.20). Such impairment of function is caused by a shock-wave concussion of the kidney.

Retroperitoneal hemorrhage results from rupture of a retroperitoneal organ or from laceration of the psoas muscle or the muscles of the abdominal wall. Major laceration of the kidney is accompanied by leakage of urine, as well as blood, into the retroperitoneal space.

Radiographically, the retroperitoneal accumulation of fluid is marked by obliteration of the renal and psoas shadows and the presence of a soft tissue density which represents the hematoma (Fig. 9.13). Lumbar scoliosis due to splinting or muscle spasm has been described as a classic radiographic sign associated with a retroperitoneal hematoma. However, scoliosis is *not* a constant roentgen sign of retroperitoneal hemorrhage. When present, the concavity is on the side of the hematoma.

Retroperitoneal hemorrhage occurring without visceral injury is most frequently the result of fracture of the lumbar transverse processes and laceration of the psoas muscle (Fig. 9.22).

When the hemorrhage associated with lumbar transverse process fracture is contained within the psoas muscle mass, the shadow of the lateral margin of the muscle may be indistinct (Fig. 9.23) or bulge laterally (18).

Injury of the ureters is rare and, when caused by external trauma, usually due to a penetrating force. The commonest injuries of the ureters are associated with instrumentation or laparotomy (15).

Nontraumatic Lesions

Inflammatory disease, neoplasia, and calculi may all produce signs and symptoms of acute urinary tract disease. The differential diagnosis of acute right ureteral colic and acute appendicitis has frequently been challenging in our experience. The diagnostic enigma arises when the inflamed appendix lies in proximity to the ureter and produces an inflammatory response of the ureter, resulting in microscopic hematuria. The puzzle has been resolved by an infusion pyelogram delineating a normal right ureter.

Inflammation

Radiographic evidence of acute pyelonephritis consists, when present, of persistent spasm of the collecting system (Fig. 9.24). This is not a pathognomonic roentgen sign. Segmental or diffuse spasm ("irritability") of the pelvocalyceal system only suggests the possibility of acute pyelonephritis. The diagnosis must be established on the basis of clinical findings and appropriate laboratory studies.

Perinephric abscess produces roentgen signs similar to a retroperitoneal hemorrhage. The margins of the renal shadow are indistinct or obliterated, the margin of the proximal portion of the psoas shadow illdefined or absent, and lumbar scoliosis with the concavity to the affected sign is common.

Calculus

In our opinion, ureteral colic constitutes a medical emergency and infusion pyelography should be performed promptly. We have observed that if the infusion pyelogram is performed within 8 hours after onset of symptoms, renal function on the involved side will still be maintained to the degree that, even in the face of complete obstruction, contrast medium will be elaborated in sufficient quantity to opacify the ureter and localize the site of obstruction within an hour following the infusion. When symptoms have been present beyond 8 hours, the elaboration of contrast material from the affected kidney decreases significantly and it requires an appreciably longer period of time to confirm the site of obstruction. Further, there seems to be a direct relationship between the duration of symptoms and the length of time required to opacify the involved ureter. The pathophysiologic basis for this roentgen observation is the effect of increased hydrostatic pressure upon renal function.

The supine radiograph of the abdomen, alone, is an

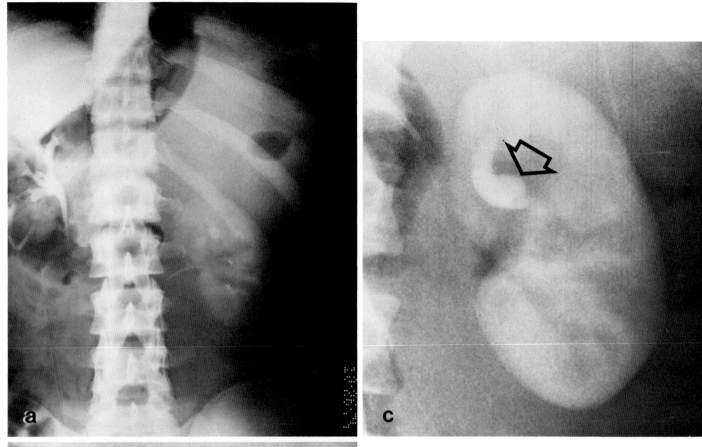

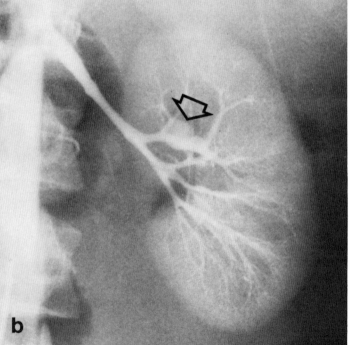

Fig. 9.18. Renal vein thrombosis. The left kidney is swollen and the nephrogram prolonged and abnormally dense. On infusion pyelography (**a**), the ureteropelvocalyceal system is incompletely opacified. A large suprarenal hematoma displaces the stomach medially and the left kidney inferiorly. In the arterial phase of the renal arteriogram (**b**), the renal artery is attenuated secondary to inferior displacement of the left kidney. The arterial pattern is normal, but an abnormal extravascular collection of contrast medium (*open arrow*) is seen in the hilum of the kidney. In the delayed phase of the arteriogram (**c**), no contrast is seen in either the renal venous system or the collecting system. The extravascular collection of contrast (*open arrow*) marks the site of the renal vein laceration.

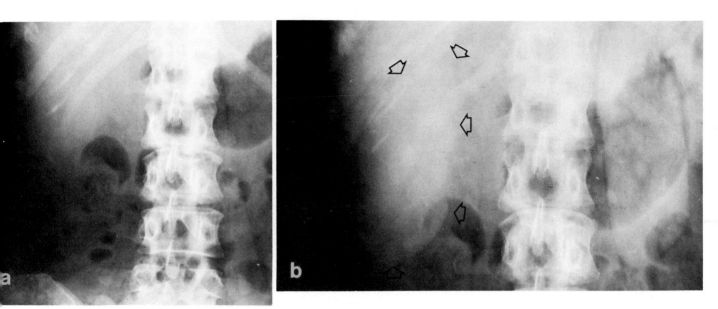

Fig. 9.19. Transected right renal pedicle. In the supine examination of the abdomen (**a**), the liver, kidney, and psoas shadows are completely obscured by a large retroperitoneal hematoma. An infusion pyelogram (**b**) was performed in the face of severe shock. Only a nephrogram was demonstrated on the left. The right kidney is very faintly opacified (*open arrows*), is laterally displaced, and is slightly rotated in a clockwise direction on its longitudinal axis. At laparotomy, the liver was extensively lacerated and the right kidney was "practically transected" from the aorta.

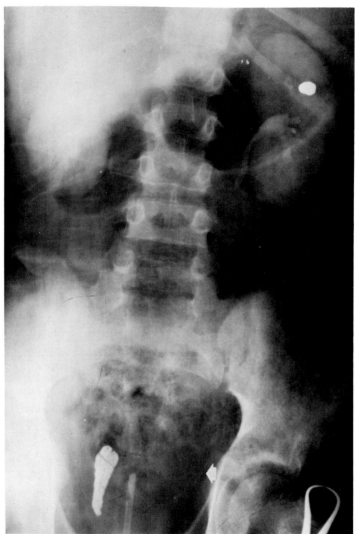

Fig. 9.20. Infusion pyelogram performed on a patient who was shot at close range with a high velocity missile. The bullet, which entered the right flank, passed through the liver, anterior to the right kidney, and lodged in the soft tissues anterior to the left kidney. At laparotomy, the right kidney was intact. The impaired right renal function is due to the blast concussion of the missile passing close to the kidney. Notice that even in the presence of severe shock (BP 60/0), infusion pyelography resulted in a diagnostic urogram. The distal portion of the left ureter is indicated by the *white arrow*.

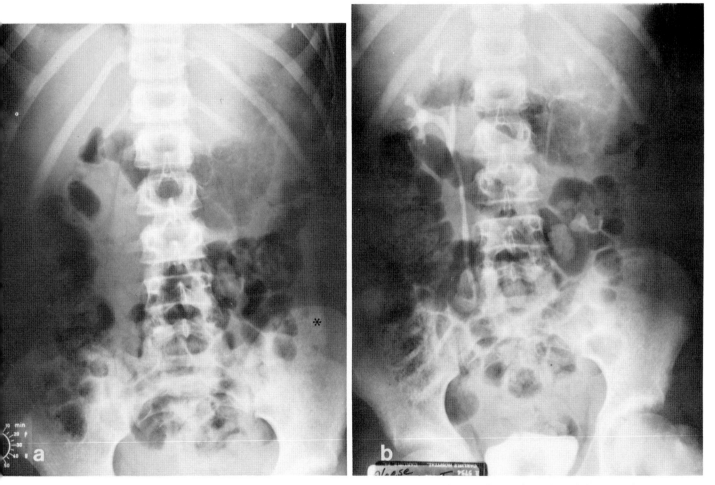

Fig. 9.21. Concomitant shattered left kidney and splenic rupture. In the plain radiograph of the abdomen (**a**), the splenic shadow is obliterated and blood is present in the left paracolic gutter, (*) indicating hemoperitoneum. The left renal and psoas shadows are obscured, indicating a large left retroperitoneal hemorrhage. The infusion pyelogram (**b**) demonstrates gross distortion of the left collecting system and extravasated contrast medium lateral to the kidney. The homogeneous density between the bladder and the pelvic ilial loops represents blood in the pouch of Douglas.

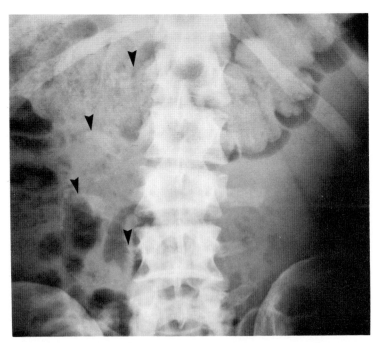

Fig. 9.22. Right retroperitoneal hematoma. The right psoas shadow is completely obliterated by blood in the retroperitoneal space and laceration of the psoas muscle. Displaced fractures involve the upper four right lumbar transverse processes (*arrowheads*).

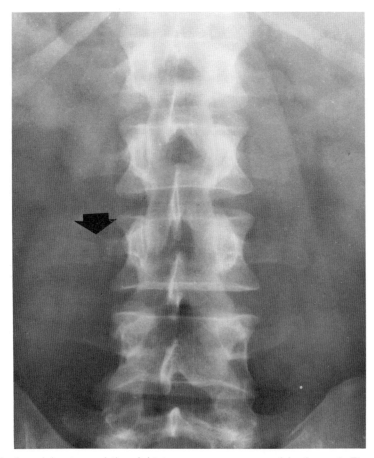

Fig. 9.23. Minimally displaced fracture of the right transverse process of L₃ (*arrow*). The right psoas shadow is indistinct. The left is sharply defined.

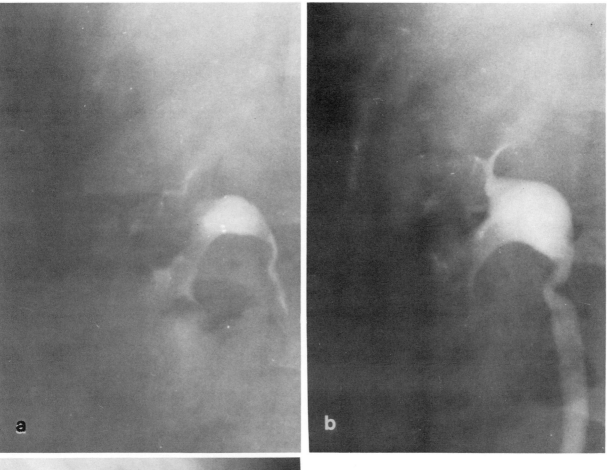

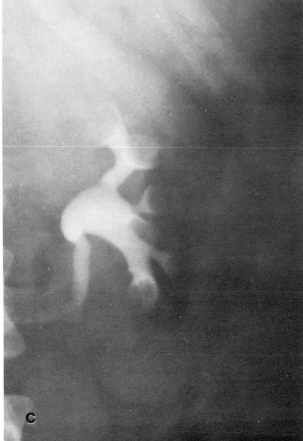

Fig. 9.24. Acute pyelonephritis. The diagnosis was established clinically. The right pelvocalyceal system was irritable and spastic throughout the urographic study (a, b) and the contrast medium in the right collecting system less dense than that in the uninvolved left (c).

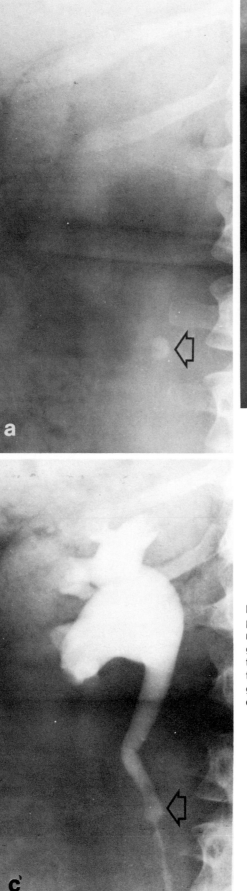

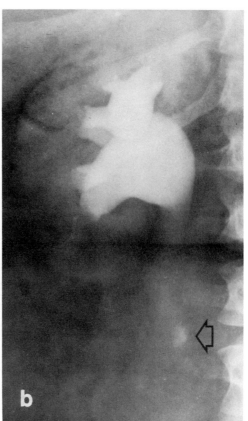

Fig. 9.25. Large round calculus in the mid-portion of the right ureter (*arrow*). The rounded density is seen on the survey radiograph of the abdomen (**a**), its location within the ureter is established by the dilatation of the right collecting system (**b**), and the degree of its obstruction is indicated in the delayed roentgenogram (**c**).

inadequate roentgen study for the evaluation of a patient with urinary colic because (1) approximately 10% of urinary calculi are nonopaque and, therefore, would not be visible on a survey radiograph of the abdomen; (2) small opaque calculi are readily obscured by intestinal artifacts or the density of lumbar transverse processes and the sacrum; and (3) calcified mesenteric lymph nodes and pelvic phleboliths may simulate ureteral calculi. For these reasons, and because antegrade urography is the only method whereby both the quality of renal function and the site and degree of ureteral obstruction can be established (Fig. 9.25), infusion pyelography should be the roentgen study requested when the clinical differential diagnosis includes urinary calculus.

Urinary calculi composed of uric acid, cystine, or xanthine crystals are radiographically nonopaque. The presence and location of these calculi is best established by antegrade pyelography.

Occasionally, a ureteral calculus will have passed through the ureterovesical junction immediately prior to or during infusion pyelography. Under such circumstances, edema and spasm of the ureterovesical orifice may result in a temporary obstruction at this site with minor ureteropelvocaliectasis. Thus, it may be very difficult, if not impossible, to radiographically distinguish between an obstruction at the ureterovesical orifice caused by edema or by a tiny calculus.

In acute ureteral obstruction, opacified urine may appear in the peripelvic and periureteral tissue during urography (Fig. 9.26) (19). This extravasation is the result of increased hydrostatic pressure causing leakage of urine from the fornices. It should not be interpreted as indicating renal or ureteral rupture.

Neoplasm

Hypernephroma, by causing costovertebral angle pain, tenderness, fever, hematuria, and ureteral colic, may simulate an acute upper urinary tract process. The roentgen signs of malignant tumor of the kidney may include the presence of a renal mass, distortion of the collecting system, including pinching off of minor calyces and infundibulae and, in 10–15% of cases, calcification within the tumor (20). The distinction between a hypernephroma and a renal cyst may be presumed on the basis of the urographic or nephrotomographic characteristics of the collecting system and the degree of opacification of the mass. The differentiation can be made, in the great majority of patients by ultrasound or computed tomography.

Ureteral displacement may indicate the size and location of a retroperitoneal tumor (Fig. 9.27), enlarged para-aortic (Fig. 9.28) or pelvic (Fig. 9.29) lymph nodes, abdominal aortic aneurysm (Fig. 9.30), and intraperitoneal masses (Fig. 9.31).

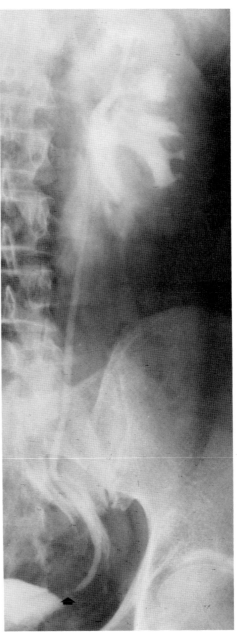

Fig. 9.26. Extravasation of opacified urine into the peripelvic and periureteral tissues during infusion pyelography in acute ureteral obstruction.

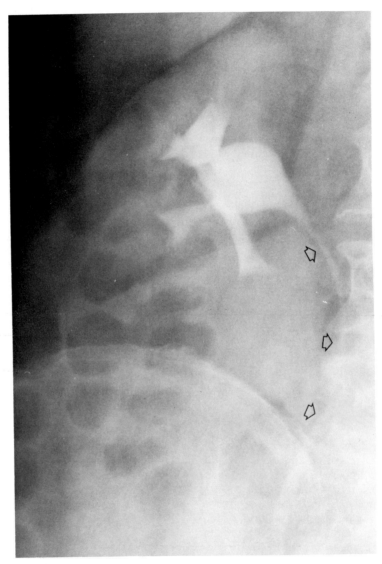

Fig. 9.27. Large hypernephroma of the lower pole of the right kidney. The outline of the lower half of the right kidney is completely lost. The middle and lower pole minor calyces are distorted. The proximal portion of the ureter is medially displaced by the tumor mass.

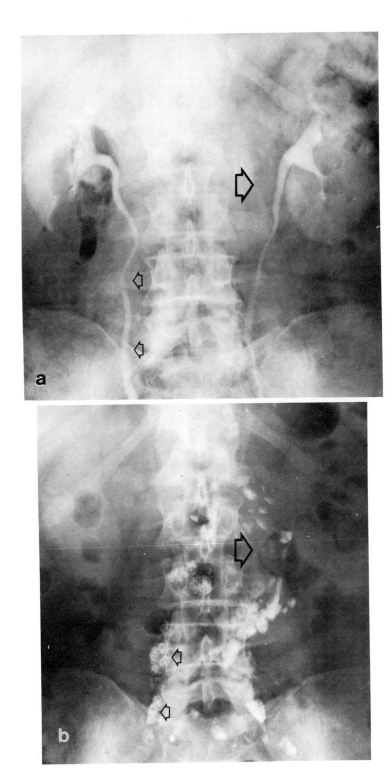

Fig. 9.28. Infusion pyelogram **(a)** demonstrating multiple sites of ureteral displacement (*open arrows*) by enlarged para-aortic lymph nodes. The lymphangiogram **(b)** performed on the same patient indicates nodal masses (*open arrows*) corresponding to the sites of ureteral displacement.

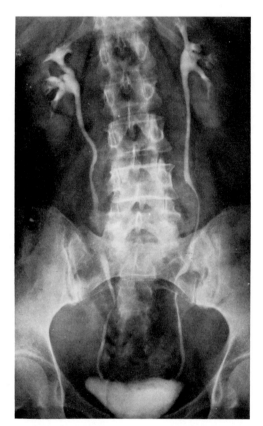

Fig. 9.29. Extensive ureteral displacement by enlarged lymph nodes. Medial displacement of the pelvic portion of each ureter indicates the presence of laterally situated pelvic masses in a patient with lymphoma.

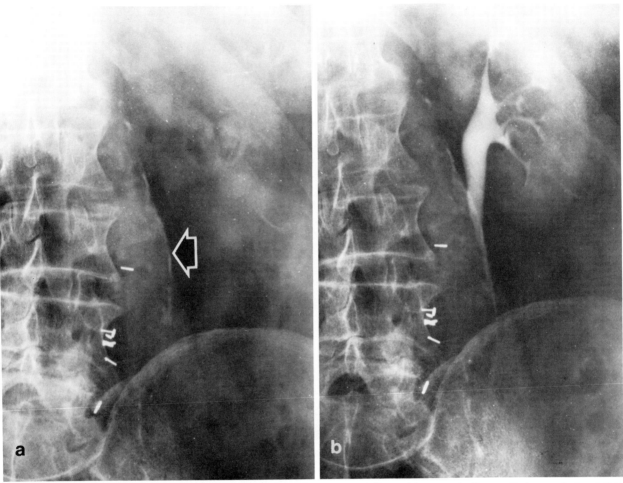

Fig. 9.30. Calcification in the wall of an abdominal aortic aneurysm (*arrow*) is seen in the preliminary study of the abdomen (**a**). The opacified left ureter is seen to be laterally displaced by the aneurysm (**b**).

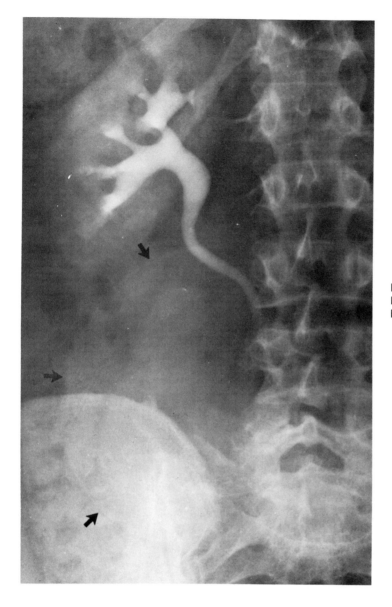

Fig. 9.31. The right ureter is medially displaced by a mesenteric cyst, the thin, sharp lateral border of which is indicated by the *arrows*.

References

1. MITCHELL JP: Trauma to the urinary tract. *New Engl J Med* 288:90, 1973.
2. SCHNECKER B: Drip infusion pyelography; indications and applications in urologic roentgen diagnosis. *Radiology* 83:12, 1964.
3. HARRIS JH, HARRIS JH JR: Infusion pyelography. *AJR* 92:1391, 1964.
4. MORSE TS: Infusion pyelography in the evaluation of renal injuries in children. *Trauma* 6:693, 1966.
5. OLSSON O, LUNDERQUIST A: Angiography in renal trauma. *Acta Radiol* 1:1, 1963.
6. HEMLEY SD, FINBY N: Renal trauma. *Radiology* 79:816, 1962.
7. COLLINS HA, JACOBS JK: Acute arterial injuries due to blunt trauma. *J Bone Joint Surg* 43-A:193, 1961.
8. JOSE JS: Angiography in renal trauma. *Br J Urol* 40:448, 1968.
9. BANOWSKY LH, WOLFEL DA, LACKNES LH: Considerations in diagnosis and management of renal trauma. *J Trauma* 10:587, 1970.
10. ELKIN M, MENG CH, DePAREDES RG: Correlation of intravenous urography and renal angiography in kidney injury. *Radiology* 86:496, 1966.
11. MEYERS MA, WHALEN JP, PEELLE K, BERNE AS: Radiologic features of extraperitoneal effusions. *Radiology* 104:249–257, 1972.
12. BASMAJIAN JV: *Grant's Method of Anatomy*, ed. 8. Williams & Wilkins, Baltimore, 1971.
13. RIESER C: Injuries of the kidney. *Am Surg* 25:657, 1959.
14. EMMETT JL, WITTEN BM: *Clinical Urography.* W.B. Saunders, Philadelphia, 1971.
15. PERSKY L: Injuries of the kidneys and ureters. *Med Sci* April: 49, 1966.
16. SARGENT JC, MARQUADT DR: Renal injuries. *J Urol* 63:1, 1950.
17. CASS AS, IRELAND GW: Management of renal injuries in the severely injured patient. *Trauma* 12:516, 1972.
18. McCORT JJ: *Radiographic Examination in Blunt Abdominal Trauma.* W.B. Saunders, Philadelphia, 1966.
19. ELKIN M: Obstructive uropathy and uremia. *Radiol Clin North Am* 10:447, 1972.
20. KINCAID CW: *Renal Angiography.* Year Book Medical Publishers, Chicago, 1966.

chapter ten

Pelvis and Hips

General Considerations

For the purpose of this discussion, the pelvis shall be determined to consist of the bony pelvis, including the sacrum and coccyx, the extraperitoneal soft tissue structures within the bony pelvis, and the hips.

Injuries involving the pelvis and its contents result in some of the most challenging and serious diagnostic problems to confront the physician involved in the practice of emergency medicine. Radiographically, this is particularly true for two reasons. First, the pelvis is the single area of the body which defies the radiologic dictum of obtaining useful roentgenograms in both frontal and lateral projections. Secondly, the soft tissue injuries frequently associated with the skeletal damage, even though radiographically much less striking than the skeletal changes, may be of far greater clinical significance than the skeletal injury.

The principal cause of death associated with pelvic trauma is hemorrhage, previously estimated to be as high as 30% in patients with major pelvic trauma. Interventional angiography (2,3) has resulted in a significant reduction in this mortality rate.

Rupture of the bladder or urethral laceration or transection occurs in approximately 20% of patients with significant anterior pelvic arch injuries. Some authors (16,23,24) believed that *all* patients with major pelvic trauma should be evaluated for bladder or urethral injury.

The proper evaluation of urethral injuries requires retrograde urethrocystography (26–33) performed under fluoroscopic control. The "diagnostic" (blind) insertion of a urethral catheter and the "single-shot" urethrogram performed in the emergency department are both to be condemned: the diagnostic catheterization because of the possibilities of iatrogenic urethral injury, introduction of infection, initiation or reactivation of bleeding, or the extension of an existing urethral laceration, and the "single-shot" urethrogram because of the probability of obtaining an inadequate or false negative study.

Insertion of a Foley catheter as an initial procedure and prior to urethrocystography should be reserved for those patients so critically injured that a urethral injury is of relatively low immediate priority. All other patients suspected of having a urethral injury, either clinically or on the basis of radiographically demonstrated anterior pelvic arch trauma, should have a retrograde cystourethrogram to establish the indication for therapeutic catheterization.

The pain that results from a fracture of the hip and the pain of a fracture of the anterior pelvic arch are quite similar and frequently the patient is unable to discern the precise location of the pain. It is frequently impossible, on the basis of the patient's symptoms and the clinical signs, to distinguish a fracture of the hip from one of the anterior pelvic arch or other adjacent skeletal parts. Therefore, in every patient suspected of having a hip fracture, the entire pelvis must be examined in frontal projection and, particularly when the femur is negative, the pubis and ischium and ileum must be carefully studied for the presence of a fracture.

Radiographic Examination

The routine radiographic examination of the pelvis is the anteroposterior view (Fig. 10.1). This projection must include the iliac crests, each hip joint, and the femur distal to the lesser trochanter.

A lateral projection of the pelvis provides little useful information because of the superimposition of very dense skeletal parts and is, therefore, rarely indicated. The spatial relationships of the pelvis can be demonstrated by special views such as oblique or tangential radiographs, anteroposterior projections of

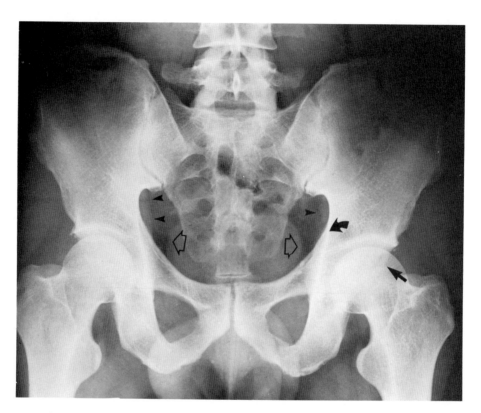

Fig. 10.1. Anteroposterior radiograph of the normal adult pelvis. This examination must include the entire bony pelvis from the iliac crests to the ischial tuberosities as well as each hip and the proximal portion of each femur. The belly of the obturator internus muscles (*arrowheads*) and the urinary bladder (*open arrows*) are soft tissue structures normally present in the pelvic extraperitoneal space and are commonly radiographically visible. The *curved arrow* indicates the ilioischial line (the cortical surface of the quadralateral plate) and the *stemmed arrow*, the posterior acetabular rim projecting through the femoral head.

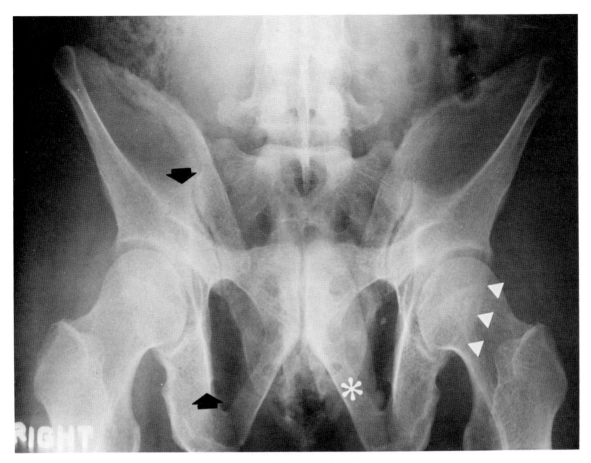

Fig. 10.2. Anteroposterior radiograph of a normal adult pelvis made with the central beam angle 35° cephalad and centered on the pubic symphysis. Although the femora are distorted, there is excellent visualization of the posterior acetabular rim (*arrowhead*), the inferior pubic rami (*), and the entire extent of the quadralateral plate (*solid arrows*) of the pelvis.

the pelvis made with the x-ray tube angled cephalically and caudally, and computed tomograms. In the interest of reducing unnecessary patient radiation and eliminating unnecessary movement of the patient required to obtain oblique or tangential views, the anteroposterior roentgenograms of the hips and pelvis should be obtained initially and carefully studied from the point of view that the pelvis is, in fact, a three-dimensional structure. Only when this "survey" radiograph of the pelvis is studied in this fashion and the examination found to be inconclusive, should additional views be obtained.

The cephalad (Fig. 10.2) and caudad (Fig. 10.3) angled anteroposterior projections of the pelvis are particularly useful in instances of trauma (Fig. 10.4) because they more accurately delineate the extent and relationship of pelvic fractures and joint disruptions.

The os pubis and the ischii are canted posteriorly approximately 30°. Consequently, the anteroposterior radiograph of the pelvis more correctly represents an oblique view of the anterior pelvic arch. It is, therefore, quite possible to overlook minimally displaced fractures of this portion of the pelvis in the straight anteroposterior radiograph. In order to thoroughly radiographically examine the margins of the obturator foramen, oblique views (Figs. 10.5 and 10.6) of the anterior pelvic arch are required (Fig. 10.7).

The iliac wing is a concave structure, and, as such, is not completely visualized in the routine anteroposterior radiograph of the pelvis. When the clinical findings suggest injury to the iliac crest or wing, oblique views of the iliac wing should be obtained.

The routine examination of the hip includes anteroposterior (Fig. 10.8a) and lateral (Fig. 10.8b) projections.

Distinction must be made between true lateral and "frog-leg lateral" projections of the hip. The true (horizontal beam, cross table, "groin") projection is obtained with the patient supine and the injured lower extremity in full extension. The opposite, uninvolved

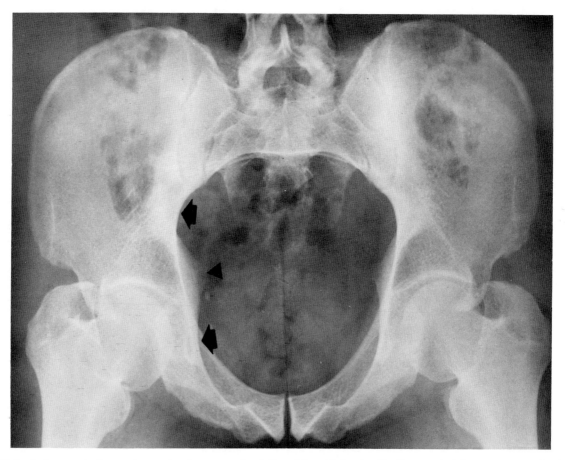

Fig. 10.3. Anteroposterior radiograph of a normal adult pelvis obtained with the central beam centered midway between the superior margin of the pubic symphysis and the umbilicus and angled 35° caudad. This projection provides excellent visualization of the pelvic inlet including the sacral promontory and the iliopectineal line (*solid arrows*), the geometry of the pubic symphysis, and the ischial spines (*arrowhead*).

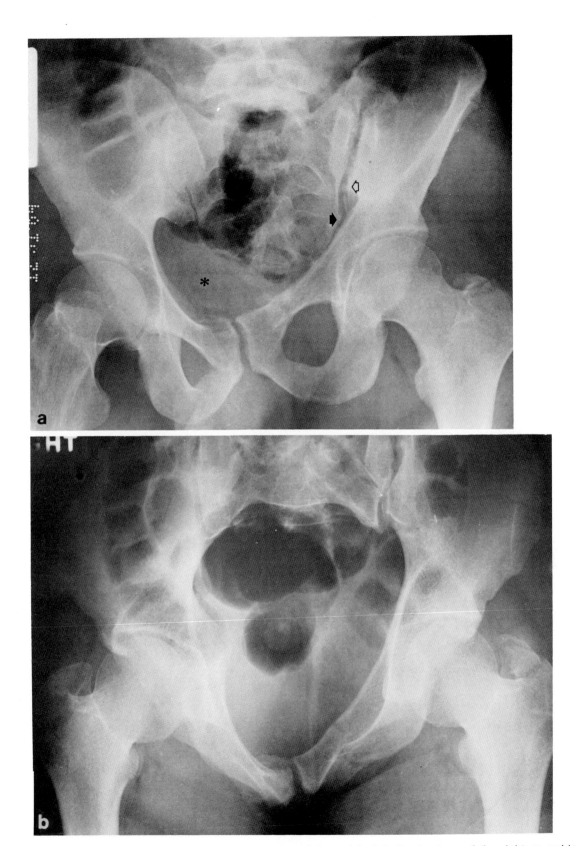

Fig. 10.4. In the straight anteroposterior roentgenogram of the pelvis **(a)**, the fracture of the right os pubis and asymmetry of the left side of the pelvis is obvious. Dislocation of the left sacroiliac joint is not readily identifiable. The *solid* and *open arrows* indicate the contiguous margins of the inferior aspect of the sacral and iliac components, respectively, of the joint. In the caudally angled frontal projection **(b)**, fractures of the left pubic rami and separation of the left sacroiliac joint are obvious.

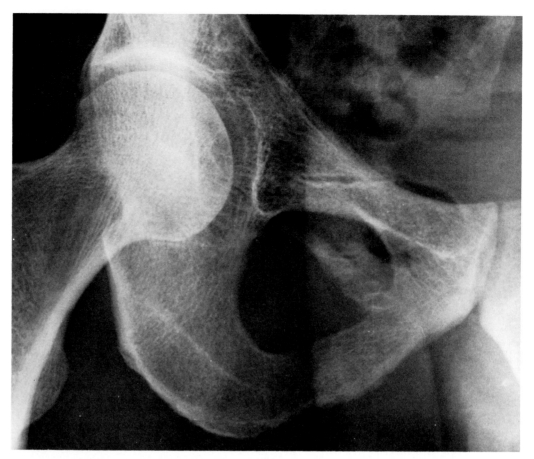

Fig. 10.5. Supine, right anterior oblique view of the obturator foramen. This examination can be obtained with the patient in the right anterior oblique projection, either prone or supine. This projection provides the true frontal examination of the os pubis and ischium. The radiolucent defect with densely sclerotic margins is the S₄-S₅ interspace superimposed upon the superior pubic ramus.

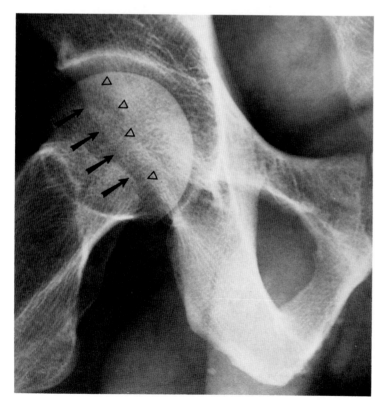

Fig. 10.6. Supine, right posterior oblique radiograph of the right hip of a normal adult. The *stemmed arrows* indicate the posterior acetabular lip and the *open arrowheads*, the anterior lip. With further posterior rotation, this relationship would be reversed.

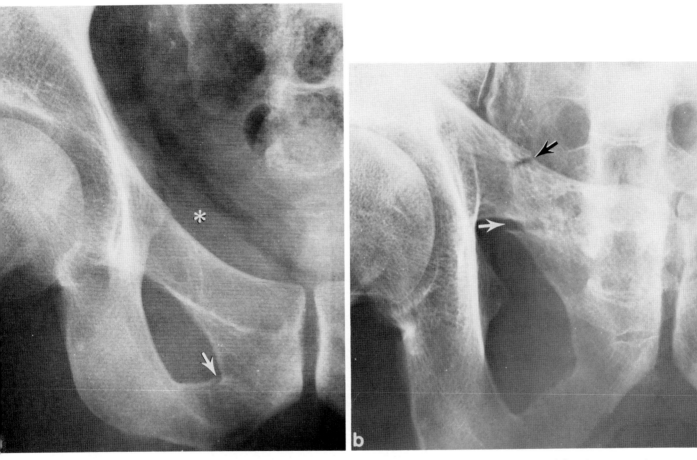

Fig. 10.7. This 63 year old man injured his right hip in a fall from a height. In the frontal projection **(a)**, a fracture at the junction of the inferior ramus and the body (*arrow*) of the right pubis is evident. No fracture is seen in the superior ramus, but the shadow of the aponeurosis of the obturator internus muscle (*) is abnormally prominent, indicative of subperiosteal hemorrhage deep to the aponeurosis which, in turn, suggests a fracture of the superior ramus. The supine, right anterior oblique projection **(b)** clearly demonstrates the superior ramus fracture (*arrows*).

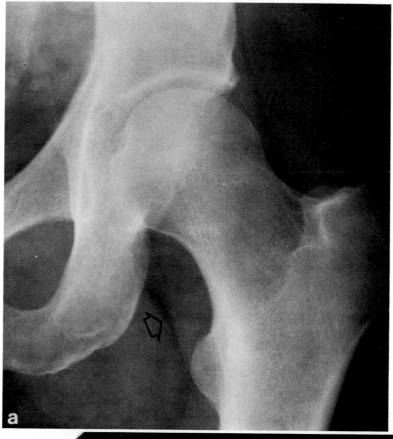

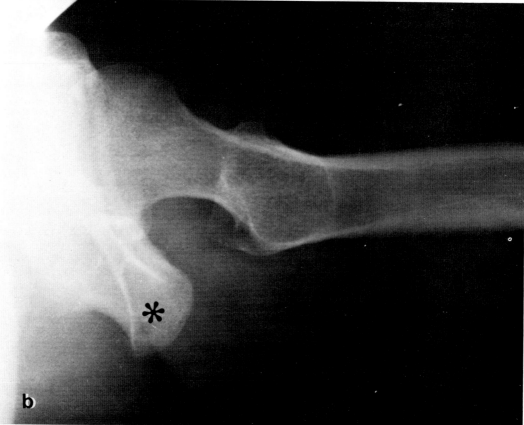

Fig. 10.8. The frontal projection of a normal adult hip is seen in **(a)**. The *superior arrow* indicates areolar tissue covering the piriform muscle. The *inferior arrow* indicates the margin of the iliopsoas muscle shadow. These muscles lie immediately upon the capsule of the hip joint. When the capsule is distended by fluid or pus, these shadows will become displaced, convex, and indistinct. The small concavity in the center of the articulating surface of the femoral head is the fovea centralis which serves for the attachment of the ligament of the femoral head (ligamentum teres). Normal horizontal beam (cross table, "groin") lateral radiograph of the hip **(b)**. The normal relationship of the femoral head to the neck, the approximate 120° posterior angulation at the junction of the neck and shaft, and the posterior aspect of the greater trochanter are all well seen. The *asterisk* indicates the ischial tuberosity.

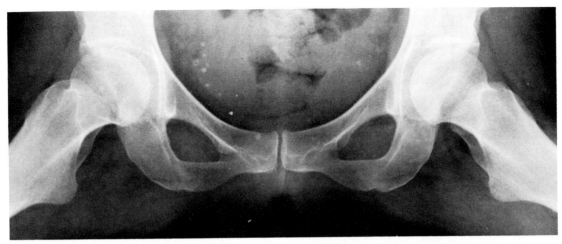

Fig. 10.9. "Frog-leg" radiograph of the hips. This projection is obtained with the femora flexed approximately 45° and maximally passively abducted. The proximal femora are, therefore, seen in *oblique*, rather than lateral, position. The greater trochanter is superimposed upon the femoral neck and the femoral neck shaft angle is not recorded. This projection is contraindicated in patients suspected of injury of the pelvis or hip.

hip and knee are each flexed approximately 90° and the ipsilateral foot supported off the radiographic table by a low stool or box. The x-ray tube is then positioned so that the beam is parallel to the table top, with the central ray directed mediolaterally parallel to and in the same vertical plane as the inguinal crease (groin). The cassette is firmly positioned against the flank between the iliac crest and the 12th rib on the *injured side*, perpendicular to the central ray. This beam cassette geometry results in the true lateral radiograph of the hip (Fig. 10.8*b*), which is essential for the complete evaluation of injuries of the proximal portion of the femur.

The frog-leg lateral, on the other hand, is actually an oblique projection of the proximal portion of the femur and is obtained with the patient supine and the femora abducted and externally rotated. The x-ray tube is vertically positioned with respect to the patient (and the radiographic table) and centered over the pubic symphysis. The resultant radiograph (Fig. 10.9) depicts the femora in midposition between true anteroposterior and true lateral positions. The frog leg lateral radiograph is *inappropriate* in the evaluation of the patient with an acute injury of the hip because of the manipulation of the hip necessary to achieve this view and because neither the femoral neck shaft angle nor the trochanters can be evaluated.

The routine radiographic examination of the sacrum and coccyx must include a straight anteroposterior projection (Fig. 10.10*a*) as well as anteroposterior views with the central beam angled cephalad (Fig. 10.10*b*) and caudad (Fig. 10.10*c*) in order to adequately visualize the concave sweep of the sacrum and coccyx. A true lateral radiograph of the sacrum and

coccyx is also required (Fig. 10.10*d*).

Retrograde urethrography, because it is not associated with the complications of catheterization and because the urethrogram provides much more information than simply whether the urethra is intact or not, is the preferred method of evaluating possible urethral or bladder injury. The purpose of infusion pyelography is to evaluate the status of the kidneys, ureters, and bladder. The location of the pelvic portion of the ureters and the configuration and position of the bladder are valuable in assessing the magnitude of pelvic effusion (1). These studies are mutually complementary.

The importance of hypogastric arteriography and the efficacy of transcatheter embolization in the localization (Fig. 10.11) and control (Fig. 10.12) of posttraumatic pelvic hemorrhage has been clearly established (2–4).

Ultrasound is very useful in the detection of intraperitoneal fluid, particularly that located in the pouch of Douglas, is sensitive, and is frequently specific in the identification of pelvic masses, cysts, and abscess. Ultrasound is valuable in the evaluation of obstetrical and gynecological emergencies such as ectopic pregnancy, missed abortion, and tubo-ovarian abscesses. However, the sonographic findings are not necessarily specific in these instances and close clinical and laboratory correlation is required to establish the precise diagnosis.

Radiographic Anatomy

The radiograph of the normal adult pelvis is seen in Figure 10.1. Figure 10.13 is the radiographic ap-

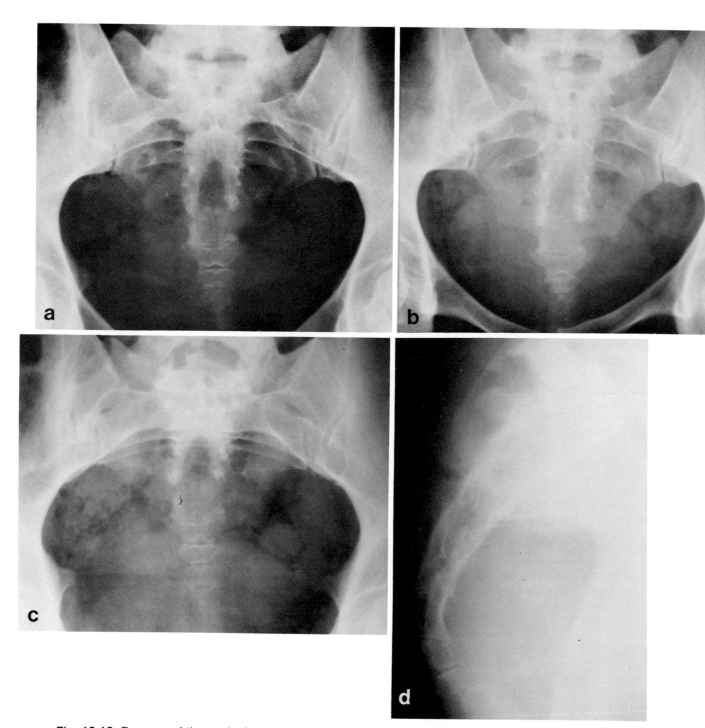

Fig. 10.10. Because of the marked concavity of the sacrum, the straight frontal projection **(a)** does not adequately visualize the superior and inferior extent of the concave arc. In order to examine these segments of the sacrum and coccyx more thoroughly in frontal projection, an anteroposterior view is obtained with the central beam angled toward the head **(b)** and toward the feet **(c)**. The lateral examination of the sacrum is seen in **(d)**.

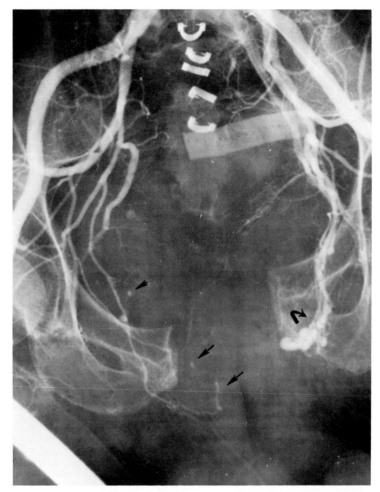

Fig. 10.11. Pelvic arteriogram demonstrating multiple points of extravasation from the pudendal artery on the right side and a traumatic arteriovenous fistula on the left. (Courtesy of Christos A. Athanasoulis, M.D.)

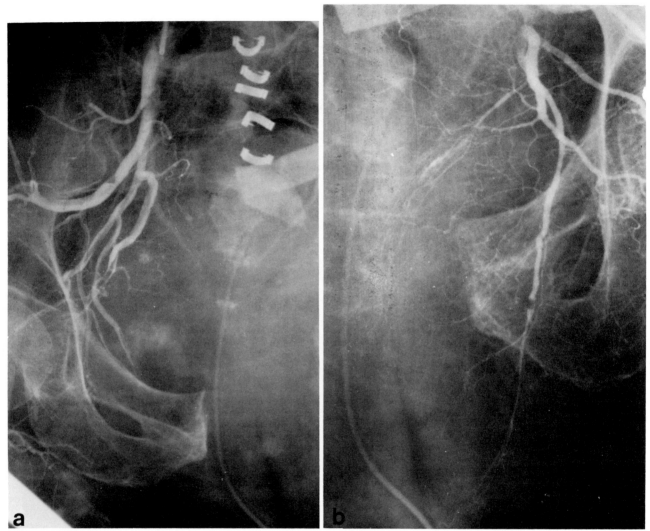

Fig. 10.12. Same patient as Figure 10.11. Selective right and left hypogastric arteriogram following embolization with autologous blood clot. On the right **(a)**, there is no further extravasation and on the left **(b)**, the arteriovenous fistula has been occluded. (Courtesy of Christos A. Athansoulis, M.D.)

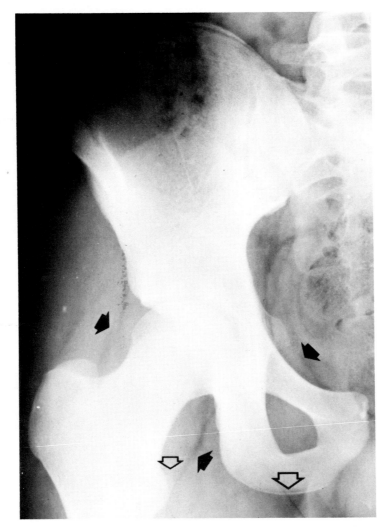

Fig. 10.13. Frontal projection of the normal pelvis of an adolescent. The *open arrows* indicate the ununited iliac crest, ischial tuberosity, and lesser trochanteric apophysis. The *solid arrows* indicate the "capsule" of the hip joint and the shadow of the aponeurosis of the obturator muscle.

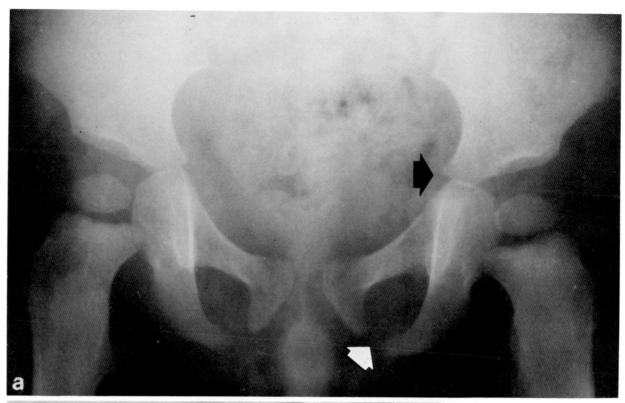

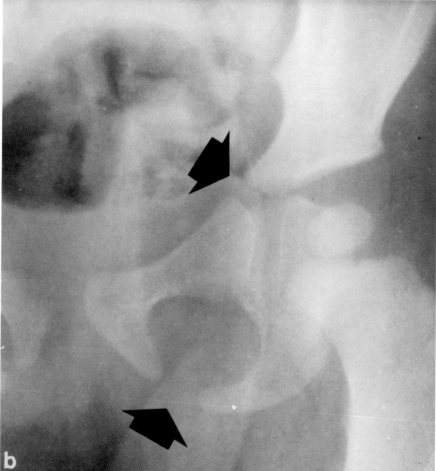

Fig. 10.14. Radiographic appearance of the normal pelvis of a child seen in straight frontal **(a)** and oblique **(b)** projections. The ischiopubic synchondrosis fuses between the ages of 4 (5%) and 12 years (82%) and the synchondrosis within the acetabulum between the ages of 13 and 16 years (5).

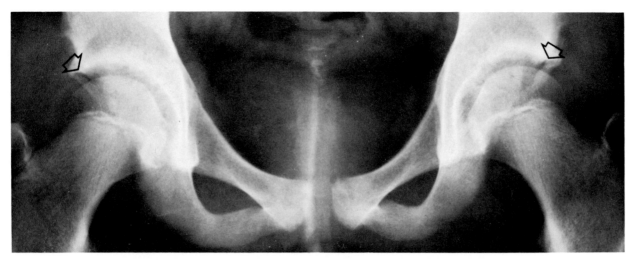

Fig. 10.15. Frontal examination of the hips of a patient who had no symptoms referable to the pelvis. The *arrows* indicate secondary ossification centers of the posterior lip of each acetabulum.

pearance of the pelvis of a normal adolescent. It is important to realize that the aponeurosis of the obturator muscle normally produces a soft tissue shadow adjacent to the superior margin of the superior pubic ramus and that the capsule of the hip joint may be made radiographically visible by the surrounding adipose tissue. The apophyses of the ischial tuberosity, the lesser trochanter, and the iliac crest remain ununited during the second decade.

The radiographic appearance of the normal pelvis of a child is seen in Figure 10.14. The cartilage separating the inferior ramus of the pubis and the ischium persists as a radiolucent space until these bones fuse at about 8 years of age. The Y shaped cartilage separating the pubis, the ischium, and the ilium at the acetabulum persists until these bones unite at the time of puberty.

The capital femoral epiphysis appears during the 1st year of life. The apophysis of the greater trochanter appears before the 5th year, and that of the lesser trochanter during the 13th year. All of these centers unite with the femoral shaft during the 18th–20th years.

A homily aptly describes the relationship of the femoral head to the femoral neck. The femoral head rests symmetrically upon the femoral neck and resembles a scoop of ice cream squarely placed in an ice cream cone. In both the anteroposterior and lateral radiographs, the sweep of the cortex extending from the neck to the head is smooth and symmetrical (Fig. 10.8). Prior to the fusion of the head with the neck, the capital femoral epiphysis sits squarely upon the metaphysis of the femoral neck. Asymmetry of the head with respect to the neck, even if seen in only one

projection, is an abnormal finding and represents either slipped capital femoral epiphysis or a subcapital fracture.

The posterior acetabular lip may arise from a separate growth center (Fig. 10.15). This normal variant, which may closely resemble a posterior hip fracture, is frequently bilateral. Therefore, during the first and second decades, the uninvolved contralateral hip must also be examined radiographically for comparison purposes.

Radiographic Manifestations of Trauma

Abnormal prominence of normally present soft tissue shadows or obliteration of normally present soft tissue structures; i.e., the obturator internus muscle or bladder, within the pelvis are valuable radiographic signs. Increase in the size of the obturator muscle shadow (Figs. 10.7 and 10.16) secondary to hemorrhage may be the most conspicuous roentgen sign of an occult fracture of the superior pubic ramus. An ill defined pelvic soft tissue density may represent a hematoma (Fig. 10.4) or indicate rupture of the bladder or urethra with resultant collection of blood, urine, or both into the pelvic extraperitoneal, perivesicular soft tissues.

In children and immature athletes, the abrupt, violent contraction of large muscles or groups of muscles may cause separation of various apophyses about the pelvis rather than the "muscle pull" which occurs in mature athletes. Regardless of the site of apophyseal avulsion, the clinical picture is similar. Apophyseal separations typically occur during events requiring

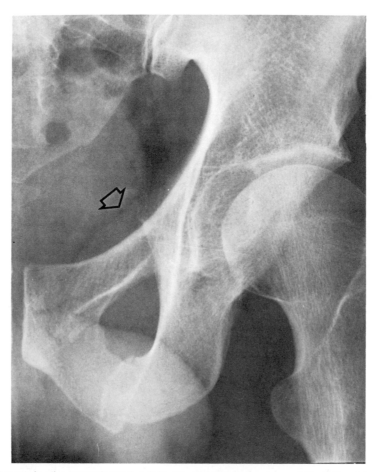

Fig. 10.16. This patient sustained a comminuted, minimally displaced fracture of the left pubic ramus and a displaced complete fracture at the junction of the inferior pubic ramus and the ischium. The *arrow* indicates the abnormally prominent obturator muscle shadow. This muscle mass is displaced medially and made radiographically more visible by the hematoma resulting from the skeletal injury.

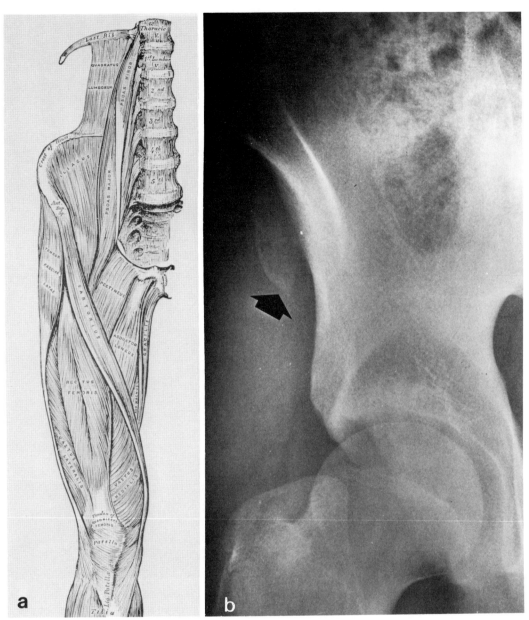

Fig. 10.17. Avulsion of the apophysis of the anterior superior iliac spine. The anatomic drawing **(a)** indicates the origin of the sartorius muscle from the anterior superior iliac spine. The radiograph **(b)** illustrates the typical location of the thin, faintly dense, avulsed anterior superior iliac spine apophysis (*arrow*).

sudden, maximum muscular effort, such as those requiring rapid acceleration (sprints) or abrupt changes of speed or direction (football, basketball, soccer, or lacrosse, for example). The athlete usually experiences a sudden, sharp pain in the area of the avulsion and a "popping" or "snapping" sensation and is abruptly incapacitated, frequently falling. Violent contraction of the sartorius may cause avulsion of the apophysis

of the anterior superior iliac spine (Fig. 10.17); the rectus femoris, the anterior inferior iliac spine apophysis (Fig. 10.18); the hamstring group of muscles, the ischial tuberosity apophysis (Fig. 10.19); and the iliopsoas, the apophysis of the lesser trochanter of the femur (Fig. 10.20).

Dislocation of the hip has increased in frequency in direct proportion to the incidence of automobile ac-

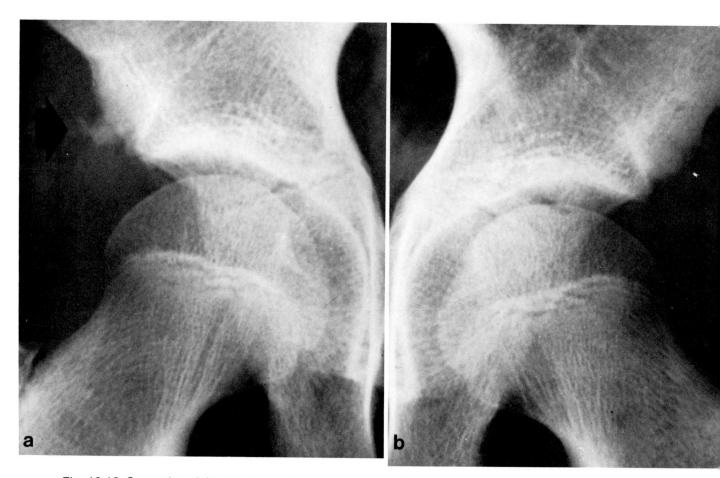

Fig. 10.18. Separation of the apophysis of the anterior inferior iliac spine on the right (**a,** *arrow*), the site of origin of the rectus femoris muscle. The roentgen appearance of the normal anterior inferior iliac spine apophysis is seen on the left (**b**).

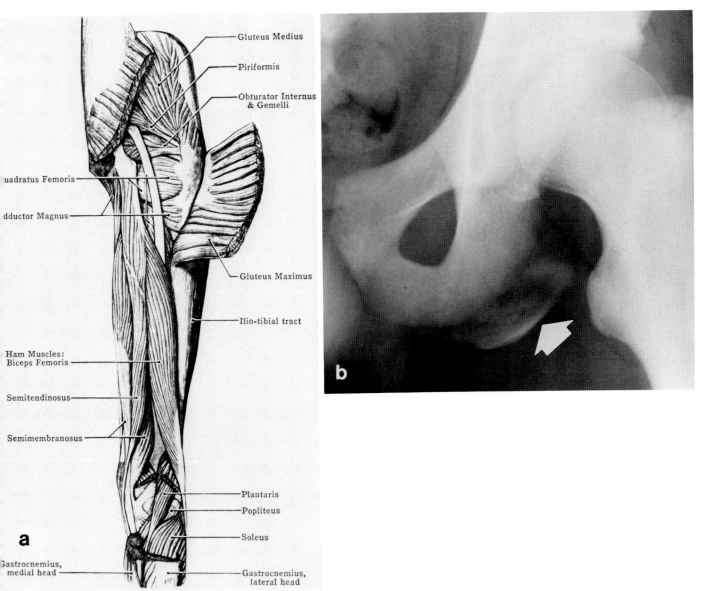

Labels in (a): Gluteus Medius, Piriformis, Obturator Internus & Gemelli, uadratus Femoris, dductor Magnus, Gluteus Maximus, Ilio-tibial tract, Ham Muscles: Biceps Femoris, Semitendinosus, Semimembranosus, Plantaris, Popliteus, Soleus, Gastrocnemius, medial head, Gastrocnemius, lateral head

Fig. 10.19. Anatomic drawing of the posterior aspect of the thigh indicating the site of origin of the hamstring muscles from the ischial tuberosity **(a)**. The roentgen appearance of avulsion of the apophysis of the ischial tuberosity (*arrow*) is seen in **(b)**.

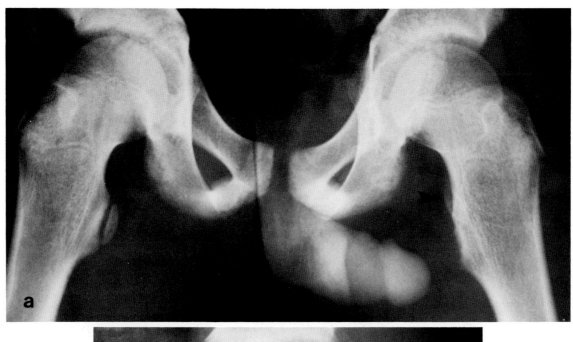

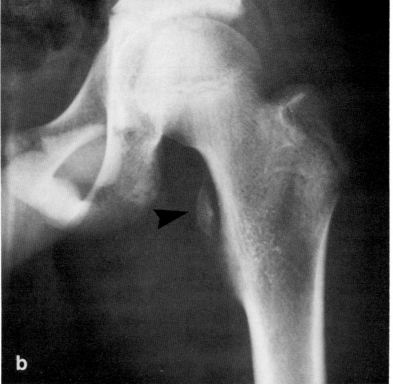

Fig. 10.20. Avulsion of the apophysis of the lesser trochanter of the femur. In the frontal projection **(a)**, the proximally retracted apophysis (*arrowhead*) is largely obscured by the femoral neck. However, comparison with the right femur indicates that the apophysis is absent from its normal position on the left side. In the externally rotated projection **(b)**, the displaced apophysis (*arrowhead*) is clearly visible.

cidents. The commonest mechanism of this injury is the result of striking the distal end of the femur against the dashboard. The force of this impact is transmitted along the femoral shaft. Depending upon the direction of this force, and the position of the femur, the femur may be driven through the posterior aspect of the hip capsule without associated fracture of the acetabulum. With this type of injury, the femoral head is usually dislocated posterior and superior to the acetabulum (Fig. 10.21). Anterior and superior (Fig. 10.22) dislocations of the femur are less common.

The fracture most commonly associated with dislocation of the hip involves the posterior acetabular lip. The fragment is usually long, thin, and vertically oriented. When only slightly displaced (Fig. 10.23), it can resemble the secondary growth center of the posterior acetabular lip (Fig. 10.15), which may persist, ununited, into adulthood. More frequently, however, the posterior acetabular lip fragment is displaced in the same direction as the femoral head, and both the fracture fragment and the defect in the posterior acetabulum are radiographically visible (Fig. 10.24).

Acute traumatic slipped capital femoral epiphysis (Fig. 10.25) occurs infrequently. It is sometimes impossible to exclude the possibility of a previously developing epiphyseal slippage being aggravated by an acute injury resulting in frank epiphyseal separation.

Complete femoral head epiphyseal separation (Fig. 10.26) may occur as the result of direct, violent trauma with the capital epiphysis completely dislocated out of the acetabulum and the femoral neck metaphysis resting against the articular surface of the acetabular fossa.

Rarely, the femoral head may be fractured while the acetabulum remains intact (Fig. 10.27).

The typical displaced femoral neck fracture is not a diagnostic problem radiographically. The less common impacted femoral neck fractures may be quite obvious or very obscure. Figure 10.28 depicts some of the radiographic pitfalls of minimally displaced fractures of the femoral neck. The abnormalities, in this example, are subtle but definite. Note the shortening of the femoral neck, the disruption of the smooth cortical line from the inferior margin of the neck to the head, and the presence of a curvilinear, broad band of increased density that extends transversely across the femoral neck from its inferior surface and is caused by impaction of the fragments and the minimal, but definite, disruption of the superior cortex of the neck, all of which establish the presence of the fracture. Any of these signs could be overlooked in a superficial or cursory review of the roentgenograms.

Ordinarily, fractures involving the trochanteric portion of the femur are obvious radiographically (Fig. 10.29). Nondisplaced or minimally displaced fractures (Fig. 10.30) at this site, however, are likely to be overlooked. Fractures of this type, in which the radio-

graph may appear negative, reinforce a basic tenet of the radiology of trauma, namely that seemingly negative roentgenograms demand stringent analysis for the presence of subtle changes. If the initial radiographic examination is indeed negative and the symptoms persist, the study must be repeated.

There is a significant group of traumatic lesions affecting structures about the hip which cause clinical symptoms suggesting "fractured hip," i.e., fracture of the femoral head, neck, or intertrochanteric region. In these patients in whom the acetabulum, femoral head, neck, and proximal shaft are intact, it is essential to critically analyze the periarticular structures for skeletal or soft tissue signs of injury, which may frequently be subtle. Avulsive apophyseal injuries about the pelvis have been previously discussed and illustrated (Figs. 10.17–10.20). Frequently, the most striking roentgen sign of minimally displaced fractures of the superior pubic ramus is abnormal prominence of the shadow of the aponeurosis of the obturator internus muscle (Figs. 10.7 and 10.16). Minimally displaced fractures of the iliac wing involving the acetabulum may be demonstrated only in oblique projections (Fig. 10.31). Subtle fractures of the pubic rami may be confirmed only in cranially or caudally angled anteroposterior radiographs of the pelvis (Fig. 10.32). Direct trauma to the lateral aspect of the hip may result in cortical fractures of the apex of the greater trochanter (Fig. 10.33) or fractures of the base of the greater trochanter in which the entire trochanter constitutes a separate fragment (Fig. 10.34).

Conwell and Reynolds (6), Judet et al. (7), and Rowe and Lowell (8) have classified the various skeletal injuries that involve the bones of the pelvis and the reader is referred to these sources for detailed descriptions. Because certain pelvic injuries have a high incidence of associated significant soft tissue damage which is usually clinically obscure, it is useful to group pelvic fractures according to the type and degree of significance of the associated soft tissue injury in order to reinforce awareness of the soft tissue components and their roentgen signs. Pelvic effusions are best detected radiographically. The characteristic plain film signs of fluid located intraperitoneally or extraperitoneally permit precise radiographic localization of the fluid.

I. Fractures that involve the anterior pelvic arch
   a. Urinary tract injury—common, significant
   b. Hemorrhage—common, frequently significant
  1. Pubic symphysis separation
  2. Single or multiple ramus fractures
  3. Malgaigne fractures
  4. Multiple, displaced fractures
II. Acetabular fractures
   a. Urinary tract injury—rare, significant

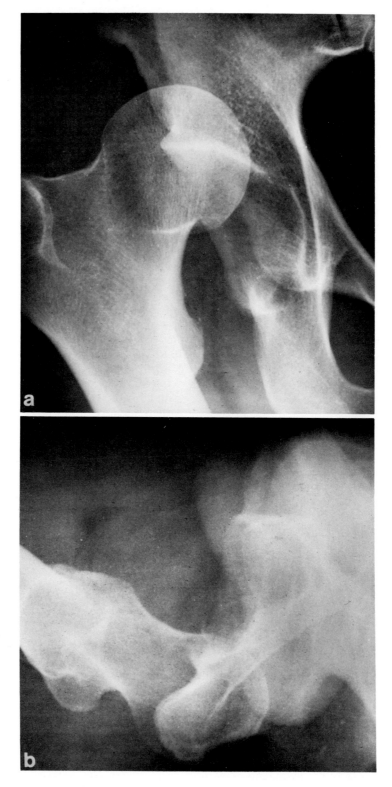

Fig. 10.21. Posterior dislocation of the right hip without associated fracture seen in frontal **(a)** and lateral **(b)** projections.

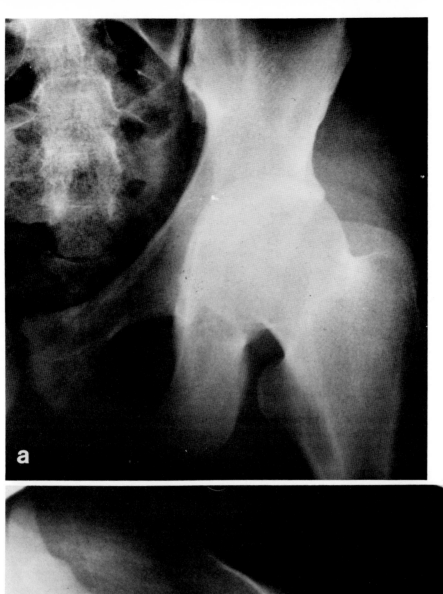

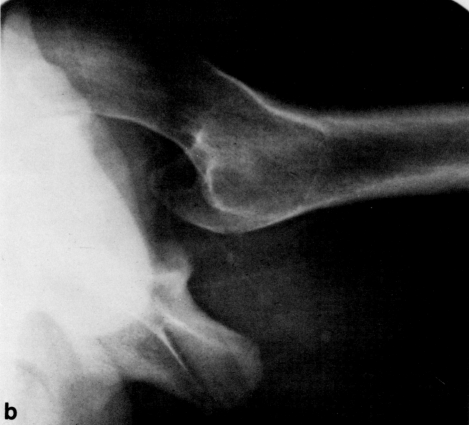

Fig. 10.22. Complete, anterior dislocation of the hip. The frontal projection **(a)** demonstrates that a dislocation exists. However, only the lateral projection **(b)** demonstrates that the femoral head is completely anteriorly dislocated out of the acetabular fossa. There is no associated fracture.

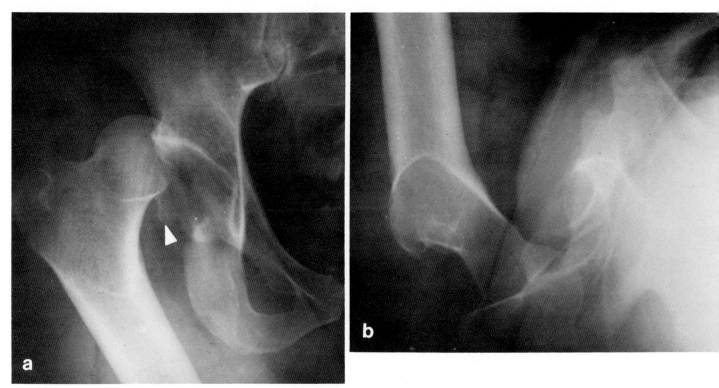

Fig. 10.23. Posterior fracture-dislocation of the right hip. In the frontal projection **(a)**, a fracture is seen in the posterior acetabular lip (*arrowhead*). The lateral projection **(b)** confirms the location of the femoral head posteriorly in the sciatic notch.

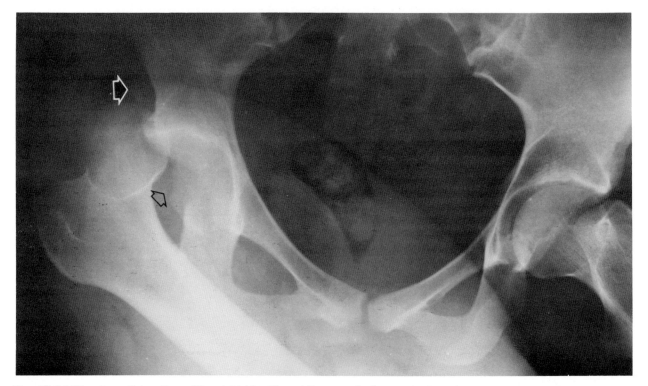

Fig. 10.24. Fracture-dislocation of the right hip. The *white arrow* indicates the location of the posterior acetabular lip fragment. The *open arrow* indicates the defect in the posterior acetabulum from which the fragment was driven by the femoral head. Compare the configuration of the posterior acetabular lip with that of the uninvolved left hip.

512

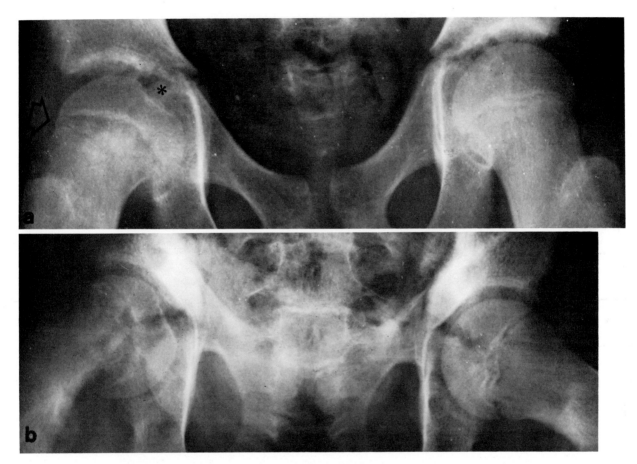

Fig. 10.25. Slipped capital femoral epiphysis. In the frontal projection **(a)**, the degree of epiphyseal slippage appears to be only minor and could be overlooked. However, careful examination of the right hip and comparison with the contralateral hip will demonstrate that the right hip joint (*) space is wider than the left and that the femoral head epiphysis no longer sits squarely atop the femoral neck metaphysis (*open arrow*). In addition, the head is flattened and irregularly calcified, and areas of subcondylar cyst formation and reactive sclerosis are present in the metaphysis of the femoral neck. **(b)** is a frontal examination of the hip made in the "frog leg" position. Here, the degree of femoral head subluxation is obvious.

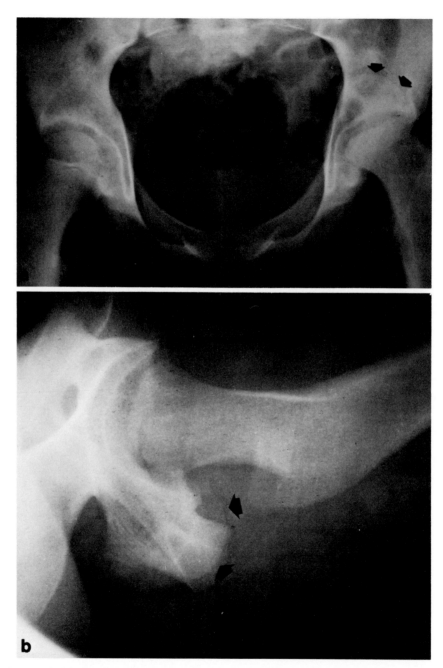

Fig. 10.26. Complete capital femoral epiphyseal separation secondary to severe acute trauma. In the frontal projection **(a)**, the *arrows* outline the articulating surface of the femoral head epiphysis. Note that the metaphyseal surface of the femoral neck articulates with the concavity of the acetabular fossa. In the lateral projection **(b)**, the *arrows* indicate the location of the capital femoral epiphysis posterior to the acetabulum and superimposed upon the ischial tuberosity.

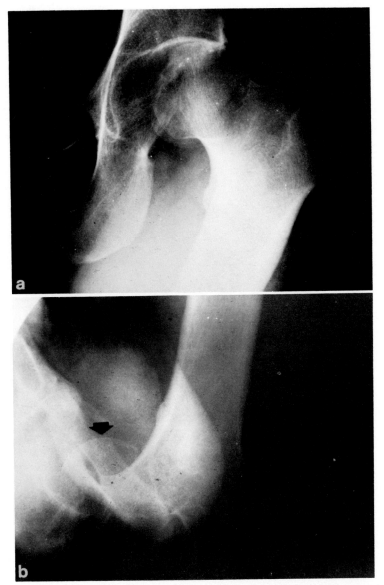

Fig. 10.27. Fracture-dislocation of the left hip. In the frontal projection **(a)**, the dislocation is obvious. In the lateral projection **(b)**, the *arrow* indicates a fragment of the femoral head that has remained within the acetabular fossa, although occupying neither a normal position nor attitude with respect to the acetabulum. The remainder of the femur is posteriorly dislocated.

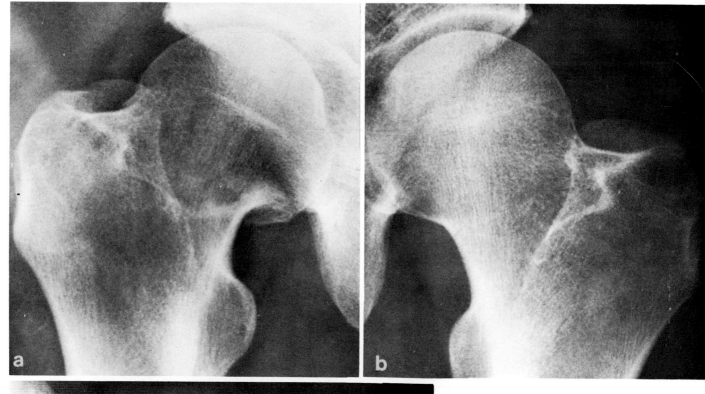

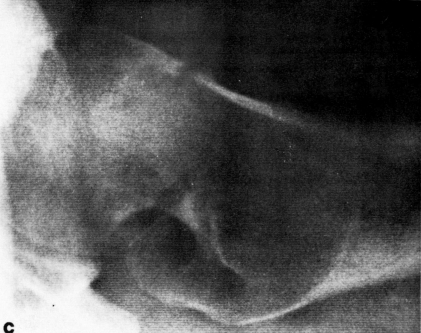

Fig. 10.28. This patient has a minimally displace
slightly impacted, obscure subcapital fracture of th
right femur. A casual observation of the frontal pr
jection of the injured side **(a)** might be interpreted a
normal. However, in comparing the injured side wi
the uninvolved left hip **(b)**, shortening of the femor
neck and disruption of the cortex of the superior ar
inferior margins of the femoral neck become appa
ent. The fracture line is clearly discernible in th
lateral projection **(c)**. In addition, the femoral hea
has slipped posteriorly with respect to the femor
neck and the "ice cream cone" sign is well demo
strated.

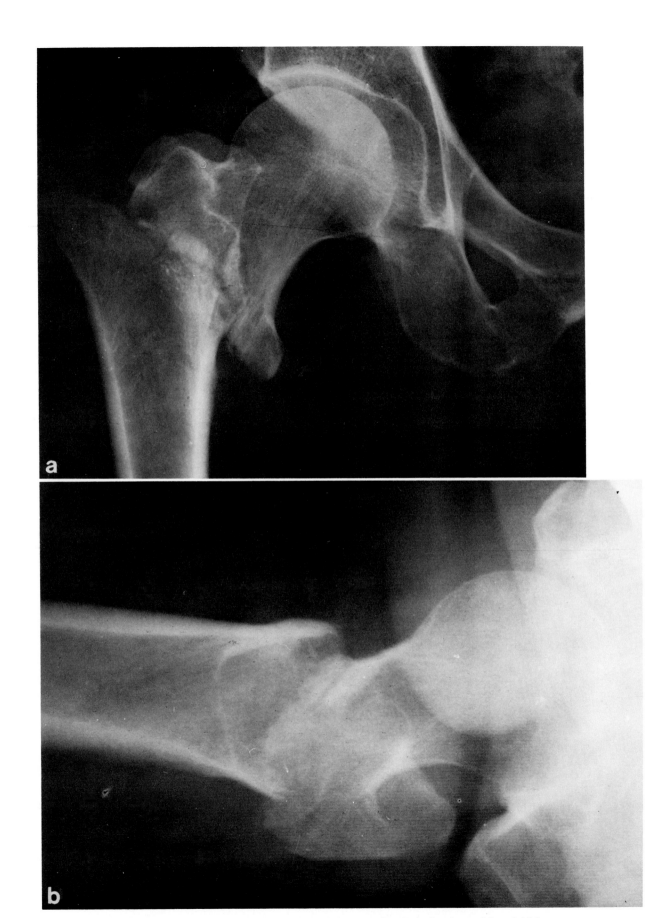

Fig. 10.29. (a, b) Complete, displaced, intertrochanteric fracture of the right femur.

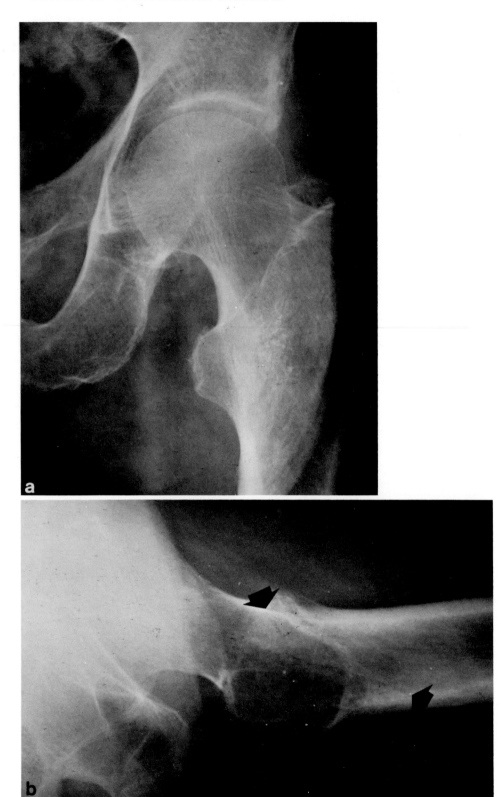

Fig. 10.30. Nondisplaced, complete, intertrochanteric fracture of the left femur. In the frontal projection **(a)**, the fracture line is practically invisible. In the lateral projection **(b)**, however, the fracture line is clearly discernible (*arrows*), even though there is no displacement of the fragments.

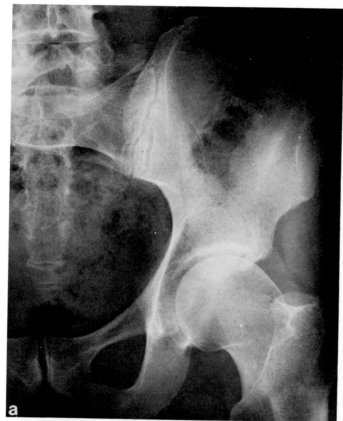

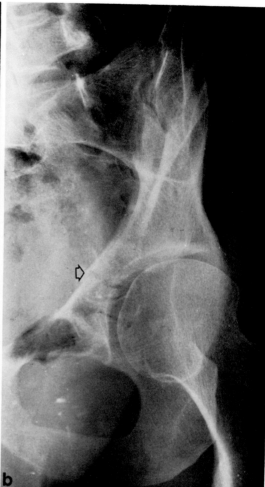

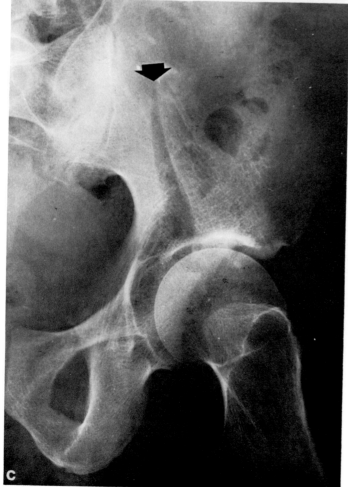

Fig. 10.31. The iliac wing fracture line is barely perceptible in the lateral aspect of the roof of the acetabulum in the routine frontal projection **(a)**. Disruption of the iliopectineal line (*open arrow*) is visible in the anteriorly rotated oblique projection **(b)**. Only in the externally rotated oblique projection **(c)** is the extent of the fracture line and the separation of the fragments accurately depicted.

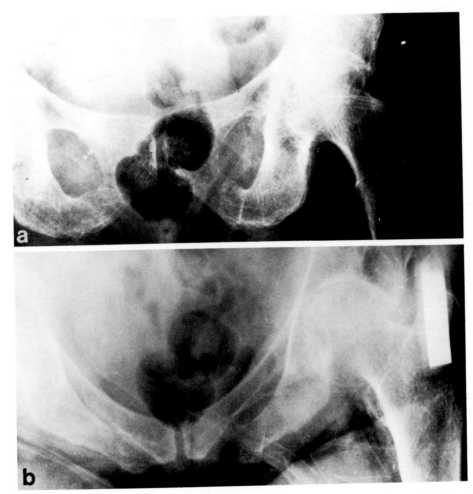

Fig. 10.32. The only suggestion of a fracture in the anterior pelvic arch is the vertical linear density at the junction of the inferior pubic ramus and the ischium on the left (**a**, *arrow*). In the frontal projection of the pelvis made with the central beam angled toward the feet (**b**), the fracture is obvious (*arrow*). In addition, this projection indicates that no other fractures exist in the anterior pelvic arch.

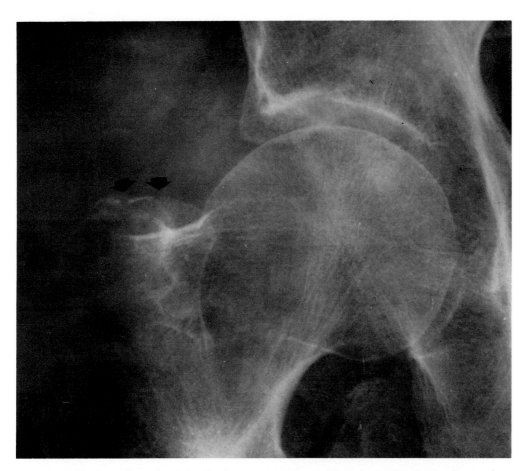

Fig. 10.33. Comminuted, minimally displaced fracture of the greater trochanter (*arrows*).

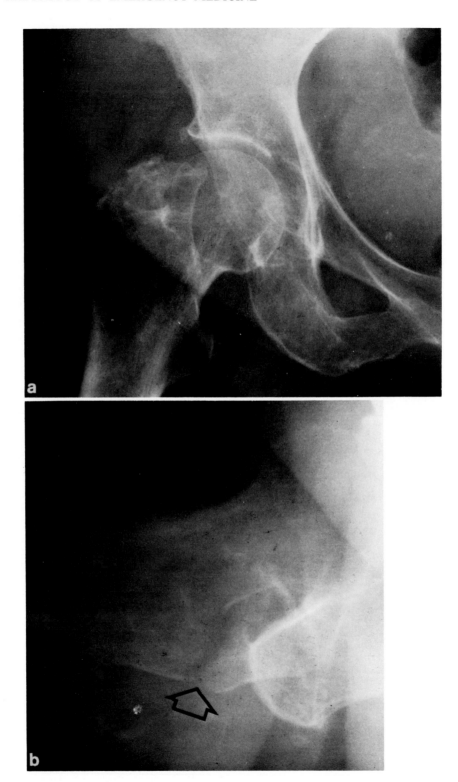

Fig. 10.34. Complete, minimally displaced fracture through the base of the greater trochanter of the right femur. In the frontal projection **(a)**, several fracture lines are seen in the superior cortex of the greater trochanter. The alignment of the fragments is satisfactory and the basilar fracture line is obscured by a soft tissue crease. In the lateral projection **(b)**, however, the fracture line through the base of the greater trochanter is evident (*arrow*).

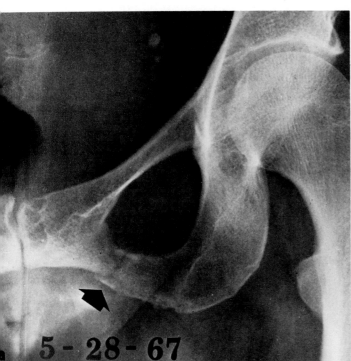 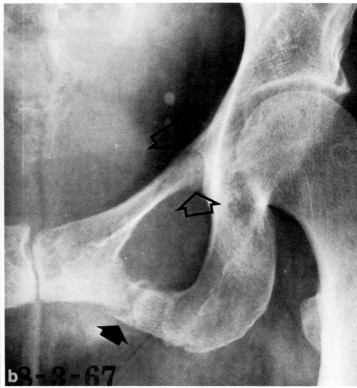

Fig. 10.35. In the frontal projection of the pelvis, made at the time of injury **(a)**, the only discernible fracture was that in the inferior pubic ramus (*arrow*). At the time of re-examination, 9 weeks later **(b)**, callous formation had developed at the inferior pubic ramus fracture (*solid arrow*). In addition, callous formation in the lateral extent of the superior pubic ramus (*open arrows*) indicates that a nondisplaced fracture was present at the site but was not discernible on the original examination.

     b. Hemorrhage—common, usually not clinically significant

     c. Sciatic nerve palsy—17% (8)

  1. Simple transverse

  2. Inner wall of acetabulum with intrapelvic displacement of femoral head

  3. Bursting

III. Isolated pelvic fractures without significant soft tissue injury

  1. Wing of ilium

  2. Ischial tuberosity

  3. Superior iliac spine

  4. Acetabular rim

  5. Sacral and coccygeal

Isolated fractures of a single component of the anterior pelvic arch may occur (Fig. 10.32). Fractures at the junction of the superior pubic ramus and the ischium may not be discernible on the routine initial radiograph. To demonstrate fractures at this location, oblique views of the anterior pelvic arch are mandatory. If these special projections are negative and if symptoms persist, the radiographic examination should be repeated in 2 to 3 weeks. A fracture may then be evident by virtue of callous formation at the fracture site (Fig. 10.35).

Caudad and cephalad angled views of the pelvis are not popular projections. Their use is, however, strongly advocated because they define the relationship of anterior arch fragments, clearly demonstrate fractures that cannot be established on the basis of routine anteroposterior radiographs alone (Fig. 10.36), and accurately demonstrate the status of the pubic symphysis, the sacroiliac joints and the presence of obscure Malgaigne fractures (Fig. 10.37). The Malgaigne injury involves a fracture of separation of both the anterior and posterior pelvic arches on the same or opposite sides, with some degree of cephalic, posterior, or lateral displacement or rotation of the separated component (9).

The "double vertical" fracture (Fig. 10.38) is a fracture of each superior and each inferior pubic

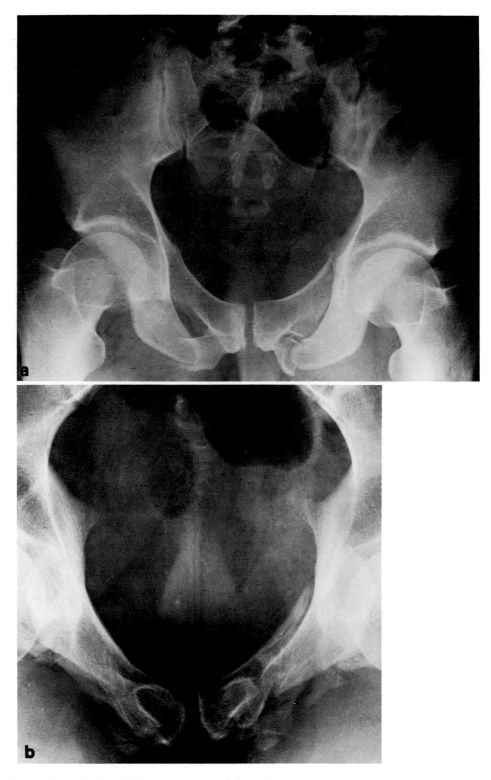

Fig. 10.36. In the routine frontal projection of the pelvis **(a)**, obvious fractures are present in each inferior pubic ramus. The complete fracture at the junction of the superior pubic ramus and the ischium, on the left, could be overlooked in the frontal projection. In the roentgenogram obtained with the central beam angled caudally **(b)**, this fracture is obvious. In addition, the posterior displacement of the comminuted left pubic fragment is apparent only in this view.

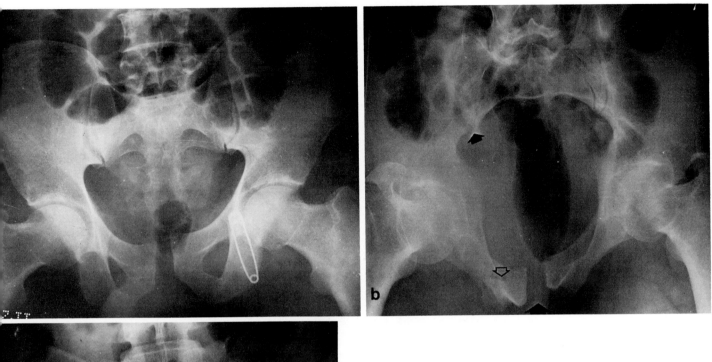

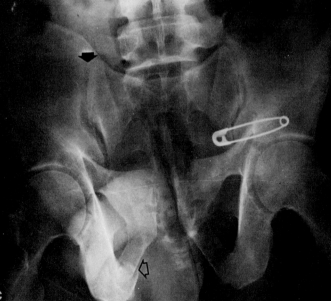

Fig. 10.37. The routine frontal projection **(a)** demonstrates pelvic asymmetry and separation of the pubic symphysis. The complete, displaced fracture in the right inferior pubic ramus is obscured. The sacroiliac joints are essentially similar in appearance. In each of the angled views of the pelvis **(b, c)**, the left inferior pubic ramus fracture is clearly visible (*open arrows*) and the characteristics of the Malgaigne fracture, on the right, are clearly evident. Anteroposterior displacement of the pubic symphysis and widening of the right sacroiliac joint is identified by the *solid arrows*.

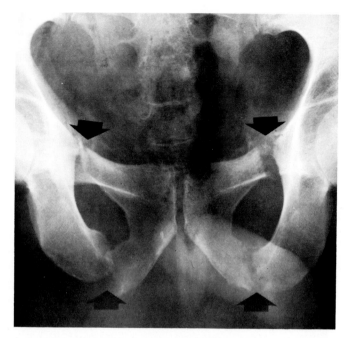

Fig. 10.38. Fractures in each superior and inferior pubic ramus (*arrows*) constitute the "double vertical" fracture of the anterior pelvic arch.

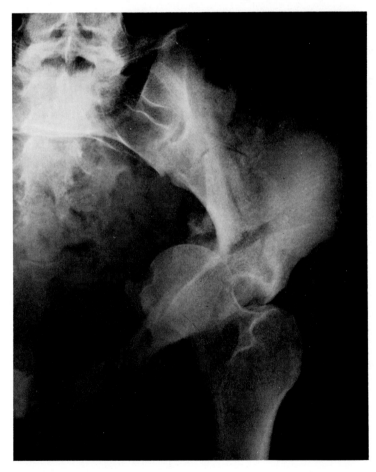

Fig. 10.39. Central fracture of the acetabulum with gross intrapelvic intrusion of the femoral head. The comminuted fracture extends into the iliac wing.

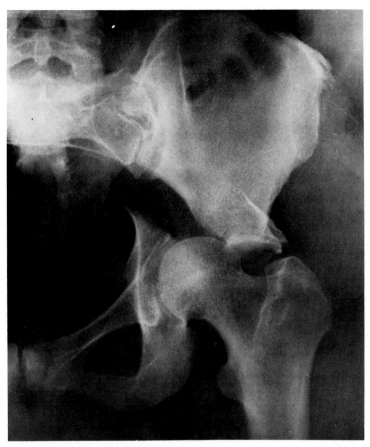

Fig. 10.40. Transverse fracture at the level of the junction of the acetabular roof and fossa with an associated fracture through the acetabular roof and separation of the sacroiliac joint.

ramus. Forces that produce the double vertical or Malgaigne fractures, or fractures or separation of the pubic symphysis, also commonly cause injury to the urinary bladder and/or urethra. Simply the presence of a major anterior pelvic arch fracture or separation should prompt consideration of a lower urinary tract injury. This relationship and the roentgen signs of pelvic effusion are discussed subsequently in this chapter.

Figures 10.39–10.41 are examples of major fractures involving the acetabulum. Urinary tract injury associated with major acetabular fractures is rare. In contrast, intrapelvic hemorrhage occurs in practically every instance, is usually venous, and, depending upon the magnitude of the injury, may be a serious complication. In a series of 93 acetabular fractures reported by Rowe and Lowell (8), sciatic nerve palsy occurred in 17%.

Simple fractures of the ilium are commonly difficult to identify and may require individualized oblique projections to confirm their presence (Figs. 10.31 and 10.42). Comminuted, displaced fractures of the iliac wing (Fig. 10.43) are usually obvious on the routine, anteroposterior roentgenogram of the pelvis.

Posterior acetabular lip fractures, which may or may not be associated with dislocation of the hip, may be very elusive or even impossible to detect in the frontal radiograph alone. The fragment, which may be comminuted, is usually small and only minimally displaced, and is frequently obscured by the density of the femoral head (10). It is imperative that a horizontal beam lateral projection be obtained routinely in every instance in which a radiographic examination of the hip is clinically indicated. Figure 10.44 illustrates the value of a horizontal beam lateral radiograph in establishing the presence of a posterior acetabular lip fracture. Oblique views of the injured hip, even in minor degrees of obliquity (Fig. 10.45), are extremely helpful in the identification of minimally displaced posterior rim fragments which may be obscure on the anteroposterior radiograph. The fragment which constitutes the posterosuperior portion of the acetabulum can be identified as such by its typical position, configuration, and triangular lucent defect in the supra-acetabular region. This type of posterior rim fracture results from a force transmitted along the femoral shaft with the shaft *ab*ducted. The greater the abduction, the larger the fragment (11).

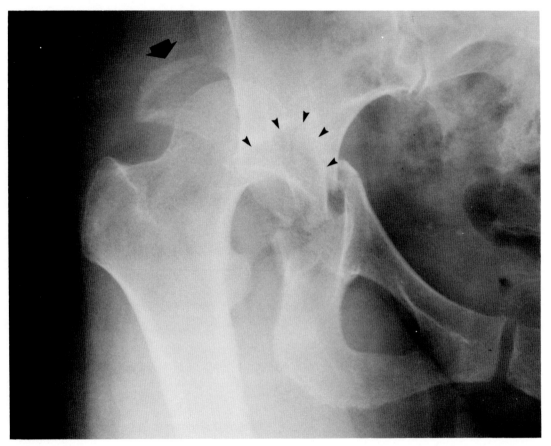

Fig. 10.41. Comminuted acetabular fracture with posterior dislocation of the femur. The acetabular fragment (*arrow*) accompanying the dislocated femur arises from the posterosuperior portion of the acetabulum. Its site of origin is indicated by the triangular lucency (*arrowheads*) above the acetabulum.

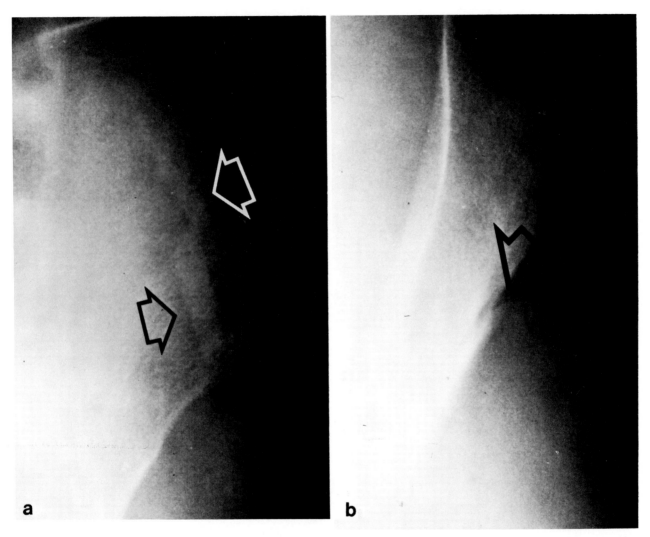

Fig. 10.42. Simple fracture of the iliac wing. In the frontal projection **(a)**, the fracture is identifiable by the broad band of increased density, caused by superimposition of the margins of the fragment. In the anteriorly rotated oblique projection, the fracture line is visible **(b)**.

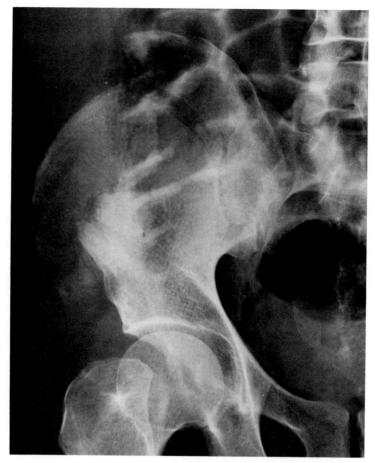

Fig. 10.43. Severely comminuted, displaced fracture of the iliac wing.

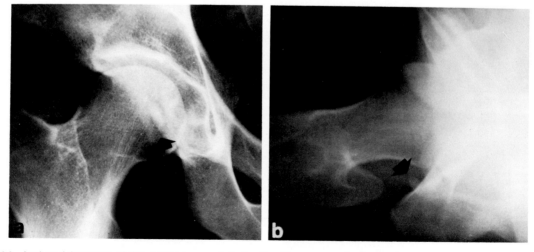

Fig. 10.44. Isolated fracture of the posterior acetabular lip. The *arrows* indicate the posterior lip fragments in both frontal **(a)** and lateral **(b)** projections. There is no associated dislocation. The femoral head is intact.

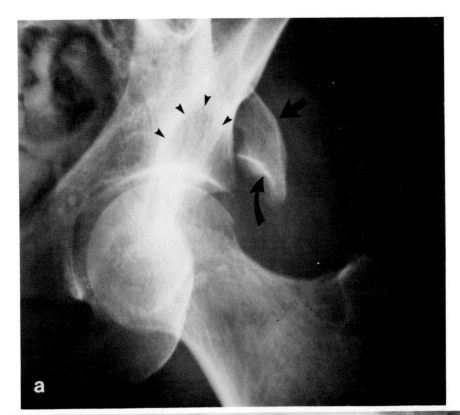

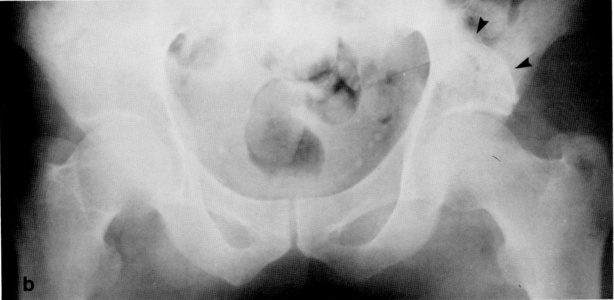

Fig. 10.45. Slightly anteriorly rotated oblique radiograph of an isolated, displaced fracture of the posterior acetabular rim **(a)**. The site of origin of the fragment is indicated by the lucent area in the supra-acetabular portion of the ilium (*arrowheads*). The *stemmed arrow* indicates the cortical surface of the fragment and the *curved arrow*, an arc of the articulating surface of the acetabular fossa. The separate fragment (*arrowheads*) was obscured by the innominate bone in the anteroposterior projection of the pelvis **(b)**.

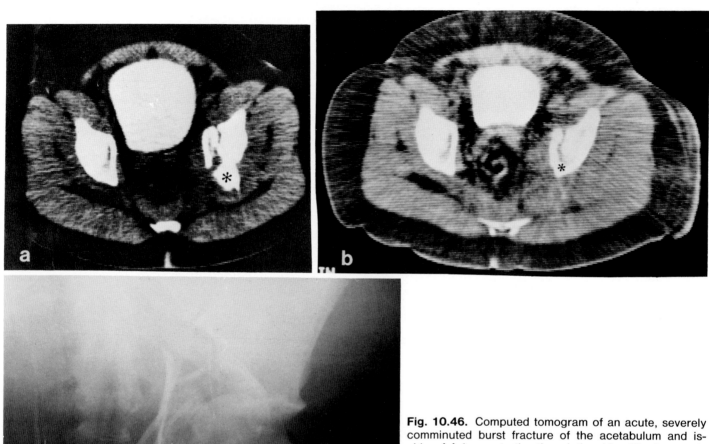

Fig. 10.46. Computed tomogram of an acute, severely comminuted burst fracture of the acetabulum and ischium **(a)** demonstrating the relationship of the fragments and the marked rotation of a large posterior fragment (*). Following reduction **(b)**, the orientation and position of the fragment is essentially anatomic. The location and rotation of this fragment could not be determined on the plain, anteroposterior radiograph **(c)**.

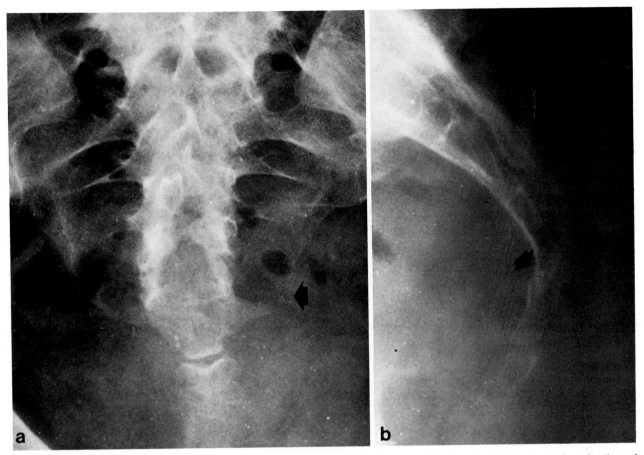

Fig. 10.47. The cortex of the left lateral margin of the fourth sacral segment is disrupted in the frontal projection of the sacrum **(a)**. In the lateral projection **(b)**, the *arrow* indicates the oblique fracture extending through the fourth sacral segment.

The separate fragment is usually superiorly and posteriorly displaced. It is characteristically triangular in shape with a posterolaterally convex cortical surface, a concave inferior surface which represents an arc of the acetabular fossa, and an irregular medial surface representing the fracture edge. If the fragment is displaced, with or without femoral dislocation, or if it remains displaced following reduction of a dislocated hip, it is an indication for open reduction and internal fixation (11). If the fragment is large and nonreduced, the hip is unstable.

Rectilinear and polydirectional tomography are useful in evaluation of acetabular fractures. Computed tomography provides invaluable, and frequently unique, data relative to the orientation and spatial relationship of complex pelvic fractures (Fig. 10.46).

The reader is referred to excellent publications by DePalma (11), Rogers et al. (12) and Thaggard et al. (13) for a more detailed description of pelvic and acetabular fractures.

Minimally displaced fractures of the sacral and coccygeal segments may be difficult to identify in the frontal projection because the fracture line is usually either not directly parallel to the x-ray beam (Fig. 10.47) or because the fracture line resembles the roentgen appearance of the rudimentary intersegmental spaces (Fig. 10.48). Fractures of the sacral segments are best seen in the lateral projection.

Soft Tissue Components of Pelvic Skeletal Injuries

Hemorrhage and lower urinary tract injury are frequent integral components of pelvic skeletal injuries and are often of greater clinical significance than the skeletal injury. Pelvic hemorrhage and lower urinary tract disruption are usually clinically silent lesions. The pelvic extraperitoneal perivesical space, into which the effusion accumulates, is practically inaccessible to clinical evaluation. Signs of extraperitoneal, perivesical effusion, indicating hemorrhage, disruption of the bladder or urethra, or both, are

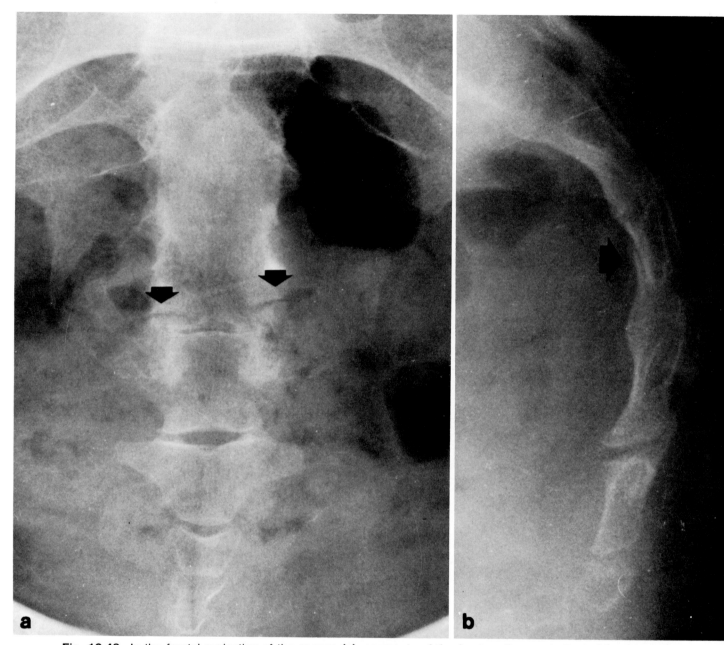

Fig. 10.48. In the frontal projection of the sacrum **(a)**, segments of the fracture line are indicated by the *arrows*. Because of the proximity of the fracture line to the intersegmental space, the fracture line could be interpreted as a portion of the intersegmental line. In the lateral projection **(b)**, however, the fracture in the body of the fourth sacral segment is evident (*arrow*).

clearly evident on the plain anteroposterior radiograph of the pelvis. The following discussion will emphasize the importance of recognizing these roentgen signs. Little attention will be placed upon the fractures beyond noting their location and the magnitude of displacement of the fragments. By relegating the fracture to a relatively minor role, we hope to direct the primary consideration of the roentgenograms away from the obvious fracture to the obscure, but clinically more significant, soft tissue injury.

Lower urinary tract injury or pelvic hemorrhage must be a diagnostic consideration even though the roentgenograms of the pelvis reveal only minor skeletal damage (Fig. 10.49).

The roentgen signs of extraperitoneal perivesical effusion are determined by the anatomy of this potential space and the radiographically discernible structures within it (Fig. 10.1). The space is bounded superiorly by the pelvic peritoneal reflection, laterally by the levator ani and obturator internus muscles,

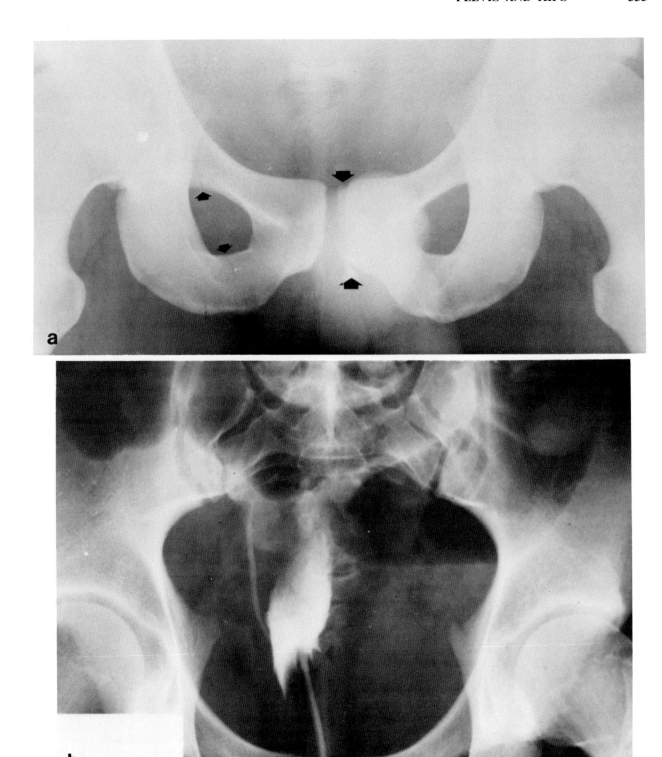

Fig. 10.49. The anteroposterior projection of the pelvis **(a)** demonstrates minimally displaced fractures of the right pubic rami and the medial surface of the left pubic body (*arrows*). The infusion pyelogram **(b)** demonstrates a small contracted, elevated bladder and diffuse soft tissue density throughout the pelvis indicative of a large extraperitoneal perivesical hematoma.

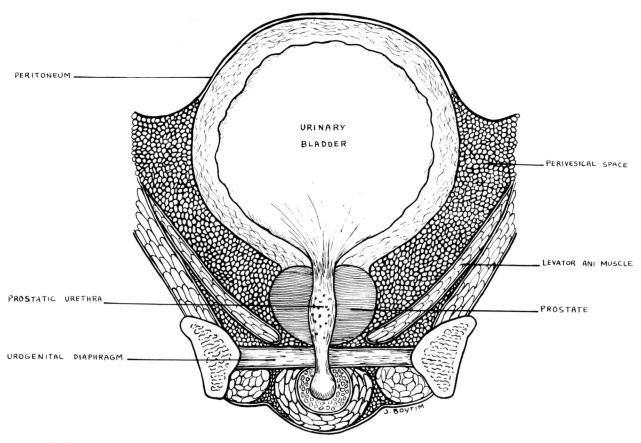

Fig. 10.50. This schematic representation of the gross anatomy of the pelvis, seen in frontal projection, demonstrates the potential space bounded superiorly by the pelvic peritoneum, laterally by the lateral pelvic wall, and inferiorly by the urogenital diaphragm. Note the relationship of the prostatic urethra to the superior layer of the diaphragm. (Reprinted with permission from E.J. Holyoke: Some anatomical considerations of pelvic injuries and their complications. *Nebraska State Medical Journal* 43: 5, 1958.)

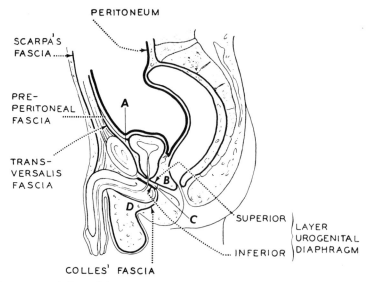

Fig. 10.51. Diagrammatic representation of the gross anatomy of the midsagittal plane of a male pelvis. The perivesical space referred to in Figure 10.50 is seen to be bounded anteriorly by the pubic symphysis and posteriorly by the anterior wall of the rectum. The urinary bladder and the prostate lie above the urogenital diaphragm. The membranous portion of the urethra lies between the superior and inferior layers of this diaphragm. (Reprinted with permission from E.J. Holyoke: Some anatomical considerations of pelvic injuries and their complications. *Nebraska State Medical Journal* 43: 5, 1958.)

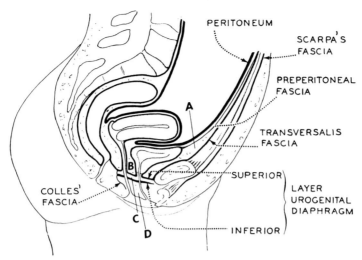

Fig. 10.52. Schematic representation of the gross anatomy of the female pelvis seen in sagittal section. Note that the urinary bladder, the proximal two-thirds of the vagina, and the uterus lie above the superior surface of the urogenital diaphragm. (Reprinted with permission from E.J. Holyoke: Some anatomical considerations of pelvic injuries and their complications. *Nebraska State Medical Journal* 43: 5, 1958.)

anteriorly by the pubic symphysis, posteriorly by the sacrum, and inferiorly by the urogenital diaphragm (Figs. 10.50–10.52). The perivesical space is filled with loose adipose tissue which is continuous with the extraperitoneal fat comprising the flank stripe. Perivesical space may accumulate as much as 2000 cc of fluid—enough blood to produce clinical shock without visible evidence of blood loss.

The signs of an extraperitoneal perivesical effusion, seen on the anteroposterior radiograph of the pelvis, include a homogenous soft tissue density which, if unilateral, obliterates the shadow of the obturator internus muscle and displaces the bladder in the opposite direction (Fig. 10.53); if in greater amounts, obliterates all soft tissue anatomy within the pelvis and displaces the pelvic ileal loops out of the pelvis (Fig. 10.54); and, when in largest amounts, extends in a retrograde fashion into the extraperitoneal space of the flank, obliterating the lucency of the flank stripe and displacing the medial wall of the stripe medially (Fig. 10.55) (14,15). It is particularly important to recognize the abnormal pelvic soft tissue density as evidence of the presence of blood (Fig. 10.56) or urine (Fig. 10.49) in the extraperitoneal perivesical space.

Injury to the bladder and urethra occurs in from 5% (16–18) to 17% (19) of patients with pelvic trauma. While there is a direct relationship between the magnitude of anterior arch fractures and disruption or separation of the pubic symphysis and lower urinary tract injury, it is sufficiently important to emphasize, by repetition, that significant urinary tract damage may also be associated with minimal skeletal changes. Lower urinary tract injuries, in civilian practice, are most commonly the result of blunt trauma. Gunshot and stabbing wounds account for the small percentage

of penetrating injuries which usually involve the bladder. Bladder injuries occur with slightly greater frequency in males (20), whereas there is a marked predilection for urethral injuries in males (21). Urethral injuries in female children (Fig. 10.57) are rare (22).

Because injury to the urinary tract is associated with such a high incidence of morbidity and mortality, because of the frequent association of injury to the urethra and bladder with anterior pelvic arch fractures and pubic symphysis separation, and because the clinical signs of lower urinary tract injury are so inconspicuous, Orkin (23) and Holdsworth (16) believe that in every case of pelvic trauma, damage to the lower urinary tract must be considered as being present until proven otherwise. Conolly and Hedberg (24) describe "major" pelvic fractures as those "which involve the line of weight transmission, from the spine to the acetabulum, or which involve the rami on both sides of the symphysis pubis" and state that "every patient with a major fracture of the pelvis should be investigated for complications that may well kill him," i.e., hemorrhage or lower urinary tract injury.

The radiographic evaluation of the lower urinary tract should be done as part of the initial radiographic examination of the patient and is indicated particularly in those patients with pelvic arch or pubic symphysis separation, hematuria, scrotal or perineal extravasation, or inability to void. Infusion pyelography and retrograde urethrography can be performed without loss of time and without unnecessary patient motion.

Lower urinary tract injuries occur commonly in severely injured patients. Obviously, in such patients, evaluation of the lower urinary tract must assume a

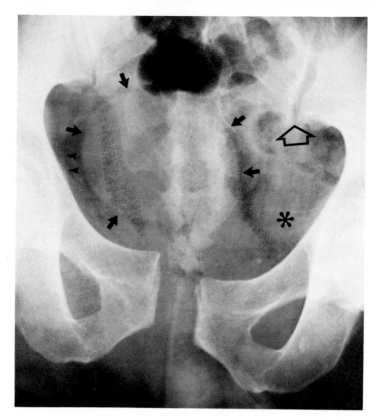

Fig. 10.53. Displacement of the bladder (*stemmed arrows*) to the right by a small left perivesical extraperitoneal hematoma (*) which also obliterates the left obturator internus muscle shadow. The obturator internus muscle is visible on the right (*arrowheads*). Separation of the pubic symphysis of the left sacroiliac joint (*open arrow*) constitutes a Malgaigne injury.

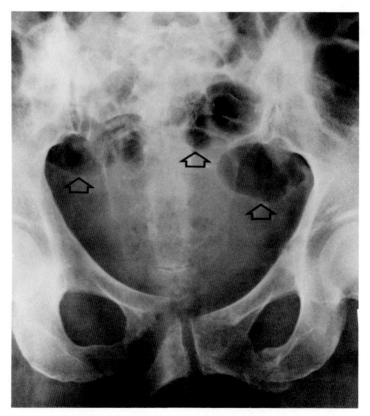

Fig. 10.54. The homogeneous soft tissue density throughout the pelvis which has obliterated the bladder and obturator muscle shadows and displaced the pelvic ileal loops (*open arrows*) upward, represents a moderate extraperitoneal perivesical effusion. An oblique fracture involves the right pubic body and minimally displaced fractures are present in each left pubic ramus.

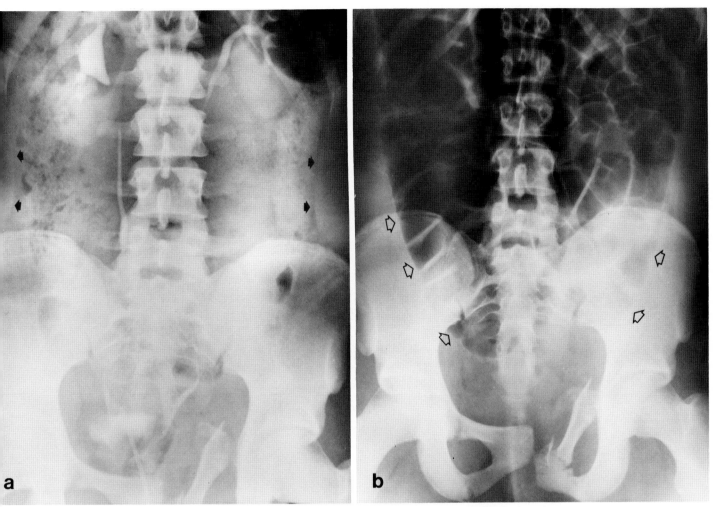

Fig. 10.55. Infusion pyelogram **(a)** obtained at the time of admission in a patient who sustained severely comminuted fractures of the anterior pelvic arch and separation of the left sacroiliac joint (Malgaigne injury). The soft tissue anatomy of the pelvis is obliterated by the large extraperitoneal perivesical hematoma which displaced the bladder to the right and the ureters medially. The extraperitoneal fat in the flank stripe (*arrows*) is normal. The anteroposterior radiograph of the pelvis and abdomen made 48 hours later **(b)** demonstrates opacification of the flank stripes and medial displacement of the medial border of each (*open arrows*) by extension of the perivesical extraperitoneal hemorrhage into the extraperitoneal fat of the flank.

lower priority to lifesaving measures. However, even in these patients, prompt evaluation of the urethra and bladder is advocated in order to reduce morbidity and mortality (20,24,25). In less severely injured patients in whom bladder or urethral injuries are suspected, radiographic examination of the lower urinary tract should be part of the initial, immediate patient evaluation. Regardless of the clinical condition of the patient, and contrary to an occasional reference advocating diagnostic ("blind") catheterization or a "single-shot" urethrogram in the emergency department, the retrograde urethrocystogram performed under flu-

oroscopic control is *the* diagnostic procedure of choice for evaluation of the urethra and bladder (24,26–33). The retrograde urethrocystogram is performed with a 50% solution of Cystokon introduced into the urethra through a bulb syringe inserted into the urethral orifice under sterile conditions. The study should be monitored fluoroscopically in order to detect small extravasations of contrast which may be visible only in the appropriate oblique position.

Reasons for condemning diagnostic (blind) catheterization for evaluation of possible urethral or even bladder injury are many (26–38). If the urethra and

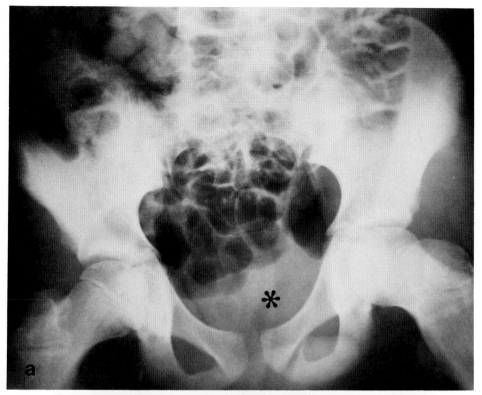

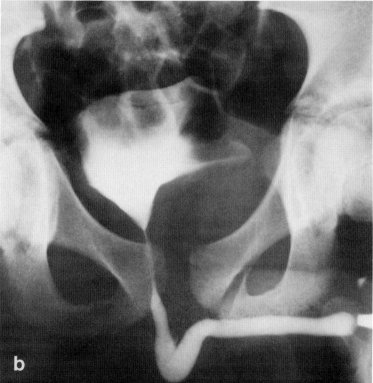

Fig. 10.56. Anteroposterior radiograph of the pelvis of a patient who sustained a left Malgaigne fracture with separation of the pubic symphysis and the left sacroiliac joint and a fracture of the left inferior pubic ramus **(a)**. The homogeneous density (*) represents an extraperitoneal perivesical effusion. The retrograde urethrocystogram **(b)** confirms the extraperitoneal hemorrhage exerting pressure upon and displacing the bladder and the periurethral hematoma which produces circumferential narrowing and attenuation of the posterior urethra.

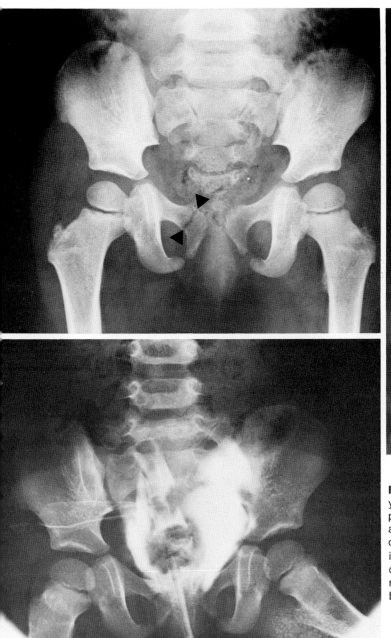

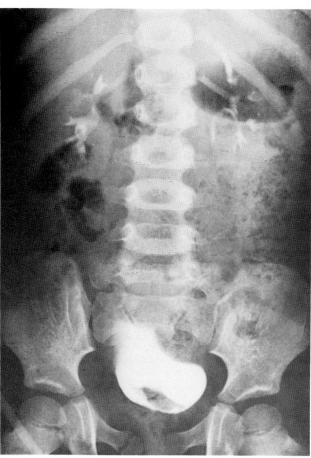

Fig. 10.57. Transection of the posterior urethra in a 6-year-old girl associated with a minimally displaced anterior pelvic arch fracture. The only visible skeletal injury in the anteroposterior radiograph of the pelvis **(a)** is the innocuous appearing fracture in the right os pubis (*arrowheads*). infusion pyelogram **(b)** demonstrated elevation of the bladder and large defect at its base. Gross extraperitoneal rupture at the urethrovesical junction was demonstrated by cystography **(c).**

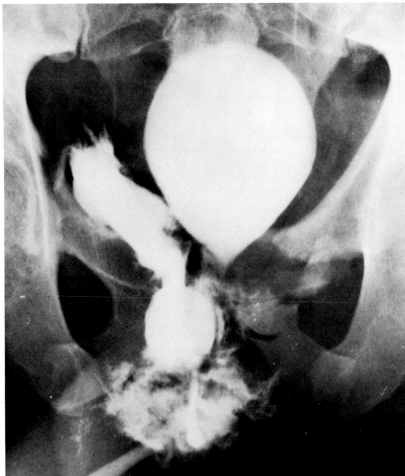

Fig. 10.58. Urethrogram performed following attempted catheterization of a patient with severe anterior pelvic arch fractures. The Foley catheter passed through the urethral tear and lodged in the periurethral soft tissues causing the round defect to the right of the midline.

bladder are not injured, the catheterization constitutes inappropriate and unnecessary instrumentation of the urinary tract. Introduction of infection, initiation or reactivation of hemorrhage, and placement of the catheter in the periurethral (Fig. 10.58) or perivesical tissues may occur. Simply the passage of a catheter into the bladder and the obtaining of clear urine, or no urine, does not exclude either a urethral or bladder injury. A cystogram performed through a Foley catheter, without antecedent urethrogram, will fail to demonstrate a urethral laceration (Fig. 10.59). McLaughlin and Pfister (34) have described a technique of performing a urethrogram around an indwelling Foley catheter by opacifying the urethral lumen with contrast introduced through a #16 gauge polyethylene tube inserted into the urethra alongside the Foley catheter. Vigorous or persistent attempts at passage of a filiform catheter may cause iatrogenic urethral laceration (Fig. 10.60).

Bladder Injuries

The most common cause of bladder injury is blunt lower abdominal or pelvic trauma. Penetrating wounds account for 9–14% of bladder injuries (25,31). Approximately 14% of patients with pelvic fractures sustain bladder injuries (33,35), while approximately 70% of patients with bladder injury have pelvic fractures, particularly fractures involving the anterior arch (31). As many as one-third of patients with extraperitoneal rupture of the bladder may also have clinically unrecognizable intraperitoneal injury (36). The distribution of intra- and extraperitoneal rupture of the bladder is approximately equal (20,25,31), with a greater incidence of intraperitoneal rupture in the absence of pelvic fracture (27). 20% of patients with pelvic fracture and extraperitoneal rupture of the bladder also have associated posterior urethral lacer-

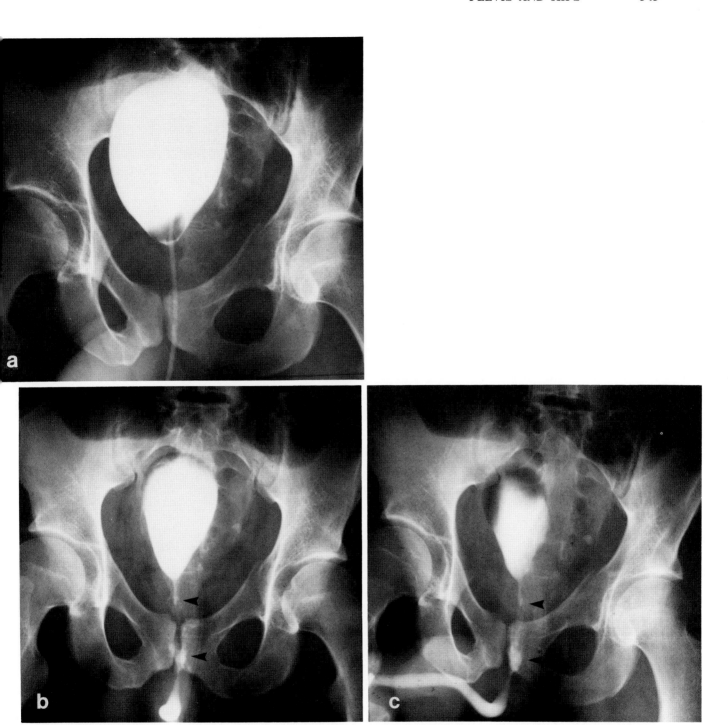

Fig. 10.59. Cystogram performed through a Foley catheter **(a)** in a patient who sustained a minimally displaced double vertical fracture of the anterior pelvic arch. The homogeneous density throughout the pelvis and compressing the bladder indicates a large extraperitoneal perivesical effusion. The high position of the bladder suggested urethral laceration. There is no evidence of contrast medium outside the lumen of the lower urinary tract. A retrograde urethrogram performed following removal of the Foley catheter **(b,c)** identified multiple sites of urethral laceration (*arrowheads*) and extravasation of contrast into the periurethral soft tissues.

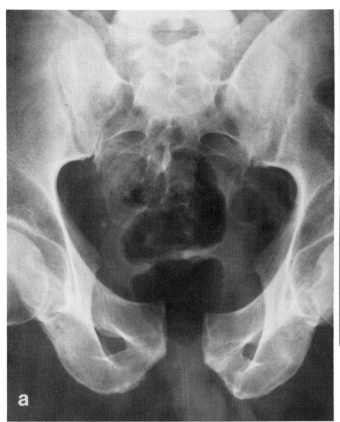
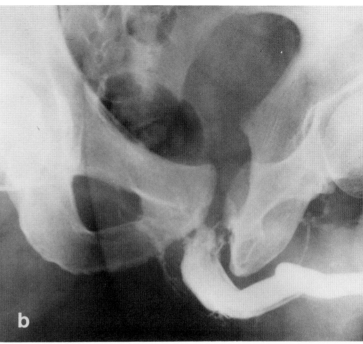

Fig. 10.60. Iatrogenic urethral lacerations. The Malgaigne injury (separation of the pubic symphysis and the left sacroiliac joint) **(a)** was sustained in an automobile accident. Attempts at catheterization were unsuccessful and a subsequent retrograde urethrogram **(b)** demonstrated complete extrinsic occlusion of the urethra and multiple sites of extravasation of contrast medium into the periurethral tissue. At laparotomy, the urethra was occluded by a massive periurethral hematoma, and multiple small, discrete, puncture wounds of the urethra, distal to the hematoma, were present.

ation (27). Bladder injuries have been described as contusion, intraperitoneal rupture, extraperitoneal rupture, and combined intra- and extraperitoneal rupture by Brosman and Fay (31).

The roentgen diagnosis of bladder injury may be made by antegrade urography but is more reliably made by retrograde urethrocystography. This is particularly true in instances of penetrating bladder injuries. Rieser (29) reported four patients with penetrating wounds of the bladder in whom the bladder laceration was not demonstrated by intravenous urography, but was by cystography.

Bladder contusion cannot be identified radiographically. Intraperitoneal rupture of the bladder is characterized by the presence of intravenously or cystographically administered contrast medium within the peritoneal space, outlining the paracolic gutters, the pelvic peritoneal recess, and surrounding loops of bowel (Fig. 10.61).

Extraperitoneal rupture of the bladder is characterized by streaky collections of contrast medium confined to the perivesical space (Figs. 10.49, 10.57, and 10.62).

Urethral Injuries

Urethral injuries caused by external violence are usually the result of blunt pelvic trauma, occur most commonly above the urogenital diaphragm at the junction of the prostatic and membranous portions of the urethra, and occur most frequently in patients with double vertical or Malgaigne fractures or fractures involving, or separation of, the pubic symphysis.

Mitchell (27) has stated that the diagnosis of urethral injury can be made on the basis of the clinical signs of blood at the external meatus, inability to void, and, subsequently, urinary retention. However, because significant injury to the lower urinary tract may

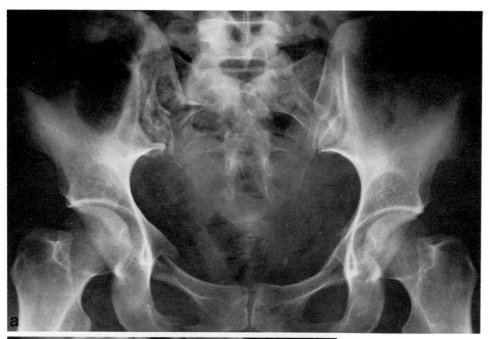

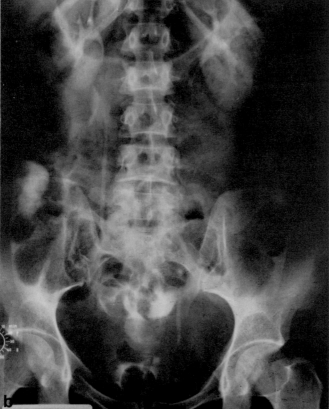

Fig. 10.61. Intraperitoneal rupture of the bladder and extraperitoneal perivesical hematoma. The plain radiograph of the pelvis **(a)** demonstrates minimally displaced, laterally situated, double vertical fractures of the anterior pelvic arch and the homogeneous soft tissue density throughout the pelvis which obliterates the normal pelvic soft tissue anatomy and has displaced the ileal loops out of the pelvis. The latter signs indicate an extraperitoneal perivesical effusion which, in the absence of contrast medium in the same space, represents hemorrhage. The infusion pyelogram **(b)** demonstrates contrast medium free in the peritoneal space, in the paracolic gutters and pelvic peritoneal recess, and in surrounding loops of bowel.

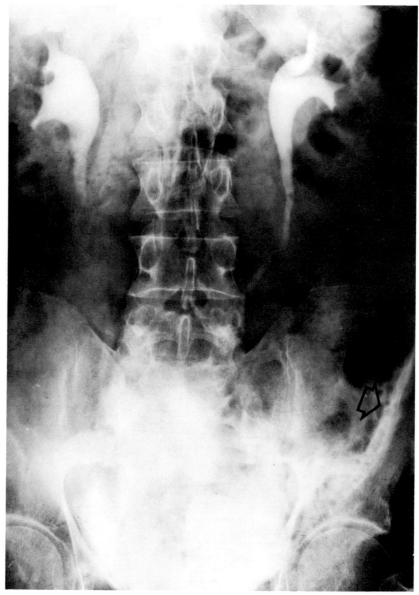

Fig. 10.62. Extraperitoneal rupture of the bladder with large amounts of contrast medium filling the perivesical space and extending retrogradely into the extraperitoneal fat of the flank stripe (*open arrow*).

occur without hematuria (33) and because there is an approximate 20% association of urethral and bladder injuries (27), retrograde urethrography is advocated in all patients suspected of having urethral injury.

Precise identification of the location and type of urethral injuries is evident on urethrography performed under fluoroscopic control. The diagnosis of urethral laceration or transection is dependent upon the demonstration of extraluminal contrast medium. Rarely, a patient with a pubic symphysis separation may have an intact urethra obstructed by a large periurethral hematoma. Such patients will be unable to void, initially, and urethrography will demonstrate circumferential, extrinsic compression of the urethra, incomplete visualization of the lumen of the compressed segment and, most importantly, absence of extravasation of contrast into the periurethral tissues (Fig. 10.63). With progressive distention of the bladder, the intravesical pressure usually overcomes the resistance of the periurethral tamponade and voiding occurs spontaneously. Catheterization is indicated if the patient does not void within 8–10 hours postinjury.

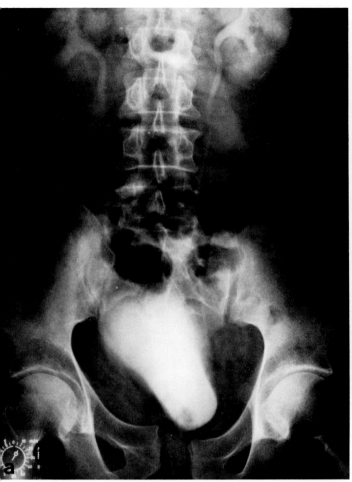
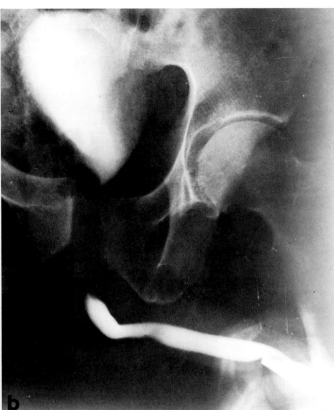

Fig. 10.63. Traumatic separation of the pubic symphysis. Opacification of the urinary bladder by means of infusion pyelography **(a)** demonstrates the typical "pear-shaped" configuration indicative of bilateral, large pelvic hematoma. The base of the bladder is displaced to the patient's left. A cystourethrogram **(b)** was performed. No contrast medium is seen in the bulbous, membranous, or prostatic portions of the urethra. The configuration of the base of the bladder and the proximal end of the column of contrast medium in the penile urethra are characteristic of extraluminal compression. None of the contrast medium was seen outside the lumen of the urinary tract. These findings are those of a massive pelvic hematoma that externally compressed the proximal urethra. The urinary tract itself is intact.

Urethral laceration is indicated by extravasation of contrast medium at the junction of the prostatic and membranous portions of the urethra (Fig. 10.59) or at the junction of the bladder and prostatic urethra (Figs. 10.64–10.66).

Transection of the urethra occurs most frequently at the junction of the prostatic and membranous portions, just above the urogenital diaphragm (Figs. 10.50–10.52). The transection is indicated by an abrupt and complete disruption of the column of contrast within the urethral lumen and gross extravasation of opaque into the periurethral tissues. Neither the urethra proximal to the level of transection nor the bladder will be opacified by the retrograde study (Fig. 10.67).

Rupture of the male urethra at the apex of the prostate, where it passes through the deep layer of urogenital diaphragm, is the commonest urologic injury associated with pelvic trauma (Fig. 10.68) (38). Digital rectal examination will reveal a defect at the site of the prostatic fossa, and the prostate, having been retracted upward with the bladder, will not be palpable.

Rupture of the membranous urethra, that portion of the urethra lying between the fascial layers of the urogenital diaphragm, results in the accumulation of blood and urine within a confined space. As the fluid continues to accumulate, usually the thin deep layer of the urogenital diaphragm breaks down and the urine then escapes into the perivesical space.

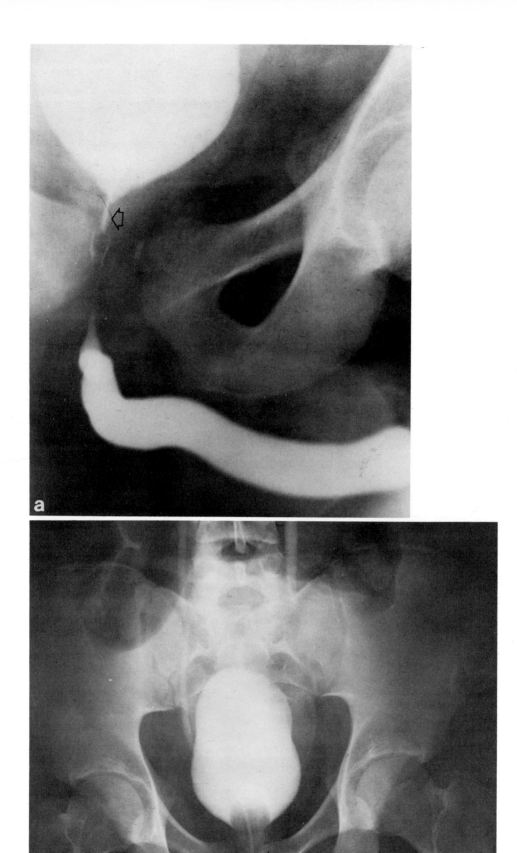

Fig. 10.64. Laceration at the urethrovesical junction demonstrated by retrograde urethrocystography **(a)** in a patient who sustained pubic symphysis separation. The short, straight collection of contrast between the veru montanum and the bladder (*open arrow*) is characteristic of the appearance of a urethral laceration at this site. Initial extravasation of contrast was prevented by the tamponade effect of the periurethral hematoma. Subsequent infusion pyelography **(b)** demonstrated the ''hour-glass'' configuration of the bladder reflective of a periurethral effusion, and contrast had diffused into the periurethral tissues (*open arrows*).

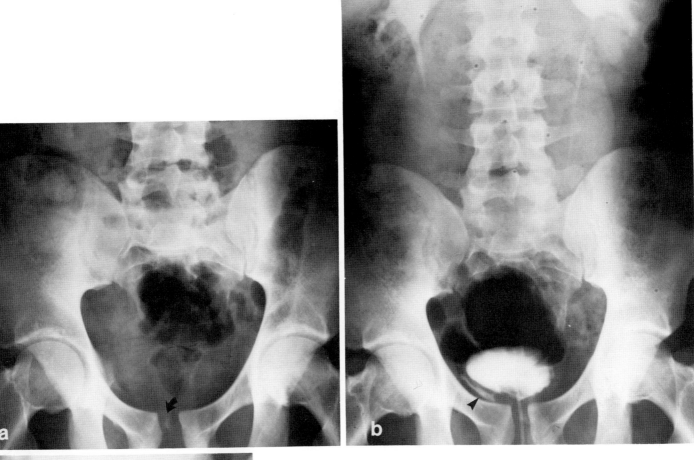

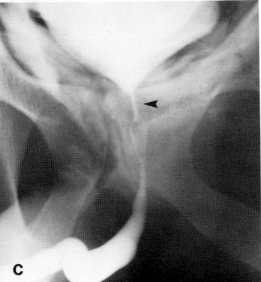

Fig. 10.65. Laceration of the urethrovesical junction. The survey radiograph of the abdomen and pelvis **(a)** reveals a pubic symphysis separation with a small avulsion fracture in the symphysis and separation of the left sacroiliac joint (Malgaigne injury) and soft tissue signs of an extraperitoneal perivesical effusion. Infusion pyelography **(b)** following insertion of a Foley catheter demonstrated contrast medium in the perivesical space (*arrowhead*) but not the site of laceration. The retrograde urethrocystogram performed following removal of the Foley catheter **(c)** identified the urethrovesical laceration (*arrowhead*).

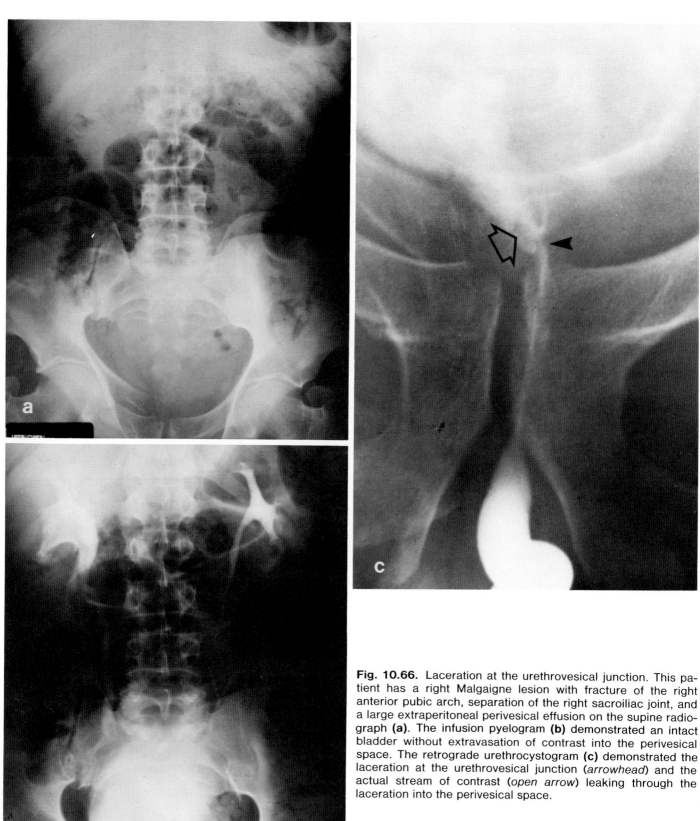

Fig. 10.66. Laceration at the urethrovesical junction. This patient has a right Malgaigne lesion with fracture of the right anterior pubic arch, separation of the right sacroiliac joint, and a large extraperitoneal perivesical effusion on the supine radiograph **(a)**. The infusion pyelogram **(b)** demonstrated an intact bladder without extravasation of contrast into the perivesical space. The retrograde urethrocystogram **(c)** demonstrated the laceration at the urethrovesical junction (*arrowhead*) and the actual stream of contrast (*open arrow*) leaking through the laceration into the perivesical space.

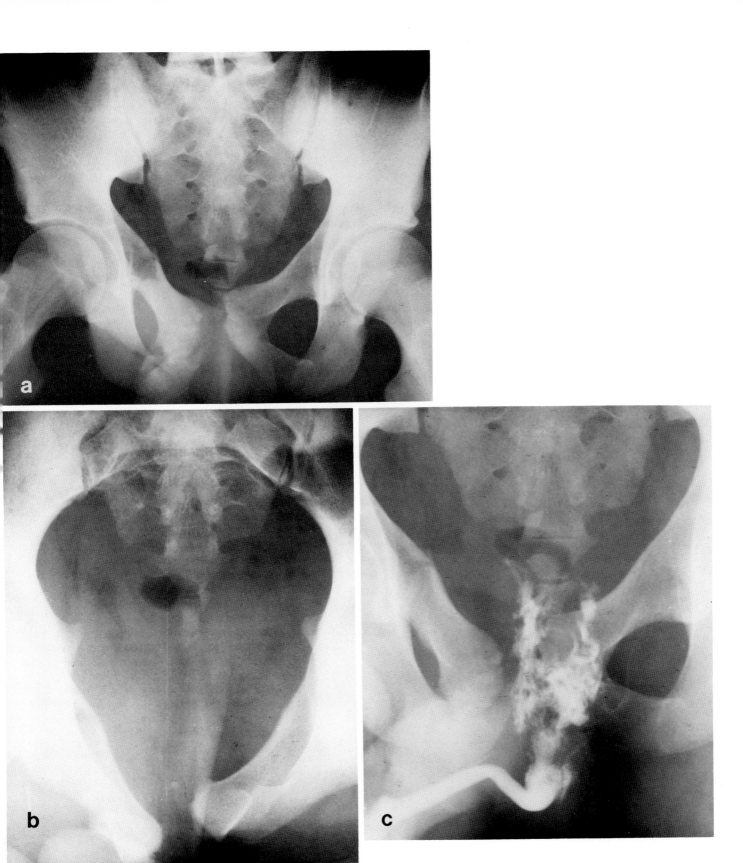

Fig. 10.67. Complete transection of the urethra. The anteroposterior radiograph of the pelvis **(a)** demonstrates a comminuted, displaced fracture of the right anterior pelvic arch and separation of the pubic symphysis. The homogeneous density in the pelvis indicates a large extraperitoneal perivesical effusion (hemorrhage). The degree of pubic symphysis separation is better appreciated in the caudally angled anteroposterior radiograph **(b)**. Urethral transection and gross extravasation of contrast medium is demonstrated on the retrograde urethrogram **(c)**.

551

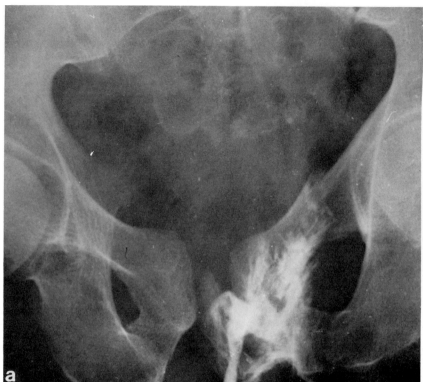

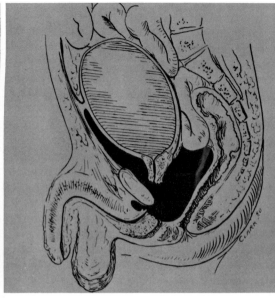

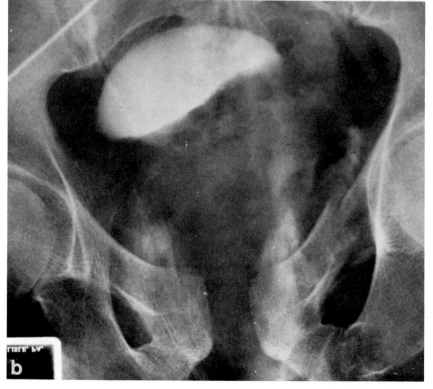

Fig. 10.68. Multiple fractures of the anterior pelvic arch associated with separation of the pubic symphysis. The retrograde urethrogram **(a)** demonstrates disruption of the posterior urethra and contrast medium into the periurethral soft tissues. An infusion pyelogram **(b)** demonstrates the marked upward displacement of the urinary bladder that has resulted from transection of the proximal urethra. Contrast medium is admixed with the large infravesical hematoma. **(c)** This schematic representation of the midsagittal plane of the male pelvis illustrates the effects of disruption of the membranous urethra. These include superior displacement of the bladder and the prostate and the accumulation of a retroperitoneal, perivesical hematoma. (Modified from J. H. Harrison: The treatment of rupture of the urethra especially when accompanying fractures of the pelvic bones. *Surgery, Gynecology and Obstetrics* 72: 622, 1941.)

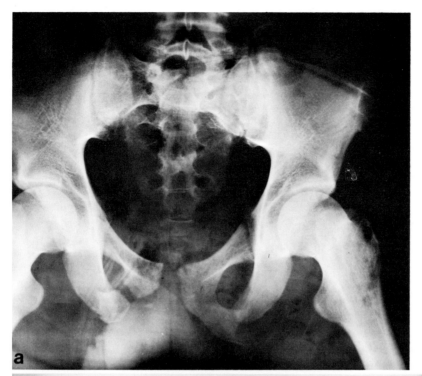

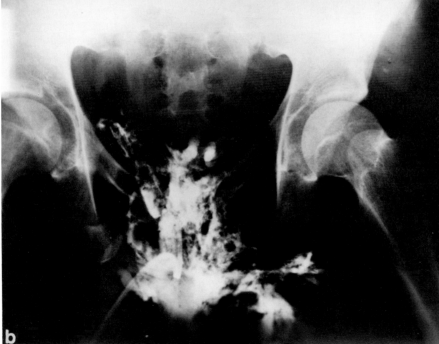

Fig. 10.69. Crushing injury of the pelvis with multiple bilateral anterior pelvic arch fractures and pubic symphysis separation. There is extensive subcutaneous emphysema of the thighs, perineum, and pelvis **(a)**. The retrograde urethrogram **(b)** demonstrates complete transection of the urethra and gross extravasation of contrast medium both within the perineum and the pelvis, indicating disruption of the urogenital diaphragm.

Disruption of the urethra superficial to the external surface of the urogenital diaphragm results in extravasation of urine and, when present, contrast medium into the perineum and scrotum (Fig. 10.69).

Prior to interventional angiography, hemorrhage into the retroperitoneal space was the most common cause of death associated with pelvic fractures. An approximate 20% mortality of patients who required laparotomy because of severe injury and massive blood loss associated with pelvic fractures has been reported (1,37). The usual sites of arterial bleeding are branches of the hypogastric artery. Extensive bleeding may also result from disruption of the rich venous plexuses deep in the pelvis related to the base of the bladder, prostate, vagina, and anterior pelvic arch. The fundamental clinical feature of this bleeding is that it is "silent." As much as 1500–2000 cc of blood can accumulate within the pelvic retroperitoneal space without any clinical sign until the patient suddenly goes into shock. Therefore, it is incumbent upon everyone involved in the management of patients with pelvic trauma to be acutely aware of the possibility of intrapelvic hemorrhage.

Insight into the soft tissue complications of pelvic fractures is predicted upon a knowledge of the soft tissue anatomy of the pelvis. The blood supply of the pelvis is shown in Figure 10.70. The hypogastric (internal iliac) artery is the source of the major blood supply of the pelvic canal via its branches, the iliolumbar, sacral, gluteal, pudendal, vesical, and obturator arteries. Of these, the iliolumbar is a major source

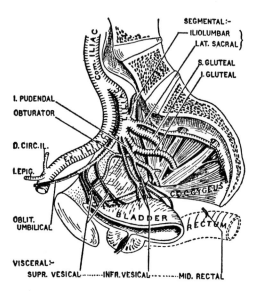

Fig. 10.70. The blood supply of the pelvis arises from the internal iliac (hypogastric) artery. Note the relationship of the obturator artery and the superior vesical artery to the anterior pubic arch. [Reprinted with permission from J. V. Basmajian (Ed): *Grant's Method of Anatomy,* ed. 8. Williams & Wilkins, Baltimore, 1971.]

of arterial bleeding caused by posterior pelvic arch fractures and the obturator artery associated with anterior arch fractures.

The rich venous plexus of the pelvis (Fig. 10.71) is a source of major bleeding with anterior pelvic arch fractures and with fractures resulting in injury to the urogenital diaphragm, the base of the bladder, the prostatic urethra, and fractures near, or separation of, the sacroiliac joint.

The plain film signs of an extraperitoneal perivesical effusion (hemorrhage) have been previously described. Figure 10.72 is an example of the roentgen appearance of a right sided extraperitoneal perivesical hematoma. The position and configuration of the bladder provides a quantitative estimate of the size and location of the extraperitoneal perivesical hematoma (Figs. 10.64, 10.73–10.75).

Nontraumatic Lesions

Slipped capital femoral epiphysis typically occurs in males between the ages of 12 and 16 years and is uncommon in children under the age of 10 years. It is usually an insidious process extending over a period of several weeks and associated with progressive discomfort and a limp. The pain associated with a slipped capital femoral epiphysis may not be experienced in the hip but is commonly referred to the knee. Therefore, it is imperative to examine the hip clinically and, if indicated, radiographically in every child with unexplained pain in the knee.

The proximal femoral epiphysis usually slips both dorsally and medially resulting in a varus deformity (Fig. 10.76), although the epiphysis may shift in either direction alone. The earliest radiographic signs of slipped capital femoral epiphysis are subtle. Depending upon the direction of movement of the epiphysis, the abnormal roentgen findings may be visible in only one projection. Straight anteroposterior and horizontal beam lateral projections should be obtained initially. If these are negative, an anteroposterior radiograph in the "frog leg" position is indicated because, in this position, the femoral head and neck are seen in the plane midway between that projected in the straight anteroposterior and the true lateral radiograph.

Distention of the capsule of the hip joint (Fig. 10.77) may be the earliest or most prominent radiographic finding of osteomyelitis of the bones of the hip or of pyarthrosis.

Frank, acute osteomyelitis of the hip may produce an ill defined area of demineralization of the involved bone (Fig. 10.78).

Aseptic necrosis of the femoral head is due to a disturbance in the blood supply of the head or its epiphysis. Loss of blood supply results in death of the involved segment. The roentgen appearance of necro-

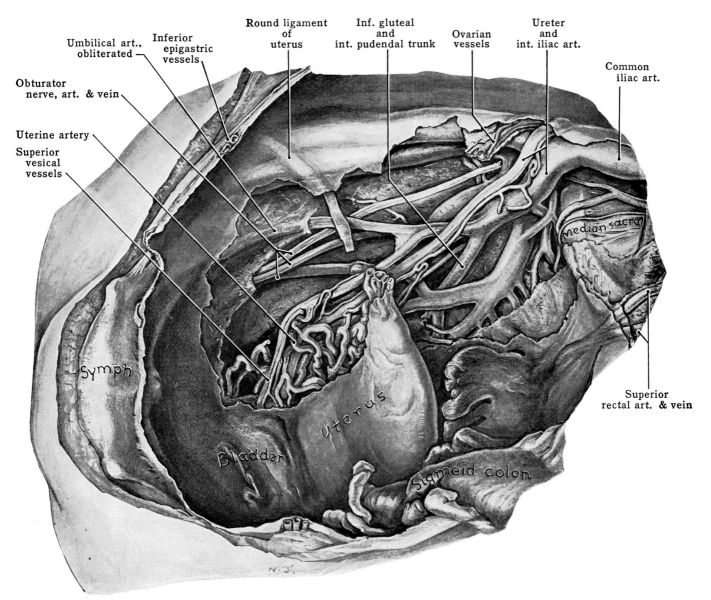

Fig. 10.71. Note the extensive venous plexuses in the floor of the pelvis. This profuse venous network is a major source of retroperitoneal intrapelvic hemorrhage associated with pelvic trauma involving the bladder, the posterior urethra, or the urogenital diaphragm. (Reprinted with permission from J.E. Anderson: *Grant's Atlas of Anatomy*, ed. 6. Williams & Wilkins, Baltimore, 1972.)

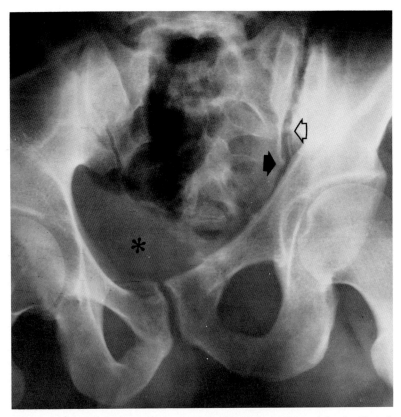

Fig. 10.72. This patient sustained a Malgaigne fracture of the left side of the pelvis. An ill defined homogeneous soft tissue density (*) involving principally the right side of the pelvis represents a hematoma in the perivesical space.

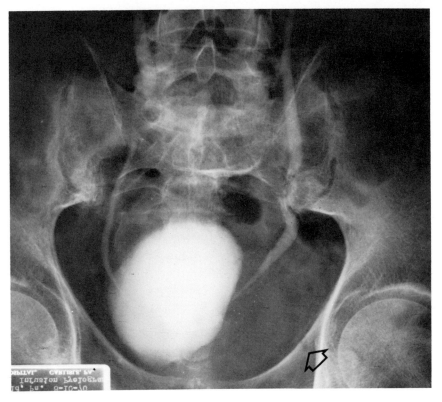

Fig. 10.73. An infusion pyelogram was performed in this patient who sustained trauma to the pelvis. The only fracture of the bones of the pelvis is indicated by the *arrow*. The amount of displacement of the urinary bladder and the pelvic portion of the left ureter indicates the size of the left-sided perivesical hematoma.

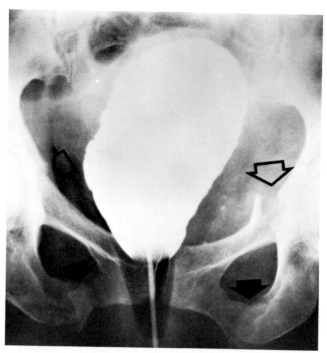

Fig. 10.74. This patient sustained bilateral fractures of each pubic ramus. The typical "pear-shaped" configuration of the urinary bladder is indicative of the presence of bilateral perivesical effusion.

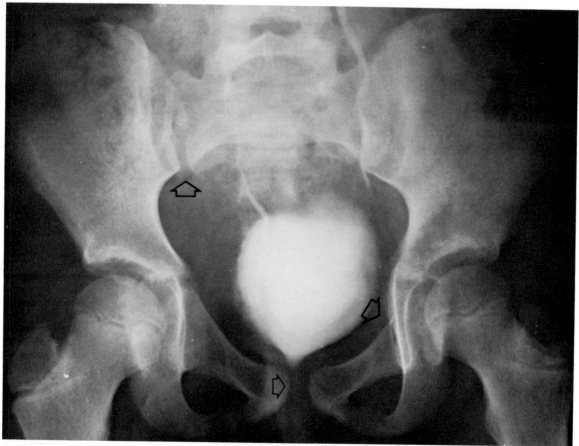

Fig. 10.75. Bilateral pelvic hematoma associated with multiple skeletal injuries, including separation of the right sacroiliac joint and pubic symphysis. The hemorrhage on the right has displaced the right ureter medially and the bladder to the left.

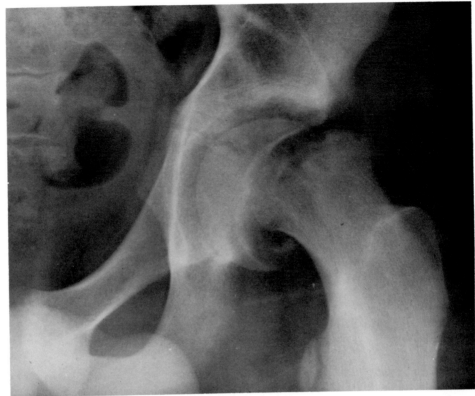

Fig. 10.76. Acute slip of the left capital femoral epiphysis. The epiphysis has slipped inferiorly while remaining within the acetabulum.

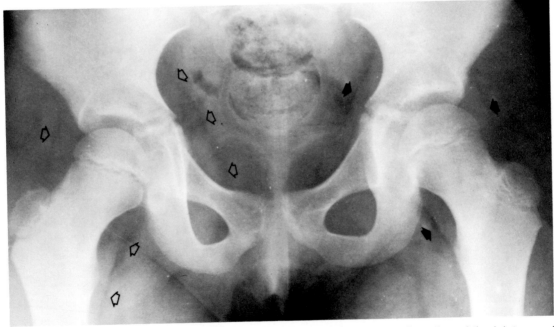

Fig. 10.77. Prominence of the soft tissue shadows about the right hip indicates distention of the joint capsule. The right obturator muscle shadow is also prominent. The contralateral, normal soft tissue shadows are indicated by *solid arrows.*

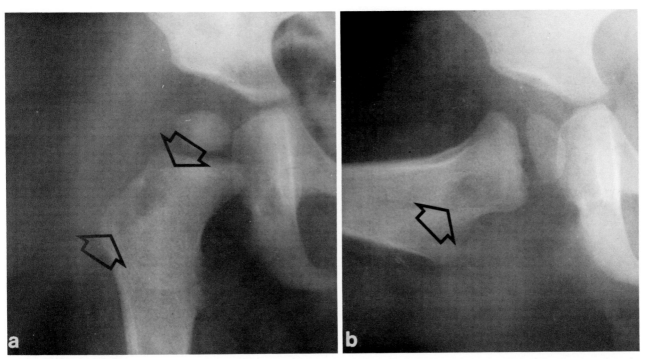

Fig. 10.78. (a, b) The *arrows* indicate ill defined, poorly marginated, radiolucent defects in the femoral neck caused by acute osteomyelitis.

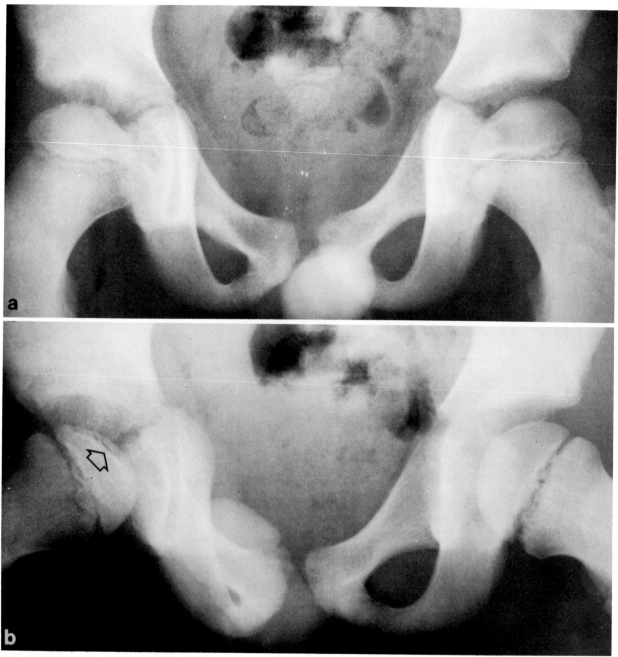

Fig. 10.79. (a) The radiographic signs of aseptic necrosis are seen in the right capital femoral epiphysis. These include widening of the joint space, flattening and irregular mineralization of the epiphysis, irregularity of its articulating surface, and fragmentation (**b**, *arrow*).

sis of the head and its reparative process may produce irregular demineralization, fragmentation, cortical disruption, and flattening or loss of structure of the femoral head or epiphysis. The latter may result in apparent widening of the joint space (Fig. 10.79).

Paget's disease of the pelvis usually involves multiple bones (Fig. 10.80), but may be limited to a single component of the pelvis. The radiographic features include irregular demineralization of the involved bones associated with cortical thickening, striations within the cortex, and prominence of the trabecular pattern.

Benign neoplasms involving the bones of the pelvis may, depending upon their cell type and location,

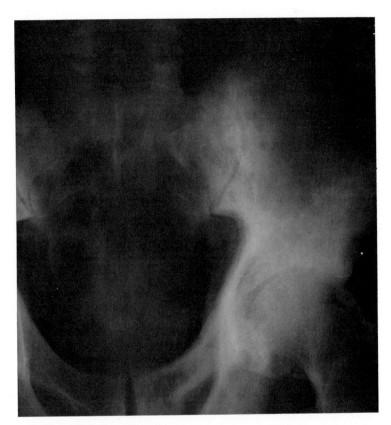

Fig. 10.80. Paget's disease of the left innominate bone. The classic radiographic findings include cortical thickening, prominence of trabecular pattern, and demineralization.

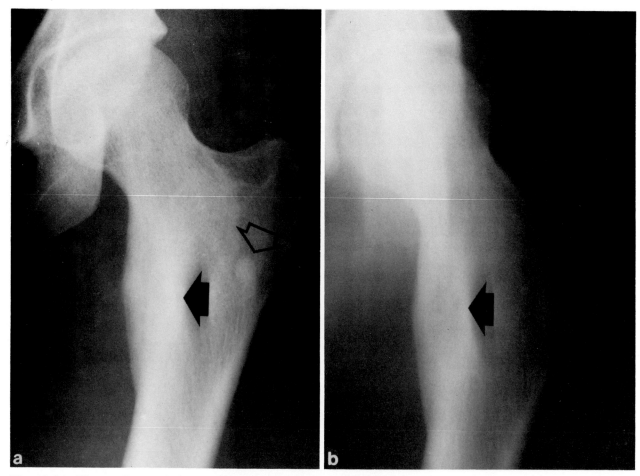

Fig. 10.81. The small, round, discrete density in the greater trochanter represents a bone ''island'' or ''infarct'' **(a)**. This is a clinically insignificant lesion of uncertain etiology. Cortical thickening in the region of the lesser trochanter and extending onto the base of the inferior aspect of the femoral neck is caused by an osteoid osteoma. The body section roentgenogram **(b)** demonstrates the radiolucent nidus (*arrow*) of the osteoma.

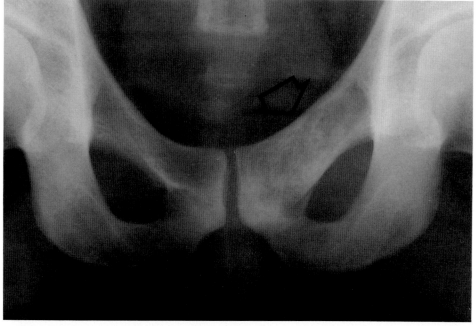

Fig. 10.82. The abnormalities of configuration, cortical thickness, and trabeculation in the left superior pubic ramus (*arrow*) of a 33-year-old female represent hemangioma of bone.

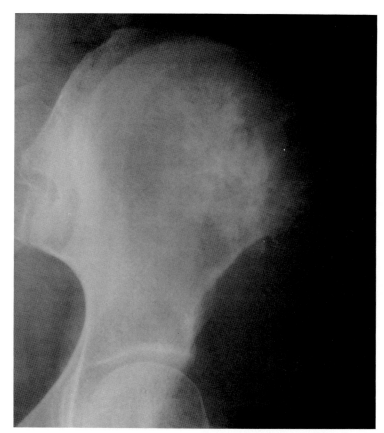

Fig. 10.83. Chondrosarcoma of the left iliac wing.

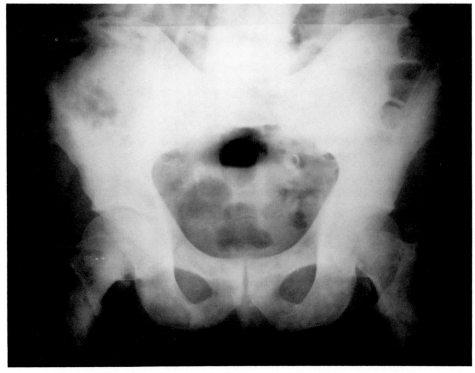

Fig. 10.84. Osteoblastic metastatic lesions of prostatic carcinoma.

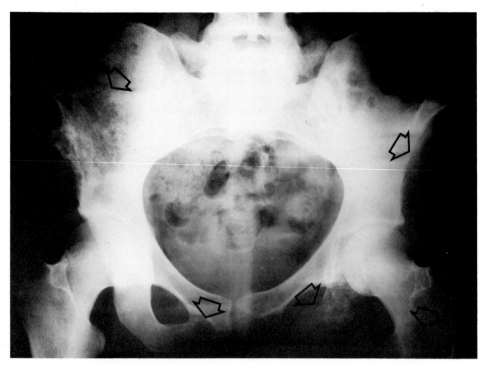

Fig. 10.85. Osteolytic metastasis from a primary breast carcinoma.

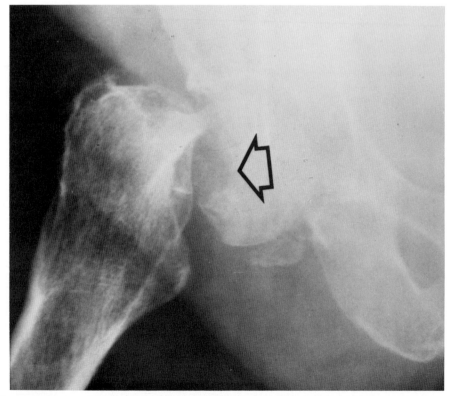

Fig. 10.86. Pathologic fracture in the neck of the right femur secondary to primary breast carcinoma. The characteristics of the margins of the fracture fragments (*arrow*) and the lytic defect with loss of trabecular pattern in the femoral neck fragment are typical signs of a metastatic lesion through which a fracture has occurred.

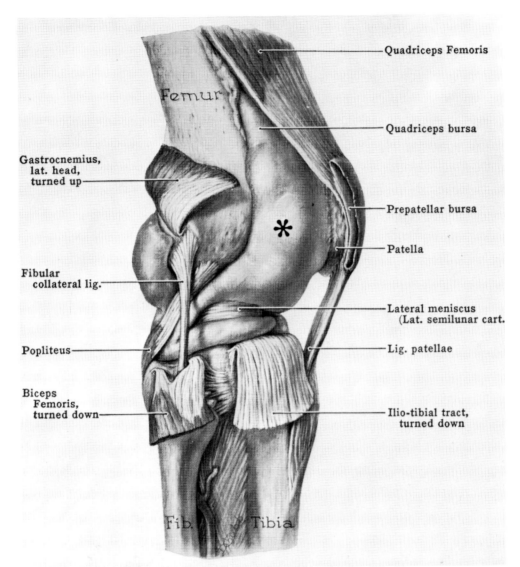

Fig. 11.6. Distention of the capsule (*) of the knee joint displaced the patella anteriorly. (Reprinted with permission from *Grant's Atlas of Anatomy*, ed. 6. Williams & Wilkins, Baltimore, 1972.)

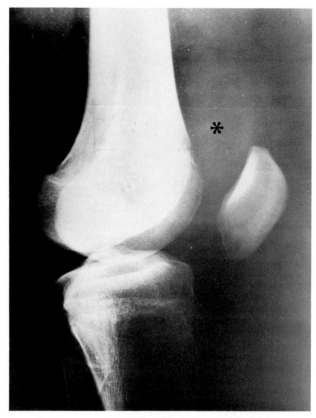

Fig. 11.7. Left knee joint effusion. The suprapatellar recess is distended by a homogeneous soft tissue density (*) which represents the joint effusion. The patella is displaced, by the distended joint capsule, anteriorly and canted inferiorly.

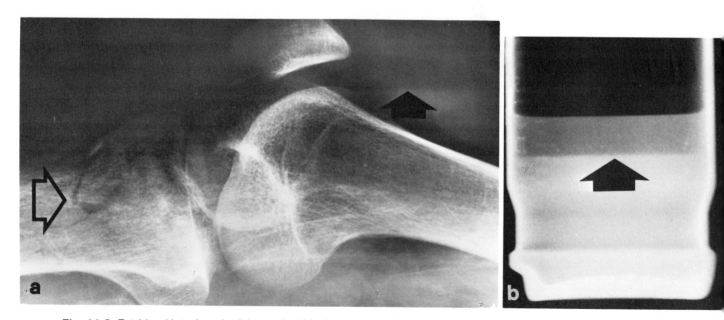

Fig. 11.8. Fat-blood interface (*solid arrow*) within the capsule of the knee joint (**a**). This sign is caused by the presence of liquid fat which has entered the joint space through a fracture involving the proximal articulating surface of the tibia (*open arrow*). (**b**) Radiographic appearance of the fluid aspirated from the knee joint. The *arrow* indicates the blood-fat interface.

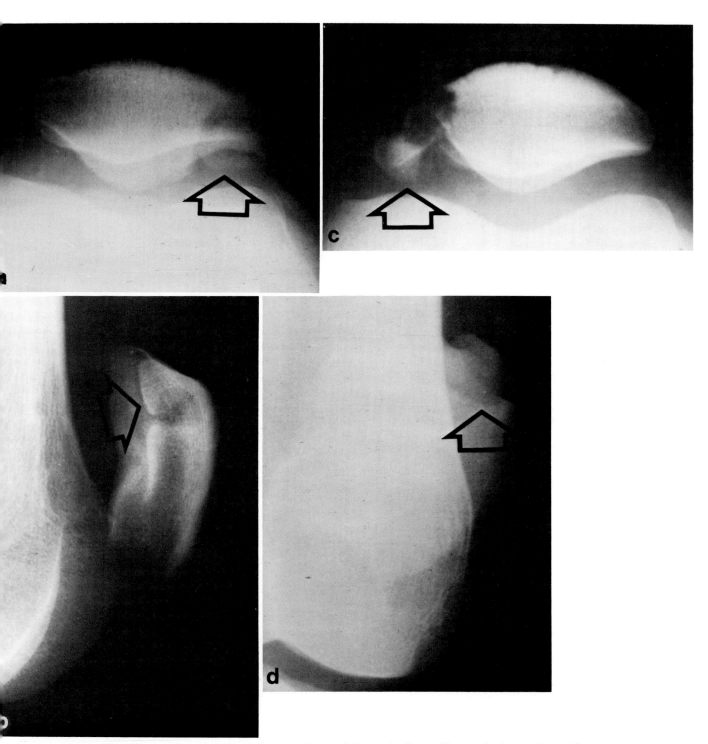

Fig. 11.17. Bipartite patella seen in axial (**a**) and lateral (**b**) projections. The cortical margins of the accessory ossification center are smooth and dense. The radiographic characteristics of this normal variant should distinguish it from a fracture of the patella (**c, d**).

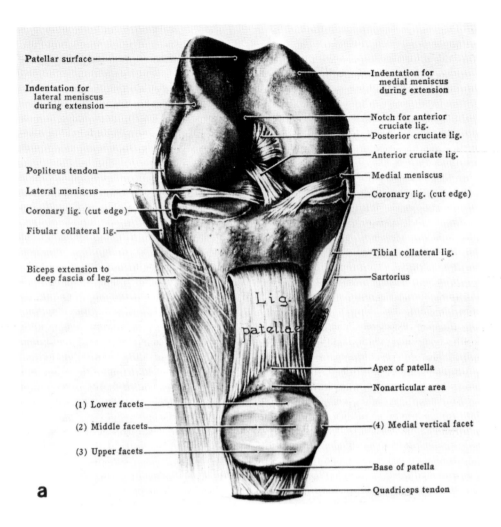

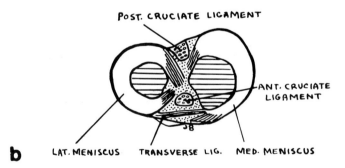

Fig. 11.18. (a) Soft tissue structures of the knee seen from the front. Observe the location of the anterior cruciate ligament. (Reprinted with permission from *Grant's Atlas of Anatomy*, ed. 6. Williams & Wilkins, Baltimore, 1972.) **(b)** Proximal articulating surface of the tibia seen from above. Note that only the anterior cruciate ligament attaches to the intercondylar eminence. (Modified from *Grant's Atlas of Anatomy*, ed. 6. Williams & Wilkins, Baltimore, 1972.)

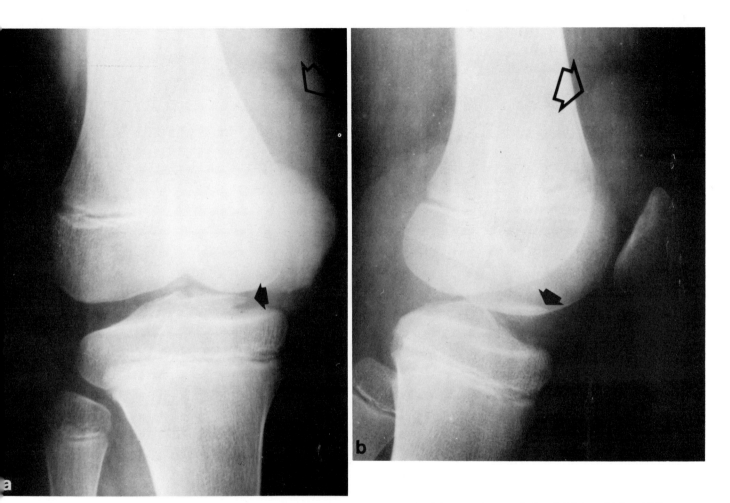

Fig. 11.19. Fracture through the base of the intercondylar eminence (*solid arrows*), seen in frontal (**a**) and lateral (**b**) projections. The location of the fracture indicates that the tibial attachment of the anterior cruciate ligament is disrupted. The soft tissue density anterior to the distal end of the femur (*open arrows*) is the hemorrhagic effusion distending the suprapatellar recess of the joint space.

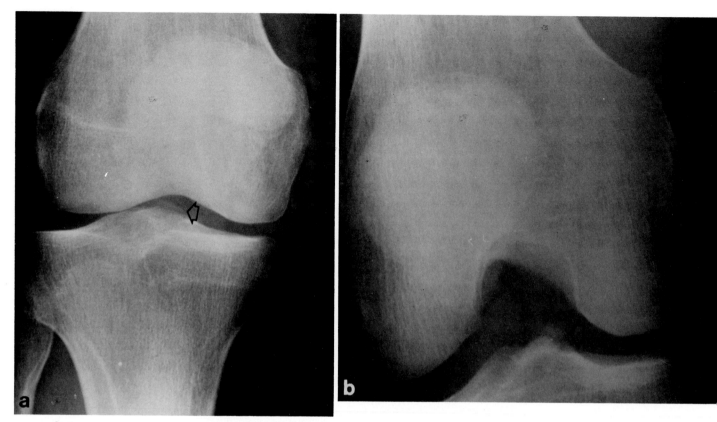

Fig. 11.20. Avulsion fracture of the medial tubercle (spine) of the intercondylar eminence, seen in the internally rotated oblique **(a)** and the ''tunnel'' (open-joint) **(b)** projections. This fracture indicates that the anterior cruciate ligament has been detached from its tibial insertion.

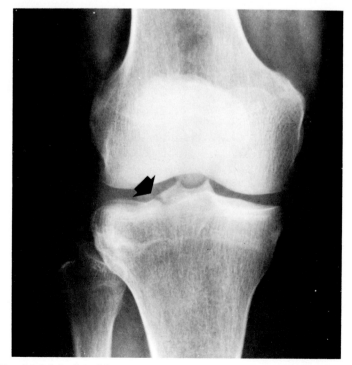

Fig. 11.21. Isolated fracture of the lateral tubercle of the tibial spine.

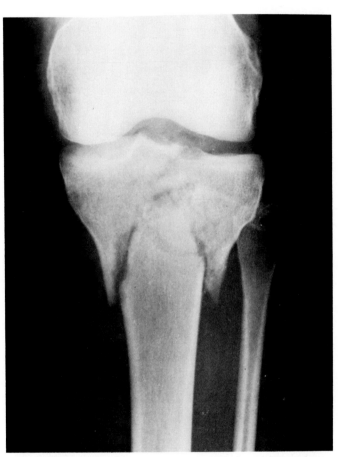

Fig. 11.26. Comminuted, minimally displaced, inverted "Y" fracture of the proximal portion of the tibia.

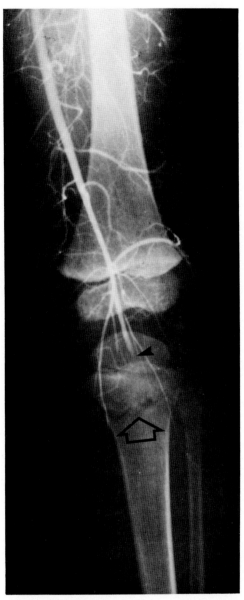

Fig. 11.27. Femoral arteriogram demonstrating complete obstruction of the popliteal artery (*arrowhead*) associated with a minimally displaced "bumper" fracture (*open arrow*) in a child.

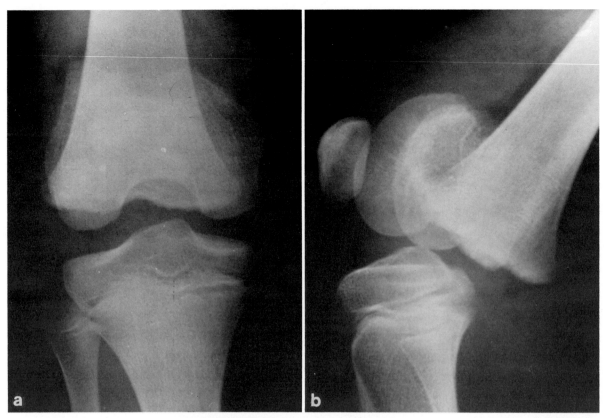

Fig. 11.28. (a, b) Distal femoral epiphyseal separation.

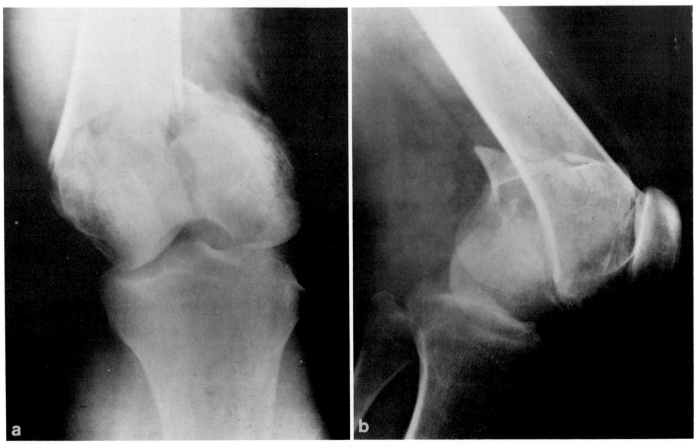

Fig. 11.29. (a, b) Comminuted, displaced intercondylar fracture.

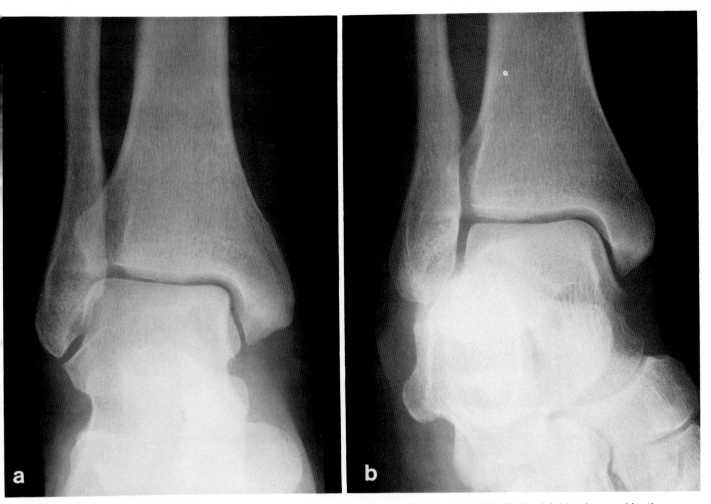

Fig. 12.5. Straight anteroposterior radiograph of the ankle **(a)**. Note that the distal tibiofibular joint is obscured by the superimposed contiguous portions of the tibia and fibula. In the mortise anteroposterior projection **(b)**, made with the leg in approximately 10° internal rotation so that the malleoli are on the same horizontal plane, the mortise is completely visualized and the distal tibiofibular joint opened.

With the foot and ankle positioned as is usually done for the anteroposterior view, i.e., with the great toe perpendicular to the plane of the table top, the ankle is actually slightly externally rotated (Fig. 12.5a). In this position, the anatomy of the mortise, the relationship of the talus to the mortise, and the distal tibiofibular articulation cannot be optimally assessed.

The correct lateral radiograph of the ankle results when the part is positioned so that the malleoli are directly superimposed upon each other (Fig. 12.6). This view should include the entire os calcis and the bones of the midfoot, including the base of the fifth metatarsal. Although neither the calcaneous nor the fifth metatarsal is a component of the ankle, each must be consciously studied for the presence of a

fracture which clinically may have been interpreted as an injury to the ankle (Figs. 12.7–12.9).

The synovial membrane of the ankle joint embraces only the talus and tibia. The distal fibula and lateral malleolus lie outside the synovium (Fig. 12.10). Therefore, distention of the capsule of the ankle joint, which is discernible radiographically only in the lateral projection, indicates an abnormality of the talus or the distal tibia.

Each oblique projection is an essential part of the routine radiographic examination of the acutely injured ankle (Fig. 12.11). These examinations are made with the patient supine and the *leg* rotated 45° internally and externally. The purpose and value of the oblique radiograph of the ankle are illustrated in Figures 12.12 and 12.13.

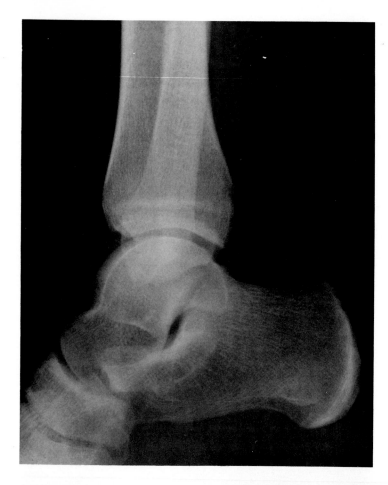

Fig. 12.6. Lateral radiograph of a normal adult ankle. The styloid processes are superimposed. The contiguous surfaces of the dome of the talus and the distal tibia are smooth and symmetrical. The subtalar joint is visible and both the talus and the os calcis are well seen in the lateral projection.

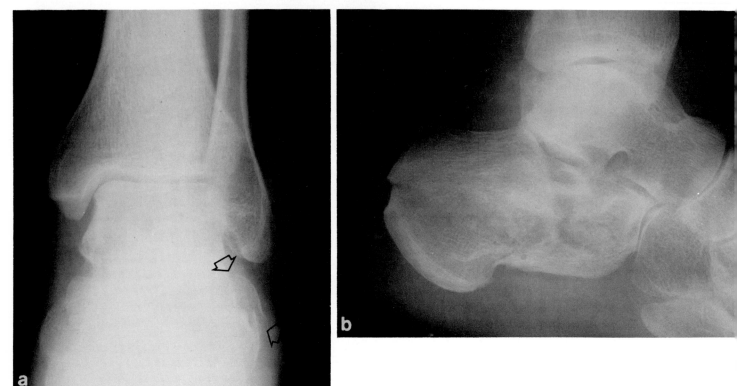

Fig. 12.7. In the frontal projection **(a)**, the bones of the ankle are normal. Soft tissue swelling is present in the inframalleolar space, and the *arrows* indicate a fracture of the calcaneus. In the lateral projection **(b)**, a severely comminuted fracture of the calcaneus is evident.

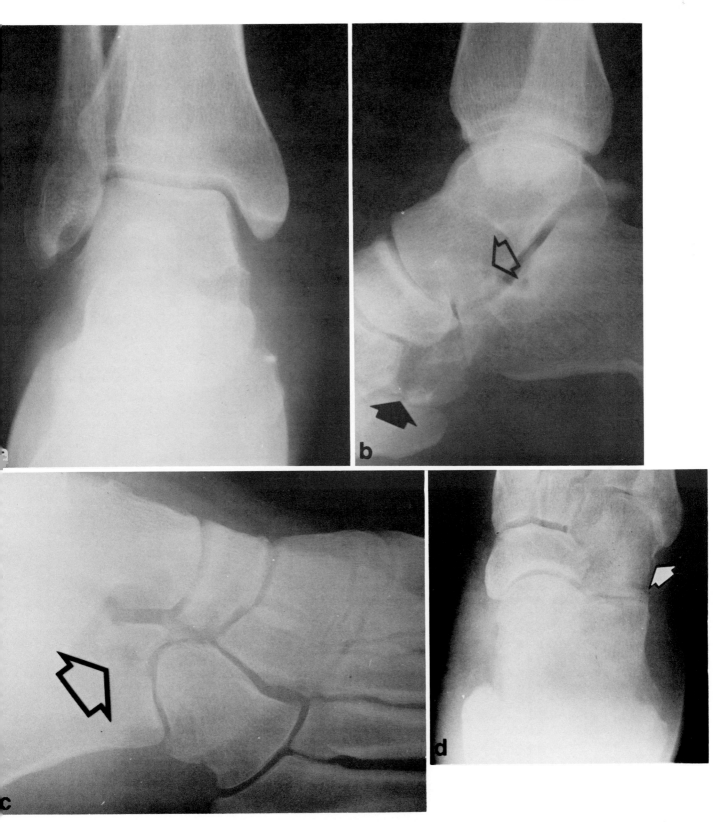

Fig. 12.8. (a) Frontal radiograph of the ankle demonstrating diffuse soft tissue swelling without evidence of fracture of the ankle. In the lateral projection (b), the *open arrow* indicates a fracture in the anterior tubercle of the os calcis and the *solid arrow* indicates a fracture in the tarsal cuboid. Oblique (c) and frontal (d) projections of the foot indicate the calcaneal (*open arrow*) and cuboid (*solid arrow*) fractures to better advantage.

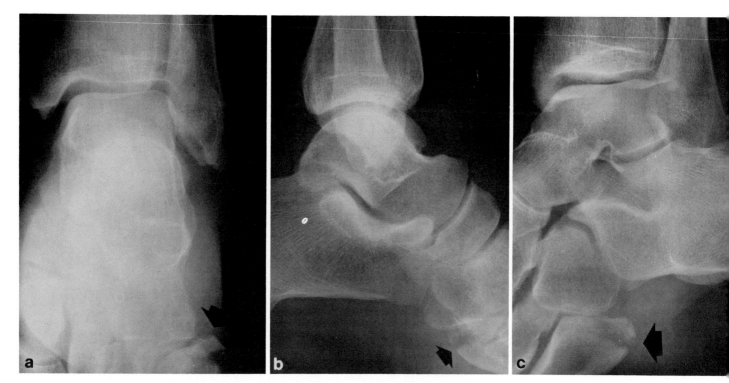

Fig. 12.9. (a) The frontal projection of the ankle is negative with exception of soft tissue swelling inferior to each malleolus. The *arrow* indicates the comminuted, displaced fracture of the base of the fifth metatarsal. **(b)** The fifth metatarsal fracture (*arrow*) can be seen in the lateral projection of the ankle but is seen to best advantage in the oblique projection **(c)**.

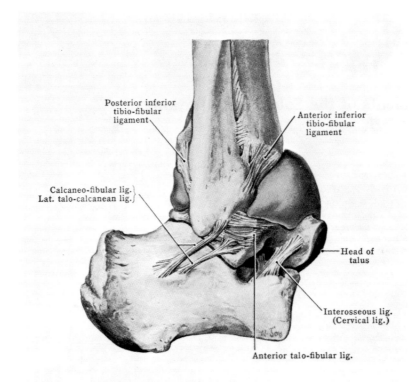

Fig. 12.10. Note the anterior bulge of the distended capsule of the ankle joint. (Reprinted from J. E. Anderson: *Grant's Atlas of Anatomy*, ed. 6. Williams & Wilkins, Baltimore, 1972.)

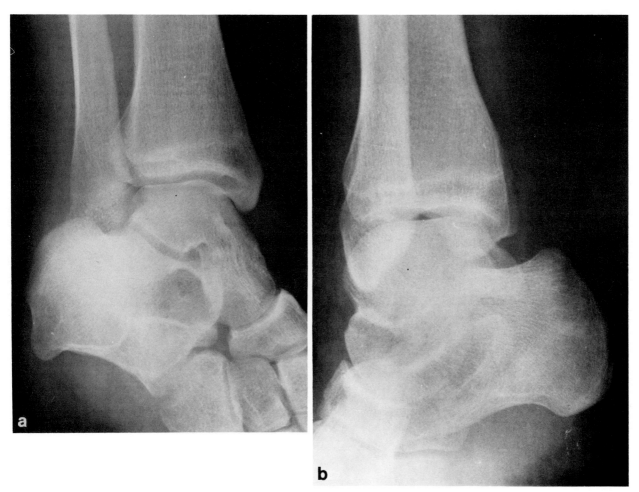

Fig. 12.11. Internally (a) and externally (b) rotated oblique projections of the ankle.

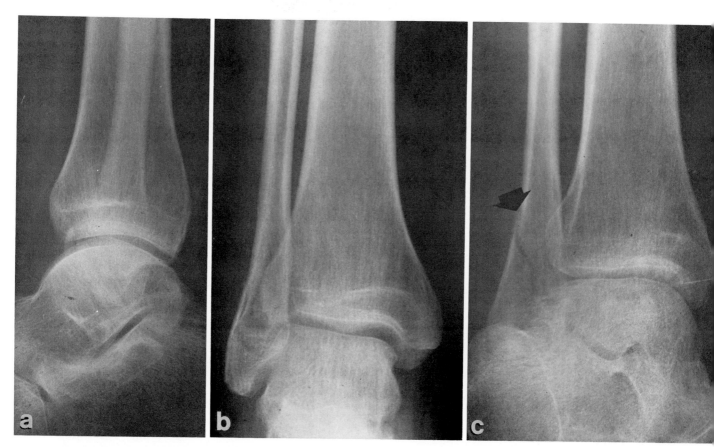

Fig. 12.12. The minimally displaced fracture in the lateral malleolus (*arrow*) is difficult to identify in the lateral (**a**) and frontal (**b**) projections and, consequently, could be overlooked. The fracture line is clearly perceptible in the internally rotated oblique projection (**c**).

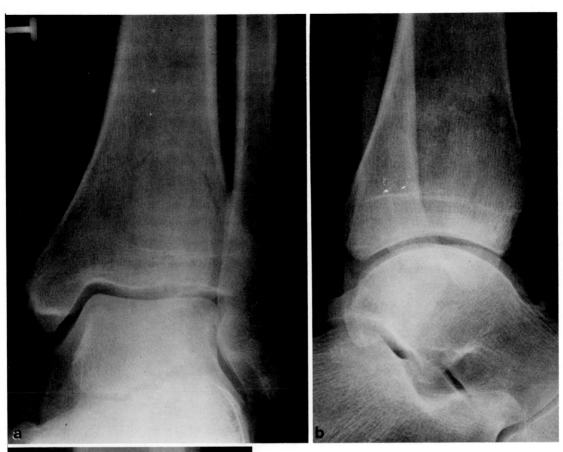

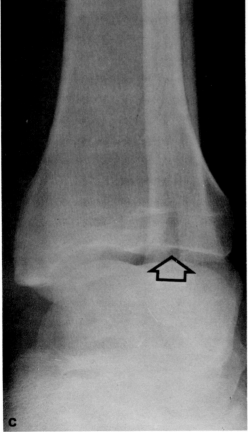

Fig. 12.13. Subtle, minimally displaced fracture in the distal tibia. The fracture line is only faintly perceptible in the frontal (**a**) and lateral (**b**) projections but is clearly evident in the externally rotated oblique projection (**c**).

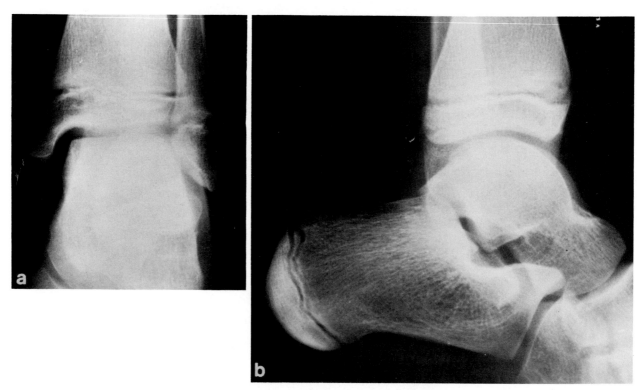

Fig. 12.14. Frontal (**a**) and lateral (**b**) radiograph of the normal child's ankle. Note the location and radiographic characteristics of the distal tibial and fibular epiphyseal lines in the frontal projection. In the lateral view, the distal fibular epiphyseal line is obscured by the density of the superimposed tibia and talus.

The roentgen appearance of the normal child's ankle is seen in Figure 12.14. The distal tibial epiphysis appears during the 2nd year of life and fuses at the 18th. The distal fibular epiphysis appears at age 2 years and fuses at age 20 years. Infrequently, the tip of the medial malleolus arises from a separate ossification center. The radiographic characteristics of this apophysis, its relationship to the epiphysis, and its frequent bilaterality help distinguish this normal variant from an avulsion fracture fragment (Fig. 12.15).

Radiographic Manifestations of Trauma

Extracapsular soft tissue swelling about the ankle joint is discernible in a properly exposed radiograph. While this is a nonspecific finding that is frequently present without an associated skeletal trauma, it may signal a subtle but significant bony injury (Figs. 12.16 and 12.17).

The roentgen significance of distention of the ankle joint capsule is illustrated in Figure 12.18.

Epiphyseal injuries, which frequently involve the ankle, are designated according to the Salter-Harris (1) classification (Table 12.1). Types III and IV occur more commonly at the ankle than any other site.

Type I epiphyseal injury, which occurs most commonly in newborns and young children, was originally described by Salter as being an epiphyseal separation without any bony fracture (Fig. 12.19). Typically, the separated epiphysis returns to a nearly anatomic position with respect to the adjacent metaphysis, and the Type I epiphyseal injury is difficult to recognize radiographically. In this instance, the most striking roentgen sign is soft tissue swelling adjacent to the epiphyseal line and minor uniform, or eccentric, widening of the epiphyseal line (Fig. 12.20). The epiphysis may not return to its anatomic position with respect to the metaphysis and, therefore, may be slightly, but definitely asymmetrically located relative to the metaphysis (Fig. 12.20). The periosteum is usually disrupted on the convex side and is invariably separated from the cortex on the concave side of the epiphyseal displacement. Occasionally, a tiny fragment of bone is pulled off from the margin of the metaphyseal or epiphyseal plate as the periosteum is stripped from the cortex. The presence of such a fragment, usually situated in the lateral aspect of the epiphyseal line between the metaphyseal and epiphyseal plates, together with widening of the epiphyseal line and adjacent soft tissue swelling, establish a Type I epiphyseal injury (Fig. 12.21).

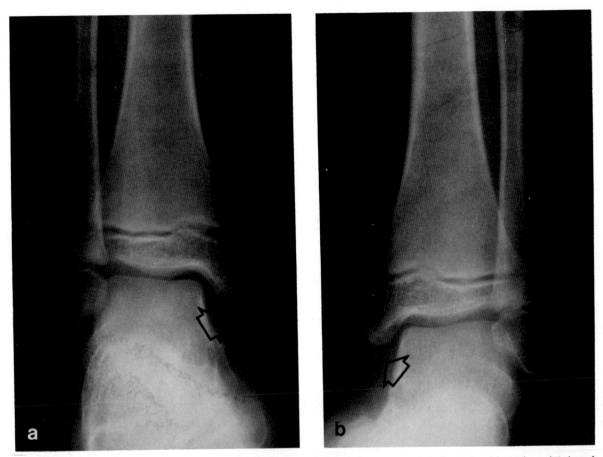

Fig. 12.15. (a, b) The *arrows* indicate medial malleolar apophyses. This normal variant should not be mistaken for an avulsion fracture fragment.

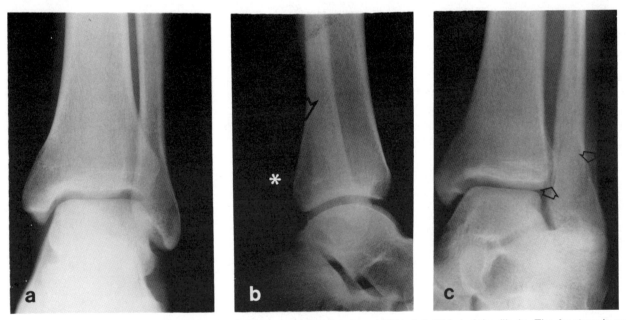

Fig. 12.16. Eversion injury with minimally displaced oblique fracture of the distal third of the fibula. The fracture is not discernible in the frontal projection **(a)** and is only faintly visible in the lateral projection **(b,** *open arrow*). Extracapsular soft tissue swelling **(*)** posterior to the distal end of the fibula is the most striking roentgen sign of this subtle skeletal injury, seen to best advantage in the internally rotated oblique projection **(c,** *open arrows*). Because of the location and direction of the distal fibular fracture line and the normal relationship between the distal end of the proximal fibular fragment and the tibia, it is reasonable to postulate that the deltoid ligament has been disrupted while the lateral collateral and tibiofibular ligaments and the interosseous membrane are intact.

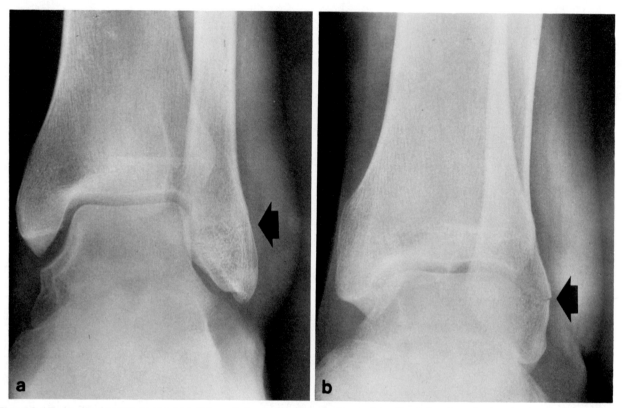

Fig. 12.17. In the frontal projection **(a)**, soft tissue swelling adjacent to the lateral malleolus is the most striking radiographic finding related to the complete, minimally displaced fracture in the lateral malleolus (*arrow*). The fracture is best seen in the oblique projection **(b)**.

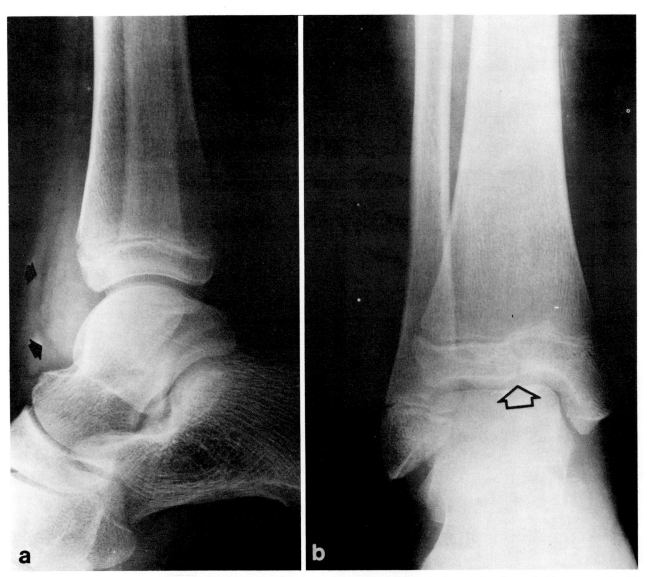

Fig. 12.18. In the lateral projection **(a)**, the *solid arrows* indicate the anterior bulge of the distended joint capsule. In the frontal projection **(b)**, there is minor separation of the lateral portion of the distal tibial physis and the *open arrow* indicates the subtle Salter-Harris III distal tibial epiphyseal injury.

Table 12.1
Incidence and Roentgen Characteristics of Physeal Injuries According to the Salter Harris Classification [a]

TYPE		ROGERS (118 fractures)	REED (33 fractures)
1		6%	5 (15%)
2		75%	17 (52%)
3		8%	7 (21%)
4		10%	4 (12%)
5		1%	

[a] From MH Reed: Fractures and dislocations of the extremities in children. Journal of Trauma *17:* 351, 1977.

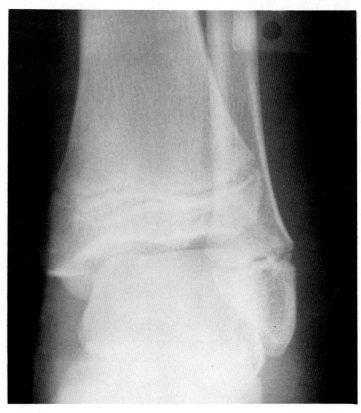

Fig. 12.19. Salter-Harris I epiphyseal injury of the lateral malleolus. The most striking radiographic sign is the diffuse soft tissue swelling about the malleolus. The physis is widened laterally.

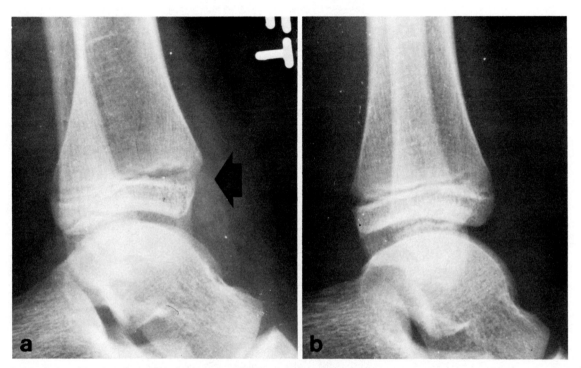

Fig. 12.20. Salter-Harris I distal tibial epiphyseal injury **(a)**. The physis is widened anteriorly and narrowed posteriorly and, consequently, is eccentrically situated with respect to the adjacent metaphysis (*arrow*). The normal side **(b)** has been reversed for ease of comparison.

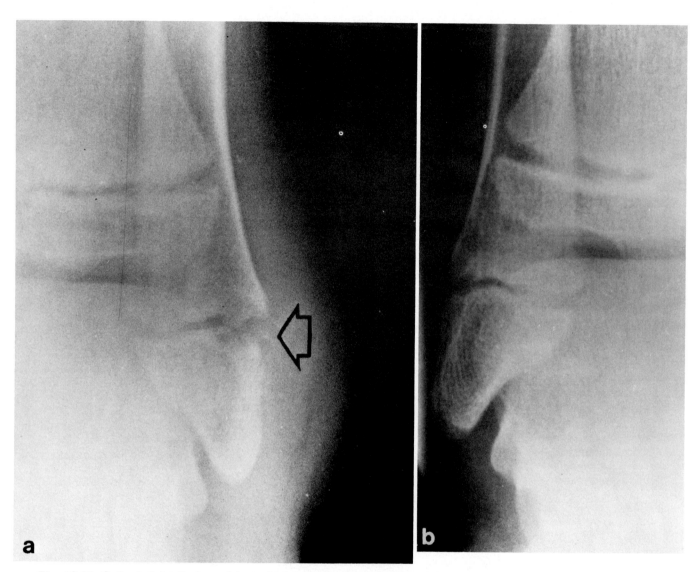

Fig. 12.21. Salter I distal fibular epiphyseal injury on the left (**a**). The epiphyseal line is widened laterally and a tiny fracture fragment (*open arrow*) has been pulled from the lateral margin of the epiphyseal plate. Diffuse soft tissue swelling is present about the lateral malleolus. The normal right ankle (**b**) is shown for comparison purposes.

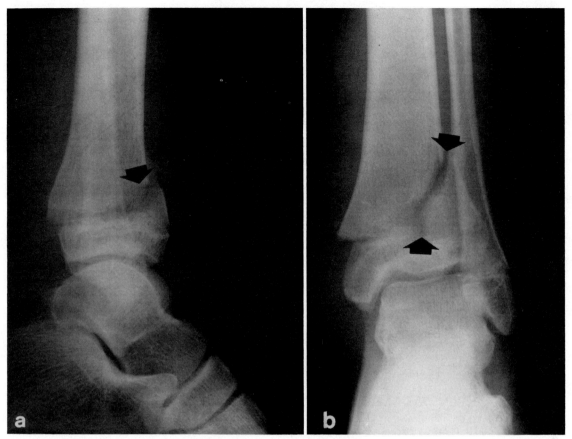

Fig. 12.22. Salter II distal tibial epiphyseal injury. The *arrows* indicate the metaphyseal fracture in both lateral **(a)** and anteroposterior **(b)** projections. Note that the resultant triangular metaphyseal fragment is normally related to the epiphysis. The epiphysis, together with the triangular metaphyseal fragment, has been separated medially and posteriorly and is displaced anteriorly and laterally relative to the metaphysis.

The Salter II ephiphyseal injury consists of an oblique fracture extending through the metaphysis into the epiphyseal line and separation through the remainder of the epiphyseal line. The triangular shaped metaphyseal fragment is not separated from the epiphysis and accompanies the epiphysis in its separation (Fig. 12.22). The Type II lesion is by far the most common of the epiphyseal injuries and usually occurs in older children, and the prognosis for normal growth is excellent.

The Salter III epiphyseal injury (Fig. 12.23) is uncommon, is usually seen in the distal tibial epiphysis, is entirely intracapsular, and the prognosis of normal growth is good provided the blood supply to the separated portion of the epiphysis has not been disrupted. Radiographically, the injury consists of a vertical fracture line which extends through the epiphysis from its articulating surface to the deep layer of the epiphyseal plate (*solid arrow*) and thence along the epiphyseal line to its margin (*open arrow*).

Figure 12.24 is an example of a Salter IV epiphyseal injury. The lesion consists of a vertical fracture that extends from the articulating surface through the entire thickness of the epiphysis, across the epiphyseal plate, and through a portion of the metaphysis (*arrows*). The mechanism of this particular fracture is schematically represented in Figure 12.35. Forced inversion of the ankle and medial rotation and displacement of the talus causes an impaction force to be exerted upon the medial malleolus, resulting in the fracture shown. In this patient, because there is no avulsion fracture of the lateral malleolus, it is reasonable to infer that the avulsion force has disrupted the lateral collateral ligament.

The Salter IV epiphyseal injury most commonly involves the elbow and is completely intra-articular, and, unless perfect reduction is obtained and maintained, the prognosis for normal growth is poor because of fracture healing across the epiphyseal plate.

The Salter V epiphyseal injury is uncommon, usually involves the ankle or the knee, is the result of severe crushing force, and is very difficult to recognize radiographically because the epiphysis is usually not displaced and there is no associated fracture. The

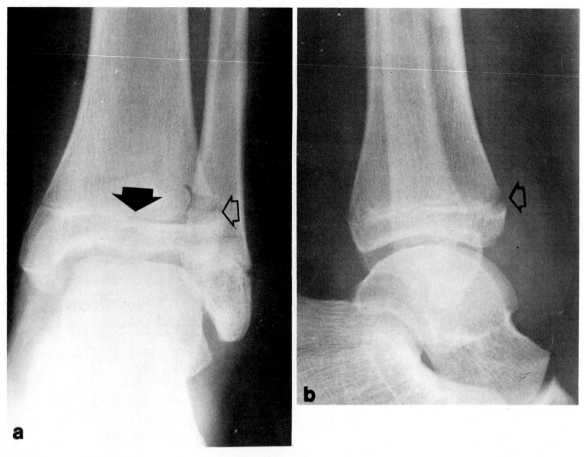

Fig. 12.23. (a, b) Salter III epiphyseal injury. The vertical epiphyseal fracture (*solid arrow*) extends through the epiphysis to the deep layer of the physis. The separated portion of the physis is indicated by the *open arrows*.

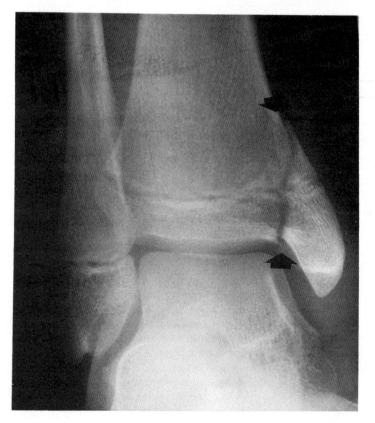

Fig. 12.24. Salter IV type epiphyseal injury. The vertical fracture line which extends through the epiphysis, the physis, and the metaphysis is indicated by the *arrows*.

prognosis for normal growth is poor because this injury is invariably associated with premature cessation of growth.

Fractures of the ankle are second only to fractures of the wrist in frequency. Since the only normal range of motion of the ankle joint is dorsi- and plantar flexion, ankle fractures are the result of severe abduction (eversion), adduction (inversion), or rotational forces. In both eversion and inversion injuries, fractures caused by both avulsion and impaction forces occur. The impaction component is caused by forceful talar shift or rotation striking the appropriate malleolus. The impaction injuries are characterized by oblique fracture lines. Horizontal fractures of the malleoli represent the effect of the avulsive force. Fractures at, and above, the level of the plafond are unstable. It must be remembered that significant ligamentous injury may occur about the ankle without associated skeletal injury. Disruption of one or more of the major ligaments at the ankle can be as important to the stability of the ankle mortise as a fracture. Therefore, it is incumbent upon the radiologist to recognize the roentgen signs of ligamentous injury and to convey that information to the attending physician. Depending upon the clinical and radiographic findings, stress views of the ankle may be indicated to determine the extent of ligamentous injury.

Classifications of ankle injuries have been presented by Ralston (2), Cave et al. (3), DePalma (4), and Salter (1). The concept of ankle injuries described by Edeiken and Cotler (5), which is based upon an understanding of the mechanism of injury, provides the most logical and practical approach to the radiologic assessment of traumatic lesions of the ankle. The following discussion of ankle injuries follows closely that of Edeiken and Cotler.

Eversion Injuries

The simplest eversion injury is a "sprain" of the ankle in which a few fibers of the deltoid ligament are disrupted. Radiographically, the only abnormality is soft tissue swelling about and distal to the medial malleolus. The bones of the ankle are intact and the anatomy of the ankle mortise is normally maintained (Fig. 12.25).

Avulsion of the deltoid ligament may be associated with cortical fractures of the medial malleolus. In this event, thin fracture fragments will be seen immediately adjacent to the styloid process of the malleolus (Fig. 12.26). Stress views are not required since the presence of the avulsion fracture fragment indicates that the deltoid ligament, together with its cortical insertion, has been disrupted. If the avulsion of the deltoid ligament is not associated with cortical fractures of the medial styloid process, stress views are

indicated to establish the avulsion of the ligament. In either instance, soft tissue swelling is present at and distal to the level of the medial malleolus.

If the force of the eversion injury is expended on the medial malleolus, a transverse (avulsion) fracture distal to the level of the plafond results (Fig. 12.27). In this injury, the medial collateral (deltoid) ligament is intact.

Eversion injuries associated with forceful lateral displacement and outward rotation of the talus have both an avulsion and an impaction component. Dispersion of the impaction force may result in any one of several different forms of injury. In Figure 12.28, the talus is laterally displaced and has impacted upon the lateral malleolus producing an oblique fracture through the distal portion of the fibula, proximal to the level of the plafond. The normal relationship between the distal end of the proximal fibular fragment and the tibia indicates that the tibiofibular ligaments and the interosseous membrane remain intact. The absence of a medial malleolar fracture, together with lateral displacement of the talus, indicates that the medial collateral (deltoid) ligament has either been disrupted or avulsed from the medial styloid process or from the talus.

In Figure 12.29, the impaction force of the talus upon the lateral malleolus has resulted in disruption of the tibiofibular ligaments and the interosseous membrane. Distal tibiofibular diastasis attests to these ligamentous injuries. The fibula is intact. The avulsive force has resulted in a transverse fracture of the medial malleolus, indicating that the deltoid ligament remains intact.

The Maisonneuve fracture (6), which is caused by the same mechanism of injury, includes disruption of the deltoid and distal tibiofibular ligaments, distal tibiofibular diastasis, disruption of the interosseous membrane, and a fracture of the neck of the fibula proximally (see Fig. 14.13).

When eversion injuries of the ankle cause transverse (Fig. 12.30) or oblique (Fig. 12.31) fractures of the distal third of the fibula, it is evident that both of the tibiofibular ligaments are disrupted and that the interosseous membrane is torn to the level of the fracture. These injuries represent the impaction component. Medially, the avulsion force may result in either disruption or avulsion of the deltoid ligament or a transverse fracture of the medial malleolus.

Inversion Injuries

Inversion injuries of the ankle also consist of an avulsion and an impaction component. The avulsion force affects the lateral structures of the ankle and may cause disruption (Fig. 12.32) or avulsion (Fig. 12.33) of the lateral collateral ligament or a transverse

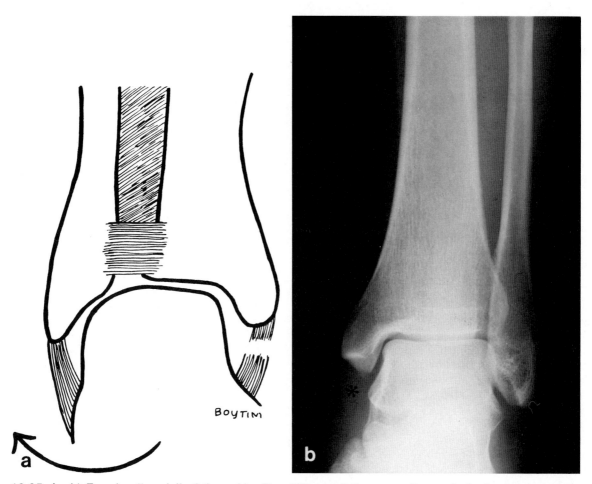

Fig. 12.25. (a, b) Eversion ''sprain'' of the ankle. The diffuse soft tissue swelling, principally distal to the medial malleolus (*), and the absence of a medial malleolar fracture, indicate that the deltoid ligament has been at least partially disrupted.

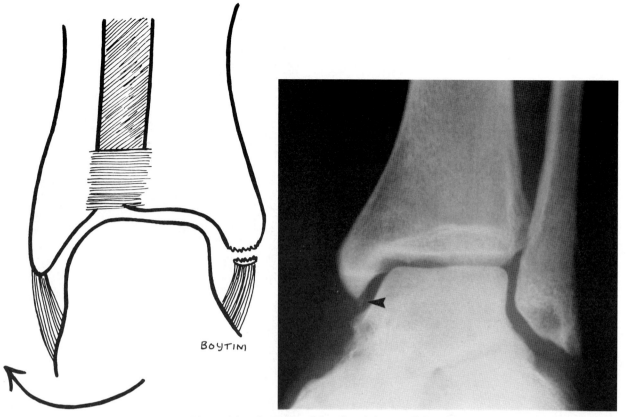

Fig. 12.26. (a, b) Eversion injury with avulsion fracture of the tip of the medial malleolus. The presence of this tiny fragment indicates that the deltoid ligament is intact, but has been separated from the medial styloid process.

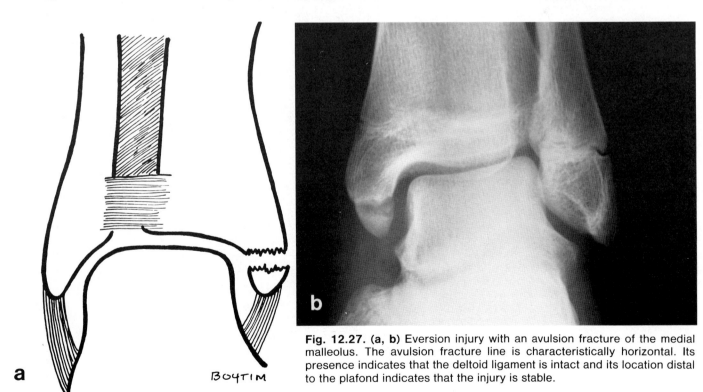

Fig. 12.27. (a, b) Eversion injury with an avulsion fracture of the medial malleolus. The avulsion fracture line is characteristically horizontal. Its presence indicates that the deltoid ligament is intact and its location distal to the plafond indicates that the injury is stable.

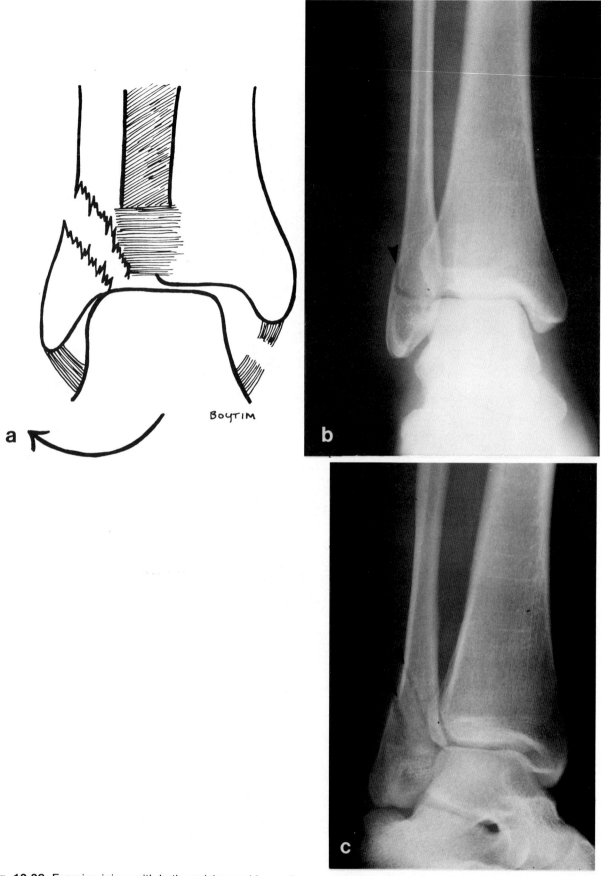

Fig. 12.28. Eversion injury with both avulsion and impaction components. The oblique fracture of the distal fibula (**b, c,** *arrowheads*) seen best in the externally rotated oblique radiograph **(c)**, represents the impaction force of the talus against the lateral malleolus. The normal relationship of the distal end of the proximal fibular fragment indicates that the distal tibiofibular ligaments are intact. The absence of a medial malleolar fracture indicates that the deltoid ligament is torn.

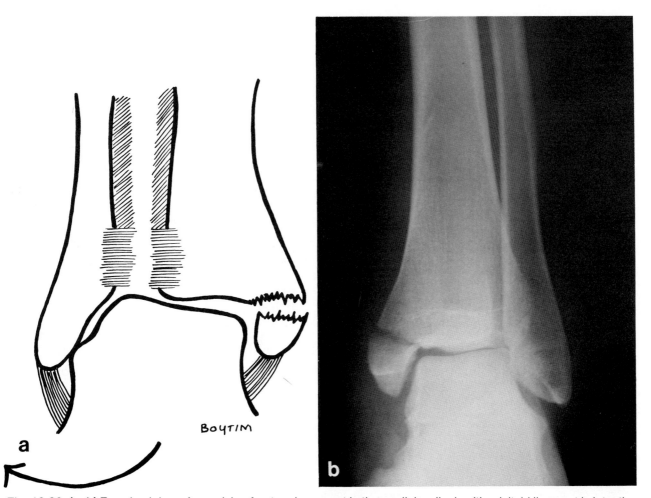

Fig. 12.29. (a, b) Eversion injury. An avulsion fracture is present in the medial malleolus (the deltoid ligament is intact). The impaction force of the laterally displaced talus upon the fibula has resulted in disruption of the distal tibiofibular ligaments and separation of the tibia and fibula distally. The lateral collateral ligament is intact as is the fibula.

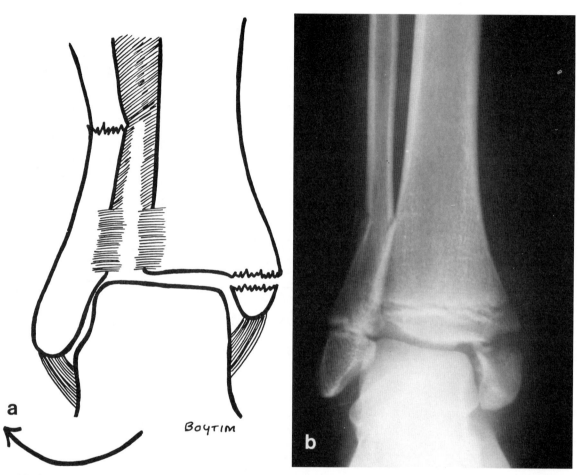

Fig. 12.30. (a, b) Eversion injury with an avulsion fracture of the medial malleolus at the level of the plafond (the mortise is unstable), widening of the distal tibiofibular joint (the distal tibiofibular ligaments are torn), and a fracture in the distal third of the fibula (the distal portion of the interosseous membrane is torn). The avulsion fracture of the medial malleolus also indicates that the deltoid ligament is intact.

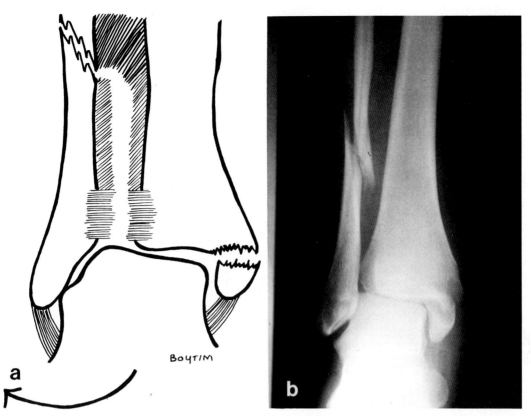

Fig. 12.31. (a, b) Eversion injury. The avulsion fracture of the medial malleolus indicates that the mortise is unstable and that the deltoid ligament is intact. Separation of the distal tibiofibular joint and the location of the distal fibular fracture indicate that the distal tibiofibular ligament and the distal portion of the interosseous membrane are disrupted. The lateral collateral ligament is intact, as evidenced by the normal relationship of the talus to the lateral malleolus.

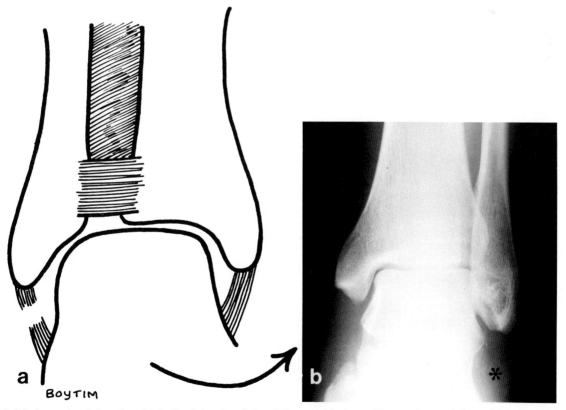

Fig. 12.32. Inversion injury in which the lateral collateral ligament is torn. Stress views of the ankle, demonstrating abnormal medial rotation of the talus and widening of the lateral aspect of the joint space, are required to confirm this injury. Note that the deltoid and the distal tibiofibular ligaments are intact. Soft tissue swelling is greatest distal to the lateral malleolus **(*)**.

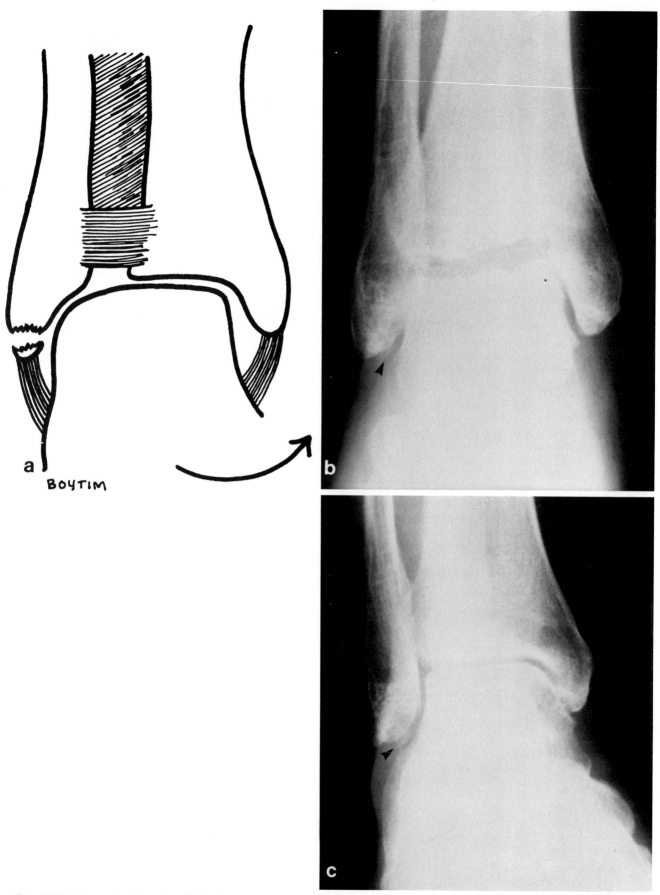

Fig. 12.33. Inversion injury in which the lateral collateral ligament remains intact and produces an avulsion fracture (**b, c**, *arrowhead*) of the styloid process of the lateral malleolus.

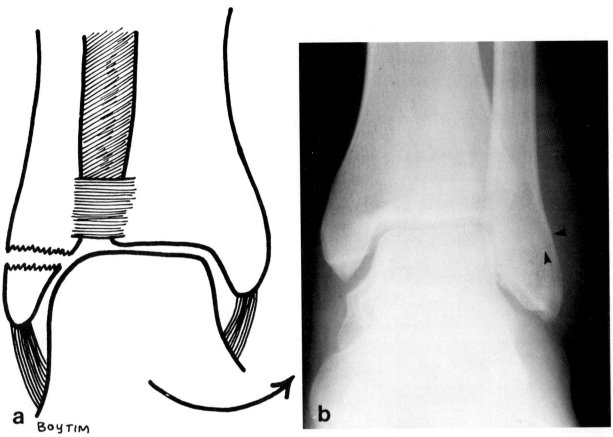

Fig. 12.34. Schematic representation **(a)** of an inversion injury in which the avulsive force, transmitted through the intact lateral collateral ligament, has resulted in a transverse fracture (*arrowheads*) of the lateral malleolus **(b)**. The deltoid ligament, the distal tibiofibular ligaments, and the interosseus membrane remain intact. Note that the soft tissue swelling is greatest lateral and proximal to the distal fibula.

fracture of the lateral malleolus distal to the level of the plafond (Fig. 12.34). The impaction force is caused by rotation and medial displacement of the talus which impinges upon the medial malleolus, producing a transverse or oblique fracture through the base of the medial malleolus (Fig. 12.35).

Bimalleolar Fracture

Bimalleolar fractures or fracture-dislocations may be the result of either an inversion (Figs. 12.36 and 12.37) or an eversion (Fig. 12.38) injury. The position of the fragments and the characteristics of the fracture lines indicate the mechanism of injury.

Trimalleolar Fracture

The trimalleolar fracture may be caused by inversion or eversion of the ankle or posterior dislocation of the talus (Fig. 12.39) (4,5). Trimalleolar indicates that a fracture of the posterior tibial margin is present in addition to the medial and lateral malleolar frac-

tures. The posterior tibial lip fracture may involve only the posterior rim of the distal tibial articulating surface (Fig. 12.40) or it may involve as much as 50% of the plafond (Fig. 12.41). Because the head of the talus is wider anteriorly than posteriorly, posterior dislocation of the talus must result in widening of the ankle mortise either by a fracture of the lateral malleolus or disruption of the tibiofibular ligament.

Figure 12.42 is an example of an eversion injury that has resulted in a fracture of the lateral malleolus proximal to the level of the tibial plafond and a fracture of the posterior tibial lip. Instead of producing a fracture of the medial malleolus (i.e., a trimalleolar fracture), the avulsion force has caused disruption of the deltoid ligament. This is indicated by the lateral displacement of the talus and the abnormal width of the space between the talus and the medial malleolus. The location of the distal fibular fracture line and lateral displacement of the lateral malleolus (tibiofibular diastasis) indicate that the distal tibiofibular ligaments have been disrupted as well. (Compare the distal fibular fracture line and the distal tibiofibular relationship in this patient in whom the tibiofibular

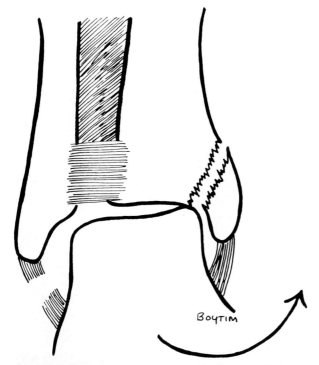

Fig. 12.35. Schematic representation of the type of injury caused by forced inversion of the ankle and medial displacement and rotation of the talus. The effect of the impaction force upon the medial malleolus resulting from the displacement of the talus is the vertical fracture through the base of the medial malleolus. The avulsion force may either disrupt the lateral collateral ligament (as depicted here) or, if the lateral collateral ligament remains intact, produce an avulsion fracture of the styloid process of the lateral malleolus. Note that the distal tibiofibular ligaments and the interosseous membrane remain intact. (Fig. 12.24 is an example of this type of inversion injury.)

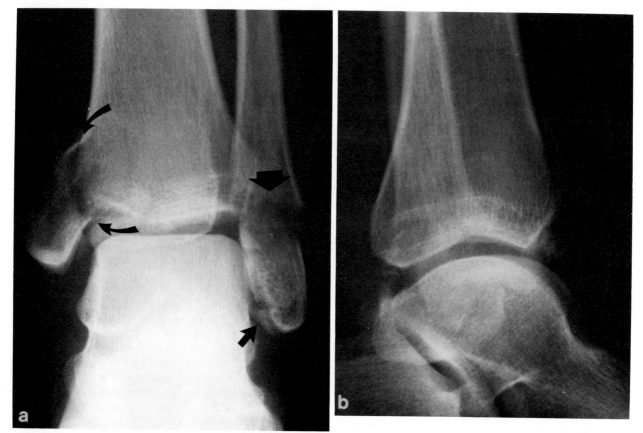

Fig. 12.36. Bimalleolar fracture caused by an inversion injury with internal rotation and displacement of the talus. The impaction force has produced the vertical fracture through the base of the medial malleolus (*curved arrows*) and the medial and proximal displacement of the distal fragment. The avulsion force caused the horizontal fracture of the base of the lateral malleolus (*arrows*). A small separate fragment arises from the medial aspect of the styloid process of the fibula (*stemmed arrow*). This also is an avulsion injury. The normal relationship at the distal tibiofibular joint indicates that the tibiofibular ligaments are intact.

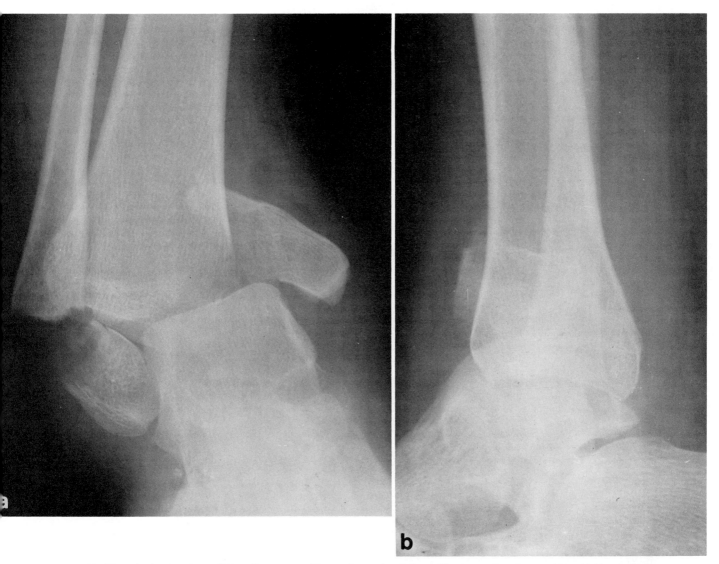

Fig. 12.37. Bimalleolar fracture-dislocation caused by an inversion injury. The impaction force of the dislocated talus striking the medial malleolus has resulted in the oblique fracture (*arrows*) of its base and the direction of displacement of the distal fragment. The distance between the medial malleolus and the medial surface of the talus indicates that the deltoid ligament is disrupted. The avulsion force transmitted through the intact lateral collateral ligament has caused the transverse fracture of the lateral malleolus (*open arrows*) at the level of the plafond. The normal relationship between the distal end of the proximal fibular fracture and the tibia indicates that the distal tibiofibular ligaments and the interosseous membrane are intact.

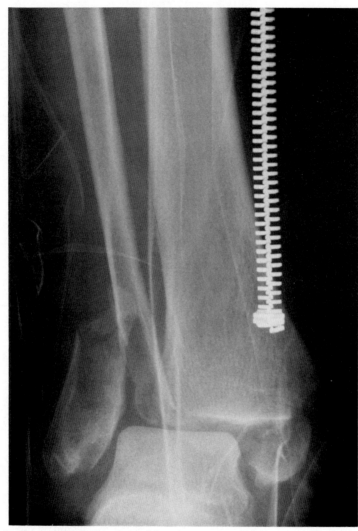

Fig. 12.38. Bimalleolar fracture-dislocation caused by an eversion injury. The impaction force has produced the oblique fracture in the distal fibula proximal to the level of the plafond. The normal relationship between the distal end of the proximal fibular fragment and the tibia indicates that the tibiofibular ligaments and the interosseous membrane are intact. The avulsion force transmitted through the intact deltoid ligament (*) has caused the transverse fracture of the base of the medial malleolus.

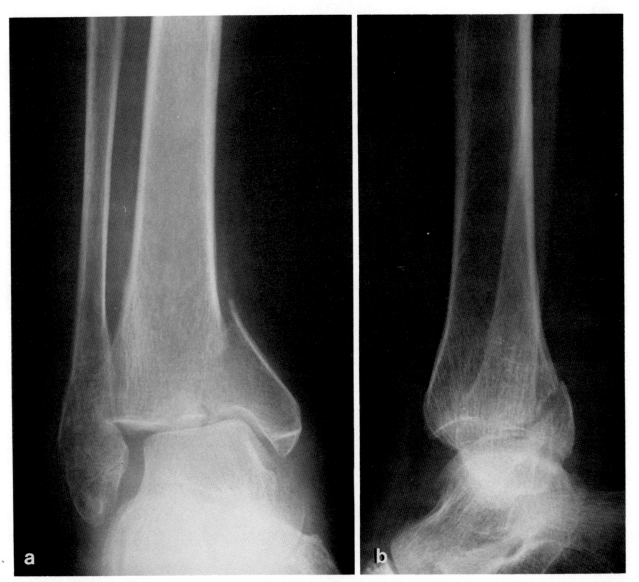

Fig. 12.39. Trimalleolar fracture-dislocation of the ankle. In the frontal projection (**a**), the signs of an inversion injury are readily apparent. Minimal posterior dislocation of the talus and the slightly displaced posterior tibial lip fracture are evident in the lateral radiograph (**b**).

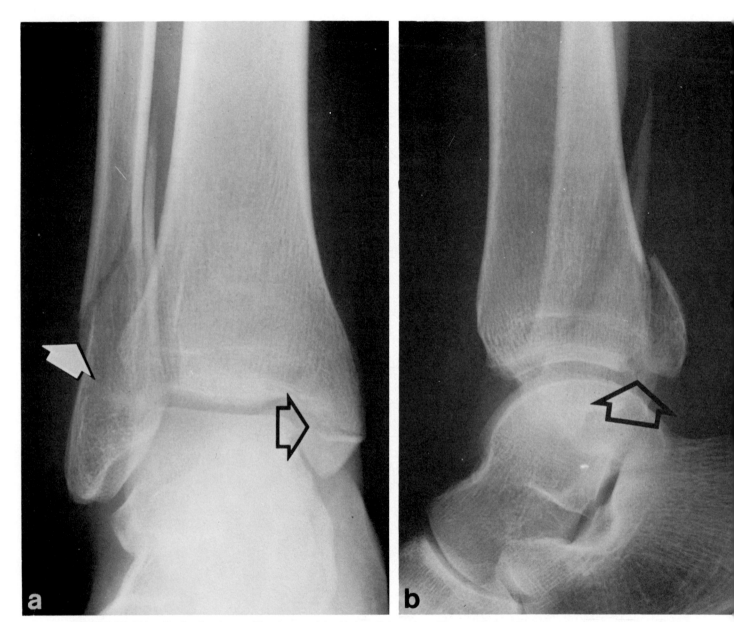

Fig. 12.40. Trimalleolar fracture without associated talar dislocation. The posterior tibial fragment comprises only the rim of the plafond. The fracture line is obscured by superimposition upon the posterior cortex of the fibula. The most striking feature of this fracture is the disruption of the distal tibial articulating surface (**b,** *open arrow*). In the frontal projection (**a**), the *solid arrow* indicates the distal fibular fracture and the *open arrow*, the medial malleolar fracture.

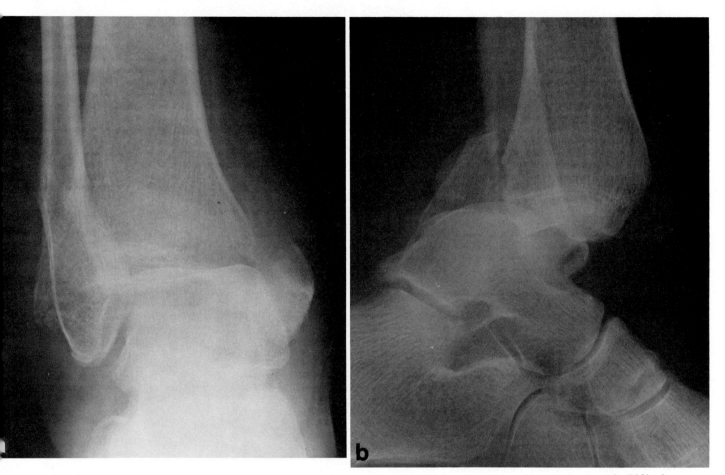

Fig. 12.41. Trimalleolar fracture-dislocation in which the posterior tibial lip fragment comprises approximately 50% of the plafond.

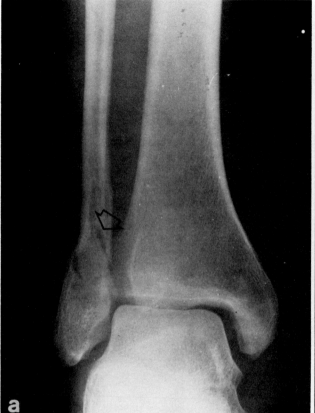

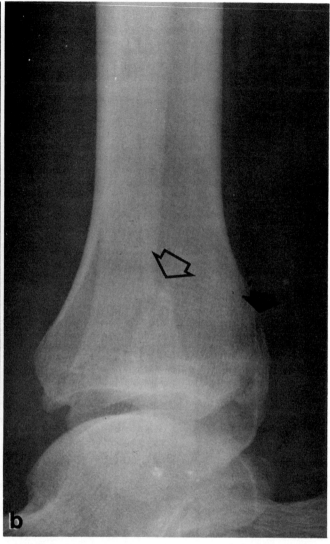

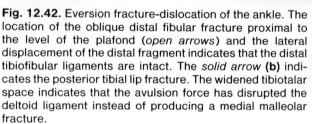

Fig. 12.42. Eversion fracture-dislocation of the ankle. The location of the oblique distal fibular fracture proximal to the level of the plafond (*open arrows*) and the lateral displacement of the distal fragment indicates that the distal tibiofibular ligaments are intact. The *solid arrow* (**b**) indicates the posterior tibial lip fracture. The widened tibiotalar space indicates that the avulsion force has disrupted the deltoid ligament instead of producing a medial malleolar fracture.

ligaments are torn with Fig. 12.28, in which the distal tibiofibular ligaments are intact.)

Posterior tibial lip fracture may occur as an isolated injury (Fig. 12.43). This fracture may be difficult to identify in a true lateral radiograph when the fracture line is superimposed upon the posterior cortex of the fibula. In this instance, the fracture may be more readily apparent in a slightly rotated, i.e., "poorly positioned," lateral projection.

Dislocation of the talus (dislocation of the ankle) occurs infrequently because of the configuration of the ankle mortise and the exceptionally strong ligamentous support of the joint. Dislocation of the talus is defined as displacement of its dome from the mortise and usually occurs in conjunction with a fracture of one or more of the components of the mortise.

Isolated dislocations are rare. Posterior dislocation is the most frequent form of this type of injury. Anterior dislocation (Fig. 12.44) is rare and is usually associated with fracture of the anterior tibial lip.

Fractures of the astragalus are rare. Isolated fractures of the talus usually involve the neck (Fig. 12.45) or the lateral (Fig. 17.46) or posterior (Fig. 12.47) talar process. These fractures may be difficult to identify on routine radiographs of the ankle because of their location and because they are frequently minimally displaced. Individualized oblique or tangential projections of the ankle or foot may be required to establish the presence of these fractures.

Fracture-dislocations of the talus, also rare, most frequently involve the neck of the talus (Fig. 12.48) but may involve the body as well (Fig. 12.49).

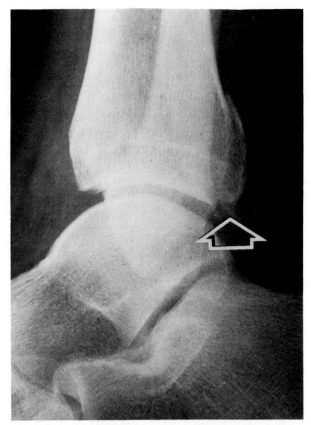

Fig. 12.43. Isolated posterior tibial lip fracture (*open arrow*).

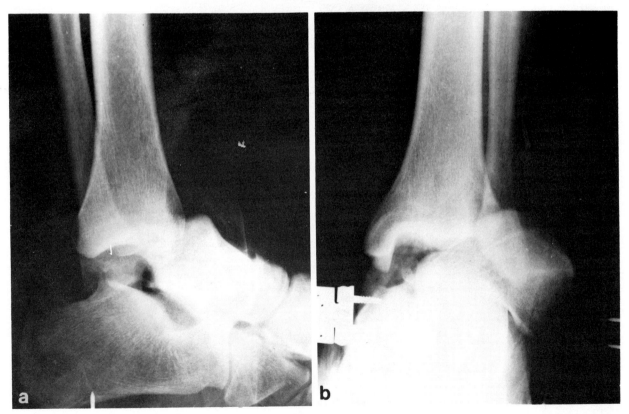

Fig. 12.44. (a, b) Anterior dislocation of the talus.

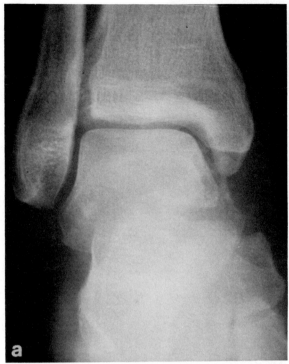

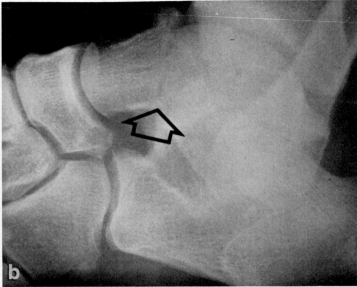

Fig. 12.45. (a, b) Isolated fracture of the neck of the talus.

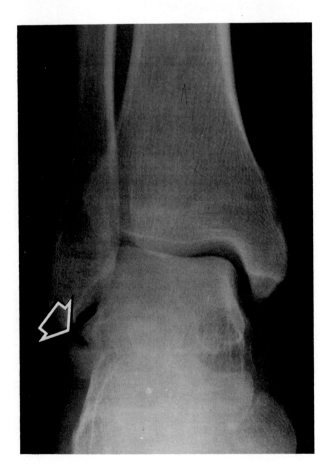

Fig. 12.46. Minimally displaced fracture of the lateral talar process (*open arrow*).

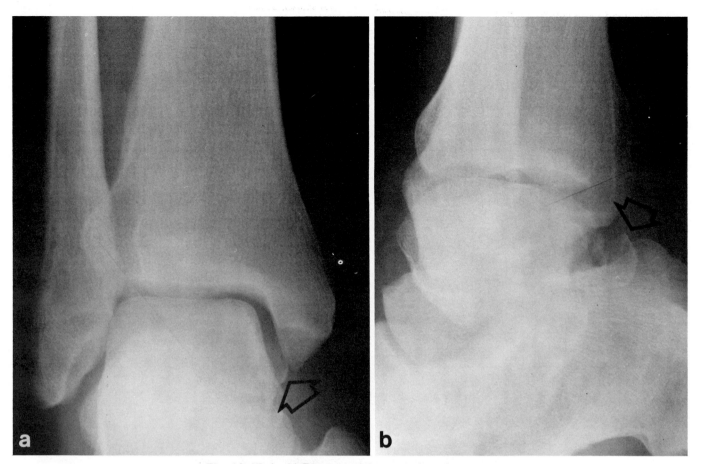

Fig. 12.47. (a, b) Fracture of the posterior talar process.

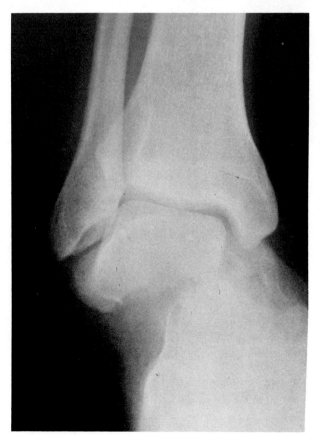

Fig. 12.48. Displaced fracture of the neck of the talus.

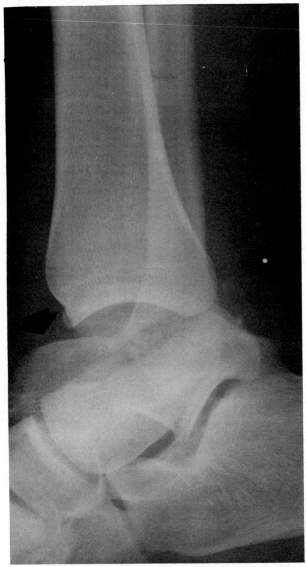

Fig. 12.49. Fracture-dislocation of the body of the talus. The superior fragment (*arrow*) is distally displaced so that it overlies the distal end of the talus and the tarsal navicular.

Nontraumatic Lesions

The os trigonum (Fig. 12.50) is a normal variant of the talus created when the posterior process of the talus arises from a separate growth center. This frequently encountered anomaly may resemble an old, ununited fracture fragment. Its location, radiographic characteristics, and the fact that it is usually bilateral should help to establish the correct identity of this variant.

Transverse linear densities seen in the metaphyses of growing long bones (Fig. 12.51) are referred to by Caffey (7) as "transverse (stress) lines of Park," after the investigator who has been primarily responsible for the present concept relative to this radiographic finding.

The transverse lines may be found in healthy or sick children and never cause local signs or symptoms. The lines, which usually are bilateral, which may be found at the ends of any long bone, and which may extend partially or completely across the metaphysis, are thought to develop during periods of accelerated growth following periods of arrested growth such as caused by fever or starvation (stress).

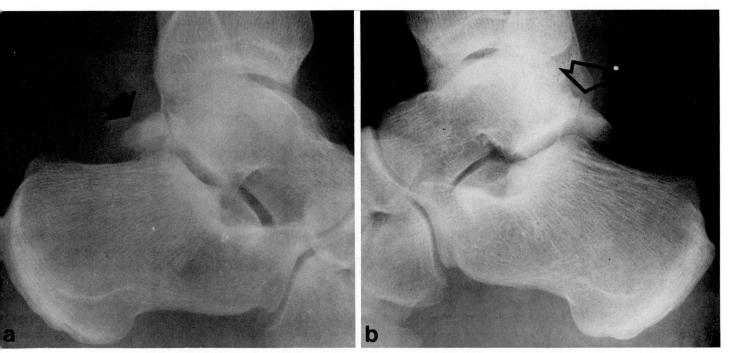

Fig. 12.50. Bilateral os trigonum. **(a)** is the injured ankle. The piece of bone posterior to the body of the talus (*solid arrow*) and separated from it by a defect with smooth sclerotic margins represents an os trigonum, a congenital variant. A similar anomaly (*open arrow*) is present on the uninjured side **(b)**.

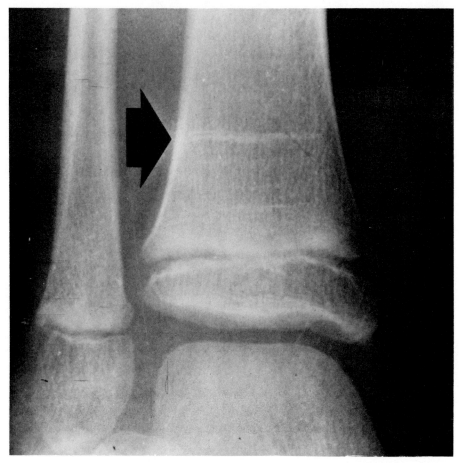

Fig. 12.51. Transverse stress line.

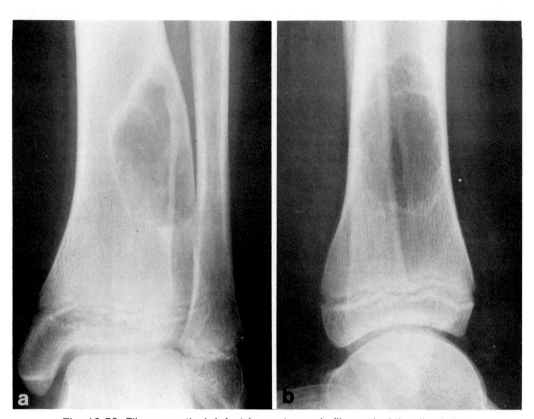

Fig. 12.52. Fibrous cortical defect (nonosteogenic fibroma) of the distal tibia.

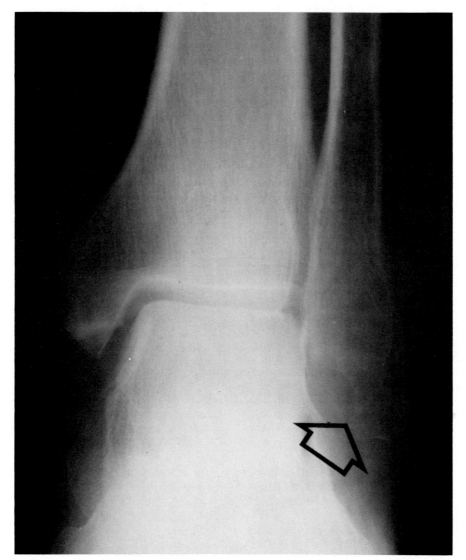

Fig. 12.53. Osteolytic metastasis of the fibular styloid process.

Fibrous cortical defect (nonosteogenic fibroma) (Fig. 12.52) is the most frequently encountered benign lesion of the long bones. The defect, which is limited to the cortex, is commonly found in the metaphysis but may be located in the diaphysis, is lobulated in configuration, may contain septa, and has faintly sclerotic margins. The cortical defect does not produce local signs or symptoms and is invariably an incidental finding on the roentgenogram.

Metastatic disease involving the ankle is uncommon but does occur (Fig. 12.53) and may be the cause of local pain, tenderness, and swelling.

References

1. SALTER RB: *Textbook of Disorders and Injuries of the Musculoskeletal System.* Williams & Wilkins, Baltimore, 1970.
2. RALSTON EL: *The Handbook of Fractures.* C. V. Mosby, St. Louis, Mo., 1967.
3. CAVE EF, BURKE JF, BOYD RJ: *Trauma Management.* Year Book Medical Publishers, Chicago, 1974.
4. DePALMA AF: *The Management of Fractures and Dislocations,* ed. 2. W. B. Saunders, Philadelphia, 1970.
5. EDEIKEN J, COTLER JM: Ankle trauma. *Semin Roentgenol* 13:145, 1978.
6. SHULTZ RJ: *The Language of Fractures.* Williams & Wilkins, Baltimore, 1972.
7. CAFFEY J: *Pediatric X-ray Diagnosis.* ed. 5. Year Book Medical Publishers, Chicago, 1973.

chapter thirteen

Foot and Heel

General Considerations

Anatomically, the foot includes all of the tarsal bones, the metatarsals, and the phalanges. The foot, therefore, includes the heel as well as the bones of the mid- and forefoot. The forefoot includes the phalanges and metatarsals; the midfoot, the three cuneiform bones, the cuboid, and the navicular; and the hindfoot, the talus and calcaneus (Fig. 13.1). The heel is occasionally referred to as the hindfoot. Radiographically, however, the heel and foot comprise separate regions requiring specific radiographic examination.

The frequency with which injuries of the heel or midfoot produce clinical signs suggesting an abnormality of the ankle has been previously discussed. However, this circumstance merits emphasis by repetition because of the likelihood of overlooking a significant abnormality when the radiographic study does not include the appropriate area.

Previously, it was a generally accepted principle that when an injury involved a peripheral part of a patient during childhood or adolescence, the opposite part should be *routinely* examined for baseline comparison purposes. In the interests of reducing radiation exposure, that principle has recently been modified to no longer obtain *routine* opposite side views. Rather, the current philosophy is that opposite side radiographic studies should be obtained only when specifically required to help distinguish between a developmental variant and a traumatic lesion.

Radiographic Examination

The routine roentgen study of the foot includes anteroposterior and internally rotated oblique views. The lateral examination of the foot, as with the lateral examination of the hand, is of limited value because of superimposition of the bones of the mid- and forefoot in the lateral projection.

There are no "special" views of the foot. However, it is frequently necessary to obtain radiographs in the externally rotated or individualized tangential projections in order to adequately visualize the complex skeletal anatomy of the mid- or hindfoot.

Routine examinations of the heel are made in the lateral and axial projections. The latter may be obtained with the patient supine or prone.

Radiographic Anatomy

In the foot, a pair of sesamoid bones is normally present on the volar aspect of the head of the first metatarsal. Either of these may be bifid developmentally. This variant may be distinguished from an acute fracture by the sclerotic parallel margins of the separate ossification centers (Fig. 13.2). When present, this variant is usually bilateral. Sesamoid bones are occasionally seen at the level of the interphalangeal joint of the great toe and the metatarsophalangeal joint of the second and little toes.

The tubercle of the tarsal navicular may constitute a separate bone (tibiale externum) (Fig. 13.3) in approximately 4% of the population (1).

The calcaneal apophysis is typically fragmented, more dense than the calcaneus, and irregular in its density (Fig. 13.4).

The apophysis of the base of the fifth metatarsal and the os secundum of the anterior tubercle of the calcaneus, both of which may resemble acute avulsion fracture fragments, will be described subsequently in this chapter.

The os trigonum, which is present in approximately 26% of individuals, has been illustrated in Chapter 12.

Figure 13.1 is an anteroposterior view of the normal adult foot. The third cuneiform and the cuboid bones are superimposed and the anatomy of the bases of the lateral four metatarsals is obscure because of super-

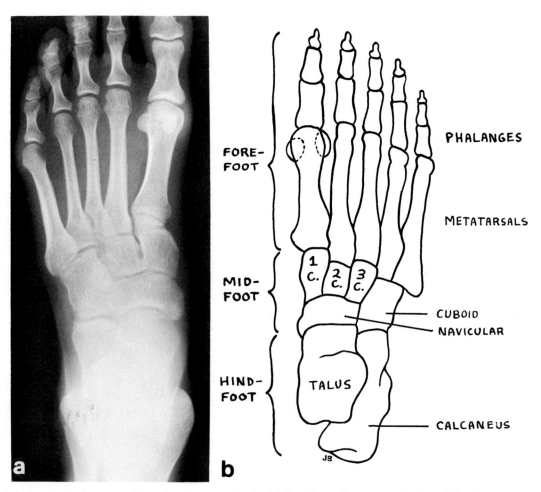

Fig. 13.1 Anteroposterior projection of a normal adult foot (**a**). Schematic representation of the bones of the foot (**b**). (Modified from R. J. Schultz: *The Language of Fractures*. Williams & Wilkins, Baltimore, 1972.)

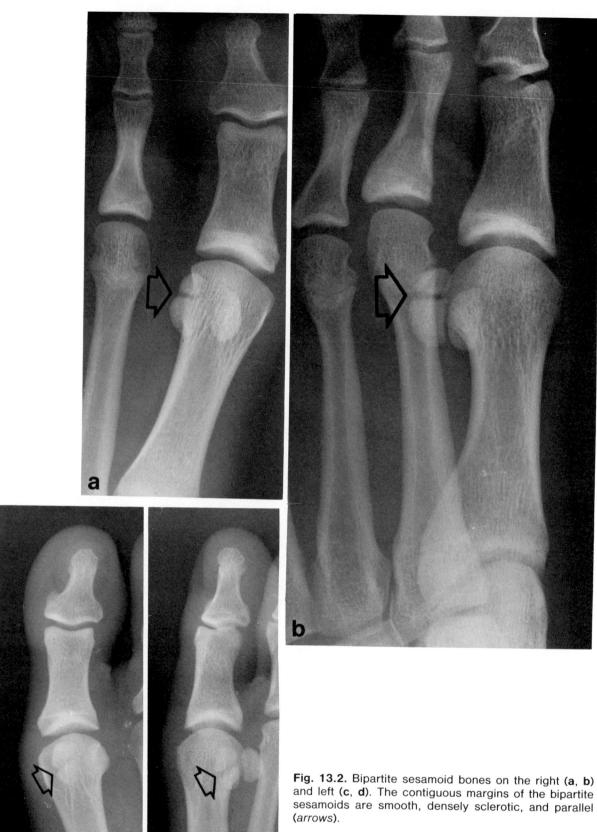

Fig. 13.2. Bipartite sesamoid bones on the right (**a, b**) and left (**c, d**). The contiguous margins of the bipartite sesamoids are smooth, densely sclerotic, and parallel (*arrows*).

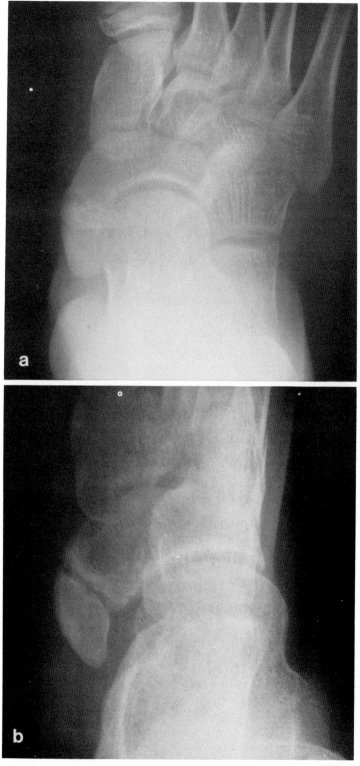

Fig. 13.3. This separate, ununited secondary ossification center of the medial aspect of the tarsal navicular is referred to as the tibiale externum.

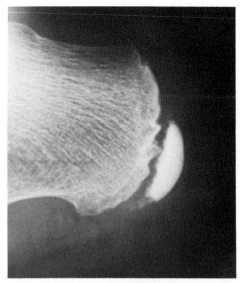

Fig. 13.4. Typical appearance of the normal calcaneal apophysis. The apparent fragmentation of the plantar aspect of the apophysis is physiologic and represents incomplete calcification of the apophyseal cartilage. This appearance and variations of it are frequently seen in the calcaneal apophysis and should not be misinterpreted as fractures. Also, the calcaneal apophysis is normally more dense than the calcaneus itself.

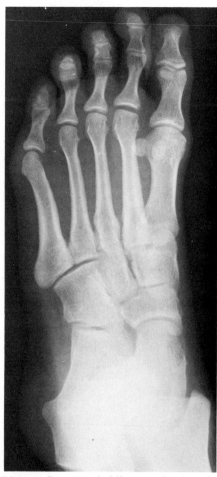

Fig. 13.5 Internally rotated oblique projection of a normal adult foot.

imposition caused by the normal transverse arch of the midfoot.

The internally rotated oblique projection (Fig. 13.5) is made with the foot internally rotated and the central beam perpendicular to the table top and centered over the third metatarsal. In this way, the third cuneiform, cuboid, and lateral three metatarsals are projected into profile.

The appearance of a normal child's foot is seen in Figure 13.6. The epiphyses of the metatarsals are distally located while those of the phalanges are proximally situated.

The lateral radiograph of the foot (Fig. 13.7) is essential in the roentgen evaluation of the heel and midfoot. The subtalar joint, the talonavicular, and calcaneocuboid joints are well seen in this projection.

The externally rotated oblique (Fig. 13.8) is designed to project the medial cortical surface of the navicular, the first cuneiform, and the base of the first metatarsal in profile.

Boehler's (the tuber joint) angle (Fig. 13.9) is formed by the intersection of a straight line extending along the superior cortex of the body of the os calcis (A - A^1) with a line extending from the dome to the anterior tubercle (B - B^1). The resultant angle is normally between 20 and 40° (2).

The axial projection of the os calcis (Fig. 13.10) demonstrates the convex lateral and concave medial surfaces of the calcaneus, and in a properly exposed roentgenogram, provides a clear view of the sustentaculum tali.

Radiographic Manifestations of Trauma

Dislocation at interphalangeal joints is usually either dorsal or volar in direction, in contradistinction to metatarsotarsal dislocation which is usually lateralward. In the frontal projections, loss of the joint space and the increased density of the superimposed phalanges (Fig. 13.11) indicate the presence of a dislocation. The direction of displacement can only be established by oblique or lateral projections of the involved digit.

Fractures of the distal phalanx of the great toe are among the most common injuries of the foot. These may involve the subungual tuft (Fig. 13.12) or the base of the phalanx (Fig. 13.13). Soft tissue swelling of the digit may be the most obvious roentgen abnormality.

The sesamoid bones along the volar aspect of the first metatarsophalangeal joint are subject to fracture and post-traumatic aseptic necrosis (Fig. 13.14).

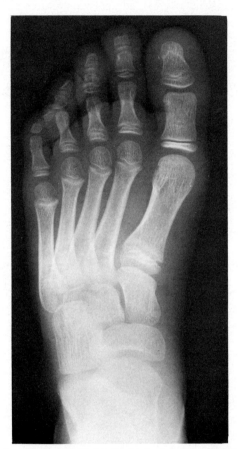

Fig. 13.6. Anteroposterior radiography of a normal child's foot. Note the location of the metatarsal and phalangeal epiphyses.

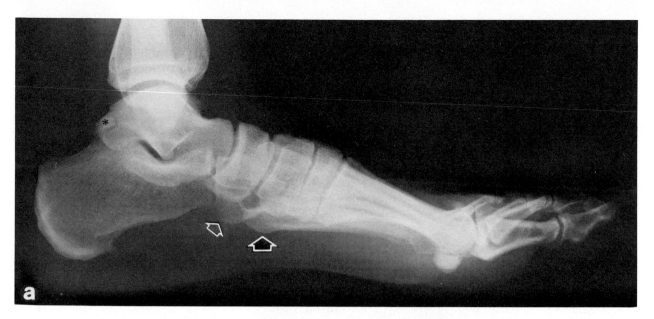

a

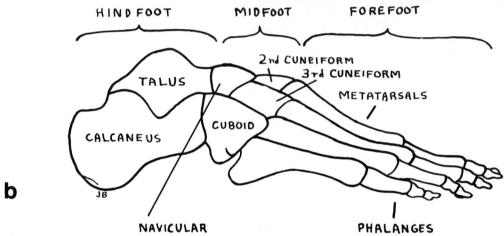

HINDFOOT · MIDFOOT · FOREFOOT

TALUS

CALCANEUS

CUBOID

2nd CUNEIFORM

3rd CUNEIFORM

METATARSALS

NAVICULAR

PHALANGES

JB

b

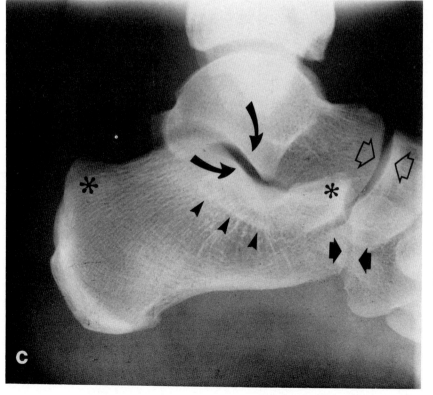

c

Fig. 13.7. Lateral radiograph of the foot (**a**). (*) The *asterisk* indicates an os trigonum. The *small open arrow* designates the lateral aspect of the cuboid and the *large solid arrow* signals the base of the fifth metatarsal. (**b**) Schematic representation of the bones of the foot as seen in the lateral radiograph. (Modified after R. J. Shultz: *The Language of Fractures*. Williams & Wilkins, Baltimore, 1972.) (**c**) Lateral projection of the hindfoot. The posterior and anterior calcaneal tubercles are indicated by *asterisks* (*). The subtalar joint (*curved arrows*), the sustentaculum tali (*arrowheads*), the talonavicular (*open arrows*), and the calcaneocuboid (*solid arrows*) joints are all well demonstrated in this view.

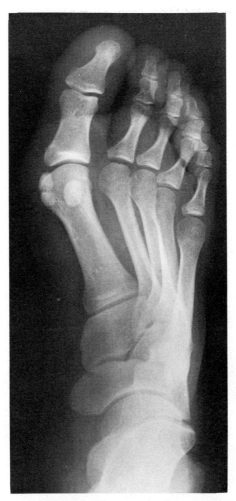

Fig. 13.8. Externally rotated oblique projection of a normal adult foot.

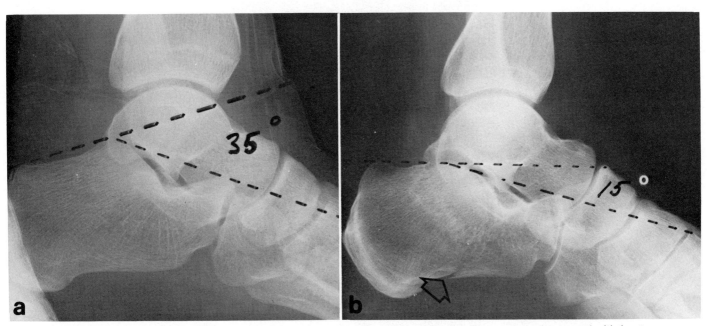

Fig. 13.9. Boehler's angle which normally ranges between 20–40° in adults (**a**). The angle is decreased with fractures of the body of the os calcis (**b**).

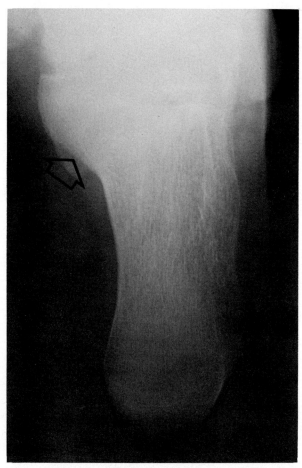

Fig. 13.10. Axial view of the os calcis. The *arrow* indicates the sustentaculum tali.

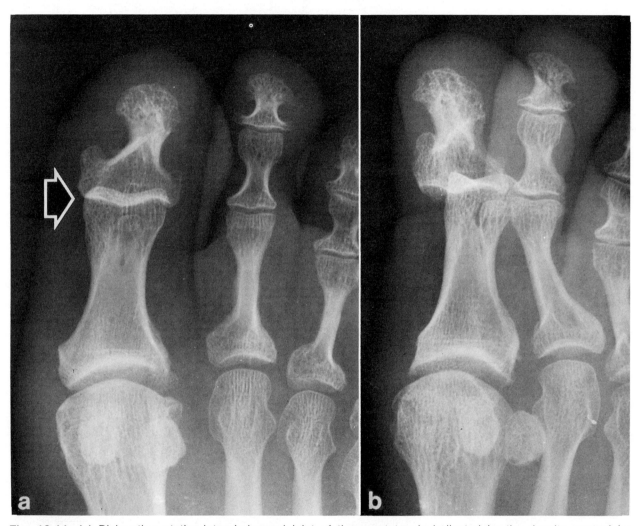

Fig. 13.11. (a) Dislocation at the interphalangeal joint of the great toe is indicated by the density caused by superimposition of the base of the distal phalanx upon the head of the proximal phalanx (*arrow*). In the oblique projection **(b)**, the dorsal direction of the dislocated distal phalanx is apparent.

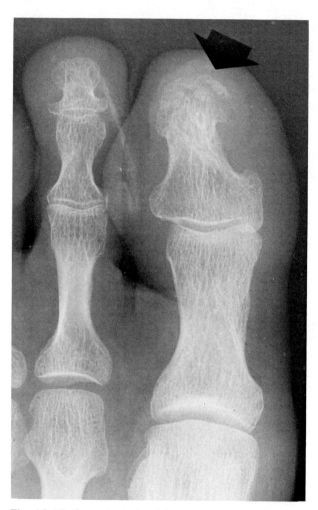

Fig. 13.12. Comminuted, minimally displaced fracture of the subungual tuft of the great toe (*arrow*). Note also the soft tissue swelling of this digit.

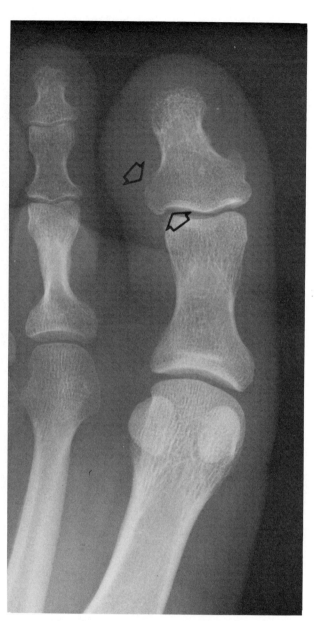

Fig. 13.13. Minimally displaced oblique fracture of the lateral aspect of the base of the distal phalanx (*arrows*). Note also the diffuse soft tissue swelling.

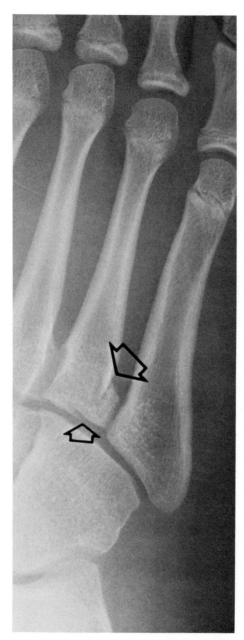

Fig. 13.18. Minimally displaced fracture in the base of the fourth metatarsal (*arrows*) which was visible only in the oblique projection.

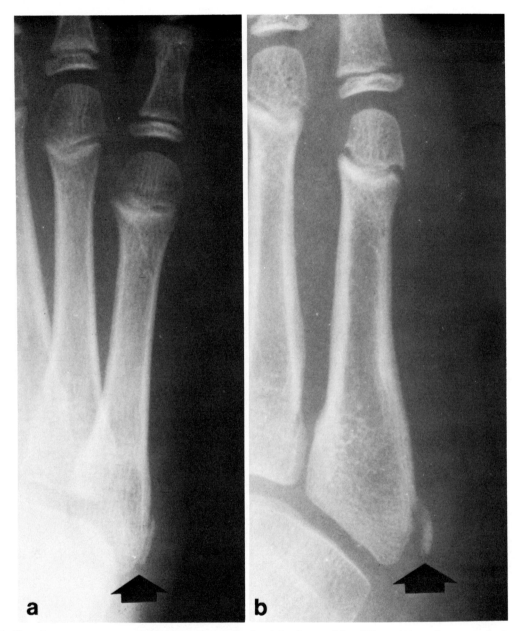

Fig. 13.19. Roentgen appearance of the normal apophysis at the base of the fifth metatarsal as seen in the frontal (**a**) and oblique (**b**) projections.

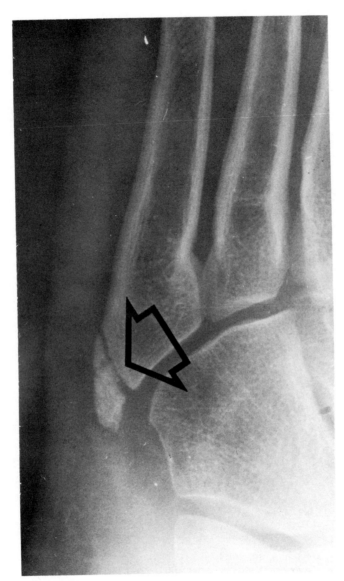

Fig. 13.20. The appearance of the apophysis of the base of the fifth metatarsal of this asymptomatic patient simulates a fracture fragment.

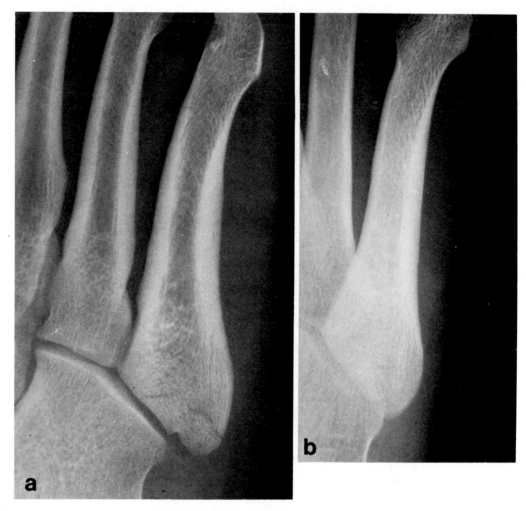

Fig. 13.21. Minimally displaced, complete, fracture of the base of the fifth metatarsal seen only in the oblique radiograph **(a)**. The fracture line was not discernible in the frontal projection **(b)**.

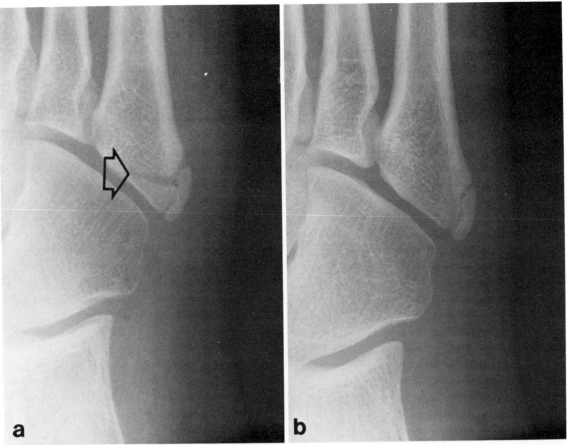

Fig. 13.22. (a) Complete, minimally displaced fracture of the base of the proximal phalanx of the fifth metatarsal (*arrow*). The fracture line is transverse. The apophyseal line is longitudinally situated. The contralateral normal side (b) has been reversed to facilitate comparison.

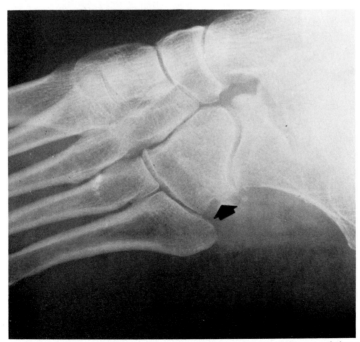

Fig. 13.23. Isolated fracture of the tarsal cuboid (*arrow*). The radiographic evidence of the presence of the fracture consists of buckling and irregularity of the lateral cortex and a vague zone of increased density through the waist of the cuboid caused by impaction of the fragments.

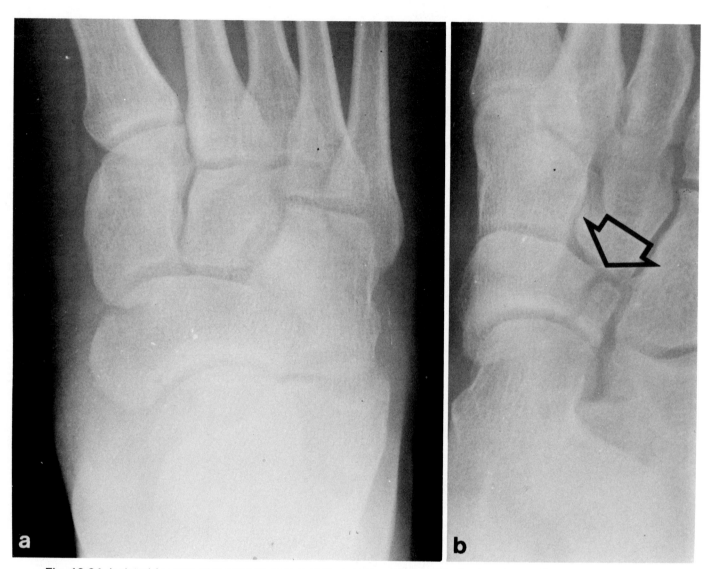

Fig. 13.24. Isolated fracture of the lateral aspect of the tarsal navicular. This fracture is not discernible in the frontal (**a**) projection of the foot, but is clearly discernible (*arrow*) in the internally rotated oblique view (**b**).

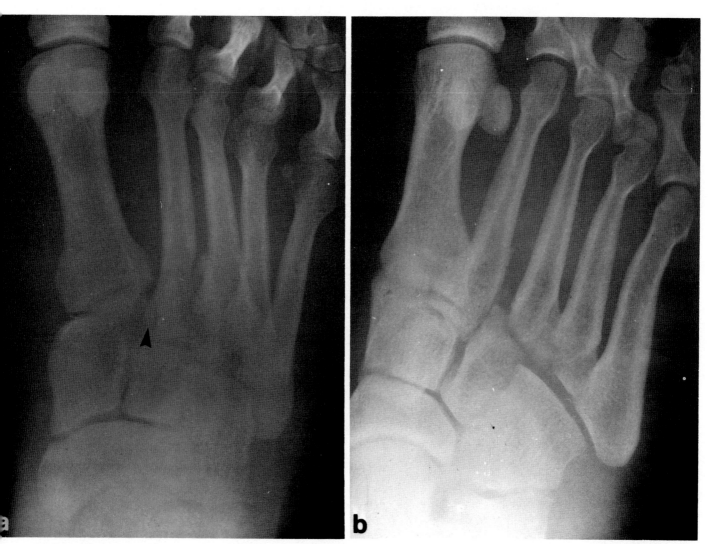

Fig. 13.25. Minimally displaced homolateral (convergent) Lisfranc fracture-dislocation. The *arrowhead* indicates the small fragment avulsed from the medial aspect of the base of the second metatarsal by the intact Lisfranc ligament. Additional comminuted fractures involve the base of the second metatarsal as well. This is an example of the homolateral, or convergent, fracture-dislocation because only the four lateral metatarsals are dislocated, while the first retains its anatomic relation to the first cuneiform. Compare with Figure 13.27, a divergent Lisfranc injury.

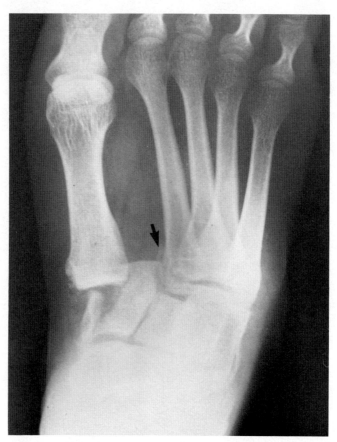

Fig. 13.26. Divergent Lisfranc fracture-dislocation. The first metatarsal is dislocated medially, dorsally and proximally. A vertical fracture involves the medial aspect of the tarsal bone. The lateral four metatarsals are slightly laterally dislocated. The tiny fragment immediately adjacent to the medial aspect of the base of the second metatarsal (*arrow*) has been avulsed by the intact Lisfranc ligament.

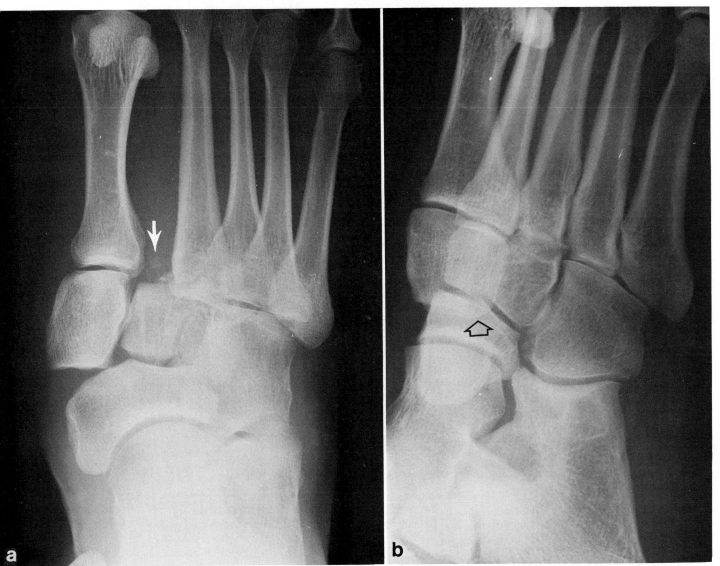

Fig. 13.27. Divergent Lisfranc injury. In the anteroposterior projection (**a**), the first cuneiform and metatarsal have been medially displaced, as a unit, as a result of dislocation between the first and second cuneiforms and at the navicular-cuneiform joint. The lateral four metatarsals are laterally dislocated. A tiny avulsion fragment (*stemmed arrow*) arises from the medial aspect of the base of the second metatarsal. In the oblique projection (**b**), the dorsal dislocation of the first cuneiform and metatarsal (*open arrow*) is evident.

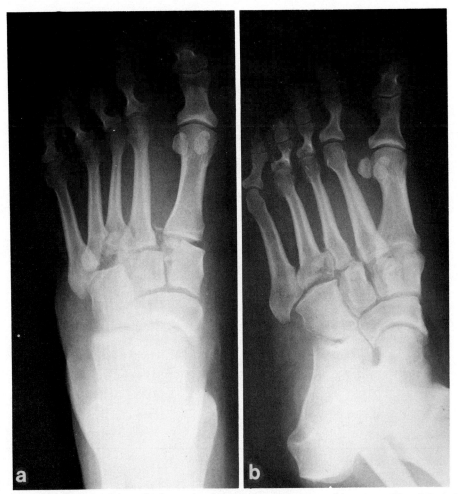

Fig. 13.28. Homolateral (convergent) type Lisfranc fracture-dislocation caused by a crushing injury. The lateral four metatarsals are laterally dislocated. There is no dislocation of the first metatarsal. Fractures involve the first and second cuneiforms and the base of the second, third, and fourth metatarsals.

Figure 13.28 is an example of a homolateral (convergent) Lisfranc lesion caused by a crushing type of injury. The lateral four metatarsals are laterally dislocated and fractures involve many of the bones of the Lisfranc area.

The preceding examples of the Lisfranc injury have all had rather obvious radiographic findings. Figures 13.29 and 13.30 are examples of Lisfranc fractures with much more subtle roentgen signs. In each of these patients, the space between the first and second metatarsal is widened and an avulsion fracture arises from either the base of the second metatarsal or the lateral aspect of the first cuneiform.

The os calcis is fractured more frequently than any other tarsal bone and accounts for 1–2% of all fractures (7). Fractures of the body represent the great majority of calcaneal fractures and are usually the result of a fall upon the heels from a height. The mechanism producing this injury is a downward force

of the body transmitted through the talus which acts as a wedge crushing and splitting the midportion of the os calcis. Because of the mechanism of this injury, calcaneal fractures are frequently bilateral and, in approximately 10% of cases, are associated with compression fractures of the thoracolumbar spine (8) (Fig. 13.31).

The majority of crushing injuries of the os calcis involve the subtalar joint, and the majority of these result in depression of the posterior facet of the calcaneus. Depression of the posterior facet produces a reduction (flattening) of Boehler's angle. Reduced Boehler's angle may be the most striking roentgen sign, in the lateral projection (Fig. 13.32a), of a subtle calcaneal fracture, and it is of considerable interest in determining the management of this fracture.

The axial projection (Fig. 13.32b) is easily obtained without patient discomfort, is essential to the complete evaluation of crushing fractures of the calcaneus and,

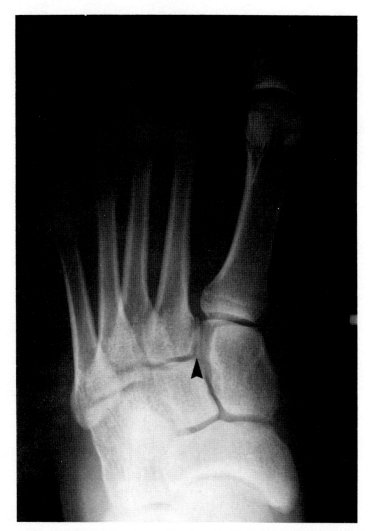

Fig. 13.29. Subtle Lisfranc fracture-dislocation. The *arrowhead* indicates the avulsion fracture fragment arising from the lateral aspect of the first cuneiform. The lateral four metatarsals are slightly laterally displaced.

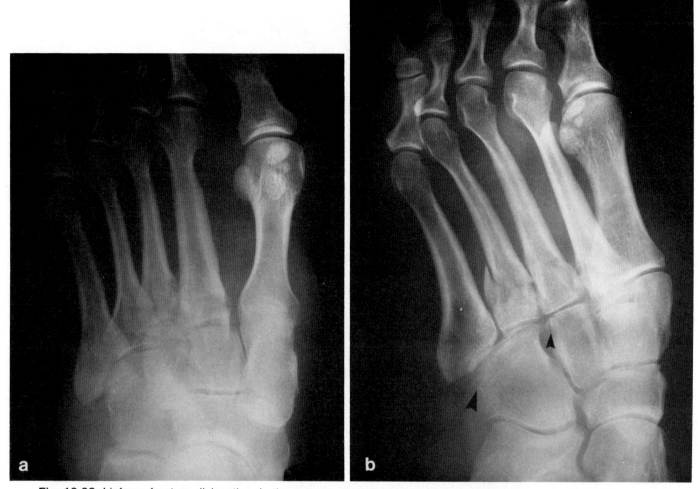

Fig. 13.30. Lisfranc fracture-dislocation. In the anteroposterior projection **(a)**, the lateral four metatarsals are slightly laterally displaced, resulting in abnormal separation between the first and second metatarsals. Comminuted fractures involve the base of the lateral three metatarsals. In the oblique radiograph **(b)**, the dislocation of the lateral four metatarsals is more apparent. In addition, an avulsion fracture of the third cuneiform and a crushing fracture of the cuboid are evident (*arrowheads*).

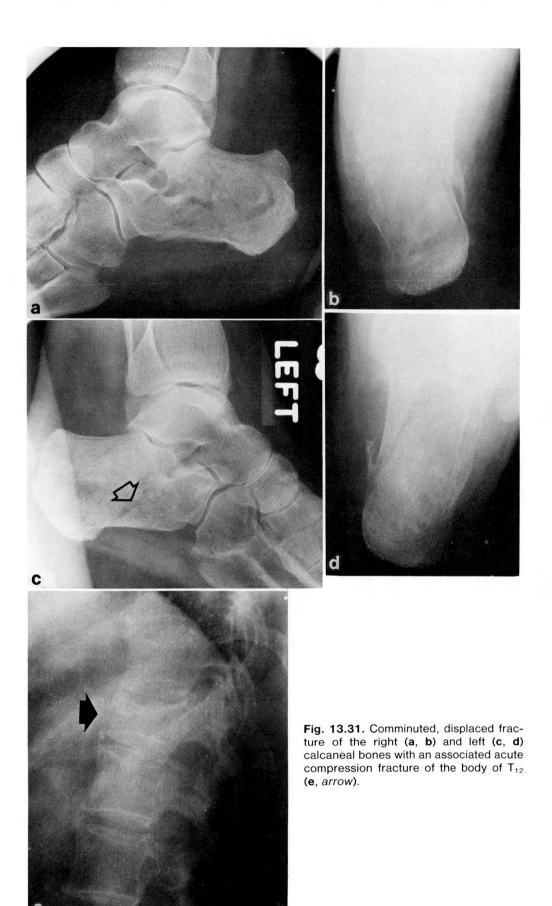

Fig. 13.31. Comminuted, displaced fracture of the right (**a**, **b**) and left (**c**, **d**) calcaneal bones with an associated acute compression fracture of the body of T_{12} (**e**, *arrow*).

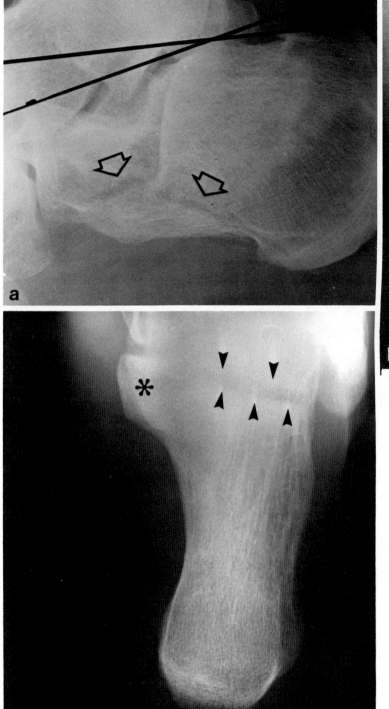

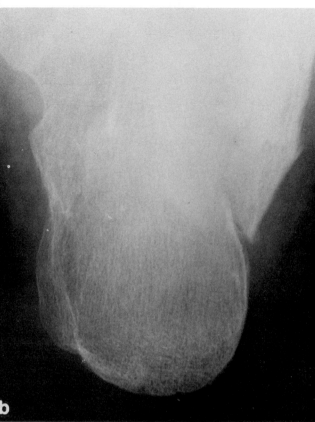

Fig. 13.32. Comminuted, minimally displaced fracture of the calcis. In the lateral projection **(a)**, the poorly defined frac lines are indicated by the *open arrows*. The most obvious ra graphic evidence of this fracture is a decrease in Boeh angle. In the axial view **(b)**, the fracture lines are more appa and the relationship of the fragments is more precisely def than in the lateral **(a)** projection. **(c)** Axial projection of a no os calcis clearly demonstrating the sustentaculum (*) and posterior aspect of the subtalar (talocalcaneal) joint (*ar heads*).

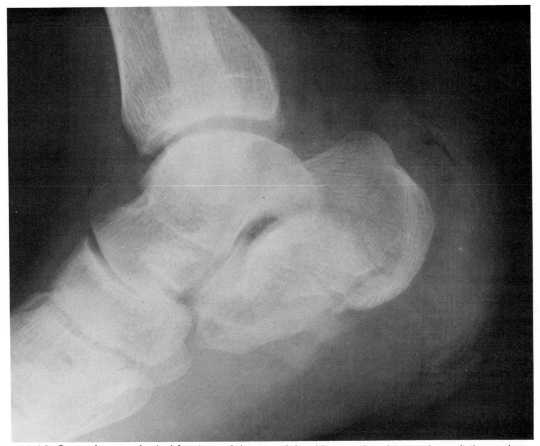

Fig. 13.33. Severely comminuted fracture of the os calcis with associated extensive soft tissue damage.

employing proper technical factors and positioning, affords excellent visualization of the sustentaculum tali and the posterior margin of the talocalcaneal joint (Fig. 13.32c).

Extensive soft tissue injury frequently accompanies severely comminuted, displaced fractures of the calcaneus (Fig. 13.33). Isolated fractures of the anterior process of the os calcis occur infrequently, may be difficult to identify radiographically (Figs. 13.34 and 13.35), and may be mistaken as the os secundum (Fig. 13.36).

Nontraumatic Lesions

Linear radiolucencies caused by normal soft tissues of the toes or foot may simulate phalangeal fractures. Extension of the radiolucency beyond the cortical margins and absence of consistency on multiple projections establishes that such shadows are not fracture lines (Figs. 13.37 and 13.38).

The epiphysis of the proximal phalanx of the great toe may be fissured by a vertical radiolucent defect (Fig. 13.39). This infrequently encountered normal variant, which is usually bilateral, but which may be unilateral, may be difficult to distinguish from a fracture radiographically. The width of the defect, its sclerotic margins, location and direction, common bilaterality, and absence of associated epiphyseal separation and soft tissue swelling should help in distinguishing it from a fracture.

Anomalies of the phalanges (Fig. 13.40) are common and may, on initial inspection, suggest a fracture. The roentgen appearance of the margins of the linear defect are usually sufficiently characteristic to exclude the probability of its representing an acute fracture.

Calcaneal "apophysitis" is not a radiologic diagnosis. The roentgen appearance of the calcaneal apophysis is extremely variable. The radiographic signs of "apophysitis," namely fragmentation, irregular calcification, and separation of the apophysis frcalcaneal tubercle, may all occur normally in asymptomatic children. If calcaneal apophysitis represents a true disease entity, its diagnosis must be made on the basis of the clinical findings.

Acute osteomyelitis produces soft tissue swelling and irregular demineralization of the affected bone (Figs. 13.41 and 13.42).

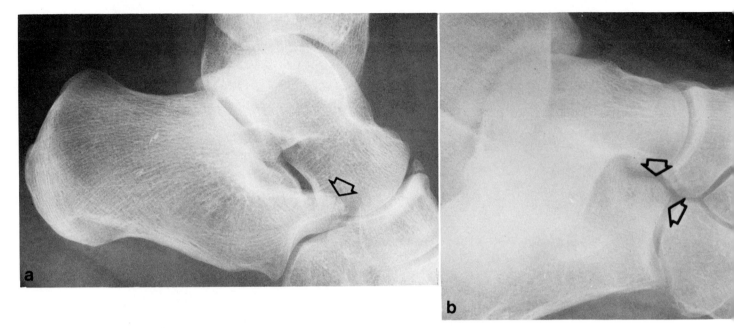

Fig. 13.34. (a, b) Minimally displaced fracture of the anterior process of the os calcis (*arrows*).

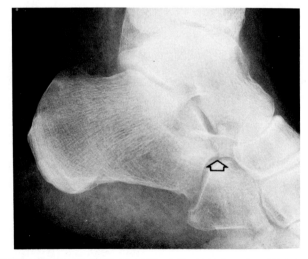

Fig. 13.35. Slightly displaced fracture of the anterior tubercle of the os calcis (*arrow*).

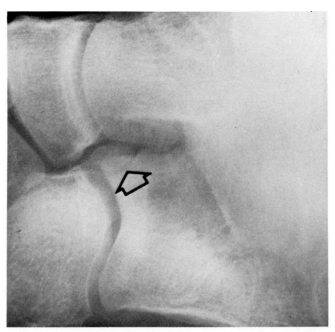

Fig. 13.36. Os secundum (*arrow*). Note the smooth, faintly sclerotic margins of this accessory growth center.

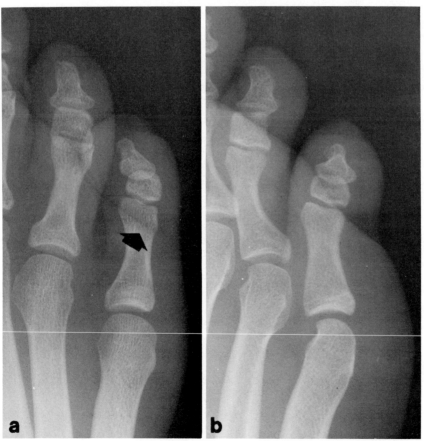

Fig. 13.37. Linear, soft tissue radiolucency extending across the head of the proximal phalanx (*arrow*) in frontal radiograph **(a)** occupies a different position in the oblique projection **(b)**.

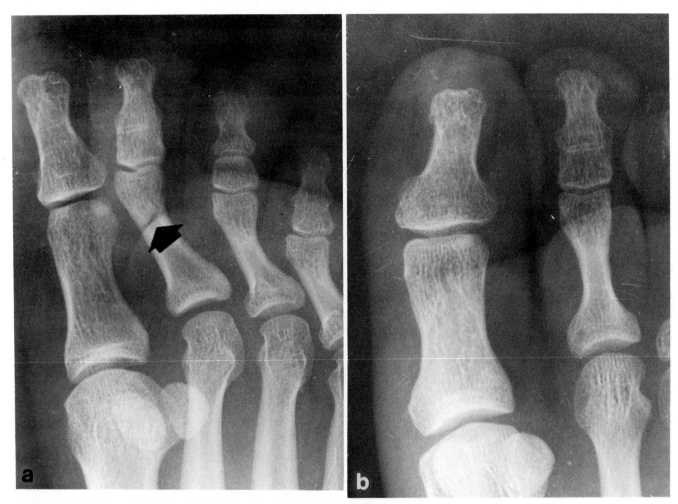

Fig. 13.38. The soft tissue radiolucency (*arrow*) across the neck of the proximal phalanx of the second toe in the oblique projection (**a**) is not seen in the same location in the frontal projection (**b**). In addition, the soft tissue density extends beyond the cortical margins of the phalanx. For these reasons, this type of soft tissue shadow should not be misinterpreted as a fracture line.

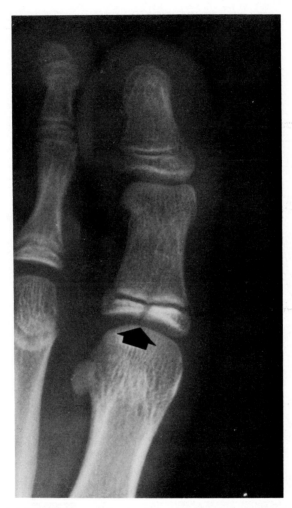

Fig. 13.39. Vertical, radiolucent defect in the epiphysis of the proximal phalanx of the great toe (*arrow*) is a normal variant that is frequently difficult to distinguish from a fracture line.

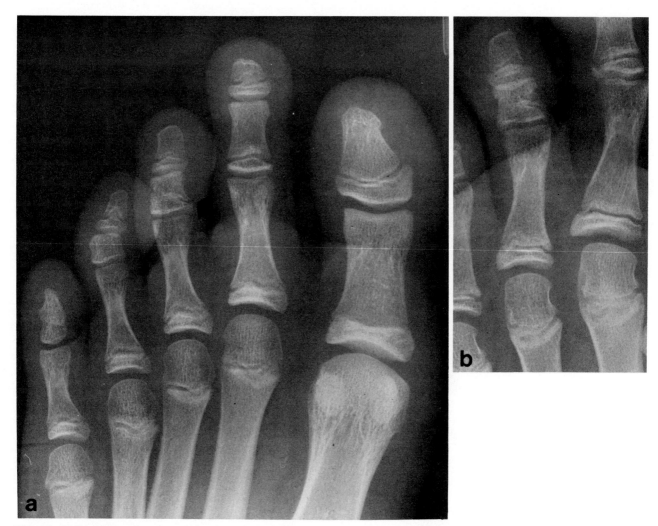

Fig. 13.40. (a, b) Developmental anomaly of the middle phalanx of the third digit (*arrows*). The broad, smooth, sclerotic margins of the linear, transverse defect should distinguish this normal variant from a fracture line.

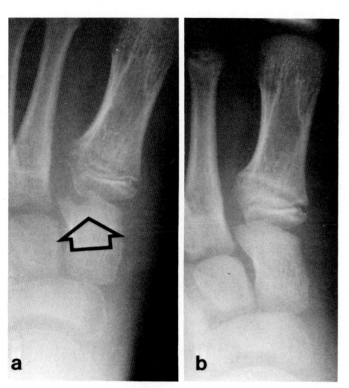

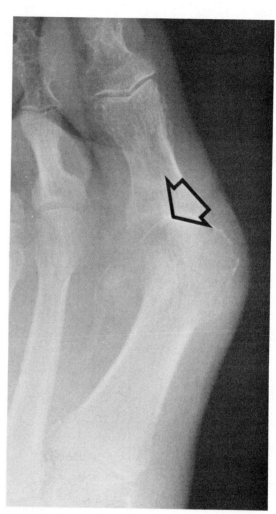

Fig. 13.41. (a) Acute osteomyelitis of the distal end of the first cuneiform (*arrow*). Note the soft tissue swelling about the first tarsometatarsal joint **(a)**. The uninvolved, contralateral foot is seen in **(b)**. The radiograph has been reversed for ease of comparison.

Fig. 13.42. Acute osteomyelitis of the first metatarsal-phalangeal joint. Note the irregular demineralization, loss of articulating cortical surface, and soft tissue swelling.

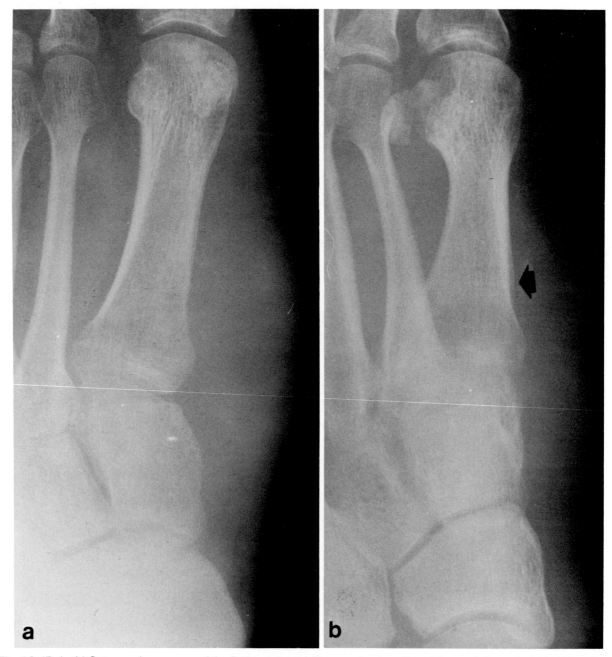

Fig. 13.43. (a, b) Osteogenic sarcoma of the first metatarsal. The proximal portion of the ray is irregularly demineralized, periosteal new bone reaction (*arrow*) and a soft tissue mass are present.

Primary malignant tumors may arise from, or involve, the bones of the foot, producing soft tissue swelling, soft tissue calcification, lysis of bone, and periosteal bone reaction (Fig. 13.43).

References

1. ANDERSON JE: *Grant's Atlas of Anatomy*, ed. 7. Williams & Wilkins, Baltimore, 1978.
2. NELSON SW: Some important diagnostic and technical fundamentals in the radiology of trauma. *Radiol Clin North Am* 4: 241, 1966.
3. SHULTZ RJ: *The Language of Fractures.* Williams & Wilkins, Baltimore, 1972.
4. O'REGAN DJ: Lisfranc dislocations. *J Med Soc NJ* 66:575, 1969.
5. LENCZNER EM, WADDELL JP, GRAHAM JD: Tarsal-metatarsal (Lisfranc) dislocation. *J Trauma* 14:1012, 1974.
6. ROGERS LF, CAMPBELL RE: Fractures and dislocations of the foot. *Semin Roentgenol* 13:157, 1978.
7. CONWELL HE, REYNOLDS FC: *Key and Conwell's Management of Fractures, Dislocations and Sprains*, ed. 7. C.V. Mosby, St. Louis, Mo., 1961.
8. MOSELEY HF: Traumatic disorders of the ankle and foot. *Ciba Found Clin Symp* 17:26, 1965.

chapter fourteen

The Diaphyses

General Considerations

Diaphyseal lesions are unique because of their location, their frequent indirect but significant bearing upon related joints, and their intimate association with peripheral arteries and nerves.

Lesions involving the diaphyseal region of all the long bones will be considered here.

Radiographic Examination

The routine radiographic examination of the long bones must include roentgenograms made in both frontal and lateral projections. A single projection of a long bone is an inadequate roentgen study (Fig. 14.1), except when the patient's condition is so precarious that only the obtaining of "survey" information can be tolerated. Prior to definitive evaluation, however, right angle radiographs of the long bones must be obtained to provide the necessary data upon which therapeutic decisions can be made.

It is equally fundamental to include the entire long bone(s) in the examination whenever possible. When not possible, for whatever reason, the joint closest to the site of injury must be included in the examination. The purpose of the "closest joint" tenet is to be able to accurately localize the injury and to identify concomitant injuries which frequently occur close to, or involve, the joint (Fig. 14.2).

Shortening of one of the bones of the forearm or leg associated with angulation or overlap of fragments can only be accommodated by either a fracture or dislocation of the other bone. Therefore, when one of the bones of the forearm or leg is shortened as the result of fracture, it is imperative to examine the entire part radiographically in order to diagnose the fracture or dislocation which must involve the other bone (Fig. 14.3).

The distal fragment of fractures of the mid- or distal third of the femur may be externally rotated as much as 90°. This feature may not be appreciated unless the entire femur is included in the roentgen study.

Peripheral arteriography plays an important role in the evaluation of traumatic lesions of the extremities. While it is the responsibility of the attending physician to specifically evaluate the circulation of an injured extremity, it is equally the responsibility of the radiologist to identify and indicate to the attending physician those injuries which, because of the normal anatomic relationship between the arteries and the bones, have the potential of associated vascular involvement.

Radiographic Anatomy

The contour of the part and the configuration of the soft tissues are important aspects of the roentgen evaluation of the extremities.

Normally, adipose or loose areolar tissue is present adjacent to or surrounding the soft tissue structures of the extremities. In properly exposed radiographs, the muscles and fascial planes may be visible as linear or curvilinear radiolucent shadows.

The anatomy of the bones of the forearm is unique in that the radius "winds around" the ulna as the wrist and hand move from supination to pronation (Fig. 14.4). Therefore, the relationship of the diaphysis of the radius and the ulna radiographically depends upon the position of the forearm when the roentgen exposures are made (Fig. 14.5). Routinely, the anteroposterior examination of the forearm is made with the part supine in order to avoid superimposition of the radial shaft upon the ulna.

673

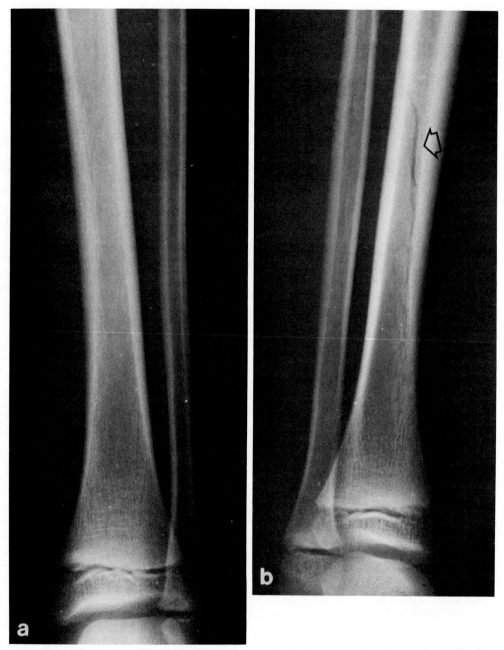

Fig. 14.1. The frontal radiograph of the leg (**a**) could very easily be interpreted as ''negative.'' The lateral projection (**b**) clearly demonstrates the minimally displaced spiral fracture in the mid-third of the tibia (*arrow*).

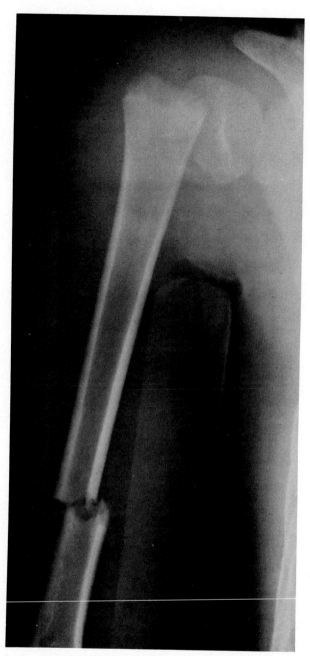

Fig. 14.2. Transverse fracture in the shaft of the humerus with an associated proximal humeral epiphyseal separation.

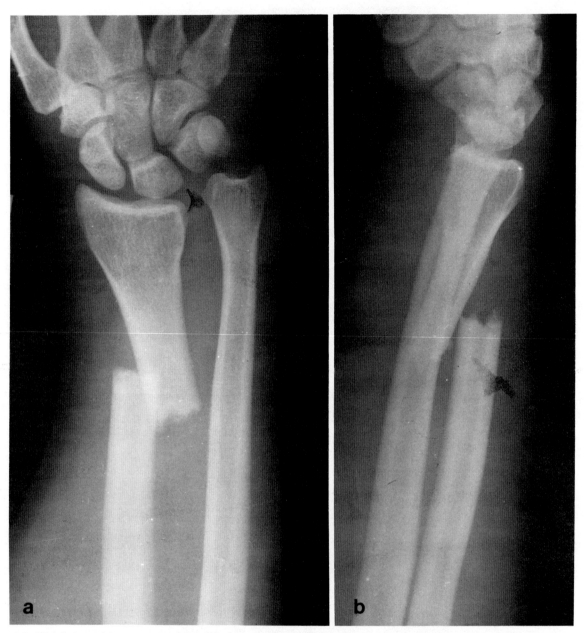

Fig. 14.3. The Galeazzi fracture, sometimes inappropriately referred to as a ''reversed Monteggia'' fracture, consists of a fracture of the distal third of the radius and dislocation of the distal radioulnar joint **(a,b)**. This injury illustrates a basic tenet relative to fractures of the forearm or leg; namely, that if angulation or overriding of fragments produces shortening of one bone, either a fracture or dislocation of the other bone must also be present.

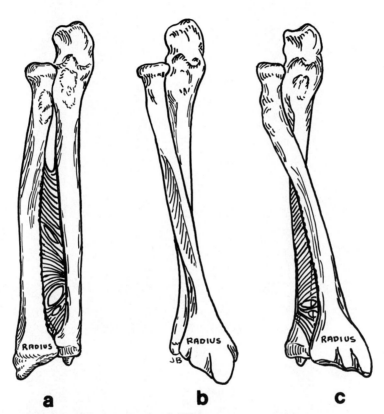

Fig. 14.4. The effect of pronation and supination of the forearm upon the radius and ulna. The radius appears to ''wind around'' the ulna as the forearm moves from the supine (**a**) through the neutral (**b**) to the prone position (**c**).

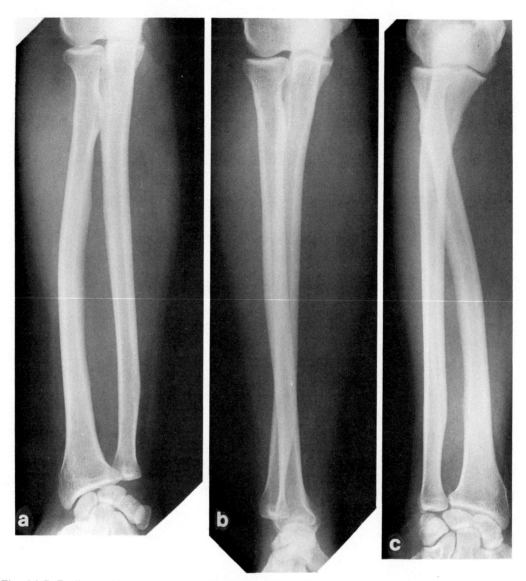

Fig. 14.5. Radiographic appearance of the forearm in supine (**a**), neutral (**b**), and prone (**c**) position.

Radiographic Manifestations of Trauma

Humerus

Fractures of the shaft of the humerus occur less frequently than fractures of the proximal end of the bone and are usually the result of direct violence. Frequently, the humerus may be fractured by indirect force, such as a fall on the hand or elbow. Fractures of the proximal portion of the humerus caused by muscular action alone occur rarely (1–3).

Humeral shaft fractures are usually either spiral (Fig. 14.6) or transverse (Fig. 14.2). Displacement of the fragments is common, with the direction and magnitude of displacement due to (1) the direction and magnitude of the force causing the injury and (2) the action of the muscles that insert upon the humerus and their relation to the fracture site. Generally, if the fracture line is located distal to the insertion of the deltoid muscle, the *proximal* fragment tends to be retracted outward while the muscles of the arm draw the distal fragment upward. When the fracture is above the insertion of the deltoid, the *distal* fragment will be drawn outward and the proximal fragment medially by the unopposed action of the pectoralis, the latissimus dorsi, and the teres major.

Because the radial nerve lies in the musculospiral groove of the humerus, radial nerve paralysis is the principal complication of humeral shaft fractures.

Radius and Ulna

The pronator quadratus sign, described in conjunction with injuries of the wrist, is extremely valuable in the detection of minimally displaced fractures of the distal diaphysis of the ulna (Fig. 14.7) or radius.

Isolated ulnar shaft fractures are usually the result of direct trauma and the alignment of the fragments reflects the direction of the causative force. The frequent association or dislocation or fracture of the proximal radius with distal ulnar fracture makes radiographic examination of the entire forearm necessary (4).

The Monteggia fracture, which consists of a displaced fracture of the proximal ulna and dislocation of the radial head, has been described in Chapter 5. Classifications of the types of Monteggia fractures and the mechanism of producing each have been described by Reckling and Cordell (5) and Bryan (6).

Isolated fractures of the radius occur less frequently than isolated ulnar fractures and may be the result of either direct or indirect trauma, such as a fall on the outstretched hand. The displacement of the fragments reflects the pull of the muscles of the forearm and the relationship of the fracture site to the insertion of the pronator teres muscle. The Galeazzi fracture (7) deserves special mention because, although not a com-

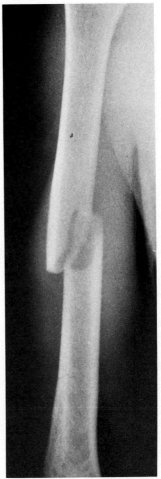

Fig. 14.6. Oblique fracture in the mid-third of the humerus. Fractures in this location may involve the radial nerve as it winds around the medial side of the mid-third of the humerus.

mon injury, it is associated with a high incidence of complication (8). This lesion consists of a displaced or shortened fracture of the distal radius complicated by dislocation of the ulna at the distal radioulnar joint (Figs. 14.3 and 14.8). Frequently, a fracture occurs at the base of the ulnar styloid process as well.

Shortening, angulation, and rotary deformity of the fragments of forearm fractures are the result of the effects of the fracturing force and muscle pull, notably that of the biceps, brachialis, pronator teres, and pronator quadratus. Displacement of the fragments is always associated with soft tissue damage including muscle tear, damage to the interosseous membrane which may heal with excessive fibrosis or calcification resulting in limitation of pronation and supination, or vascular disruption or compression resulting in Volkmann's ischemic contracture.

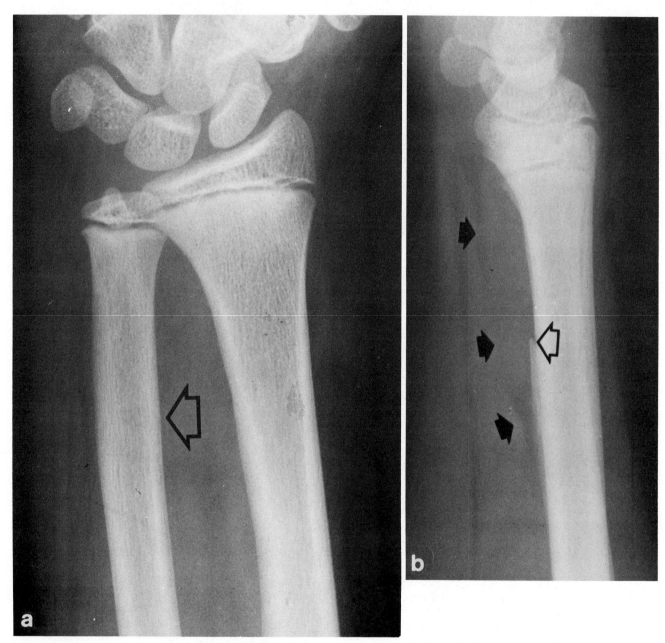

Fig. 14.7. The minimally displaced fracture in the distal third of the ulna (*open arrow*) is almost imperceptible in the frontal projection (**a**). The obvious pronator quadratus sign (*solid arrows*) signals the cortical disruption of the ulnar fracture (*open arrow*) in the lateral radiograph (**b**).

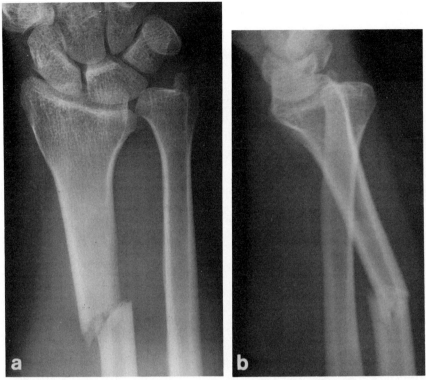

Fig. 14.8. Galeazzi fracture, consisting of a complete, displaced fracture in the distal radius and dislocation at the distal radioulnar joint seen in frontal (**a**) and lateral (**b**) projections. The slightly displaced fracture of the ulnar styloid process seen in the frontal (**a**) projection is a frequently associated, but incidental, fracture.

Femur

The femur is the largest and heaviest long bone of the skeleton. It is protected by heavy, thick musculature, which in turn is invested in dense fascia. Thus, severe force is required to produce a fracture of the femur and femoral fractures are usually associated with significant soft tissue injury which may obliterate the normal soft tissue planes of the thigh (Fig. 14.9).

Femoral fractures are usually displaced by the force of the injury and the effect of the thigh muscles upon the fragments. Both anteroposterior and lateral roentgenograms are mandatory to establish the degree and direction of displacement (Fig. 14.9) and the degree of rotation of the distal fragment (Fig. 14.10).

Fractures of the proximal third of the femoral shaft may cause disruption of the deep femoral artery or its branches. The superficial femoral artery, as it leaves the adductor canal and passes through the popliteal space, is immediately adjacent to the femur and may be injured by displaced fractures of the distal femoral shaft. Percutaneous femoral arteriography should be considered in all patients with displaced distal femoral shaft fractures, and particularly in those patients with

clinical evidence of diminished or absent peripheral circulation.

Tibia and Fibula

Fractures of the tibial shaft are usually the result of direct trauma, are commonly associated with fractures of the fibula, and are frequently open.

The popliteal artery and its branches may be injured by the force causing the proximal tibial fracture or by the fracture fragments themselves. In addition, the lumen of these vessels may be compromised by the hematoma confined within the closed space of the calf (Fig. 14.11). Because clinical appraisal of the status of the anterior and posterior tibial and peroneal arteries may be difficult, percutaneous femoral arteriography should be seriously considered in the evaluation of comminuted, displaced proximal tibial shaft fractures.

Distal tibial fractures may be associated with proximal fibular fractures (Fig. 14.12). The tibial fracture, being the major and most symptomatic injury, tends to mask the proximal fibular fracture.

The combined injury just described, although it

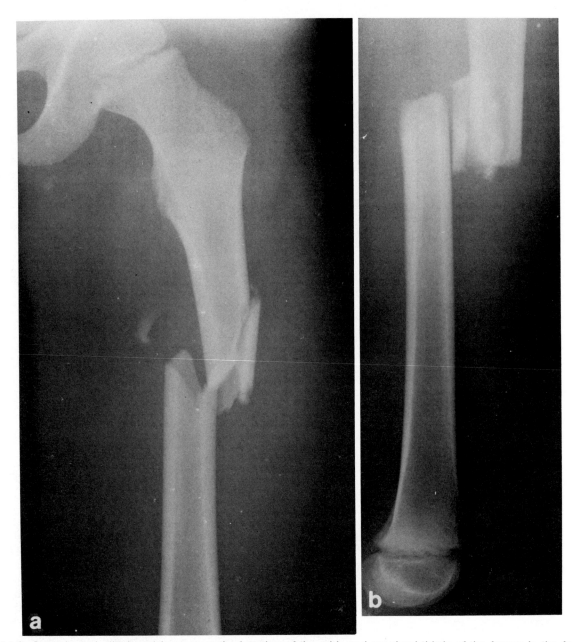

Fig. 14.9. Comminuted, displaced fracture at the junction of the mid- and proximal thirds of the femur. In the frontal projection **(a)**, the normal soft tissue planes of the thigh have been obliterated by the hematoma. There is little indication of the magnitude of displacement of the fragments in this projection. The horizontal beam lateral radiograph **(b)** of the femur delineates the degree of posterior and proximal displacement of the distal fragment.

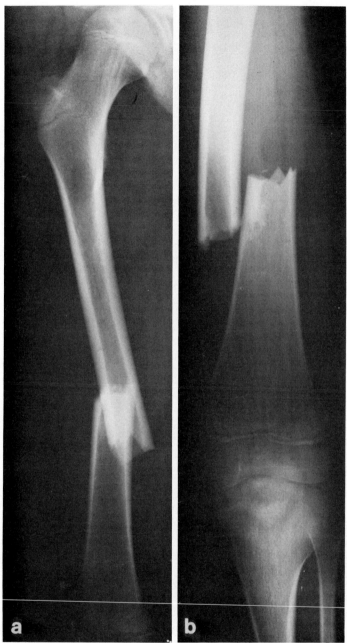

Fig. 14.10. Complete, displaced fracture of the distal third of the femur with approximately 90° rotation of the distal fragment. In the frontal projection **(a)**, the distal fragment is obviously displaced laterally and proximally. The external rotation of the distal fragment is not well appreciated. In the lateral radiograph **(b)**, however, in which the proximal fragment is seen in lateral view and the distal fragment is seen in frontal projection, the rotation of the distal fragment is obvious. In order to recognize the commonly occurring external rotation of the distal femoral fragment, it is necessary to include the entire femur in both frontal and lateral projections.

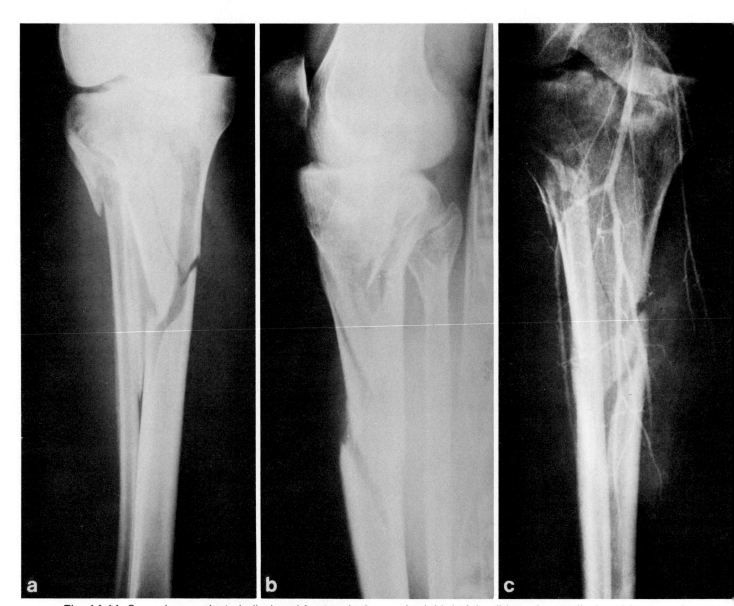

Fig. 14.11. Severely comminuted, displaced fracture in the proximal third of the tibia and a nondisplaced fracture of the fibular neck seen in frontal (**a**) and lateral (**b**) projections. The femoral arteriogram (**c**) demonstrates impaired run-off of the contrast medium in the calf caused by the tamponade effect of the hematoma which developed in the confined space of the calf.

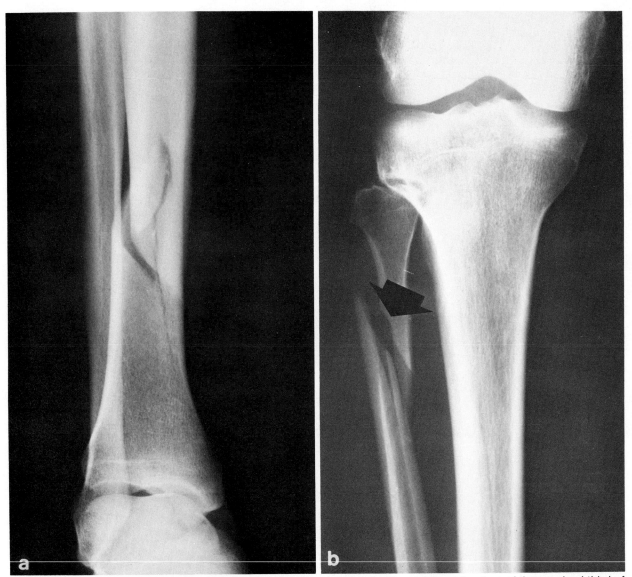

Fig. 14.12. Spiral fracture of the distal third of the tibia (**a**) associated with an oblique fracture of the proximal third of the fibula (**b**). Because the distal tibiofibular joint and its ligaments are intact, the injury does *not* meet the criteria of a Maisonneuve fracture.

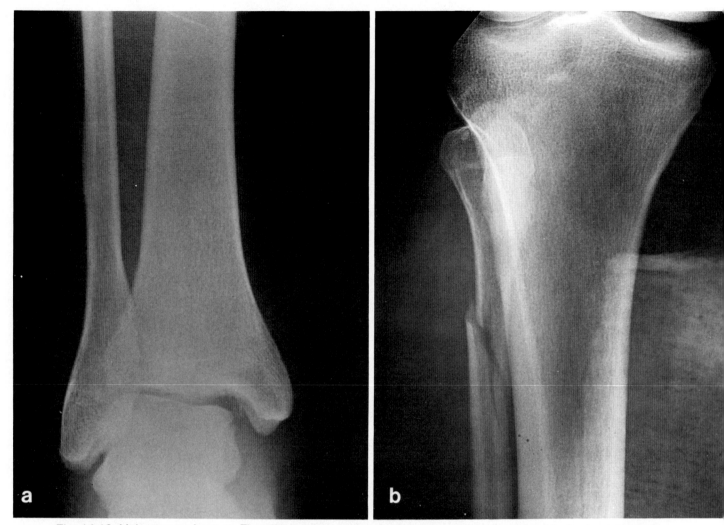

Fig. 14.13. Maisonneuve fracture. The effects of an eversion injury of the ankle are recorded in the frontal projection **(a)**. The talus is laterally displaced with respect to the distal tibia and, consequently, the distal tibiofibular ligaments must be disrupted, thereby fulfilling one of the criteria of the Maisonneuve fracture. The fracture in the proximal third of the fibula **(b)** completes the definition of this lesion. (Courtesy of Robert E. Campbell, M.D., Pennsylvania Hospital, Philadelphia.)

involves the distal tibia and proximal fibula, is not a Maisonneuve fracture. The latter, as originally described by Maisonneuve in 1812 (7), is a fracture of the proximal fibula associated with rupture of the distal tibiofibular ligaments and the interosseous membrane (Fig. 14.13). This injury is caused by an eversion mechanism involving the ankle in which the talus is displaced laterally and the impaction force upon the distal fibula, instead of fracturing the malleolus, displaces the fibula laterally, causing disruption of the distal tibiofibular syndesmosis and the interosseous membrane. As the fibula continues to be laterally displaced and freed from the tibia, the proximal fibula fractures as the proximal tibiofibular joint remains intact.

Isolated fractures of the fibula occur infrequently,

are usually located in the distal third of the shaft, are usually nondisplaced, and are the result of direct trauma to the lateral aspect of the leg (Fig. 14.14). The clinical signs of these fractures are commonly minimal and the acute fracture is frequently not appreciated clinically.

Stress (fatigue) fractures of the proximal tibia occur most commonly in overweight, generally sedentary adolescents. When symptoms first appear, the fracture may not be radiographically visible. Periosteal new bone reaction or endosteal callous formation (Fig. 14.15) producing a broad band of increased density appear within 2–3 weeks following onset of symptoms and establish the diagnosis (9–12).

The major arteries of the leg may be avulsed by severe injuries of the ankle or hindfoot (Fig. 14.16).

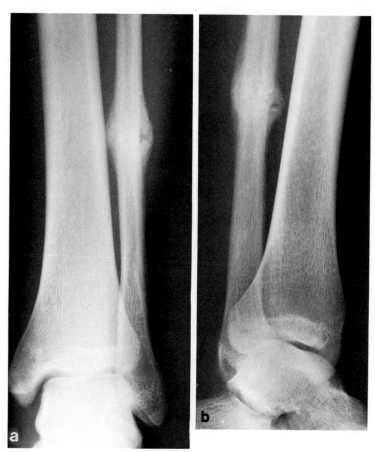

Fig. 14.14. (a, b) Nondisplaced, isolated fracture of the distal third of the fibula. The fracture was not appreciated clinically until the callous became palpable.

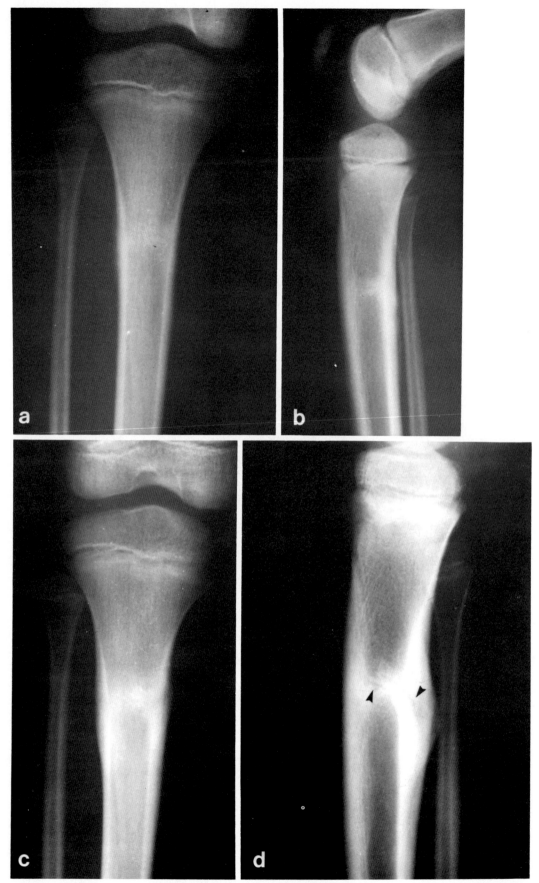

Fig. 14.15. Stress fracture of the proximal tibia. In the initial radiographs (**a, b**), the minimal periosteal new bone reaction, laterally and posteriorly, and the broad, ill defined band of increased density in the proximal third of the tibia indicate the fracture site. Subsequent radiographs (**c, d**) reveal solid periosteal reaction at the fracture site and, in the lateral projection, sclerotic margins of the fracture line (*arrowheads*).

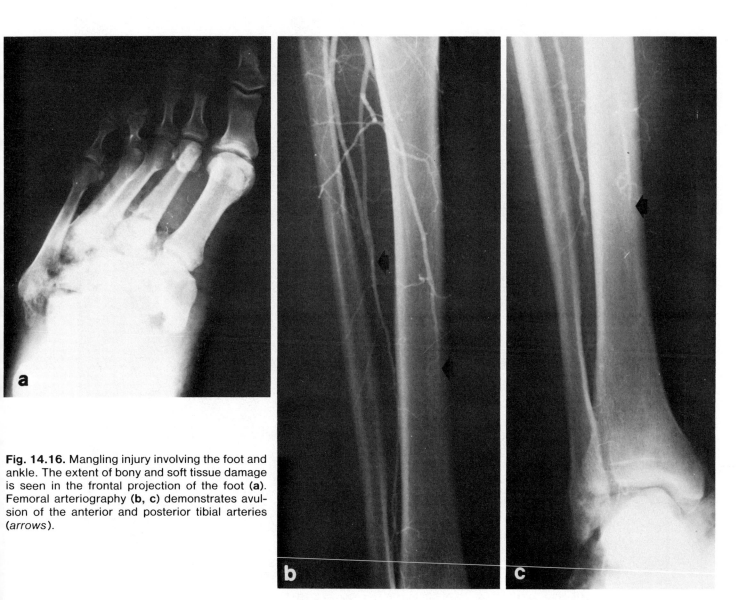

Fig. 14.16. Mangling injury involving the foot and ankle. The extent of bony and soft tissue damage is seen in the frontal projection of the foot **(a)**. Femoral arteriography **(b, c)** demonstrates avulsion of the anterior and posterior tibial arteries (*arrows*).

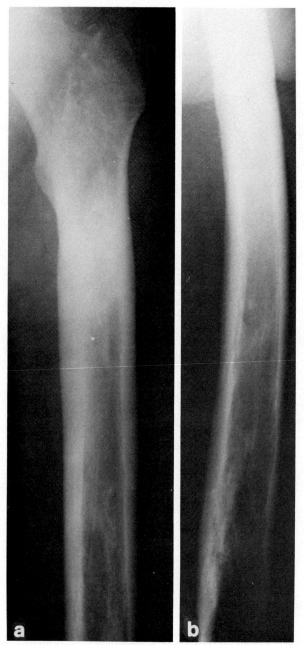

Fig. 14.17. (a, b) Chronic osteomyelitis of the femur.

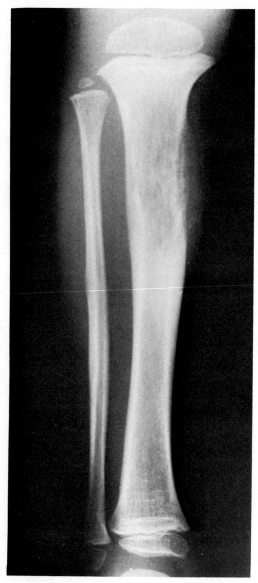

Fig. 14.18. Ewing's sarcoma of the proximal third of the tibia.

Nontraumatic Lesions

The edema associated with cellulitis results in increase in size and distortion of the contour of the involved part, increase in soft tissue density, and loss of soft tissue planes. All of these signs are discernible on a properly exposed radiograph.

The roentgen signs of osteomyelitis are protean and depend largely upon the stage of the inflammatory process. The roentgen appearance of acute osteomyelitis has been illustrated elsewhere. Sclerosis and cortical thickening of chronic osteomyelitis are seen in Fig. 14.17.

Benign tumors rarely involve the diaphyses of long bones and are rarely symptomatic.

Primary (Fig. 14.18) or metastatic (Figs. 14.19 and 14.20) tumors of long bones may be the etiology of pain, tenderness, the presence of a mass, or a pathologic fracture (Fig. 14.21).

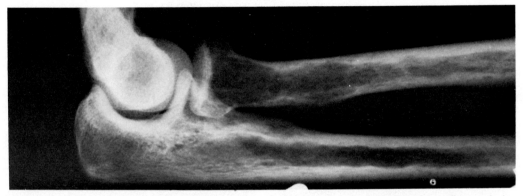

Fig. 14.19. Osteolytic metastasis from a primary breast carcinoma involving the radius and ulna.

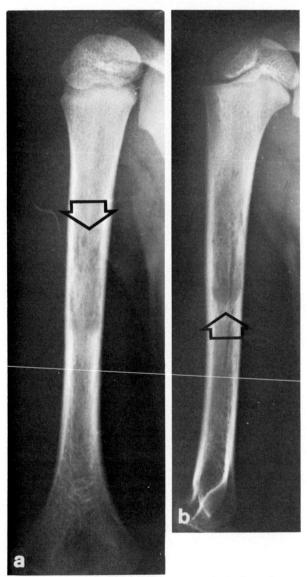

Fig. 14.20. (a, b) Osteolytic metastatic lesions from a primary neuroblastoma involving the midshaft of the humerus.

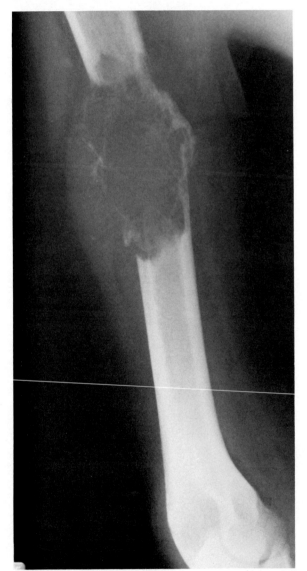

Fig. 14.21. Pathologic fracture through an osteolytic metastatic lesion from a primary carcinoma of the kidney.

References

1. TULLOS, HS, KING, JW: Lesions of the pitching arm in adolescents. *JAMA* 220:264, 1972.
2. BINGHAM, EL: Fractures of the humerus from muscular violence. *US Armed Forces Med J* 10:22, 1959.
3. O'DONOGHUE, DH: *Treatment of Injuries to Athletes.* W. B. Saunders, Philadelphia, 1962.
4. RALSTON, EL: *Handbook of Fractures.* C. V. Mosby, St. Louis, Mo., 1967.
5. RECKLING, FW, CORDELL, LD: Unstable fracture-dislocation of the forearm. *Arch Surg* 96:999, 1968.
6. BRYAN, RS: Monteggia fracture of the forearm. *J Trauma* 11: 992, 1971.
7. SHULTZ, RJ: *The Langugage of Fractures.* Williams & Wilkins, Baltimore, 1972.
8. HUGHSTON, JC: Fracture of the distal radial shaft: Mistakes in management. *J Bone Joint Surg* 39–A:249, 1957.
9. SALTER, RB: *Textbook of Disorders and Injuries of the Musculoskeletal System.* Williams & Wilkins, Baltimore, 1970.
10. SALTER, RB (Ed): *Care for the Injured Child.* Williams & Wilkins, Baltimore, 1975.
11. GRUSD, R: Gamut: Pseudofractures and stress fractures. *Semin Roentgenol* 13:81, 1978.
12. SWISCHUCK, LE: *Emergency Radiology of the Acutely Ill or Injured Child.* Williams & Wilkins, Baltimore, 1979.

Index